SHAW'S TEXTBOOK OF GYNAECOLOGY

DEDICATION

*This revised edition is dedicated to
the memory of Wilfred Shaw,
a great teacher.*

G. 2
1

7.00

Shaw's Textbook of
GYNAECOLOGY

NINTH EDITION

Revised by

JOHN HOWKINS

MD, MS, FRCS, FRCOG

Honorary Obstetric & Gynaecological Surgeon,
St. Bartholomew's Hospital, and Hampstead General Hospital
(Royal Free Group), London.
Gynaecological Surgeon, Royal Masonic Hospital, London.
Examiner in Midwifery to the Universities of London and Cambridge,
and to the Royal College of Obstetricians & Gynaecologists.
Examiner to the Conjoint Board of England.

and

GORDON BOURNE

FRCS, FRCOG

Obstetric & Gynaecological Surgeon, St. Bartholomew's
Hospital, London. Lecturer to the City University, London.
Examiner in Midwifery & Gynaecology to the Universities
of London and Oxford, and to the Royal College of Obstetricians
& Gynaecologists. Examiner to the Conjoint Board of England.

with 431 illustrations

CHURCHILL LIVINGSTONE

EDINBURGH LONDON AND NEW YORK

1971

CHURCHILL LIVINGSTONE

Medical Division of Longman Group Limited

Distributed in the United States of America by Longman Inc., New York and by associated companies, branches and representatives throughout the world.

First Edition	. .	1936
Second Edition	. .	1938
Reprinted	. .	1939
Third Edition	. .	1941
Reprinted	. .	1943
Fourth Edition	. .	1945
Reprinted	. .	1946
Fifth Edition	. .	1948
Reprinted	. .	1949
Sixth Edition	. .	1952
Seventh Edition	. .	1956
Reprinted	. .	1959
Eighth Edition	. .	1962
Reprinted	. .	1964
Reprinted	. .	1965
Ninth Edition	. .	1971
Reprinted	. .	1975

First published 1936

ISBN 0 7000 1475 6

Printed in Great Britain

Preface to the Ninth Edition

The ninth edition of Shaw's Textbook of Gynaecology is the first in the series to be published under joint authorship. The choice of Mr. Gordon Bourne will I feel sure be acknowledged as a natural and logical step. Obviously as an author of Recent Advances in Obstetrics and Gynaecology his editorial capacity is established and his position as a consultant and teacher at St. Bartholomew's Hospital respects the wishes of Wilfred Shaw that this publication should continue as a product of his own Hospital. It would moreover have pleased the original author that his latest successor was one of his own pupils.

The purpose of the book remains unchanged. Safe standard orthodoxy that is acceptable to candidate, tutor and examiner has been our object and we have endeavoured to incorporate those recent trends that have been developed since the last edition. Every word of the previous text has been scrutinised and all dead wood ruthlessly pruned. The chapters on physiology, endocrinology and birth control have been almost completely rewritten and a new chapter on the proctological aspects of gynaecology incorporated. We are again indebted to Dr. Claude Nicol for his authoritative chapter on sexually trans-mitted diseases and we welcome Dr. David Skeggs as contributor of the excellent chapter on radiotherapy. Many new illustrations have been added and those that we consider inadequate eliminated. Although much new text has been written the total length of the book remains much as before.

We are grateful to Mr. Bert Cambridge and the staff of the Williamson Laboratory at St. Bartholomew's Hospital, and also to Mr. Tredinnick and Mr. Cull (Directors of the Department of Medical Illustration at St. Bartholomew's Hospital) whose guidance has been invaluable and whose staff have provided most of the new illustrations.

I acknowledge the generosity of friends and colleagues in this and other countries who have allowed me to reproduce illustrations from their own publications, of which acknowledgement has been made in the text. Sincere thanks are also extended to Mr. J. Rivers and Mr. G. J. Hooton, of Churchill Livingstone, for encouragement and generous help.

J. H.

Contents

1 Anatomy

THE VULVA

The **vulva** is an ill-defined area which in gynaecological practice comprises the whole of the external genitalia and conveniently includes the perineum. It is, therefore, bounded anteriorly by the mons veneris, laterally by the labia majora and posteriorly by the perineum. The **labia majora** pass from the **mons veneris** to end posteriorly in the skin over the perineal body. They consist of folds of skin which enclose a variable amount of fat and are best developed in the child-bearing period of life. In children before the age of puberty, and in post-menopausal women the amount of subcutaneous fat in the labia majora is relatively small and the cleft between the labia is therefore conspicuous. At puberty the pudendal hair appears on the mons veneris, on the outer surface of the labia majora and in some cases on the skin of the perineum as well. The inner surfaces of the labia majora are hairless and the skin of this situation is softer, moister and pinker than over the outer surfaces (see Fig. 1). The labia majora are covered with squamous epithelium

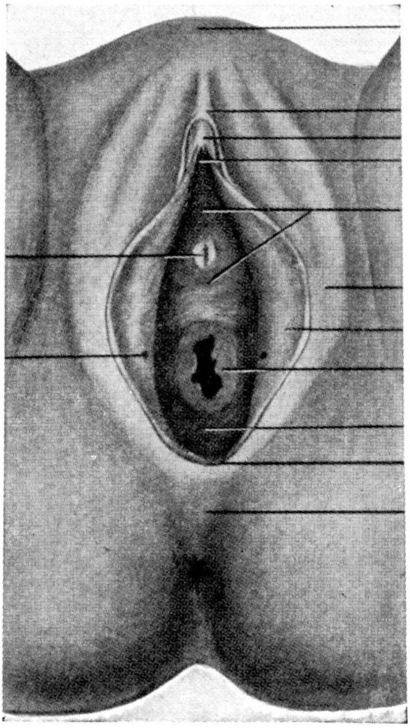

FIG. 1.   Anatomy of the vulva.

1

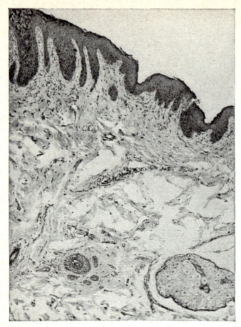

Fig. 2. Section of labium majus showing squamous epithelium with, at bottom left, a hair follicle cut transversely and, at bottom right, a sebaceous gland. (×55.)

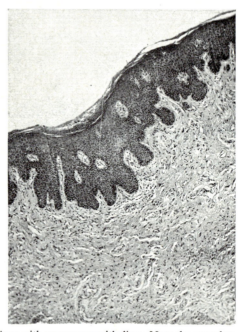

Fig. 3. Section of labium minus with squamous epithelium. Note the complete absence of hair follicles, sebaceous and sweat glands. Contrast this picture with that of the labium majus.

and contain sebaceous glands, sweat glands and hair follicles. There are also certain specialised sweat glands called apocrine glands which produce a characteristic aroma and from which the rare tumour of hidradenoma of the vulva is probably derived. The presence of all these structures in the labia majora renders them liable to the common skin infections, folliculitis, boils and sebaceous cysts. The masculine counterpart is the scrotum (Figs. 2 and 3).

Bartholin's gland lies postero-laterally in relation to the vaginal orifice, deep to the bulbospongiosus muscle and superficial to the outer layer of the triangular ligament. It is embedded in the erectile tissue of the vestibular

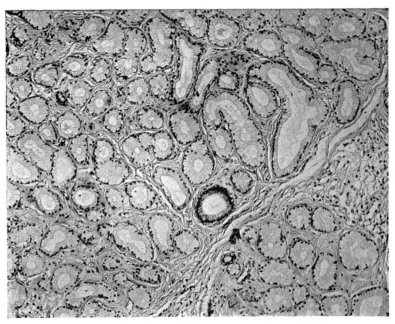

FIG. 4. Bartholin's gland. Low power section.   (×92.)

bulb at its posterior extremity. It is normally impalpable when healthy but can be readily palpated between finger and thumb when enlarged by inflammation. Its vascular bed accounts for the brisk bleeding which always accompanies its removal. Its duct passes forwards and inwards to open, external to the hymen, on the inner side of the labium minus. The gland measures about 10 mm. in diameter and lies near the junction of the middle and posterior thirds of the labium majus. The duct of the gland is about 25 mm. long and a thin mucous secretion can be expressed from it by pressure upon the gland. Bartholin's gland and its duct are infected in acute gonorrhea, when the reddened mouth of the duct can easily be distinguished on the inner surface of the labium minus to one side of the vaginal orifice below the level of the hymen. Bartholin's gland belongs to the compound racemose type and the acini are lined by low columnar epithelium (see Fig. 4). The epithelium of the duct is cubical near the acini, but becomes transitional and finally squamous near the mouth of the duct. The function of the gland is to secrete a lubricating mucus during coitus. The labia majora join at the posterior commisure and merge imperceptibly into the perineum.

The **labia minora** lie on the inner aspect of the labia majora. Anteriorly they enclose the clitoris to form the prepuce on the upper and the frenulum on the under surface: posteriorly they join to form the fourchette. The **fourchette** is a thin fold of skin, identified when the labia are separated, which is often torn during parturition. The **fossa navicularis** is the small hollow between the

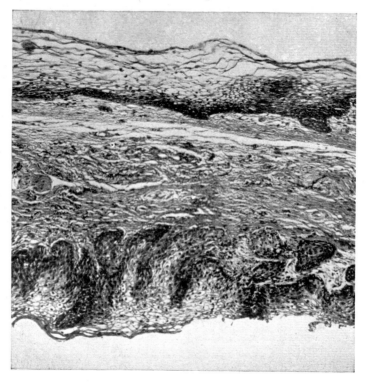

FIG. 5. The normal hymen showing the squamous epithelium of both surfaces. (×110.)

hymen and the fourchette. The labia minora are thin folds of skin which enclose veins and elastic tissue; they are, therefore, erectile under sexual activity. They do not contain any sebaceous glands or hair follicles (see Fig. 3).

The **clitoris** consists of a glans, covered by the prepuce, and a body which is subcutaneous; it corresponds to the penis and is attached to the under surface of the symphysis pubis by the suspensory ligament. Crura cavernosa attach the clitoris to the inferior margin of the pubic rami. The clitoris is well supplied with nerve endings and is extremely sensitive. During coitus it becomes erect and plays a considerable part in inducing the orgasm of the female.

The **vestibule** is the space lying between the anterior and inner aspects of the labia minora and is bounded posteriorly by the vaginal introitus. The **external urinary meatus** lies immediately posterior to the clitoris: its shape varies from a circular opening to a slit with lateral lips. The **vaginal orifice** or introitus vaginae lies posterior to the meatus and is surrounded by the **hymen.** In virgins the hymen is represented by a thin membrane covered on each surface by squamous epithelium (Fig. 5), and has a small eccentric opening which is not usually wide enough to admit the finger-tip. Coitus results in rupture of the hymen and the coital lacerations are radially arranged and are multiple. Occasionally coital rupture can cause quite a brisk haemorrhage. During child-birth further lacerations occur: the hymen is widely stretched and subsequently is represented by the tags of skin known as the **carunculae myrtiformes.** The hymen varies considerably in shape even in virgins, and annular, cribriform, falciform and imperforate are all known. Furthermore hymen rigidus may prevent penetration of the penis in attempted coitus, while on the other hand, even in virgins, the hymen may be sufficiently patulous to admit two fingers. Since the popularity of internal sanitary tampons, the loss of integrity of the hymen is no longer evidence of loss of virginity.

THE VAGINA

The lower end of the **vagina** lies at the level of the hymen and of the introitus vaginae. It is surrounded at this point by the erectile tissue of the **bulb** which corresponds to the corpus spongiosum of the male. The direction of the vagina is approximately parallel to the plane of the brim of the true pelvis: the vagina is slightly curved forwards from above downwards and its anterior and posterior walls lie in close contact. It is not of uniform calibre, being nearly twice as capacious in its upper part and somewhat flask shaped. The vaginal portion of the cervix projects into its upper end and leads to the formation of the anterior, posterior and lateral fornices. The depth of the fornices depends upon the development of the portio vaginalis of the cervix: in girls before the development of the portio vaginalis at puberty and in elderly women in whom the uterus has undergone post-menopausal atrophy the fornices are shallow, while in congenital vaginal elongation of the cervix, the fornices are particularly well marked. The vagina is attached to the cervix at a higher level posteriorly than elsewhere and this makes the posterior fornix the deepest of the fornices and the posterior vaginal wall longer than the anterior. The posterior wall is $4\frac{1}{2}$ in. (11·5 cm.) long, the anterior $3\frac{1}{2}$ in. (8·9 cm.). Transverse folds which are present in the vaginal walls of nulliparae allow the vagina to stretch and dilate during coitus and parturition. They are never well defined in women who have borne many children. In the anterior vaginal wall three sulci can be distinguished. One lies immediately above the meatus and is called the *submeatal sulcus* (see Fig. 6). About 35 mm. above this level in the anterior vaginal wall is a second sulcus, known as the *transverse vaginal sulcus*, which corresponds approximately to the junction of the urethra and the bladder. Further upwards is the *bladder sulcus* which indicates the limit of the attachment of the bladder to the anterior vaginal wall. Near the submeatal sulcus on each side is an oblique vaginal fold.

The vagina is lined by squamous epithelium which consists of a basal layer of cuboidal cells, a middle layer of prickle cells and superficial layers of corni-fied cells (see Fig. 7). It is, therefore, incorrect and indefensible ever to use the term vaginal mucosa in reference to a strictly squamous epithelial struc-ture. It should be called vaginal skin. The epithelium is much more delicate than that of the skin and is softer and pinker. In the new-born the epithelium is almost transitional in type and cornified cells are scanty until puberty is reached. No glands open into the vagina, and the vaginal secretion is derived

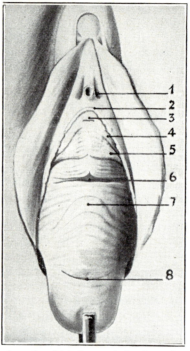

FIG. 6. A case of prolapse in which the cervix has been drawn down. (1) Para-meatal recess. (2) Hymen. (3) Submeatal sulcus. (4) Para-urethral recess. (5) Oblique vaginal fold. (6) Transverse sulcus of the anterior vaginal wall. (7) Arched rugae of the vaginal wall. (8) Bladder sulcus, see p. 5. (*By kind permission of Brit. Med. Jnl.*)

partly from the mucous discharge of the cervix and partly from a transudation through the vaginal epithelium. The sub-epithelial layer is vascular and con-tains much erectile tissue (see Fig. 7). A muscle layer consisting of a complex interlacing lattice of plain muscle lies external to the sub-epithelial layer, while the larger vessels lie in the connective tissues surrounding the vagina. The **vaginal secretion** is small in amount in healthy women, and consists of white coagulated material. When it is examined under the miscroscope, squamous cells which have been shed from the vaginal epithelium and **Döder-lein's bacilli** alone are found. Döderlein's bacillus is a large Gram-positive rod-shaped organism which grows anaerobically on acid media. It appears in the vagina during the first week of extrauterine life. The vaginal secretion is acid due to the presence of lactic acid and this acidity inhibits the growth of pathogenic organisms. The pH of the vagina averages about 4·5 during reproductive life. The acidity, which is undoubtedly oestrogen dependent, falls after the menopause to neutral or even alkaline. Before puberty the pH is about 7. This high pH before puberty and after the menopause explains the tendency for the development of mixed organism infections in these age groups.

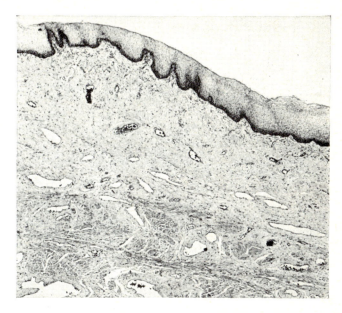

FIG. 7. The normal vagina. (×36.) Vaginal wall showing the corrugated squamous epithelium, while below are bundles of plain muscle cells.

The synthesis of lactic acid is probably effected either by enzyme or bacterial activity (Döderlein) on the glycogen of the epithelial cells which is itself dependent on the level of oestrogen so that a deficient acidity can be boosted by the administration of oral or local oestrogen. During the puerperium and also in cases of leucorrhoea the acidity of the vagina is reduced and pathogenic organisms are then able to survive. The squamous cells of the vagina and cervix stain a deep brown colour after being painted with iodine, owing to the presence of glycogen in healthy cells. If this reaction is not given, it suggests that the cells are abnormal and may possibly be malignant.

The relations of the vagina are as follows:

(1) *Anterior.* In its lower half the vagina is closely related to the urethra and the para-urethral glands (Skene's tubules), so closely in fact that the urethro-vaginal fascia is a fused structure and only separable by sharp dis-

section. In its upper half the vagina is related to the bladder in the region of the trigone and here the vesical and vaginal fasciae are easily separable via the vesico-vaginal space by blunt dissection. There is a considerable vascular and lymphatic intercommunication between the vesical and vaginal vessels, a sinister relationship in the surgery of malignant disease of this area.

(2) *Posterior*. The lower third of the vagina is related to the perineal body, the middle third to the ampulla of the rectum and the upper third to the anterior wall of the pouch of Douglas and its contained large and small bowel. This partition dividing the vagina from the peritoneal cavity is the thinnest area in the whole peritoneal surface and, therefore, a site of election for the pointing and opening of pelvic abscesses or the production of a hernia or enterocele.

(3) *Lateral*. The lateral relations from below upwards are: the cavernous tissue of the vestibule, the superficial muscles of the perineum, the triangular ligament and at about 2·5 cm. from the introitus the levator ani, lateral to which is the ischio-rectal fossa. Above the levator lies the paravaginal extension of Mackenrodt's ligament usually called the paracolpos and the parametrium of the vaginal vault. The paracolpos, parametrium and Mackenrodt's ligament are all really one structure—the endopelvic cellular tissue. The ureter traverses this tissue in the ureteric canal and is about 12 mm. antero-lateral to the lateral fornix.

(4) *Superior Relations*. The cervix with its four fornices—anterior, posterior and two lateral. These last are related to the uterine vessels, Mackenrodt's ligament and the ureter. Posteriorly in the floor of Douglas' pouch lie the uterosacral ligaments and these can be identified on vaginal examination especially if thickened by disease. The uterus if retroverted becomes a posterior superior relation of the vaginal vault and the appendages are then readily palpable lateral to the uterus.

(5) *The inferior relation* is the hymen.

THE UTERUS

The **uterus** is pyriform in shape and measures approximately $3\frac{1}{2}$ in. (9 cm.) in length, $2\frac{1}{2}$ in. (6·5 cm.) in width and $1\frac{1}{2}$ in. (3·5 cm.) in thickness. It is divided anatomically and functionally into body and cervix. The line of division corresponds to the level of the internal os and here the mucous membrane of the body becomes continuous with that of the cervical canal. At this level the peritoneum of the front of the uterus is reflected on to the bladder, and the uterine artery, after passing almost transversely across the pelvis, reaches the uterus, turns at right angles and passes vertically upward along the lateral wall of the uterus. The **cervix** is divided into vaginal and supravaginal portions. The **vaginal portion** of the cervix projects into the vagina and in virgins is conical in shape; in multiparae it is shorter and squatter. The **fundus** of the uterus is that part of the corpus uteri which lies above the insertion of the Fallopian tubes. The cavity of the uterus is constricted at the level of the internal os where it passes into the cervical canal. Above, the cavity of the uterus communicates with the openings of the Fallopian tubes, and by way of the Fallopian tubes and their abdominal ostia is in direct

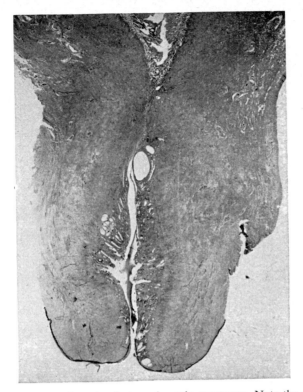

FIG. 8. Isthmus and cervix of uterus in early pregnancy. Note the cervical glands penetrating direct into the cervical muscle.

continuity with the peritoneal cavity. The cervical canal extends from the **internal os** above to the **external os** below where it opens into the vagina; it is spindle shaped, as both ostia are narrower than the rest of the canal (Fig. 9). In nulliparous women the external os is circular, but vaginal delivery results in the transverse slit which characterises the parous cervix. The mucous membrane of the body of the uterus is smooth and glistening except during menstruation when it becomes dull and finely irregular. The mucous membrane of the cervical canal, like the skin of the lower part of the vagina, is thrown into folds, and oblique furrows pass away from anterior and posterior vertical ridges (arbor vitae) (Fig. 9).

The wall of the uterus consists of three layers, the peritoneal covering or perimetrium, the muscle layer or myometrium and the mucous membrane or endometrium.

Perimetrium

The peritoneal covering of the uterus is incomplete. Anteriorly the whole of the body of the uterus is covered with peritoneum. The peritoneum is reflected on to the bladder at the level of the internal os, which indicates the

Fundus   Cornu

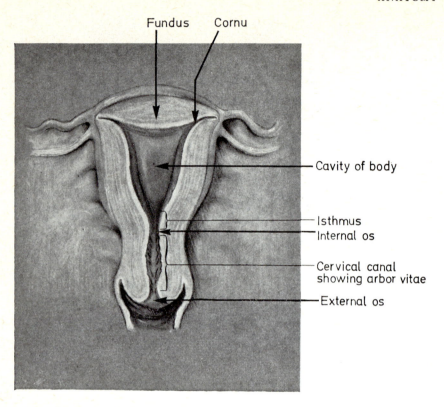

Cavity of body

Isthmus
Internal os

Cervical canal
showing arbor vitae

External os

FIG. 9. A nulliparous uterus showing the anatomical structures.

junction of the body with the cervix of the uterus. The cervix of the uterus
has therefore no peritoneal covering anteriorly. Posteriorly the whole of the
body of the uterus is covered by peritoneum, as is the supravaginal portion of
the cervix. The peritoneum is reflected from the supravaginal portion of the
cervix on to the posterior vaginal wall in the region of the posterior fornix.
The peritoneal layer is incomplete laterally because of the insertion of the
Fallopian tubes, the round and ovarian ligaments into the uterus, and below
this level the two sheets of peritoneum which constitute the broad ligament
leave a thin bare area on each side. This extraperitoneal area widens as it
descends and is, therefore, triangular in shape from above downwards; at the
level of the cervix Mackenrodt's ligament is inserted over a broad area into
the uterine wall.

Myometrium

The **myometrium** is the thickest of the three layers of the wall of the uterus.
In the cervix the myometrium consists of plain muscle tissue together with a
large amount of fibrous tissue which gives it a hard consistence. The muscle

fibres and fibrous tissue are mixed together without orderly arrangement. In the body of the uterus the myometrium measures about 10–20 mm. in thickness, and three layers can be distinguished which are best marked in the pregnant or puerperal uterus. The external layer lies immediately beneath the peritoneum and is longitudinal, the fibres passing from the cervix anteriorly over the fundus to reach the posterior surface of the cervix. This layer is thin and cannot easily be identified in the nulliparous uterus. The main function of this layer is a detrusor action during the expulsion of the foetus. The middle layer is the thickest of the three and consists of bundles of muscle separated by connective tissue the exact amount of which varies with age: plain muscle tissue is best marked in the child-bearing period, especially during pregnancy, while before puberty and after the menopause it is much less plentiful. There is a tendency for the muscle bundles to interlace, and, as the blood vessels which supply the uterus are distributed in the connective tissues, the calibre of the vessels is in part controlled by the contraction of the muscle cells. The purpose of this layer is therefore in part haemostatic, though its expulsive role is equally important. The inner muscle layer consists of circular fibres. The layer is never well marked and is best represented by the circular muscle fibres around the internal os and the openings of the Fallopian tubes. It can be regarded as sphincteric in action.

Endometrium

The **endometrium** of the body of the uterus has a different structure from that of the cervix. In the body of the uterus it measures about 3 to 4 mm. in thickness and consists of a surface epithelium, glands and stroma. The endometrium of the body varies in its structure and in its thickness during the menstrual cycle, becoming hypertrophied in the premenstrual phase and showing necrosis of the superficial layers during menstruation. In pregnancy it hypertrophies much more and forms the decidua of the uterus. The cells of the surface epithelium are cubical or low columnar in shape, with centrally placed nuclei and faintly granular cytoplasm. They are ciliated and the direction of ciliary movement is downwards towards the internal os. The surface epithelium is sometimes high columnar in cases of myomata and uterine hyperplasia. The glands of the endometrium of the body are simple tubules during the post-menstrual phase of the cycle (see Fig. 10) but become hypertrophied as menstruation approaches, changing from simple tubules to sinuous and finally corkscrew-shaped glands (see Fig. 36). The glandular epithelium resembles the surface epithelium but is subject to great variation during the menstrual cycle. The stroma intervenes between the surface epithelium and the myometrium; it is richly cellular and consists of spindle-shaped cells, blood vessels and lymphatics. A few small lymph follicles are scattered over the basal part of the endometrium in the vicinity of which lymphocytes can be distinguished amongst the spindle cells of the stroma. Similar follicles are found in the endometrium of the uterus of primates. Normally the endometrium is sharply demarcated from the underlying myometrium, but in the pathological condition of adenomyosis interna, both stroma and glandular tissue from the endometrium invade the myometrium. The endometrium possesses remarkable powers of rapid regeneration, as repair is complete within three weeks of parturition and within a few days of menstruation.

The **mucosal lining of the cervix** differs fundamentally from that of the body of the uterus by the absence of a submucosa. The epithelium of the cervical canal and of its glands comes directly into contact with the myometrium of the cervix. The glands of the cervix are acinar in type (see Fig. 11), and much

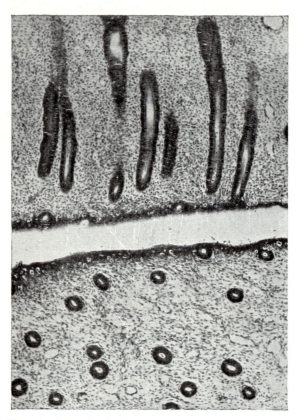

FIG. 10. Normal endometrium in the proliferative phase. The glands are simple tubules and are shown in longitudinal and transverse section.   (×66.)

more complex than those of the body. They secrete mucus with a high carbohydrate content, probably fructose. This secretion is alkaline and its pH and carbohydrate content render it attractive to ascending spermatozoa. This secretion collects as a plug in the cervical canal and possibly hinders ascending infections. In gonococcal infections of the cervix the organisms collect amongst the intricate crypts of the cervical glands. The epithelium of the cervical glands and of the cervical canal is high columnar in type with spindle-shaped nuclei lying adjacent to the basement membrane. The cells of the cervical canal are mostly ciliated, and the direction of ciliary movement is

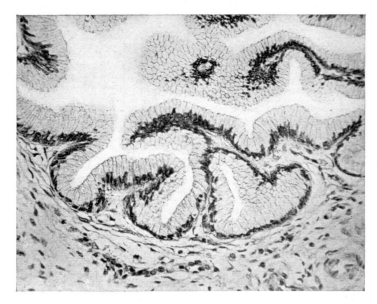

FIG. 11. Normal cervical glands. These are of the racemose type and are lined by high columnar epithelium which secretes mucus. (×250.)

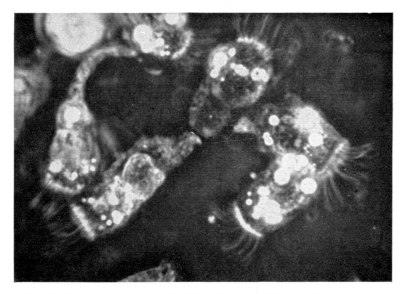

FIG. 12. High power photograph of the ciliated epithelium of the endo cervix showing ciliae.

downwards towards the external os (Fig. 12). The basement membrane of the epithelium of the cervical glands and cervical canal lies in contact with the myometrium of the cervix and there is no intervening stroma. The cervical canal is bounded above by the internal os and below by the external os, and measures 2·5 cm. or a little more.

The **vaginal portion of the cervix** is that part of the cervix which protrudes into the vaginal vault and comprises the lower half of the cervix; the upper half is termed the **supravaginal cervix.** The vaginal portion is covered by squamous epithelium which becomes continuous with the columnar cells of the cervical canal at the external os. This territorial boundary is called the squamo-columnar junction and it is believed that here most carcinomata of the cervix arise. The squamous epithelium is similar to that of the vagina and is more delicate than that of the skin. It consists of a basal layer, one cell thick, a middle layer of prickle cells, and superficial layers of cornified cells (see Fig. 13). The surface of the portio vaginalis of the cervix is normally salmon pink in colour, but it is not uncommon for the columnar epithelium of the cervical canal to replace the squamous epithelium in the vicinity of the external os to produce the condition of erosion of the cervix. Because of the translucency of the columnar cells these erosion areas appear bright red in colour in marked contrast to the normal salmon pink tint of the squamous covering of the portio vaginalis.

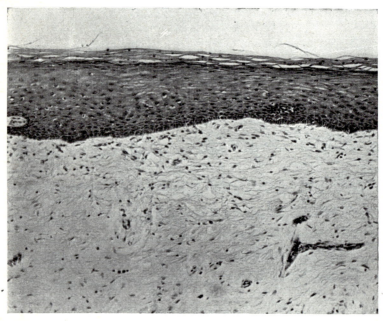

FIG. 13. Normal cervix showing the squamous epithelium of the portio vaginalis. The epithelium consists of a single basal layer of cubical cells, above which lies the prickle cell layer, and superficially the desquamating cornified cell layer. The stroma consists mainly of connective tissue. (×125.)

In nulligravidae the vaginal portion of the cervix is conical with a circular aperture, the external os, at the apex of the cone. A few circular muscle fibres surround the external os. During labour these fibres are split on each side, the tear being usually on the left so that the external os becomes a transverse slit. As a result of this tearing of the circular muscle fibres, the anterior and posterior lips of the cervix become differentiated: they cannot be distinguished in the nulliparous cervix. This is of medico-legal importance.

Structurally and functionally the body and cervix of the uterus are in marked contrast. The cervical endometrium shows no periodic alteration during the menstrual cycle, and the decidual reaction of pregnancy is seen only rarely in the cervix. Similarly, in malignant disease of the uterus, there are well-marked differences: carcinoma of the body of the uterus is an adenocarcinoma of relatively low malignancy, while carcinoma of the cervix is usually a squamous-celled growth of high malignancy.

Although it is convenient for descriptive purposes to divide the uterus into body and cervix, the line of division is not so clear-cut as the above description suggests. It was pointed out by Aschoff, and subsequently confirmed by his pupils, that an intermediate zone, the **isthmus uteri,** lies between the endometrium of the body and the mucous membrane of the cervical canal. This area is limited above by the anatomical internal os and below by the histological internal os and its length is probably about 6 mm. Its endometrium resembles that of the body more than that of the cervical canal, not only structurally but because it displays changes during the menstrual cycle and its stroma undergoes decidual reaction during pregnancy. This histological differentiation of the isthmus uteri may have some bearing on the line of demarcation between the upper and lower uterine segments during labour. One of the unusual features of the isthmus uteri is that its glands frequently show cystic dilatation which may be visible to the naked eye. These follicles are also found in the cervical canal and in follicular erosion of the cervix they can be seen beneath the epithelium of the vaginal portion of the cervix in the vicinity of the external os as translucent pearl coloured protuberances.

The relationship in the length of the cervix and that of the corpus of the uterus varies with age. During the first ten years of life the cervix to corpus ratio is 2:1. At puberty this ratio is reversed so that the cervix: corpus ratio is 1:2 while the mature organ shows a cervix: corpus ratio of 1:3 or even 1:4. After the menopause a progressive atrophy of the whole organ occurs and the portio vaginalis eventually disappears. Anteversion and anteflexion do not fully develop until sexual maturity, the undeveloped uterus being more or less straight.

Relations of the uterus:

Anterior. The base of the bladder at the level of the cervix, uterovesical pouch at the level of the internal os, and bladder or small gut above this.

Posterior. The pouch of Douglas at the level of the cervix with contained small and large gut.

Lateral. From below upwards. Mackenrodt's ligament, the uterine vessels and the ureter at the level of the cervix and above this the broad ligament, ovary, Fallopian tube and round ligament anterior to these.

THE UTERINE APPENDAGES

The uterus projects upwards from the pelvic floor into the peritoneal cavity and carries on each side of it two folds of peritoneum which pass laterally to the pelvic wall and form the **broad ligaments.** The Fallopian tubes pass outwards from the uterine cornua and lie in the upper border of the broad ligaments. The ovarian ligaments posteriorly, and the round ligaments anteriorly, also pass into the uterine cornua, but at a slightly lower level than the Fallopian tubes. Both these ligaments and the Fallopian tubes are covered with peritoneum.

The **round ligaments** pass from the uterine cornua beneath the anterior peritoneal folds of the broad ligaments to reach the internal abdominal rings. In this part of their course they are curved and, lying immediately beneath

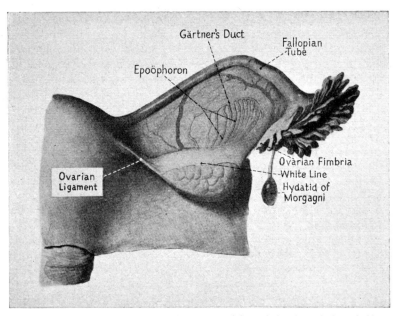

Fig. 14. The right uterine appendages viewed from behind. (Veit-Stoeckel.)

the peritoneum, are easily distinguished. The round ligaments pass down the inguinal canals and finally end by becoming adherent to the skin of the labia majora. The ligaments consist of plain muscle and connective tissue and vary considerably in thickness. They hypertrophy during pregnancy. The round ligaments are much better developed in multiparae than in virgins. They are most remarkably hypertrophied in the presence of large fibroids when they may attain a diameter of 1 cm. They correspond developmentally to the gubernaculum testis and are morphologically continuous with the ovarian ligaments, as during intrauterine life the ovarian and round ligaments are continuous and connect the lower pole of the primitive ovary to the inguinal canal. The round ligaments are lax, and, except during labour, are free of tension. There is no evidence that the normal position of anteflexion and anteversion of the uterus is produced by contraction of the round ligaments. The ligaments, however, may be shortened by operation or they may be attached to the anterior abdominal wall, both procedures being used to cause anteversion in a uterus which is pathologically retroverted. The round ligaments are supplied by a branch of the ovarian artery derived from its anastomosis with the uterine artery, hence the necessity for ligation of the round ligament during hysterectomy. Along it pass lymphatic vessels from the fundus which connect with those draining the labium majus into the inguinal glands. This explains the possibility of metastases in these glands in late cases of cancer of the endometrium of the fundus.

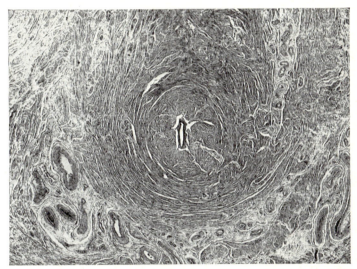

FIG. 15. Interstitial part of Fallopian tube. Note complete absence of plicae and the narrow calibre of the canal. (×22).

The **ovarian ligaments** pass upwards and inwards from the inner poles of the ovaries to reach the cornua of the uterus (see Fig. 14) below the level of the attachment of the Fallopian tubes. They lie beneath the posterior peritoneal fold of the broad ligament and measure about an inch in length. Like the round ligaments they consist of plain muscle fibres and connective tissue, but they are not so prominent because they contain less plain muscle tissue. They are morphologically a continuation of the round ligament.

The Fallopian Tubes. Each Fallopian tube is attached to the uterine cornu and passes outwards and backwards in the upper part of the broad ligament. The Fallopian tube measures 4 in. (10 cm.) or more in length and approximately 8 mm. in diameter, but the diameter diminishes near the cornu of the uterus. The Fallopian tube is divided anatomically into four parts:

(1) *The Interstitial Portion.* This is the innermost part of the tube which traverses the myometrium to open into the endometrial cavity. It is the short-

est part of the tube, its length being the thickness of the uterine muscle, about 18 mm. It is also the narrowest part, its internal diameter being 1 mm. or less so that only the finest cannula can be passed into it during salingostomy operations. There are no longitudinal muscle fibres here but the circular fibres are well developed (Fig. 15).

(2) *The isthmus* comprises the next and inner part of the tube and represents about one-third of the total length, i.e. 35 mm. It is narrow but a little wider than the interstitial part and its lumen has a diameter of 2 mm. Its muscle

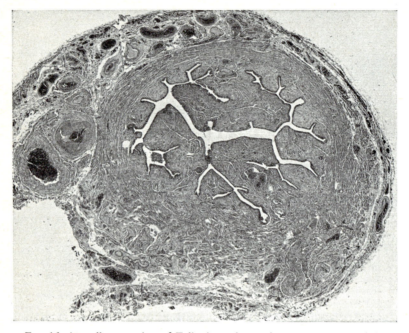

Fig. 16. Ampullary portion of Fallopian tube to show arrangement of the plicae. (×18).

wall contains both longitudinal and circular fibres and it is covered by peritoneum except for a small inferior bare area related to the broad ligament. it is relatively straight.

(3) *The ampulla* is the lateral, widest and longest part of the tube and comprises roughly two-thirds of the tube, measuring $2\frac{1}{2}$–3 inches (60–75 mm.) in length. Here the mucosa is arborescent with many complex folds (Fig. 16).

(4) *The fimbriated extremity* or *infundibulum* is where the abdominal ostium opens into the peritoneal cavity. This opening was likened to a trumpet by the old anatomists who called the tube the trumpet or salpinx. Actually the infundibulum more closely resembles a sea anemone in its appearance and behaviour since the fimbriae are motile and almost prehensile, and enjoy a considerable range of movement and action. One fimbria—the ovarian

fimbria—is larger and longer than the others and is attached to the region of the ovary.

The Fallopian tube represents the cranial end of the Müllerian duct and its lumen is continuous with the cavity of the uterus. Consequently spermatozoa and the fertilised ovum can pass along the tube. Fluids such as Diodone and gases such as carbon dioxide may be injected through the uterus and by way of the Fallopian tubes into the peritoneal cavity, and by these means the patency of the Fallopian tubes can be investigated clinically. The Fallopian tubes lie in the upper part of the broad ligaments and are covered with peritoneum except along a thin area inferiorly, which is left bare by the reflection of the peritoneum to form the two layers of the broad ligament. The blood supply of the Fallopian tube is mainly derived from the tubal branches of the ovarian artery, but the anastomosing branch of the uterine artery supplies its inner part. Unlike the vermiform appendix the Fallopian tube does not become gangrenous when acutely inflamed, as it has two sources of blood which reach it at opposite ends. The lymphatics of the Fallopian tube communicate with the lymphatics of the fundus of the uterus and with those of the ovary and they drain along the infundibulo-pelvic ligament to the aortic glands near the origin of the ovarian artery from the aorta.

The Fallopian tubes have three layers: serous, muscular and mucous. The serous layer consists of the mesothelium of the peritoneum. Intervening between the mesothelium and the muscle layer is a well-defined subserous layer in which numerous small blood vessels and lymphatics can be demonstrated. The muscle layer consists of outer longitudinal and inner circular fibres. The circular fibres are best developed in the isthmus and are thinned out near the fimbriated extremity. The mucous membrane is thrown into folds or plicae. Near the isthmus three folds can be recognised, but when traced laterally they divide and subdivide so that in the ampullary region they become highly complex. Each plica consists of stroma which is covered by epithelium. The stroma is cellular and its cells are in some ways similar to those of the endometrium. The blood vessels of the stroma are plentiful and are particularly well marked in the ampullary region. The epithelium of the mucous membrane consists of several types of cell. The commonest is ciliated, and is either columnar or cubical in type. Its function is to propel a fluid current towards the uterus which plays some part in the transport of the inert ovum which, unlike the sperm, has no motive power of its own. Next in order of frequency is a goblet-shaped cell, not ciliated, which does not give the histochemical reactions for mucin. Its function is lubricant and possibly nutritive to the ovum. A cell intermediate in type to the two already mentioned can be distinguished, and small rod-shaped cells are also present (Fig. 421). These are the so-called "peg" cells whose purpose is not known. It has been possible to demonstrate differences in the histological appearances of the epithelium of the Fallopian tubes during the menstrual cycle.

Anatomical relations of the Fallopian tube:

(1) *Medial*. The uterus.
(2) *Lateral*. The pelvic wall, with the hypogastric vessels.

(3) *Superior*. Coils of small gut, caecum and appendix on the right and sigmoid on the left.

(4) *Inferior*. A thin area of retroperitoneal connective tissue with branches of the ovarian and tubal vessels in the mesosalpinx which is the highest level of the broad ligament and its contents. Below lie the vestigial structures of Gaertner's duct and below these the ovary.

(5) *Anterior*. The bladder covered with utero-vesical peritoneum.

(6) *Posterior*. The pouch of Douglas and whatever it may contain—small and large bowel and omentum.

THE OVARIES

Each **ovary** measures about 35 mm. in length, 25 mm. in width and 18 mm. in thickness. The ovaries are roughly almond-shaped but there is much variation both in their shape and size at different stages of the menstrual cycle. The colour is pearly grey, due to a compact tunica albuginea, and the surface is slightly corrugated. The ovaries undergo atrophy after the menopause when they become shrivelled and shrunken and the grooves and furrows on the surface become well marked. Before puberty the ovaries are small and more elongated than in the adult, but even before puberty small follicles are frequently present. The ovary is attached to the back of the broad ligament by a thin mesentery, the **mesovarium.** This area is called the hilum and is the point of entry and exit for all the ovarian vessels, lymphatics and nerves. The ovary is covered by an imperfect layer of cubical cells which become continuous with the mesothelial cells of the peritoneum of the mesovarium along the white line, so that the actual surface of the ovarian cortex is devoid of true peritoneum. In this respect the ovary is unique compared with all the other organs in the abdominal cavity.

Anatomical Relations. The normal position of the ovary is such that its convex border is directed posteriorly, while its attachment to the mesovarium is in front. Laterally the ovary is related to the fossa below the bifurcation of the common iliac artery and the ureter. The Fallopian tube passes backwards and outwards from the uterus above the level of the ovary. The ovarian fimbriae stretch from the fimbriated extremity of the tube downwards and then inwards to come in contact with the ovary. Medially the ovary is attached to the cornu of the uterus by the ovarian ligament; in front it is fixed to the back of the broad ligament by the mesovarium. The ovario-pelvic fold (infundibulo-pelvic) is the outer border of the broad ligament and contains the ovarian vessels, nerves and lymphatics. This fold of peritoneum is brought into prominence when either the Fallopian tube or the ovary is raised out of the pelvis. It has no suspensory action. The position of the ovary is subject to some variation, depending partly upon the length of the ovarian ligament but more particularly upon the position of the uterus. Its position should not be regarded as in any way static.

When the uterus is retroverted the ovaries are prolapsed into the pouch of Douglas, in which position they are clinically palpable on vaginal examination via the posterior fornix. When occupying this position the ovaries are liable to produce pain on intercourse, especially if fixed by adhesion from chronic pelvic inflammatory disease or endometriosis.

Structure of the Ovary. When the ovary is incised a cortex and a medulla can be distinguished. The cortex is firm and fibrous while the medulla is softer and contains small vessels. Primordial follicles, Graafian follicles, corpora lutea and such structures as corpora albicantia are found in the cortex of the ovary. These structures are described in detail in chapter 2 page 48

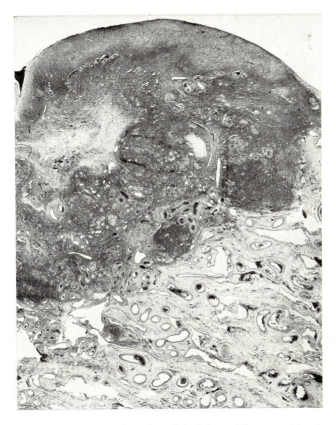

FIG. 17. Cortex and medulla in region of the hilum of the ovary. Note intense vascularity of medulla and relative avascularity of the cortex.

et seq. The stroma of the cortex consists of interlacing spindle cells which are packed closely together. The **tunica albuginea** lies immediately beneath the surface epithelium. The **surface epithelium** consists of an incomplete layer of cuboidal cells. Not uncommonly a thin layer of hyaline tissue intervenes between the cells and the tunica albuginea.

The medulla contains a large number of small arterioles, veins and lymphatics (Fig. 17). Structures derived from the follicle system do not develop in the medulla although it is quite common for such structures as corpora lutea, when they are fully developed, to spread inwards to invade the medulla. The lymphatics in the medulla of the ovary are numerous and the channels are wide. In the cortex the lymphatics are again very numerous but here they are small. The distribution of the lymphatics of the ovary can be demonstrated very clearly in early metastatic ovarian carcinoma.

The epithelial structures found in the normal ovary are restricted to the surface epithelium and a few tubules of the epoöphoron which invade the hilum of the ovary to a slight degree. No other epithelial structures are found. In consequence there is considerable difficulty in explaining the origin of the common ovarian tumours, most of which are epithelial in type. It is incorrect to use the term germinal epithelium as synonymous with surface epithelium, as it is almost certain that it does not produce the germ cells of the ovum.

The Epoöphoron. The epoöphoron, sometimes called the organ of Rosen-müller, represents the cranial end of the Wolffian body. It consists of a series of vertical tubules in the mesosalpinx and mesovarium between the Fallopian tube above and the ovary below. The tubules can usually be seen without difficulty if the mesosalpinx is stretched out and examined by transmitted light. Each tubule is surrounded by plain muscle and is lined by cubical cells.

The Paroöphoron. The paroöphoron represents the caudal end of the Wolf-fian body. It consists of a few vertical tubules in the mesosalpinx medial to the position of the ovary and internal to the tubules of the epoöphoron.

The Wolffian Duct. The Wolffian duct, or Gärtner's duct, is represented by an imperfect duct which runs parallel to the Fallopian tube in the mesosalpinx a little below the level of the tube. Medially Gärtner's duct passes downwards by the side of the uterus to the level of the internal os where it passes into the tissues of the cervix. It then runs forwards to reach the antero-lateral aspect of the vaginal wall and in some cases can be distinguished as far down as the level of the hymen. Gärtner's duct is imperfectly developed except in the mesosalpinx part of its course. It is rare for distention cysts to arise from Gärtner's duct. Cysts are sometimes found between the anterior vaginal wall and the urethra which are believed to arise from remains of Gärtner's duct.

The tube and ovary are so closely related anatomically and surgically that they are frequently referred to collectively as the appendage or adnexum. Hence the terms right or left adnexal inflammation or tumour.

THE URETHRA

The urethra measures 35 mm. in length and passes downwards and forwards from the base of the bladder behind the symphysis pubis to end in the external urinary meatus. It has an epithelial lining consisting of squamous epithelium at the external meatus which becomes transitional in the canal. Deep to the epithelium is a layer rich in small veins and connective tissue.

The urethra is surrounded by a complicated system of specially arranged, smooth muscle fibres and, when it pierces the triangular ligament 12 mm.

from the external meatus, it is surrounded by the voluntary compressor urethrae muscle.

THE EXTERNAL URINARY MEATUS

The external meatus lies in the vestibule below the clitoris and consists of two lateral lips. It is partly concealed by the upper ends of the labia minora which should be parted by the fingers in order to demonstrate its opening. Numerous periurethral glands surround the urethra and open by tiny ducts into its lumen: these are the analogue of the prostate in the male. The paraurethral glands of Skene are paired structures which lie alongside the floor of the urethra and open by two tiny ducts close to the external meatus. All these glands can be the site of acute and chronic inflammation and may form periurethral abscesses and cysts. Occasionally stones form in these inflamed structures.

THE BLADDER

The bladder lies between the uterus and the symphysis pubis, being separated from the body of the uterus by the uterovesical pouch of peritoneum. The anteverted uterus lies in contact with the top of the bladder so that when the bladder is empty its upper surface is concave. The bladder is covered by peritoneum on its upper surface and on each side.

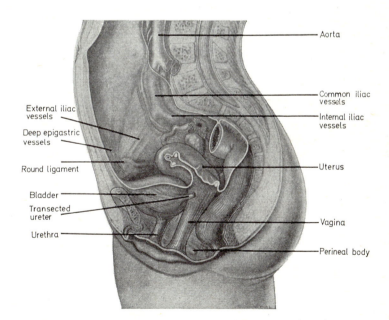

FIG. 18. Pelvic organs seen laterally in a left off-central saggital plane. In the mid-line the Pouch of Douglas is deeper than illustrated with its anterior wall more obviously related to the upper third of the vagina.

The **urachus** passes from the apex of the bladder extraperitoneally to the umbilicus. When the bladder is empty the mucosa of the bladder is thrown into folds as the result of laxity of the tissues of the submucosa. Few folds are found over the trigone. The trigone of the bladder is demarcated by the two ureteric orifices and by the internal urethral meatus. The interureteric bar passes between the two ureters while posterior to the bar lies the **retroureteric recess.** The importance of the retroureteric recess is that it is the part of the bladder which first prolapses in the presence of cystocele. The bladder consists of three layers, peritoneal, muscular and mucous, with a submucosa intervening between the mucous membrane and the muscle wall. The lining epithelium of the bladder is transitional as far as the external urethral meatus, where it becomes stratified. The bladder empties itself by contraction of the muscle wall which forms the **detrusor vesicae** muscle.

Sphincter Mechanism of the Bladder

(1) In the region of the bladder neck at the urethro-vesical junction, there is a complicated arrangement of smooth muscle fibre slings which encircle the bladder neck and the upper part of the urethra to form a smooth muscle sphincter. These involuntary muscle fibres are relaxed during micturition and the upper urethra becomes dilated by urine.

(2) The urethra itself is surrounded by spirally arranged smooth muscle slings whose function is similar to (1) above.

(3) The compressor urethrae is a voluntary muscle situated in the layers of the triangular ligament and its supposed function is to arrest the passage of urine and to empty the urethra at the end of micturition. This is sometimes called the external sphincter as opposed to the internal sphincter at the bladder neck. A similar arrangement is seen in the anal canal. The sphincteric action of this voluntary muscle is of very small importance compared with the involuntary sphincter.

(4) The anterior fibres of the pubo-rectalis when contracted draw the vagina and urethra forwards towards the symphysis and in this way somewhat help to control micturition.

All these structures may be distorted during pregnancy or injured by childbirth and their damage contributes to the causation of stress incontinence of urine.

The mechanism of micturition and its sphincteric control can be best studied by taking a lateral cystogram with a contrast medium in the bladder. In the normal bladder at rest when distended moderately, there is a well-marked posterior urethro-vesical angle of 100° between the bladder base and the posterior wall of the urethra. During micturition this is obliterated. It is also partly or completely obliterated in most patients with stress incontinence.

The normal capacity of the bladder is roughly 500 ml. The intravesical pressure is maintained by bladder muscular tone at 10 cms. of water irrespective of its capacity. In an untrained bladder at 250 ml. capacity the stretch receptors in the bladder muscle initiate a reflex process of micturition. In the normal adult trained bladder this reflex can be inhibited and some women are capable of holding urine at a capacity far greater than the normal complement of 500 ml. In spite of the increased distension the intravesical pressure remains remarkably constant at 10 cms. of water and it only becomes raised when full capacity signals an urgent desire to void. Contraction of the abdominal muscles either voluntary during the act of micturition or involuntary during coughing raises the intravesical pressure to 50 or even 100 cms. of water. The urethro-vesical sphincter mechanism, if normal, can resist pressures well above 50 cms. of water and the urethra remains watertight. If, however, this mechanism is damaged stress incontinence occurs often at quite low pressures.

The events of normal micturition can be summarised as follows. When the bladder fills to 500 ml. the stretch receptors register a desire to void. If the time and place is inconvenient the higher centres via the hypothalamus and sacral nerves 2, 3 and 4 inhibit the detrusor reflex. When the patient is able to initiate micturition she disinhibits the muscle and raises her intra-abdominal pressure partly by the position she adopts for micturition and partly by voluntary contraction of the abdominal muscles.

This voluntary bearing down, somewhat similar to defaecation and childbirth, relaxes her levators and the bladder descends so that the urethro-vesical angle is obliterated. The resultant raised intravesical pressure, 50–100 cms. of water, opens the sphincter and forces urine into the urethra which is dilated from above downwards. The compressor urethrae is either voluntarily relaxed or overwhelmed by the raised intra-urethral pressure and voiding now ensures. When the act is complete the urethra closes from below upwards and any residual urine in it is milked back into the bladder.

It is hoped that this explanation will help the reader to understand some of the problems of urge and stress incontinence, which will be further discussed in a later chapter.

The blood supply of the urethra is from the terminal branches of the internal pudendal artery. The bladder neck is supplied by the inferior vesical artery, a branch of the hypogastric, and by anastomotic vaginal and cervical vessels. Venous plexuses drain to the hypogastric vein. The lymphatics of the urethra drain to the superficial inguinal group of glands and those of the bladder to the hypogastric group.

Anatomical Relations

Anterior. The urethra is related to the cave of Retzius above the triangular ligament and the back of the symphysis in the region of the bladder neck. Above this the bladder is similarly related in its lower aspects while the dome of the bladder, when full, is in direct contact with the muscles of the anterior abdominal wall.

Posterior. The urethra is related to the lower half of the anterior vaginal wall, the trigone and bladder neck to the upper half of the anterior vaginal wall. The bladder is then closely related to the cervix, the utero-vesical fold of peritoneum and the utero-vesical pouch possibly containing small bowel.

From below upwards the urethra is related to the bulbo-spongiosus muscle, the vestibular bulb, the inferior layer of the triangular ligament, the compressor urethrae, the superior layer of the triangular ligament, the puborectalis somewhat laterally, the pubo-cervical fascia and the vesical plexus of veins around the bladder neck.

THE URETER

The course of the ureter in the pelvis is important, for the ureter has to be dissected clear during Wertheim's operation and it may run in close relation to broad ligament cysts or myomata. The ureter passes over the bifurcation of the common iliac artery and runs downwards and forwards in the ovarian fossa deep to the peritoneum. Where it enters the true pelvis at the brim it is

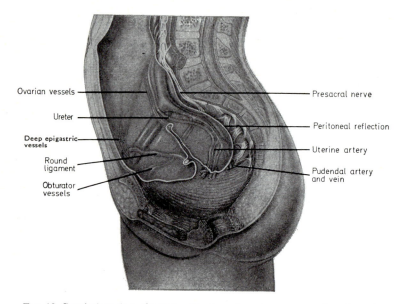

Ovarian vessels

Ureter

Deep epigastric vessels

Round ligament

Obturator vessels

Presacral nerve

Peritoneal reflection

Uterine artery

Pudendal artery and vein

FIG. 19. Saggital section of pelvis with visceral contents removed to show the structures of the lateral pelvic wall.

crossed by the ovarian vessels and, on the left side, the mesosigmoid is an anterior relation. In this situation the obturator vessels and nerve lie laterally, and the hypogastric lymphatic glands are closely related. The course of the ureter is then downwards and forwards immediately beneath the peritoneum to which it is always closely attached (Fig. 19).

The ureter pierces Mackenrodt's ligament where a canal, the ureteric canal, is developed. It is obvious that the ureter must have room in which its peristaltic movements can be carried out without pressure from surrounding structures, and it is for this reason that the ureteric canal is present. In its passage through the ureteric canal the ureter is crossed by the uterine artery and the uterine plexus of veins. After leaving the ureteric canal the ureter passes forwards and medially to reach the bladder, being separated from the cervix by a distance of 1 to 2 cm. The course of the ureter through the pelvis is not always constant, and there is a variation also in the origin of the uterine artery. At operation the ureter is recognised by its pale glistening appearance and by a fine longitudinal plexus of vessels on its surface, but more particularly by its peristaltic movements. It can be readily recognised by palpation between finger and thumb as a firm cord which, as it escapes, gives a characteristic snap. Absence of pulsation does not serve to identify a structure as the ureter. Veins do not pulsate, nor does the umbilical artery when obliterated. The ureter is sometimes duplicated, and in instances of carcinoma of the cervix with extensive involvement of the parametrium, dilatation of the ureter is frequently present. The ureter derives its blood supply from the common, external and internal iliac arteries in addition to a constant vessel from the uterine artery. It also receives blood from the inferior vesical artery. The vessels form a longitudinal anastomosis up and down the ureter, and damage or ligation of several of these vessels at operation may result in avascular necrosis and the production of a ureteric fistula.

THE RECTUM AND ANAL CANAL

The rectum proper starts at the level of the third sacral vertebra and measures about 12·5 cm. in length. Its ampulla is directly related to the middle third of the posterior vaginal wall. In the upper third its front and sides are covered by peritoneum; in the middle third its front only and in the lower third all the surfaces are devoid of peritoneal covering. It, therefore, has no mesentery and is directly related posteriorly to the hollow of the sacrum and the coccyx. The rectum ends in the anal canal which measures 2·5 cm. in length.

The blood supply of the rectum is from (1) the superior haemorrhoidal branch of the inferior mesenteric artery; (2) the middle haemorrhoidal branch of the hypogastric artery; (3) the inferior haemorrhoidal branch of the internal pudendal artery. The venous drainage follows the arteries and consequently supplies a portal-systemic anastomosis.

The anatomical relations of the rectum and anal canal are of considerable gynaecological importance.

Anterior Relations. The upper part of the rectum is related to the posterior wall of the pouch of Douglas and its contents; the ampulla is related to the vagina while its lowest part and the anal canal are in direct contact with the posterior aspect of the perineal body.

Lateral relations are the utero-sacral ligaments, levator ani (pubo-rectalis) of which fibres are inserted into the rectum and anal canal, and the ischio-rectal fossae.

Posterior relations. The lower sacrum and coccyx with its emergent nerve trunks, the middle sacral artery and venous plexus and a loose cellular connective tissue which permits easy surgical separation.

THE PELVIC MUSCULATURE

The pelvic muscles which are of importance in gynaecology are those of the pelvic floor. These muscles are grouped into three layers: (*a*) those of the

pelvic diaphragm, (*b*) those of the urogenital diaphragm, and (*c*) the superficial muscles of the pelvic floor.

(*a*) The **pelvic diaphragm** consists of the two levator ani muscles. Each
levator ani muscle consists of three main divisions, the pubococcygeus, the
iliococcygeus and the ischiococcygeus. The **pubococcygeus** muscle arises from
the posterior surface of the body of the pubic bone and passes backwards,
lateral to the vagina and rectum, to be inserted into the anococcygeal raphe
and into the coccyx. The inner fibres which come together posterior to the
rectum are known as the **puborectalis** portion of the muscle: they sling up

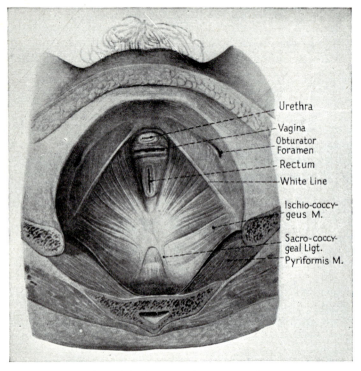

Fig. 20. The muscular pelvic floor seen from above after the removal of the
pelvic viscera and pelvic fascia .(Peham-Amreich.)

and support the rectum. Some of the inner fibres of the puborectalis fuse with
the outer wall of the vagina as they pass lateral to it. Other fibres decussate
between the vagina and rectum in the situation of the perineal body. These
decussating fibres divide the space between the two levator ani muscles into
an anterior portion, the **hiatus urogenitalis,** through which passes the urethra
and vagina, and a posterior portion, the **hiatus rectalis,** through which passes
the rectum. The dimensions of the hiatus urogenitalis depend upon two main
factors: the tone of the levator muscles and the existence of the decussating
fibres of the puborectalis muscle. Perineal tears occurring during parturition

may divide these decussating fibres, causing the hiatus urogenitalis to become patulous and leading to a tendency to prolapse. In visceroptosis and asthenic states the levator muscles become lax, the dimensions of the hiatus urogenitalis are increased, and there is a tendency for the pelvic viscera to prolapse. In virgins the hiatus urogenitalis is small, and its maximum width is less than the width of the uterus. The **iliococcygeus** is a fan-shaped muscle arising from a broad origin along the white line of the pelvic fascia and passing backwards and inwards to be inserted into the coccyx. The **ischiococcygeus** or coccygeus muscle has a narrow origin from the ischial spine and spreads out posteriorly to become inserted into the front of the coccyx (see Fig. 20).

The levator muscles together constitute the pelvic diaphragm and support the pelvic viscera: contraction of the levator muscle pulls the rectum and vagina towards the symphysis pubis; the rectum is thereby kinked and closed, and the vagina narrowed anteroposteriorly. The origin of the levator muscle is fixed because the muscle arises anteriorly either from bone or from fascia which is attached to bone: posteriorly the insertion is either into the ano-coccygeal raphe or into the coccyx, both of which are movable. It follows that contraction of the levator muscles leads to these posterior attachments being pulled towards the symphysis pubis. The movement of internal rotation of the presenting part during parturition is assisted by this property of the levator muscles. Uterine contractions push the presenting part down upon the levator ani and cause the muscle to contract as a result of the direct pressure of the presenting part. The lowest part of the foetus is carried forwards during the contraction of the levator muscles, and as the anterior fibres of the muscle are directed inwards as well as forwards the presenting part becomes rotated forwards and inwards.

The superior and inferior surfaces of the levator muscles are covered by the pelvic fascia which separates the muscles from the cellular tissue of the parametrium above and from the fibrous and fatty tissue of the ischiorectal fossa below.

(b) The **urogenital diaphragm** (also called the triangular ligament) is not so well developed in the female as in the male. It extends from the pubic arch anteriorly to the central point of the perineum posteriorly and consists of two layers of fascia through which pass the vagina and urethra. The central point of the female perineum lies between the vagina and the rectum. Within the two fascial layers of the urogenital diaphragm lies the **deep transverse perineal** muscle which extends laterally on each side to reach the ramus of the pubic bone. This muscle is so poorly developed that it is difficult to dissect in anatomical specimens and needs a special histological technique for its demonstration. Its functional significance is dubious. The striped muscle or voluntary sphincter of the urethra also lies between the two layers of the triangular ligaments.

(c) **The Superficial Muscles.** Four muscles are identified in this layer. The **external sphincter** muscle of the anus is attached anteriorly to the central point of the perineum and surrounds the anus. The **bulbospongiosus** muscle or, as it is sometimes called, the sphincter vaginae, extends from the central point of the perineum along each side of the vagina to be attached anteriorly to the symphysis pubis. It lies around and lateral to the urethral bulb. The **ischio-cavernosus** muscle extends on each side from the ischial tuberosity in relation to the crus of the clitoris to reach the clitoris in the mid-line. The **superficial transverse** muscle of the perineum passes laterally on each side from the central point of the perineum to the pubic ramus (see Fig. 21). Deep to these superficial muscles and between them and the inferior layer of the triangular ligament lie the vestibular bulb and the greater vestibular glands of Bartholin.

The **perineal body** intervenes between the posterior vaginal wall and the anal canal. It is pyramidal in shape with its apex on a level with the junction of the middle and lower thirds of the posterior vaginal wall. The three layers

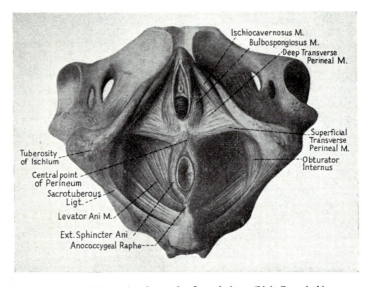

Fig. 21. The perineal muscles from below. (Veit-Stoeckel.)

of muscles of the pelvic floor are represented in the perineal body, and the intervening tissue consists of fat and fibrous tissue. Superficially, passing from the central point of the perineum, are the external sphincter of the anus, the bulbospongiosus and the superficial transverse muscle of the perineum. Deep to this layer lie the fascial layers of the urogenital diaphragm (triangular ligament) enclosing the deep transverse muscle of the perineum. Deeper still the pelvic diaphragm is represented by the fibres of the levator ani muscles which decussate between the vagina and rectum. Tears of the perineal body occur during parturition, and lacerations of the decussating fibres of the levator ani muscle widen the hiatus urogenitalis and produce a tendency to subsequent prolapse. The perineal body is examined by inspection and by palpation. Two fingers are placed in the vagina and flexed laterally, the thumb being applied externally over the perineal body. In this way the amount of muscle tissue in the perineal body can be determined and the technique affords a convenient method of estimating the tone of the levator muscles.

If the fingers are placed in the vagina and flexed laterally, the thumb being applied externally over the labium majus, the levator muscles can be palpated with remarkable ease and the size of the hiatus urogenitalis can be estimated. This method of examination demands no especial skill: all that is required is a knowledge of the anatomy of the pelvic muscles.

POSITION OF THE UTERUS

The uterus lies normally in a position of **anteversion** and **anteflexion.** The body of the uterus is bent forwards on the cervix approximately at the level of the internal os, and this forward inclination of the body of the uterus on the cervix constitutes anteflexion. The direction of the axis of the cervix depends upon the position of the uterus. In anteversion, the external os is directed downwards and backwards so that on vaginal examination the examining fingers find that the lowest part of the cervix is the anterior lip. When the uterus is retroverted the cervix is directed downwards and forwards and the lowest part of the cervix is either the external os or the posterior lip. As a result of its normal position of anteflexion the body of the uterus lies against the bladder. The pouch of peritoneum which separates the bladder from the uterus is the **uterovesical pouch.** The peritoneum is reflected from the front of the uterus on to the bladder at the level of the internal os.

Posteriorly a large peritoneal pouch lies between the uterus and the recto-sigmoid. If the uterus is pulled forwards, two folds of peritoneum can be seen to pass backwards from the uterus to reach the parietal peritoneum lateral to the rectum. These folds, the **uterosacral folds,** lie at the level of the internal os and pass backwards and upwards. The uterosacral folds should be clearly distinguished from the **uterosacral ligaments.** The uterosacral ligaments are condensations of the pelvic cellular tissues and lie at a lower level and within the uterosacral folds. The pouch of peritoneum below the level of the utero-sacral folds, which is bounded in front by the peritoneum covering the upper part of the posterior vaginal wall and posteriorly by the peritoneum covering the sigmoid colon and the upper end of the rectum, is the **pouch of Douglas.** The posterior fornix of the vagina is in close relation to the peritoneal cavity, as only the posterior vaginal wall and a single layer of peritoneum separate the vagina from the peritoneal cavity. Collections of pus in the pouch of Douglas can therefore be evacuated without difficulty by incising the vagina in the region of the posterior fornix. On the other hand the uterovesical pouch is approached with difficulty from the vagina; first the vagina must be incised and then the bladder separated from the front of the cervix and the vesicocervical space traversed before the uterovesical fold of peritoneum is reached.

THE PELVIC CELLULAR TISSUE

The pelvic cellular tissue consists of loose areolar tissue which intervenes between the peritoneum above and the pelvic fascia below. It is continuous with the subperitoneal connective tissue and with the loose tissue of the perinephric region. The areolar tissue is loose, and when inflamed in the condition of pelvic cellulitis may lead to the formation of a palpable swelling. As there is a direct continuation between the perinephric and pelvic cellular tissues effusions arising in either of these situations may track to point as an abscess in the other. In the pelvis, the pelvic cellular tissue is bounded above by the peritoneum and below by the fascia which covers the upper surface of the levator ani muscles. Laterally it is bounded by the pelvic wall, mainly by the fascia which covers the inner surface of the obturator internus, while medially it comes into contact with the uterus and the upper part of the vagina.

The **parametrium** is that part of the pelvic cellular tissue which surrounds the uterus. It is by definition extraperitoneal, and is most plentiful on each side of the uterus below the level of the internal os. Above this level, the presence of the broad ligaments reduces the amount of parametrium to a minimum. It should be remembered that the level of the levator ani muscles is well below the level of the cervix, being more than half-way down the vagina. The pelvic cellular tissue is usually very plentiful on each side of the vagina, where it is called the **paravaginal cellular tissue,** or paracolpos.

A distinction is drawn between the **pelvic fascia** and the **endopelvic fascia.** The pelvic fascia consists of the dense connective tissue which covers the surfaces of the levator ani and the obturator internus muscles. The endopelvic fascia on the other hand forms the connective tissue coverings for the vagina, the supravaginal portion of the cervix, the uterus, the bladder, the urethra and the rectum. In addition, condensed bands of endopelvic fascia pass from these movable organs to the back of the pubic bones, to the lateral walls of the pelvis and to the front of the sacrum. The function of the endopelvic fascia is partly to convey blood vessels to the pelvic organs and partly to support them. Between the different layers of the endopelvic fascia are bloodless spaces which it is important to identify in vaginal plastic operations. The term **pelvic cellular tissue** should be restricted to the cellular tissue which intervenes between the different layers of the endopelvic fascia and which lies between the peritoneum above and the true pelvic fascia below.

Anteriorly, the bladder is covered by an endopelvic fascial layer called the vesical fascia, while behind it lie the vagina and supravaginal portion of the cervix covered by their own endopelvic fascial layers.

Immediately behind the uterus and vagina the peritoneum which covers the back of the uterus and the posterior vaginal fornix reduces the pelvic cellular tissue to a minimum in these situations. Deep to the uterosacral folds of peritoneum the endopelvic fascia is plentiful, and here it is condensed to form the **uterosacral ligaments** which pass backwards and upwards from the uterus in front to reach the sacrum lateral to the recto-sigmoid. The uterosacral ligaments help to support the uterus and prevent it from being forced down by intra-abdominal pressure. By their tone they also tend to pull back the cervix and thereby antevert the uterus. Plain muscle fibres can be demonstrated in them.

The endopelvic fascia of the parametrium is also condensed to form a ligament on each side of the cervix, immediately below the level of the internal os. Three names have been given to this ligament, namely, **Mackenrodt's ligament,** the **cardinal ligament of the uterus** and the **transverse cervical ligament.** Mackenrodt's ligament spreads outwards in a fan-shaped manner from the cervix and upper part of the vagina to extend as far as the wall of the pelvis. It lies below the level of the uterine artery, but is pierced by the ureter where a canal known as the ureteric canal is formed. Mackenrodt's ligament like the uterosacral ligament, helps to support the uterus and prevents it from being forced down when the intra-abdominal pressure is raised. It is composed almost entirely of connective tissue and contains very little plain muscle (see Fig. 22).

A third and equally important part of the supporting mechanism of the pelvic viscera is the pubo-vesico-cervical fascia or pubo-cervical fascia. This is a condensation of the endopelvic fascia which passes from the antero-lateral aspect of the cervix to be attached to the back of the pubic bone lateral

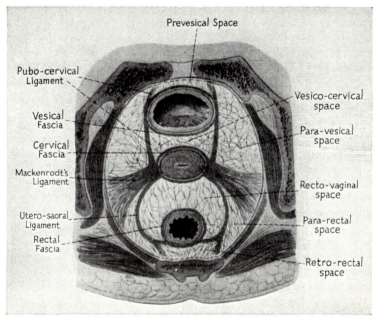

Fig. 22. The pelvic cellular tissue shown in cross-section of the pelvis. (Peham-Amreich.)

to the symphysis. Some of its cervical attachment fans out laterally and imperceptibly into the transverse cervical or Mackenrodt's ligament. It can, therefore, be regarded as morphologically and functionally a part of this structure.

If Fig. 22 is studied the supports of the uterus and bladder are seen to be a tri-radiate condensation of endopelvic fascia:

(1) The anterior spoke is the pubo-cervical fascia or so-called pubo-cervical ligament.

(2) The lateral spoke is Mackenrodt's ligament.

(3) The posterior spoke is the utero-sacral ligament.

All these three embrace and insert into the cervix and, when intact, operate on it like the strings of a hammock, preventing descent. If one or two strings are torn the contents of the hammock prolapse with resulting descent of the bladder and uterus.

The endopelvic fascial tissues contain the uterine arteries and veins, together with the venous plexuses around the cervix and the lateral fornices of the vagina. The lymphatics from the upper two-thirds of the vagina, from the uterus, from the ovaries and Fallopian tubes also pass through the pelvic cellular tissue. On each side of the uterus there is sometimes a small inconstant lymphatic gland known as the gland of the parametrium, about the size of a pin's head, near the ureteric canal. The ureter passes through the parametrium via the ureteric canal in an antero-posterior direction, about 1 cm. lateral to the cervix to reach the bladder. It passes below the level of the uterine vessels, which cross it as they run transversely through the pelvis to reach the uterus. Sympathetic nerve ganglia and nerve fibres are plentiful in the parametrium (Frankenhauser's plexus).

In the condition of parametritis the parametrium is inflamed and thickened. Rarely a large swelling is present which illustrates the anatomy of the parametrium. It extends as far down as the fascia covering the levator ani muscles and medially it comes directly into contact with the uterus and the upper part of the vagina. Laterally it extends as far out as the pelvic wall. Posteriorly it extends along the uterosacral ligaments in close relation to the recto-sigmoid. Such a swelling may track upwards out of the pelvis to reach the subperitoneal tissues of the iliac region when the effusion may point above Poupart's ligament lateral to the great vessels. In other cases, the swelling may track upwards to the perinephric region. In advanced cases of carcinoma of the cervix, the cancer cells infiltrate the parametrium when they spread either laterally along Mackenrodt's ligaments or posteriorly along the uterosacral ligaments. Clinically, infiltration of the parametrium is detected by determining the mobility of the cervix and body of the uterus, by palpating in the situation of Mackenrodt's ligament through the lateral fornix of the vagina and by examining the uterosacral ligaments by rectal examination.

THE PELVIC BLOOD VESSELS

The **ovarian arteries** arise from the aorta, just below the level of the renal arteries. They pass downwards to cross first the ureter and then the external iliac artery, and then they pass into the infundibulopelvic fold. The ovarian artery sends branches to the ovaries and to the outer part of the Fallopian tube; it ends by anastomosing with the terminal part of the uterine artery (see Fig. 23) after giving off a branch to the cornu and one to the round ligament.

The **uterine artery** arises from the anterior trunk of the internal iliac or hypogastric artery. Its course is at first downwards and forwards until it reaches the parametrium when it turns medially towards the uterus. It reaches the uterus at the level of the internal os, where it turns upwards, at right angles, and follows a spiral course along the lateral border of the uterus to the region of the uterine cornu; here it sends a branch to supply the Fallopian

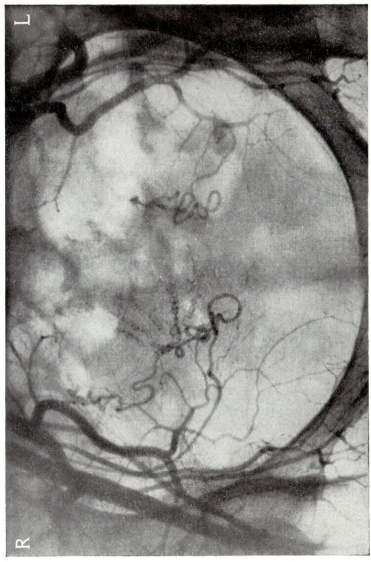

FIG. 23. Arteriogram showing the pelvic blood supply. Note the coiled uterine arteries and the anastomosis with the ovarian artery on the right side. (With acknowledgement to Drs. Borell and Fernström, Stockholm.)

tube and ends by anastomosing with the ovarian artery. The tortuosity is lost when the uterus enlarges during pregnancy. During the vertical part of its course branches, which run transversely, pass into the myometrium. These are called the arcuate arteries and from them arise a series of radial arteries almost at right angles. These radial arteries reach the basal layers of the endometrium where they are termed the basal arteries. From these are derived the terminal spiral and straight arterioles of the endometrium. The least vascular part of the uterus is in the midline: in consequence a midline incision is made in the uterus during the classical Caesarean section operation. The vaginal branch of the uterine artery arises before the uterine artery passes vertically upwards at the level of the internal os. It passes downwards through the parametrium to reach the vagina in the region of the lateral fornix. This descending vaginal artery is of great importance during the operation of total hysterectomy since, if not separately clamped and tied, it may give rise to dangerous post-operative haemorrhage. The arcuate arteries which supply the cervix are sometimes called the circular artery of the cervix. From these or the descending vaginal branches are derived the anterior and posterior azygos arteries of the vagina.

The branches of the uterine artery are:
(1) Ureteric.
(2) Descending vaginal ⎫ These unite to form the anterior and posterior
(3) Circular cervical ⎭ azygos artery of the vagina.
(4) Arcuate → radial → basal → spiral and straight arterioles of the functional layer of the endometrium.
(5) Anastomotic with the ovarian artery.

The relation of the uterine artery to the ureter is of great importance. The uterine artery crosses above the ureter in the parametrium where it gives off an important ureteric branch to that structure. The artery runs transversely while the ureter runs approximately antero-posteriorly through the ureteric canal of the parametrium.

The Vaginal Arteries

Usually the blood supply of the upper part of the vagina is derived from the vaginal branch of the uterine artery. This vessel reaches the lateral fornix of the vagina and then passes downwards along the lateral vaginal wall. It sends branches transversely across the vagina, which anastomose with branches on the opposite side to form the azygos arteries of the vagina, which run down longitudinally, one in front of the vagina and one behind. These small vessels are encountered in the operations of anterior and posterior colporrhaphy. In some cases the vaginal artery does not arise direct from the uterine artery but arises from the anterior division of the hypogastric artery, when it corresponds to the inferior vesical artery in the male.

The Arteries of the Vulva and Perineum

The blood vessels of the perineum and external genitalia are derived from the internal pudendal artery. The main vessel passes forwards in the ischiorectal fossa adjacent to the obturator internus muscle in Alcock's canal. It gives off the inferior haemorrhoidal artery and the transverse perineal artery which supplies the perineum and the region of the external sphincter. It then pierces the urogenital diaphragm and sends another transverse branch to supply the posterior part of the labia and to supply the erectile tissue which surrounds the vaginal orifice. The internal pudendal artery ends, as the dorsal artery of the clitoris, by supplying the clitoris and vestibule. The tissues around the vaginal orifice, the clitoris and the crura of the clitoris contain a large amount of erectile tissue. Lacerations of the anterior part of the vulva during childbirth which involve these areas may be followed by severe bleeding.

The terminal branches of the internal pudendal anastomose with superficial and deep pudendal arteries which are branches of the femoral artery. This anastomosis is important as it provides an alternative blood supply to the bladder in extended pelvic surgery when the vesical branches of the hypogastric are tied off or even the main trunk of the hypogastic itself may have been ligated at its source.

The Pelvic Veins

The left ovarian vein ends by passing into the left renal vein. The right ovarian vein terminates in the inferior vena cava. The most important feature of the pelvic veins is that they form plexuses. These are well marked in the case of the ovarian veins in the infundibulo-pelvic fold where they form a pampiniform plexus. Occasionally this plexus becomes varicose and the large dilated veins form a varicocele similar to the condition commonly seen in the male. The uterine plexus is found around the uterine artery near the uterus; the vaginal plexus around the lateral fornix of the vagina. These venous plexuses are well developed in the presence of large myomata and also during pregnancy when a venous plexus can be distinguished between the base of the bladder and the uterus.

There are two additional channels of venous drainage which are of interest in explaining unexpected sites of metastases in malignant disease of the genital tract:

(1) A portal systemic anastomosis exists between the hypogastric vein and the portal system via the middle and inferior haemorrhoidal veins of the systemic and the superior haemorrhoidal vein of the portal system. This accounts for some liver metastases.

(2) A communication between the middle and lateral sacral and lateral lumbar venous system and the vertebral plexus, which may explain some vertebral and even intracranial metastases, sometimes but rarely seen in genital tract cancers. In such patients the lungs may escape metastases as they are by-passed by the malignant emboli.

THE LYMPHATIC SYSTEM

The lymphatics and lymphatic glands which drain the female genital organs are of especial importance in malignant disease.

The Lymphatic Glands or Nodes

The lymphatic glands which drain the female genital organs are as follows:

The Inguinal Glands. This group of glands consists of a horizontal and a vertical group. The horizontal group lies superficially, parallel to Poupart's ligament, while the vertical group, otherwise known as the deep femoral glands, follows the course of the saphenous and femoral veins. The uppermost of the deep femoral glands, called the gland of Cloquet, or the gland of

Rosenmüller, lies beneath Poupart's ligament in the femoral canal between Gimbernat's ligament and the femoral vein. Inconstant deep inguinal nodes are found in the inguinal canal, along the course of the round ligament, and inconstant nodes are found in the tissues of the mons veneris. In such conditions as primary sore and Bartholin's abscess, the horizontal inguinal group becomes inflamed. There is some evidence that lymphatics from the fundus of the uterus pass along the round ligament and drain into this horizontal inguinal group. It is more likely that these glands will become involved after the appearance of the late suburethral metastasis seen in advanced carcinoma corporis uteri, where the growth has spread down the vagina by retrograde lymphatic spread.

The Gland of the Parametrium. This is a small lymphatic gland about the size of a pin's head which sometimes lies in the parametrium near the situation where the uterine artery crosses the ureter. It is inconstant.

The Hypogastric Glands. The hypogastric group contains all the regional glands for the cervix, the bladder, the upper third of the vagina, and also for the greater part of the body of the uterus. This group of glands may be extensively involved in carcinoma of the cervix and of the vagina. The glands are most numerous immediately below the bifurcation of the common iliac where they are sometimes called the glands of the bifurcation. The lymphatics from the hypogastric lymphatic glands pass to the common iliac group. A further group of these glands situated in the obturator fossa is often called the obturator glands and is frequently the most obviously involved in carcinoma of the cervix.

External Iliac Glands. This group of glands, several in number, is situated in relation to the external iliac artery and vein. A clean dissection of the external iliac glands can only be made if both vessels are completely mobilised as some of the glands lie lateral to the vessels between them and the lateral pelvic wall. These glands receive drainage from the obturator and hypogastric glands and are always involved in late cervical cancer.

Common Iliac Glands. This group is the upward continuation of the external and hypogastric group and, therefore, involved next after these glands in genital tract cancer.

The Sacral Group. These glands lie on each side of the rectum and receive lymphatics from the cervix of the uterus and from the upper third of the vagina which have passed backwards along the uterosacral ligaments. Two groups of glands can be recognised, a lateral group lying lateral to the rectum and a medial group lying in front of the promontory of the sacrum. The lymphatics from these glands pass directly either to the inferior lumbar group or to the common iliac group.

The Lumbar Group of Glands. These lymphatic glands are divided into an inferior group which lies in front of the aorta below the origin of the inferior mesenteric artery and a superior lumbar group which lies near the origin of the ovarian arteries. The superior group of lumbar glands receives lymphatics from the ovaries and Fallopian tubes as well as from the inferior lumbar glands. The lymphatics from the fundus of the uterus join the ovarian lymphatics to pass to the same group.

The lymphatic glands already mentioned, viz., the glands of the para-metrium, the superficial inguinal, the hypogastric, external and common iliac, the sacral and the lumbar receive lymphatics "direct" from the female generative organs and are known as the "regional lymphatic glands" of the female genitalia.

The Lymphatics of the Uterus. Two main plexuses of lymphatics can be demonstrated in the uterus, one in the basal layer of the endometrium and the other immediately beneath the peritoneum. The lymphatics of the myometrium are small channels in close relation to the small blood vessels.

The Lymphatics of the Cervix. The lymphatics of the cervix pass upwards from the cervix along the course of the uterine veins. They then pass direct to the following glands: (a) the gland of the parametrium, (b) the hypogastric group, and (c) backwards along the uterosacral ligaments to the lateral sacral group. In addition, lymphatics from the cervix pass to the lymph glands found in the obturator fossa and to the external iliac group.

The lymphatics from the lower part of the body of the uterus pass outwards to join the hypogastric group. The lymphatics from the fundus of the uterus anastomose with the ovarian lymphatics to end in the superior lumbar group. A few lymphatics may perhaps pass along the round ligament to terminate in the horizontal inguinal group, though this pathway is inconstant.

The Lymphatics of the Fallopian Tubes and Ovary. A subperitoneal and a mucosal plexus can be distinguished in the Fallopian tube. The lymphatics pass upwards to end in the superior lumbar group. The small lymphatics of the ovarian cortex drain into large channels in the medulla and via the hilum reach the infundibulo-pelvic fold to end in the superior lumbar group. There is free inter-communication between the ovarian lymphatics of each side across the fundus of the uterus and via the uterosacral lymphatics.

The Lymphatics of the Vagina. The lymphatics of the lower third of the vagina pass externally to end in the horizontal inguinal group. The lymphatic drainage of the upper third of the vagina is the same as that of the cervix. The lymphatics from the middle third of the vagina pass to the hypogastric group.

The Lymphatics of the Vulva. The lymphatics of the labia minora inter-communicate in the vestibule with lymphatics from the opposite side, and the lymphatics from the upper parts of the labia majora intercommunicate in the region of the mons. In this way a carcinoma of one side of the vulva may produce a metastasis in the glands of the opposite side. The lymphatics from the labia, together with the lymphatics from the prepuce of the clitoris, pass into the superficial inguinal glands. The lymphatics from the glans of the clitoris pass to the pubic plexus and subsequently to both groups of the inguinal glands and to the external iliac group as well. It has been shown by Stanley Way that there is a direct lymphatic pathway from the clitoris to the gland of Cloquet. The lymphatics from Bartholin's glands pass both to the superficial inguinal glands and to the anorectal group which lie behind the rectum. The lymphatics from the superficial inguinal group pass to the deep femoral group, and by way of the gland of Cloquet to the external iliac glands. The lymphatic pathways of the female genital tract can be studied *in vivo* by injecting a dye called Pontamine Sky Blue. This demonstrates that, if there is unilateral obstruction of the normal ovarian lymphatic vessels, the dye will pass mostly by the uterosacral channels to the opposite ovary. This is of importance in understanding the bilateral nature of ovarian cancer. This technique of dye injection can be used to demonstrate the spread of corporeal and cervical cancers.

NERVES

The **ilio-inguinal nerve,** derived from the first lumbar, pierces the external abdominal ring and supplies the skin of the mons and upper part of the labium majus. The genital branch of the genito-femoral (derived from L.1 and L.2) supplies the inner side of the thigh and the outer part of the labium majus, while branches from the posterior femoral cutaneous nerve supply the outer aspects of the posterior part of the labia majora and the perineum.

The **pudendal nerve,** derived from the second, third and fourth sacral segments, runs in Alcock's canal in the ischiorectal fossa where it gives off the inferior haemorrhoidal nerve. It divides into two terminal branches: the perineal nerve, the larger of the two, which supplies the posterior part of the labia and the muscles of the perineum, and the dorsal nerve of the clitoris, which passes laterally forwards to reach the dorsum of the clitoris.

The **levator ani muscle** receives its nerve supply direct from the third and fourth sacral. The muscles of the urogenital diaphragm and the superficial muscles of the perineum are supplied either directly from the pudendal nerve or from its perineal branch.

The Sympathetic Nerve Supply

Both sympathetic and parasympathetic systems supply the female genital organs.

The **sympathetic system** in the abdomen consists of the abdominal sympathetic trunk together with the nerve ganglia which lie in front of the aorta. These ganglia are the coeliac, the renal, the superior mesenteric and the inferior mesenteric. In addition to the trunks and ganglia a plexus of sympathetic nerves can be distinguished in front of the aorta. Fibres from the aortic plexus pass downwards in the midline crossing the bifurcation and are identified in front of the promontory of the sacrum by a well-defined plexus which constitutes the **presacral nerve.** The presacral nerve, or, as it is sometimes called, the superior hypogastric plexus, measures between 5 and 6 cm. in length and is roughly triangular in shape with its apex near the bifurcation of the aorta. Its main supply is from the aortic plexus, but it also receives fibres directly from the sympathetic trunk. Below, the presacral nerve divides into two branches, the hypogastric nerves, which pass downwards laterally along the pelvic wall and terminate in the inferior hypogastric plexus. This plexus is diffuse, but it lies in the situation of the uterosacral ligaments above the level of the pelvic fascia. Most of the fibres passing to the inferior hypogastric plexus are derived from the hypogastric nerve. It is also supplied by a few fibres direct from the sacral ganglia and some fibres from the superior haemorrhoidal plexus, while the remainder of the nerve is derived from the nervus erigens, which belongs to the parasympathetic system. This is called by some writers the **pelvic nerve** and is derived from sacral 2, 3 and 4. From the hypogastric ganglia nerve fibres pass to the ureter, bladder, rectum, uterus and the vagina. The cervix is surrounded by the utero-vaginal plexus of Frankenhauser which can be considered to be an anterior extension of the inferior hypogastric plexus.

The ovarian plexus, derived from the coeliac and the renal ganglia, consists of fibres which follow the course of the ovarian vessels to reach the ovary, Fallopian tubes and also the fundus of the uterus.

The operation of presacral sympathectomy consists in excising the presacral nerve. The nerve fibres are easily displayed below the bifurcation of the aorta in front of the promontory of the sacrum lying deep to the peritoneum. The operation used to be performed for the treatment of intractable spasmodic dysmenorrhoea but it is now seldom indicated.

Although the nerve supply of the uterus has not been finally agreed, certain facts have now been confirmed:

(1) The motor supply is entirely sympathetic and is derived from D.5 and 6. The contractions of labour can be modified or inhibited by a spinal or epidural anaesthetic which reaches this level.

(2) The segments responsible for uterine sensation are D.10 or D.11 down to L.1. A spinal or epidural as high but no higher than D.10 renders labour painless.

(3) The somatic distribution of uterine pain is that area of the lower abdomen supplied by D.10 to L.1.

(4) Parasympathetic fibres carried in S.2, 3 and 4 which pass to the plexus of Frankenhauser are largely sensory to the cervix. Their motor function is not understood and is probably minimal.

(5) The sensory and motor supply of the bladder is derived from the nervi erigentes (S.2, 3 and 4) and the inferior hypogastric plexus. In a radical Wertheim's operation when the pelvic cellular tissue is properly cleared, the sensory and motor function of the bladder is bound to be impaired. Bladder insensitivity and incomplete voiding or residual urine are, therefore, common complications of this operation.

(6) Inflammatory conditions of the cervix which cause parametritis, may irritate the sensory fibres of S.2, 3 and 4 and refer pain to the mid-sacral region of the back.

(7) The sensory supply of the tube and ovary is D.10 to D.12 and painful lesions of the appendages are normally projected to a somatic area of the lower abdominal quadrant above the middle point of Poupart's ligament.

(8) Both the uterus and bladder possess intrinsic powers of contraction and can act reasonably well when denervated. For example, labour proceeds painlessly but with effective contractions after bilateral ovarian denervation and presacral neurectomy and the bladder retains reasonable function after the most extensive Wertheim's operation even if it is insensitive and has a greatly impaired motor function.

(9) Like most abdominal viscera the uterus is insensitive to pinching, cutting or burning, and the cervix can be painlessly cauterised without

anaesthesia. The cervix is, however, most resentful of stretching by dilators and distension of the uterus by gas, especially if the tubes are blocked, can cause painful colicky spasm.

(10) The ovary is sensitive to distension especially if the capsule is resistant, hence the appreciation of follicular distension just before ovulation by some women—the so-called ovulation pain. Like the testicle, the ovary is acutely conscious of compression—hence the pain of dyspareunia when the ovary is prolapsed into Douglas' pouch by a retroverted uterus.

The **parasympathetic system** is represented by the **nervus erigens,** or the pelvic nerve, as it is sometimes called, which obtains fibres from the second, third and fourth sacral segments. The nervus erigens passes to the hypogastric plexus.

Development of the Female Generative Organs

There is a close relation between the genital glands, the urinary organs, and the uterus and its appendages during early intrauterine life. If a transverse

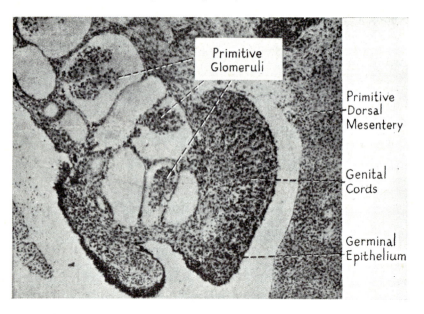

FIG. 24. The genital ridge. On the extreme right lies the mesentery of the primitive intestine. In the middle of the photograph the intermediate cell mass projects into the coelom. The genital ridge is differentiated on the inner aspect of the intermediate cell mass near the primitive mesentery. The surface epithelium together with the primitive genital cords is indicated. Primitive glomeruli lie in the deeper portion of the intermediate cell mass.

section is cut through the upper part of the coelomic cavity of an embryo of eight weeks' development, the primitive mesentery is seen to project into the coelomic cavity posteriorly near the midline. On each side of the primitive mesentery another projection, the **intermediate cell mass,** can be distinguished.

On the inner side of the intermediate cell mass, by the end of the eighth week, a ridge has appeared, the **genital ridge**. The **Wolffian body** with primitive tubules and primitive glomeruli occupies the rest of the intermediate cell mass (see Fig. 24).

The **primitive urinary system** consists of the pronephros, the mesonephros, or Wolffian body, and the metanephros, which gives rise to the permanent kidney. Each of these systems is derived from the urogenital plates of the primitive somites. The pronephros corresponds to the hinder cervical, the Wolffian body to the dorsal and lumbar, while the metanephros is sacral in origin. Each system consists of a series of tubules and a collecting tubule or duct. In the human female the pronephros disappears, and the Wolffian body is represented by the straight tubules of the epoöphoron, or organ of Rosen-müller, found in the mesosalpinx of the adult, while the tubules of the paroöphoron represent the relics of the renal tubules of the Wolffian system, Gärtner's duct representing the Wolffian duct. The metanephros gives rise to the tubules of the permanent kidney, while the ureter and renal pelvis are formed from a diverticulum from the lower end of the Wolffian duct. The uterus and Fallopian tubes and most of the vagina are derived from the **Müllerian ducts.** The Müllerian duct is formed as a result of invagination of the mesothelium of the coelomic cavity on the ventral part of the intermediate cell mass. The invagination extends from the pronephros region above to the sacral region below, and both ducts terminate in the primitive cloaca. The position of the Müllerian duct is of importance, for it lies ventral to the Wolffian duct on the outer surface of the intermediate cell mass. In the human embryo the caudal parts of the two Müllerian ducts fuse to form the uterus, while the upper parts remain as the Fallopian tubes. The significance of the development of the Müllerian ducts is of great importance in gynae-cological pathology, for a similar process of downgrowth and metaplasia may develop in adults. If it arises in the ovary it may produce endometriomata or chocolate cysts, and it is believed that many ovarian neoplasms arise from somewhat similar downgrowths. Similar changes may develop on the surface of the uterus and pelvic peritoneum to produce endometriosis.

The uterus itself can be identified as early as the end of the third month. The upper end of the Müllerian duct becomes the abdominal ostium of the Fallopian tube and it is not uncommon for small accessory ostia to be found.

In its early stages of development the **human uterus** is bicornuate, corresponding in form to the uterus of lower mammalia. Later, as the result of fusion of the two Müllerian ducts, a single uterus with a midline septum remains. During the 5th month of intrauterine life the septum disappears, and all that is left of it in the adult uterus are the anterior and posterior columns of the mucous membrane of the cervical canal. The muscle wall of the uterus is differentiated from mesoblastic tissues, and during the 5th month a circular layer of muscle can be distinguished. The longitudinal muscles of the uterus can be recognised during the 7th month, and this muscle layer is con-tinuous morphologically with the plain muscle tissue of the ovarian ligament, the round ligament and the muscle fibres found in the uterosacral ligaments.

The **primitive cloaca** is divided by the formation of the urorectal septum into a ventral part, the **urogenital sinus,** and a dorsal part, the rectum. The urorectal septum ultimately develops into the perineal body. The lower ends of the Müllerian ducts terminate in the urogenital sinus into the posterior part of which they project as a solid Müllerian tubercle. Around this Müllerian tubercle there is a solid proliferation of the urogenital sinus on each side, called the sinovaginal bulbs. By canalisation of the sinovaginal bulbs, the lower quarter to one-third of the vagina is formed and the hymen represents the remnants of the sinovaginal bulb. Incomplete breakdown is one cause of congenital vaginal atresia.

The vagina is, therefore, developed in its upper three-quarters from Müller's duct and represented at its lower end by the solid Müllerian tubercle which subsequently becomes canalised. The lower quarter of the vagina is developed from the sinovaginal bulbs of the urogenital sinus which also becomes canalised. The epithelium of the vagina and the portio vaginalis of the cervix, since it is stratified, is derived from an upgrowth of the epithelium of the urogenital sinus. This is comparable to the stratified epithelium of the anal canal.

Just as in the case of the cervix, anterior and posterior columns can be recognised in the adult vagina which represent the remains of the septum between the two Müllerian ducts.

In the early stage of development the cervix of the uterus is longer and thicker than the body, and this proportion persists until puberty. The proportions may persist in adult life, when the uterus is described as infantile in type. The cervical glands can be recognised during the 6th month, while the glands of the body of the uterus develop only during the last month of intrauterine life though primitive glands are present at the 4th month.

The Urogenital Sinus and the External Genital Organs. The cloaca becomes divided into two parts through the development of the **urorectal septum,** which originally consists of two folds which project on each side and then fuse caudally to divide the cloaca into a dorsal part, the rectum, and a ventral portion, the urogenital sinus. The primitive cloaca is closed by the cloacal membrane, which can be recognised very early in the development of the embryo and from which the vessels of the allantois are developed. The primitive intestine enters the dorsal part of the cloaca. Both Wolffian ducts, both Müllerian ducts and the allantois from which the bladder and urethra are differentiated, enter the urogenital sinus. Originally the ureter arises from the lower end of the Wolffian duct near the opening of the duct into the urogenital sinus. Subsequently, as the result of the growth of the surrounding mesoblastic tissues, the ureter is displaced cranially so that it enters the urogenital sinus independently of the Wolffian duct. This displacement of the ureter explains the aberrant types of ureter which are sometimes encountered in gynaecological surgery. The part of the urogenital sinus which lies ventral to the mouths of the Wolffian ducts becomes differentiated into the bladder, while the allantois is represented by the urachus passing upwards from the apex of the bladder to the umbilicus.

The clitoris is developed from the genital tubercle which appears about the 5th week and is originally a bilateral structure derived from mesoderm. From

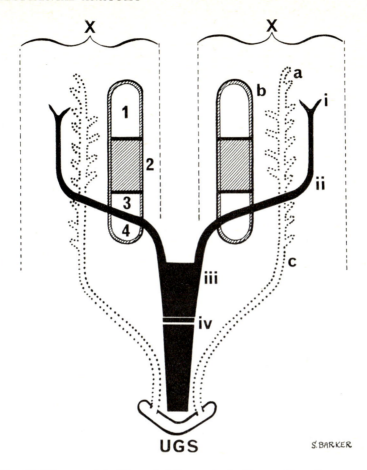

FIG. 25. Diagram of the Urogenital System in the 20 mm. (7 week) Human Embryo.

X—Intermediate Cell Mass.

Shaded areas—Genital Ridge: 1 *Infundibulo pelvic Ligament*. 2 *Ovary*. 3 *Ovarian Ligament*. 4 *Round Ligament*.

Dotted outline—Wolffian Duct (Gärtner's Duct): a Pronephric Tubules. b Genital Tubules (*Epoöphoron*). c Mesonephros.

Solid black—Müllerian Ducts: i *Fimbriae*. ii *Fallopian Tube*. iii *Uterus*. iv *Vagina* (*upper* 3/4).

UGS —Urogenital Sinus.

(Italics used for adult structures.)

the region of the genital tubercle a genital fold passes backwards lateral to the urogenital sinus to form the labium majus (scrotum in the male). Between the genital folds lies the urogenital or anterior part of the cloacal membrane which breaks down to form the labia minora (6th week). The vestibule and urethra are thus derived from the anterior part of the urogenital sinus and Bartholins' glands and Skene's paraurethral glands are developed from down-growths of the urogenital sinus. The female urethra represents the upper part of the male urethra and the para- and peri-urethral glands are the homologous of the male prostate.

Development of the Ovary

The genital ridge extends from the pronephric region above to the sacral region below, and in its earliest form is represented by an elongated vertical prominence. Very soon it develops a mesentery of its own, the mesovarium, by which it is attached to the intermediate cell mass. The infundibulopelvic fold passes upwards from the upper pole of the ovary and contains the ovarian vessels. The ovarian vessels of the adult, arising from the abdominal aorta, illustrate the original lumbar position of the upper part of the genital ridge. The genital fold of peritoneum passes downwards from the lower pole of the ovary to the region of the internal abdominal ring. The Müllerian duct originally lies on the outer aspect of the genital ridge, but it crosses the genital fold below. As the Müllerian duct crosses the genital fold the two structures fuse, and after muscle tissue has formed around the Müllerian duct, it passes into the tissues of the genital fold. The part of the genital fold lying proximal to its point of intersection with the Müllerian duct becomes the ovarian ligament, while the distal portion becomes the round ligament (see Fig 25). This corresponds to the gubernaculum of the male.

The ovary descends from its original lumbar position so that at term it lies at the level of the pelvic brim with its long axis directed vertically.

The sex cells first appear in the genital ridge. It is accepted at the present day that the cells originate from the hind gut of the embryo and migrate to the genital ridge. At first, the sex cells are arranged in columns perpendicular to the surface. These columns are called **primary sex cords** and they lie deeply in the substance of the genital ridge. At a later date, **secondary cords** develop nearer to the surface epithelium. Both primary and secondary cords consist of cells derived, in the main, from the local stroma of the genital ridge. The egg cells or **primordial ova** are distinguished by their large size and peculiar mitochondria. It is believed that the sex cells act as organisers to the adjacent stroma cells which then become converted into **granulosa cells.** In the male, the cells of the primary cords predominate, while in the ovary the secondary cords are most marked. Nevertheless, relics of the primary cords may persist under exceptional conditions in the hilum of the ovary. One theory of the aetiology of the virilising ovarian tumours is that the tumours are derived from these rudiments.

2 Normal Histology

THE FOETAL OVARY

The ovary is developed from the extra-coelomic mesenchyme of the genital ridge. The surface epithelium can be distinguished quite early in intrauterine life. The secondary sex cords which are arranged perpendicular to the surface epithelium, consist of primordial egg cells together with stroma cells which have become differentiated into prospective granulosa cells. The sex cords have been recognised for many years and have been called the Waldeyer or Pflüger tubules. It is now believed that the egg cells are not derived from the surface epithelium, but by the ingrowth of extra-embryonic yolk sac entoderm. In other words, the ova themselves are of extra-ovarian origin.

In the next stage of development, connective tissues and blood vessels break up the germinal sex cords into egg nests, while other connective tissues burrow circumferentially beneath the surface epithelium to form the primitive tunica albuginea of the ovary. The egg nests are gradually broken down into smaller pieces until finally each egg cell lies separate and surrounded by a single layer of prospective granulosa cells.

THE OVARY OF THE NEW-BORN

At term the foetal ovary measures 10–16 mm. in length and is situated at the level of the brim of the pelvis. If a section is taken through the ovary and examined histologically the following divisions can be recognised:

(1) The **surface epithelium.** This is a single layer of cuboidal cells, which gives rise later to the surface epithelium of the adult ovary, and which is morphologically continuous with the mesothelium of the peritoneum.

(2) The **subepithelial connective tissue layer.** This layer gives rise to the tunica albuginea of the adult ovary and to the basement membrane beneath the surface epithelium.

(3) The **parenchymatous zone.** This area is the most important, as it contains the sex cells. It can be subdivided into three zones:

(*a*) Immediately beneath the surface epithelium the sex cells are still grouped together in bunches to form egg nests.

(*b*) Below this area the sex cells take the form of **primordial follicles** and are packed together without orderly arrangement (see Fig. 26).

(*c*) In the deepest part of the parenchymatous zone developing follicles can be recognised.

(4) The **zona vasculosa.** This area contains the blood vessels which pass into the ovary from the mesovarium. It constitutes the medulla of the ovary, the other layers forming the cortex.

The Primordial Follicle

The **primordial follicle** consists of a large cell, the **primordial ovum,** which is surrounded by flattened cells, best termed the **follicle epithelial cells.** The follicle epithelial cells give rise to the granulosa cells of the Graafian follicle.

The primitive ovum is roughly spherical in shape and measures 18–24μ in diameter, the nucleus 12μ and the nucleolus 6μ. It has a well-defined nuclear membrane and its chromatin stains clearly.

The ovary of the new-born is packed with primordial follicles, and a computation of their number, due to Häggeström, gives an estimate of approximately 200,000 to each ovary though more recent estimates have

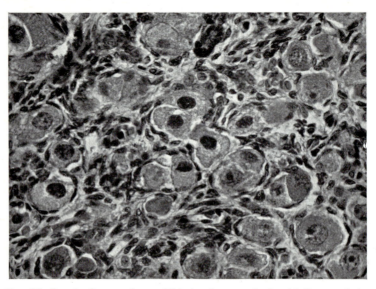

FIG. 26. Ovary of a new-born child showing germinal epithelium and the stroma packed with primordial follicles.

raised this figure to 700,000. One of the most curious features of the ovary is the tendency of the sex cells to undergo degeneration. An enormous number disappear during intrauterine life, and this process of degeneration continues throughout childhood and the child-bearing period, with the result that no ova can be detected in the ovaries of a woman who has passed the menopause. Häggeström showed that of 200,000 ova in the ovary of a child aged 3 years 8 months, 37,000 were degenerate.

The Graafian Follicle

The **Graafian follicle,** described by Regnier de Graaf in 1672, is a vesicle whose size measures on the average between 12 and 16 mm. in diameter after puberty. Before then it seldom reaches more than 5 mm. in diameter.

The mature Graafian follicle is spheroidal or ovoid in shape and contains pent-up secretion, the liquor folliculi. The lining consists of two layers. The outer, or **theca interna** layer, consists of cells which are derived from the stroma cells of the cortex. As a result of recent work the theca cell has become acknowledged to be of increasing importance in the production of ovarian hormones, both oestrogen and progesterone. These stromal cells are activated by the proximity of the ova and their granulosa cells. Their versatility in hormone activity is sometimes extended to the production of androgens. Within the theca interna layer lies the **granulosa cell** layer which consists of cells which have a characteristic appearance. The cells are 8–10μ in diameter.

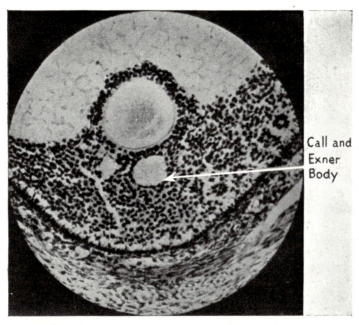

Call and Exner Body

FIG. 27. Graafian follicle. Discus proligerus showing granulosa cells, the ovum, and the membrana limitans externa. Theca interna cells are few.

The nuclei always stain deeply and the cells contain relatively little cytoplasm. In one area, the granulosa cells are collected together to form a projection into the cavity of the Graafian follicle. This projection is referred to as the **discus proligerus** or **cumulus oöphorus.** The ovum itself lies within the discus proligerus. With the exception of the area around the discus proligerus, the peripheral granulosa cells form a layer only a few cells in thickness, whereas at the discus the cells are between twelve and twenty layers thick. The granulosa layer itself is non-vascular and capillaries cannot be identified in it. Scattered amongst the granulosa cells, particularly in the vicinity of the discus proligerus, are small spherical globules around which the granulosa cells are arranged radially. These structures form the **bodies of Call and Exner.** The formation of Call and Exner bodies is a distinct feature of granulosa cells and can be readily recognised in certain types of granulosa cell tumour. Between the granulosa layer and the theca interna is a basement membrane called the **membrana limitans externa** upon which lies the basal layer of granulosa cells (see Fig. 27).

The mature ovum measures 120–140μ in diameter, its nucleus 20–25μ. At the periphery of the deutoplasm is a clear translucent capsular layer known as the zona pellucida. The granulosa cells surround the entire periphery of the ovum. Those which are immediately adjacent have a radial arrangement and form the **corona radiata.** The corona radiata remains attached to the ovum after its discharge into the peritoneal cavity at ovulation. Sometimes more than one ovum is found in a single follicle. The theca interna cells enlarge during the maturation of the follicle and shortly before ovulation they are larger than the granulosa cells. In animals, a third layer, the theca externa, is well defined but the layer is not distinguished in the human ovary.

The liquor folliculi is a clear fluid containing protein which coagulates after formalin fixation. It is secreted by the granulosa cells and contains the ovarian hormone oestrogen.

The Fate of the Graafian Follicle. The process whereby a primordial follicle is converted into a Graafian follicle—follicularisation—can be recognised as early as the 32nd week of intrauterine life. Until puberty all Graafian follicles in the ovary undergo retrogression by a process which is termed **follicle atresia. Ovulation,** whereby the follicle discharges its ovum into the peritoneal cavity, is first seen at puberty, and is restricted to the child-bearing period of life. The development of a primordial follicle into a Graafian follicle is under the control of Follicle Stimulating Hormone secreted by the anterior part of the pituitary gland. Several follicles commence to develop in each menstrual cycle. They secrete oestrogen as they mature and the gradual rise in oestrogen level in the blood stream causes a gradual reduction in secretion of Follicle Stimulating Hormone (F.S.H.) by the pituitary gland. The diminution of F.S.H. production results in only one follicle being selected for complete maturation whilst the remainder undergo gradual atrophy. A high oestrogen level inhibits F.S.H. secretion, but the delicate balance between F.S.H. production and oestrogen level is not properly understood.

Follicle Atresia. Atresia may affect a follicle at any stage in its development. The first signs of degeneration are seen in the ovum itself, which swells and undergoes hyaline and fatty degeneration. Subsequently the granulosa cells retrogress. The theca interna cells, however, do not atrophy at the same rate, so that in the early stages of atresia the theca interna cells are larger and much more conspicuous than the cells of the granulosa layer. Hyaline tissue is now deposited beneath the membrana limitans externa to form the **glass membrane,** and the presence of the glass membrane in any follicle is a certain sign of degeneration. As atresia proceeds the liquor folliculi is gradually absorbed, while more and more hyaline tissue is deposited in the glass membrane. Ultimately the ovum, the discus proligerus and the granulosa cells disappear, so that the atretic follicle is surrounded only by the hyaline tissue of the glass membrane with deeply pigmented theca interna cells at the periphery. Eventually the follicle collapses, its cavity is obliterated and the opposing surfaces of the glass membrane come into contact, so that the end result is a tortuous laminated hyaline body with large deeply staining cells—originally theca interna cells—at the periphery. These large brown cells are the **interstitial cells** of the ovary (see Fig. 28).

Interstitial cells are specialised theca cells. They are the main source of oestrogen and are therefore responsible for the secondary sex characteristics in the female. The cells are however also present in the ovary of the newborn, becoming more noticeable at puberty and particularly obvious during reproductive life especially in pregnancy in the region of the retrogressing corpus luteum. After the menopause they atrophy and disappear.

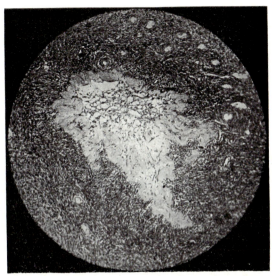

FIG. 28. Corpus atreticum. The end-result of atresia of a Graafian follicle. The granulosa cells have disappeared and a hyaline lamina has been deposited. The follicle is in process of collapse.

The Ripening Follicle. Ripening follicles can be demonstrated in the ovaries during the post-menstrual phase when they can be seen with the naked eye, for they often reach a size of 10 mm. in diameter. The characters of the process of ripening have already been described on p. 49. At the beginning of ripening the discus proligerus is directed towards the medulla of the ovary, and the mechanism whereby a follicle penetrates through the cortex and discharges its ovum into the peritoneal cavity is remarkable. As the follicle hypertrophies, more and more liquor is secreted, and the direction in which the follicle develops is determined by a rapid growth of the theca interna cells in that part of the follicle which is directed towards the surface epithelium. If a ripening follicle is examined the advancing cone of theca interna cells can be demonstrated in this part of the follicle. The cells burrow through the cortex of the ovary, so that as the follicle enlarges it develops towards the surface and not towards the medulla. In addition the discus proligerus rotates, so that when the follicle is on the verge of rupture it lies immediately beneath the surface of the ovary. Throughout the process of ripening the granulosa layer is non-vascular, but because of the hyperaemia of the theca interna layer it is not uncommon for interstitial haemorrhage to occur.

THE MENSTRUAL CYCLE

In healthy women the menstrual cycle is one of about twenty-eight days and covers the time between the first day of one menstrual period and the first day of the next. The average duration of menstrual bleeding is between three and five days. It has been found most convenient to describe the phases of the menstrual cycle in terms of the number of days after the first day of the last period.

No explanation has been given of the control of the rhythm of the menstrual cycle. It is probable that the anterior lobe of the pituitary dominates the sexual cycle, but as yet rhythmical changes in the anterior lobe of the pituitary have not been found. In the Middle Ages the rhythm of twenty-eight days was attributed to lunar influences, and there is some evidence that ultra-violet light induces sexual activity in lower animals, thus explaining the summer breeding seasons. Amongst the Esquimaux, menstruation is restricted to the time of the midnight sun and amenorrhoea is the rule during the winter months. Similar alterations in the menstrual cycle are common when European women visit tropical climes.

The menstrual cycle is the outward and visible sign of the periodic activity of the ovaries. This point is of clinical importance, for an alteration in the menstrual rhythm can only be due to a disturbance of ovarian activity. Diseases of the uterus itself cannot alter the rhythm of the menstrual cycle.

OVULATION

Immediately before rupture the ripening follicle lies near the surface of the ovary with the discus proligerus directed towards the peritoneal cavity. The theca interna layer is full of dilated capillaries, and a plug of coagulated plasma now appears in the most advanced part of the theca interna layer. The process of ovulation can be studied in such animals as the rabbit and ferret, where ovulation occurs at a fixed time following coitus. In these animals an elevation develops on the surface of the ovary, upon which conspicuous radially arranged capillaries can be distinguished. Probably a similar mechanism obtains in the human ovary. The ovum is discharged into the peritoneal cavity when the intrafollicular pressure is sufficient to burst through the intervening tissues. The corona radiata of granulosa cells accompanies the ovum during its discharge into the peritoneal cavity. The aperture through which the ovum is discharged, called the stigma, is closed almost immediately after ovulation by a plug of plasma. Prior to ovulation the granulosa layer is non-vascular and the capillaries and interstitial haemorrhages of the theca interna layer are separated from the cavity of the follicle by the membrana limitans externa. Consequently, in spite of the sudden release of intrafollicular pressure as the result of ovulation, blood is not effused into the cavity of the

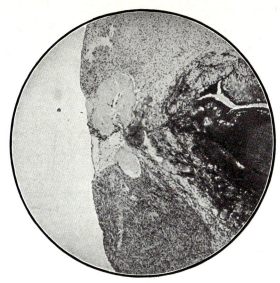

Fig. 29. A recently ruptured follicle. The surface of the ovary lies on the left and the cavity of the follicle is represented by the longitudinal space extending to the right edge of the field. The stigma has been closed by a plug of plasma. The dark area represents haemorrhage into the theca interna layer.

follicle. The ruptured follicle collapses and its opposing surfaces come together; there is also some distortion of the wall so that there is a tendency for small convolutions to be present (see Fig. 29).

Before ovulation occurs the cells of the granulosa layer rapidly divide and subdivide to produce a layer of proliferating cells. The theca interna cells also increase in size and show some degree of luteinisation even prior to ovulation.

Timing of Ovulation

Although an enormous amount of work has been carried out to determine the timing of ovulation, there is still dispute as to the correct date. Healthy women show some variation in the rhythm of their menstrual cycles and accurate dating of specimens, though scientifically essential, is often impracticable. There is no doubt that ovulation is normally restricted to approximately half-way between the first days of two successive menstrual periods in the normal twenty-eight-day cycle. Rock and Hertig have corroborated the opinion of Ogino and Knaus that ovulation usually occurs fourteen days before the onset of the next menstrual period irrespective of the length of the menstrual cycle. It seems to be more accurate to date ovulation with relation to the first day of the next period. In a twenty-eight-day cycle this is immaterial, but with irregular cycles it may be of the greatest importance.

Various methods have been employed to determine the timing of ovulation. Operation material is the most valuable, since follicles on the verge of rupture and recently ruptured follicles obviously indicate most accurately the approximate timing of ovulation. Rock and Hertig particularly have used this method with greater refinement than the older workers, Robert Meyer, Schröder, and Wilfred Shaw. Ova have also been obtained by washing out the Fallopian tube following the method originated by Allen.

Other methods are indirect. A competent histologist can detect the degree of secretory hypertrophy of the endometrium with sufficient accuracy to state how many days after ovulation the specimen was obtained. Clearly, the detection of early secretory hypertrophy of the endometrium indicates that ovulation must have occurred shortly before the specimen was obtained. The administration of progestogens for contraceptive or other purposes will cause secretory changes in the endometrium and must therefore always be remembered.

It has been shown that if women take their morning temperature throughout the menstrual cycle, before getting up, eating or drinking, the time of ovulation is indicated by a slight fall in temperature, after which, during the secretory phase the body temperature rises by about 1°F due to the effect of progesterone. The method is of clinical value in infertility but it must be remembered that the temperature may also rise as a result of electric blankets, alcohol intake, illness or physical activity. Some women experience slight spotting of blood from the vagina exactly fourteen days before the onset of the next menstrual period, from which it is concluded that the uterine haemorrhage is coincident with ovulation. Similarly, intermenstrual pain, or Mittelschmerz, often develops fourteen days before the period is due in ovular cycles.

Studies of the vaginal epithelium by Dierk, and by Rakoff particularly, have shown that cyclical changes can be demonstrated in the vaginal epithelium, which imply that ovulation occurs about fourteen days before the onset of the next period. Similar results are obtained from the study of pregnandiol excretion in the urine, and from the amount and viscosity of cervical mucus. The excretion values of oestrogens offer additional evidence and it may soon be possible to foretell ovulation by accurate measurements of the leuteinising hormone levels.

It is fair to say that all workers who have concentrated upon the ovaries of healthy women with regular cycles maintain that the timing of ovulation is fourteen days before the onset of the next menstrual period. This view is, however, by no means universally accepted, for there is clinical evidence that women may conceive either immediately after menstruation or just before the next menstrual period is due. The same view is taken by Grosser as a result of his investigation of embryological material. Some gynaecologists have maintained that ovulation can be provoked by coitus, but these clinical impressions await scientific corroboration.

Anovular Menstruation

Corner was able to demonstrate with the Macaque monkey that the animals sometimes develop rhythmical bleeding without the development of the premenstrual or secretory phase of the endometrium. He showed that the ovaries contained no corpora lutea and that, in spite of regular uterine bleeding of the same rhythm as the normal menstruation for the Macaque, ovulation had not occurred. Corner introduced the term anovular menstruation for these cases. Anovular bleeding usually develops in the Macaque at the time of year when menstruation is irregular. It is also well known that a corpus luteum is not formed in the ovaries in certain types of abnormal uterine haemorrhage in the human subject, notably metropathia haemorrhagica. The incidence of anovular menstruation in the healthy human female is unknown though it commonly occurs just after the menarche and just before the menopause. The most accurate methods are those of Rock and his colleagues, who found an incidence of 9·1% in 392 patients suffering from sterility and infertility. The cause of the uterine bleeding, both in anovular menstruation and in ovular cycles, is not known with certainty, though it is presumed to be oestrogen and progesterone withdrawal bleeding.

Usually only a single ovum is discharged from one or other ovary at the time of ovulation, but sometimes two recently ruptured follicles are found in the same ovary. If both discharged ova become fertilised, binovular twins will develop. It has been shown that the distribution of corpora lutea between the two ovaries is even, which implies that ovulation alternates between the two ovaries. Probably the alternation is not invariable, not more so than can be accounted for by the law of chance.

The Corpus Luteum

After ovulation the ruptured follicle develops into a corpus luteum. The term corpus luteum is in some ways a misnomer, for the colour is grey or greyish yellow until the onset of the next menstrual period. The yellow colour is characteristic of the retrogressing corpus luteum and of the corpus luteum of pregnancy.

Immediately after ovulation the granulosa cells undergo hypertrophy and hyperplasia and mitotic figures are numerous. The cells become larger, stain paler and more eosinophilic with bigger but less well defined nuclei. This process is called luteinisation. Instead of being two or three cells thick as in the ripening follicle, as many as eight or ten cell layers can soon be recognised. Simultaneously there is hypertrophy of the theca interna cells, so that in the early stages of development of the corpus luteum the theca interna cells outstrip the granulosa cells in size. The majority of the lutein cells of the corpus luteum are derived from the granulosa layer and form the granulosa lutein cells. The theca interna cells persist at the periphery and in the septa of the corpus luteum, and are sometimes termed **paralutein cells** (see Fig. 30).

Proliferation of the corpus luteum continues until about the twenty-second day of the menstrual cycle. The granulosa lutein cells at first become spindle-shaped with the long axis of the cells directed radially. The cells hypertrophy and the protoplasm becomes pigmented. It is unknown what happens to the bodies of Call and Exner; they can be detected in the early stages of development, but they disappear before the stage of maturity is reached. The convolutions of the corpus luteum are produced almost entirely as the result of proliferation of the granulosa lutein cells. The convoluted body has a much larger surface than one which is smooth and spherical. The theca interna cells do not invade the granulosa lutein layer, but are restricted to the periphery.

Before rupture of the follicle the granulosa layer is not vascularised, but small capillaries grow into the granulosa layer within twenty-four hours of rupture. The capillaries are numerous and grow between small bunches of cells. Connective tissue cells penetrate together with the capillaries into the

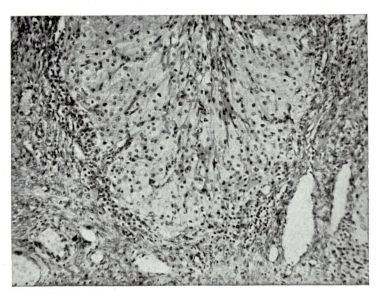

Fig. 30. Mature corpus luteum of the menstrual cycle. The photograph illustrates the convex border of a convolution of the corpus luteum. The small dark cells at the periphery are paralutein cells, while the larger cells with a tendency to a radial arrangement consist of granulosa lutein cells. The corpus luteum is approaching maturity, so the cells stain fairly uniformly.

granulosa-lutein layer. After about ten days of life the amount of blood contained in the capillaries is much reduced and only an occasional capillary contains blood. In the corpus luteum of pregnancy the vascularisation is not hindered but is continuous so that the granulosa-lutein cells are surrounded by a loose network of distended capillaries.

During the development of the granulosa lutein layer some of the young capillaries may rupture, so that blood may be discharged into the cavity. It has already been pointed out that haemorrhage into the cavity is not the normal sequel of ovulation: on the other hand, haemorrhage into the cavity during the stage of proliferation is relatively common, particularly when the ovaries are hyperaemic.

The corpus luteum attains its stage of maturity by the twenty-second day and persists as such until the onset of menstruation. The granulosa lutein cells stain uniformly and pigmentation of their cytoplasm is not so well

marked as during the stage of proliferation. The old views of the stage of
maturity of the corpus luteum, or the phase of blossom or bloom as it is
sometimes called, have been sharply criticised in recent years by Brewer.
Brewer maintains that the active secreting phase of the corpus luteum is
restricted to the first eight to ten days of its development, during which its
cells are surrounded by capillaries. Obviously some degree of functional
activity of the corpus luteum persists until gross degeneration develops just
before the onset of menstruation. On the other hand, regressive changes such
as atrophy, fatty degeneration and increase of cholesterol esters all imply
that retrogression starts after the eighth to tenth days of the corpus luteum's
existence. This view is in agreement with the modern work of Rock, who
maintains that if implantation of the ovum has not occurred by the eighth

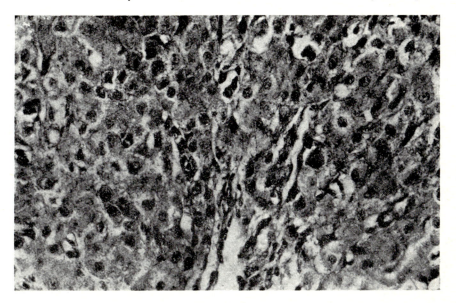

FIG. 31. Corpus luteum of the menstrual cycle on the first day of the period of
bleeding. The lutein cells are shrunken and there are spaces between the individual cells.

day, the ovulatory cycle will be non-fertile. The implication is therefore that
if the ovum is not fertilised and imbedded by the eighth day after ovulation,
the corpus luteum ceases to proliferate and assumes its state of maturity or
bloom until shortly before menstruation, when gross degenerative changes
can be demonstrated. There is additional confirmation of this point of view
from the work of Markee on the endometrium. The fully formed granulosa
lutein cell is a large cell between 13 and 14μ in diameter, and its cytoplasm
is faintly granular. The cells have a somewhat bloated appearance due to
the increase of cytoplasm and a corresponding diminution in the size of
the nucleus. This cytoplasmic increase is due to the uptake of water and
the contents contain phospho-lipid, carotene and cholesterol. The yellow

colouration of the mature corpus luteum is due to the presence of the carotene. The theca interna or paralutein cells are now much smaller than the granulosa lutein cells. Their cytoplasm is densely pigmented and during the stage of maturity contains lipoids. Lipoids do not appear in the protoplasm of the granulosa lutein cells until eight days after ovulation. Small spherical colloid bodies which stain brown with Van Giesen's stain appear amongst the cells of the granulosa lutein layer during the stage of maturity, but they become much more numerous and larger in the corpus luteum of pregnancy. The cavity of the corpus luteum during the stage of maturity contains a few connective tissue cells together with a layer of fibrin which lies immediately adjacent to the granulosa lutein layer: red blood corpuscles are also found when the ovaries are hyperaemic (Fig. 31).

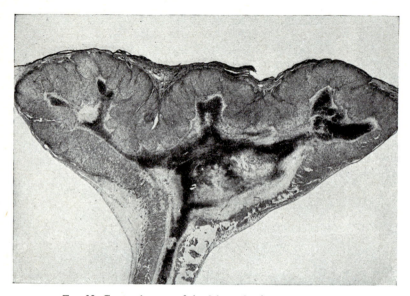

Fig. 32. Corpus luteum of the 8th week of pregnancy.   (×6.)

Retrogression of the Corpus Luteum. Unless the ovum discharged at ovulation is fertilised, the corpus luteum starts to retrogress on the 24th day of the menstrual cycle. Firstly the vascularity of the corpus luteum is reduced. Next, simple atrophy and fatty degeneration can be demonstrated in the granulosa lutein cells where large vacuolated cells, together with deeply pigmented degenerate cells, can be distinguished. By the third day of the menstrual haemorrhage retrogression is well marked. Fatty infiltration is well shown in the paralutein cells, but the paralutein cells do not atrophy at the same rate as the granulosa lutein cells, and they persist at the periphery of the retrogressing corpus luteum even after all the granulosa lutein cells have disappeared. It should be remembered that the excretion of pregnandiol in the urine decreases as soon as the early signs of degeneration of the corpus luteum appear.

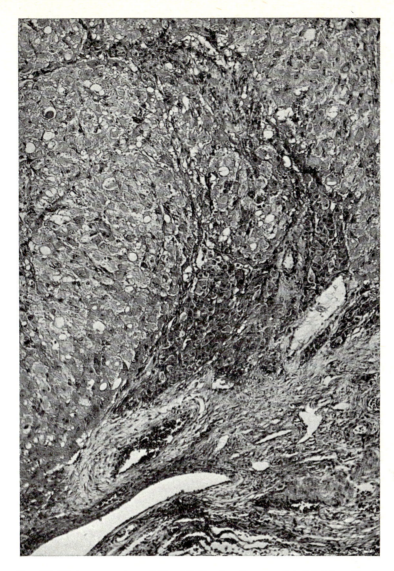

FIG. 33. High power view of Fig. 32 showing the vacuolated lutein cells. A septum of dark paralutein cells enters from below between the convolutions. (×115.)

The other characteristic feature of retrogression is the deposition of hyaline tissue amongst the granulosa lutein cells. The hyaline tissue resembles that found in the glass membrane of atretic follicles, and as retrogression proceeds more and more hyaline tissue is deposited, while scattered at the periphery are interstitial cells derived from the paralutein cells. The hyaline body is termed the **corpus albicans** and differs from the other hyaline atretic bodies of the ovaries in its size and in the thickness of the hyaline layer.

Retrogression of the corpus luteum is a slow process and it has been calculated that nine months elapse before the corpus luteum is completely replaced by hyaline tissue.

Corpus Luteum of Pregnancy. If the ovum discharged from the Graafian follicle is fertilised and embeds in the endometrium, the resulting corpus luteum of pregnancy develops certain features which are not seen in the corpus luteum of the menstrual cycle. The corpus luteum of pregnancy is larger and

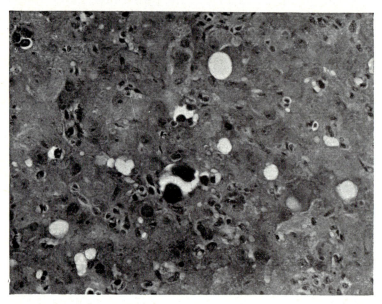

FIG. 34. Corpus luteum of pregnancy, 20th week, showing that the cells are conjoined. There are still large spaces full of secretion, while the dark rounded bodies are colloid.

is almost invariably cystic in the early months, when it contains clear yellow fluid. It may attain a size of 2·5 cm. The convolutions are larger and more intricate. Moreover, the individual granulosa lutein cells are much more hypertrophied and measure between 40 and 50μ. In early pregnancy the protoplasm of the granulosa lutein cells is packed with secretion globules and clear spherical spaces, full of secretion, appear between the individual cells. Colloid bodies are always more numerous than during the menstrual cycle. The colloid material is probably secreted by some of the granulosa lutein cells and is most plentiful about the 24th week of pregnancy. The paralutein cells hypertrophy in the early weeks of pregnancy, but they disappear at about the 20th week and cannot be demonstrated in the latter half of pregnancy. Already at the 20th week, hyaline tissue is being deposited in the cavity of the corpus luteum adjacent to the lutein cells and a small amount has appeared around the capillaries of the granulosa lutein layer. The structure of the corpus luteum remains stationary until near term, when deposits of calcium in the form of psammoma bodies staining deeply with haematoxylin can be recognised. There is much variation amongst individual specimens in the lipoid content of the lutein cells. The cells of the corpus luteum of pregnancy contain, on the whole, very little fat (see Figs. 32, 33 and 34).

It is possible to trace the transition between the corpus luteum of the menstrual cycle and the corpus luteum of pregnancy. Both structures arise in the same way, but the features of the corpus luteum of pregnancy indicate that it secretes more actively than the corpus luteum of the menstrual cycle.

The presence of granulosa lutein cells in the latter part of pregnancy indicates that some function is still exercised by the corpus luteum. On the other hand, the corpus luteum of pregnancy is most active in the early weeks, and reaches its maximum peak of functional activity at the 8th to 9th week of pregnancy. The retrogression of the corpus luteum of pregnancy during the puerperium has not been studied, for such specimens are rarely obtained. There is some evidence that retrogression is rapid, but the precise mechanism is unknown.

It is interesting to note that the ovary containing the corpus luteum can be removed after the 14th–16th week of pregnancy without necessarily interrupting the pregnancy. This suggests again that its main functional activity occurs in the first three and a half months of pregnancy, after which the placenta takes over the main production of progesterone and oestrogen.

It is the event of fertilisation and implantation of the fertilised ovum which determines the life span of the corpus luteum, since the trophoblast of the ovum is already active after its first week of life and the secretion of chorionic gonadotropin ensures the continuance of corpus luteum activity. This activity like that of synthetic oral progestogen is inhibitory to the follicle stimulating hormone of the pituitary and consequently ovulation ceases. If fertilisation does not occur the corpus luteum degenerates and the menstrual cycle continues.

THE ENDOMETRIUM OF THE UTERUS

The endometrium of that part of the uterus which lies above the level of the internal os consists of a surface epithelium, glands and a stroma. It was not until 1907 that the variations in the histological structure of the endometrium during the menstrual cycle were established by Hitschmann and Adler. They examined specimens of the endometrium at different stages of the menstrual cycle and showed conclusively that the structure was not constant, but was subject to variations which were physiological.

This work not only revolutionised the previous conception of endometrial histology, but formed the basis upon which much of the modern work on the sex hormones rests.

The endometrium of the body of the uterus can be divided into two zones: a superficial, termed the **functional,** and a deeper layer, termed the **basal layer** which lies adjacent to the myometrium. The stroma cells of the basal layer stain deeply and are packed closely together. Islands of lymphoid tissue are found in the basal layer.

The vascular system of the endometrium is of great importance. Two types of arteries supply the endometrium. One of these is restricted to the basal third and consists of small straight short arteries. The superficial two-thirds of the endometrium are supplied by coiled arteries.

The Proliferative Phase. The phase of the menstrual cycle which starts when regeneration of the menstruating endometrium is complete and lasts until the fourteenth day of a twenty-eight day cycle is referred to as the **proliferative or oestrogenic phase.** At the end of menstruation which may occupy from three to five days the necrotic superficial layers have been discharged and the endometrium is represented by only the deep or basal layer. The coiled arteries have been lost and the terminal ends of the straight arteries sealed off by fibrin. The stroma is heavily infiltrated with leucocytes and red cells. Regeneration is remarkably rapid and all elements of the endometrium including glands and new sprouting vessels are present at the end of 48 hours. The proliferative phase therefore starts and proceeds rapidly about three to five days, and not later than seven, after the start of the menstrual cycle. During proliferation the functional and basal layers are well defined. The basal layer measures 1 mm. in thickness, while the functional layer, commencing with an average of 2·5 mm., reaches about 3·5 mm. by the fourteenth day, and during the secretory phase hypertrophies still further, so that immediately before menstruation its average thickness is between 3·5 and 4 mm. There is much variation in the thickness of the functional layer, and it is not uncommon to see specimens in which it is as much as 8 mm. During the proliferative phase the glands of the functional layer are simple tubules with regular epithelium (see Fig. 10). About the tenth day of the cycle the glands become slightly sinuous and their columnar epithelium becomes taller than before. The glands sometimes show a characteristic appearance in the late proliferative phase as if the glandular epithelium had been telescoped into the lumen, rather like an intussusception. This appearance is false and this telescoping is in reality due to a tuft of epithelium which has budded off from the gland wall. It is, therefore, merely evidence of oestrogenic activity in the glandular epithelium. The stroma becomes extremely oedematous with wide separation of individual cells. During the first postmenstrual week the coiled arteries extend only half-way through the endometrium. Afterwards they grow more rapidly than the endometrium so that they become more coiled and spiralled. In some cases the vascularity is so intense that blood oozes into the cavity of the uterus at the time of ovulation to be discharged from the vagina. Regular intermenstrual bleeding of this kind is a well-known clinical symptom and is due to the intense hyperaemia at the end of the proliferative phase. It almost certainly indicates that ovulation has occurred.

The Secretory Phase. The secretory phase of the endometrium begins on the fifteenth day and persists until the onset of menstruation. The most characteristic signs of this phase are found in the glands. Their epithelial cells develop spherical translucent areas between the nuclei and the basement membrane

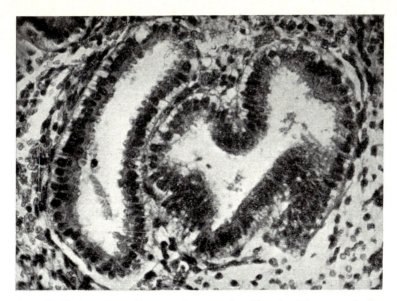

Fig. 35. Endometrium. Secretory hypertrophy. The gland is crenated, the lumen contains mucous secretion, and the inner border of the cells is irregular. Subnuclear vacuolation is well seen. The surrounding stroma is oedematous and the hypertrophied stroma cells are widely separated from each other. (×300.)

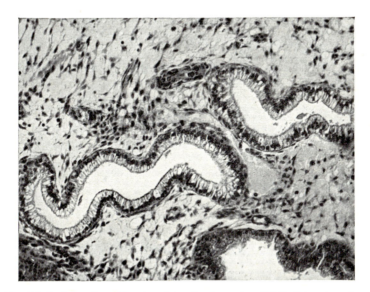

Fig. 36. Endometrium. Secretory hypertrophy—at a slightly later stage than Fig. 35. The secretory vacuoles are now near the apex of the cell. (×124.)

which contain the precursors of the glandular secretion and which persist until about the twenty-first day of the cycle. This characteristic appearance is called subnuclear vacuolation and is presumptive evidence of progesterone activity and, therefore, of ovulation. The fluid in these subnuclear vacuoles consists of mucin and glycogen (Fig. 35), the function of which is presumably nutritive to the fertilised ovum if it should become implanted. The phase of subnuclear vacuolation is rapidly followed by an increase in intracellular secretion which pushes the nuclei to the basement membrane and fills the cell. The subnuclear vacuole later migrates past the nucleus to the surface of the cell. In the latter part of the secretory phase the inner border of the epithelial cells becomes irregular through the discharge of secretion into the lumina of the glands, while shortly before menstruation the glands are full of coagulated secretion which stains deeply with eosin. The glands become crenated and assume a characteristic corkscrew-shaped form (Fig. 36). The stroma of the functional layer remains oedematous, but further interstitial haemorrhage is rare except immediately prior to the onset of menstruation. The coiled arteries become more spiral and form closely wound perpendicular columns through the mucosa. The stroma cells become swollen, and after the twenty-first day of the cycle they tend to be collected immediately beneath the surface epithelium, where they surround the ducts of the glands in such a way that the functional layer can be subdivided into two zones: the **superficial or compact** and a **deeper spongy layer.** The swollen stroma cells of the compact part of the functional layer represent young decidual cells, and in every respect the reaction of the compact zone corresponds to what is found in this part of the endometrium during pregnancy. The islands of lymphoid tissue in the basal layer of the endometrium scatter lymphocytes into the functional layer in the last few days of the menstrual cycle, so that, at this stage, there is a well-marked lymphocytic infiltration of the whole of the endometrium.

In spite of the intense secretory activity of the functional layer, the basal layer glands are not similarly affected and retain a non-secretory pattern.

The secretory phase has reached its peak by the twenty-second day of the cycle and no further growth ensues in the normal cycle of the non-pregnant. About the twenty-fourth day of the cycle some shrinkage of the glands is apparent, partly due to the loss of their secretion into the lumen and partly due to dehydration of the stroma. The corkscrew pattern has now become saw toothed. No superficial necrosis has yet occurred but the superficial layers are noticeably less vascular. Just before menstruation there is a well marked local leucocytic infiltration.

The Menstruating Endometrium. The menstrual changes in the endometrium are essentially degenerative. The coiled arteries undergo vasoconstriction a few hours before the onset of menstrual bleeding. It is believed that the ischaemia thereby produced leads to necrosis of zones in the walls of small arteries in the superficial part of the endometrium. In addition, the buckling of the coiled arteries produces blood stasis which may also cause necrosis. This buckling is resultant from the decrease in the depth of the endometrium as a whole and causes a tightening of the arterial coils. Several additional

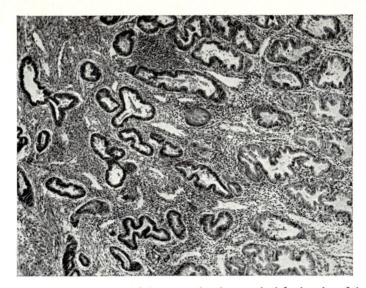

FIG. 37. The endometrium of the uterus showing, on the left, the edge of the myometrium and the basal zone of endometrium which does not assume a secretory pattern. On the right of the illustration is the spongy zone of the endometrium in which the glands show well marked secretory activity. These two areas are well contrasted in this photograph. (×52).

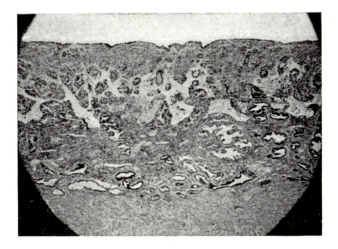

FIG. 38. Endometrium on the first day of the menstrual bleeding. The patient started to menstruate half an hour before the commencement of operation. The superficial layers are degenerate, while below secretory hypertrophy of the glands can be seen. The photograph illustrates approximately how much of the endometrium is shed during menstruation.

coils may be detected in a single vessel. Bleeding from the endometrium is restricted only to the times when the coiled arteries relax and when blood is discharged from the artery through the damaged necrotic areas in its wall. The straight arteries immediately beneath the coiled arteries undergo vasospasm at the time of menstrual bleeding and thereby provide a simple safety factor of haemostasis. This vasospasm limits the menstrual loss and when deficient may account for some forms of menorrhagia. The vasospasm is selective as it only affects the superficial layers and does not extend to the basal, which is thereby assured of an adequate blood supply necessary for regeneration. The compact zone of the functional layer becomes infiltrated with a large

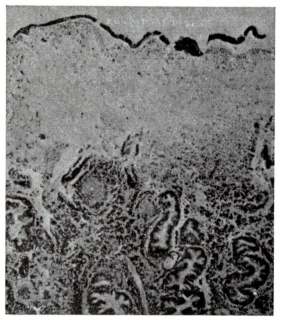

Fig. 39. The menstruating endometrium, first day, illustrating the degeneration of the superficial layers. Below lie corkscrew-shaped glands.

number of cells and the surface epithelium may be pushed away from the subjacent stroma. A little later the glands of the spongy zone of the functional layer disintegrate so that the epithelial cells separate from each other and become scattered amongst the red blood cells, leucocytes and the cells of the stroma (Figs. 37 and 38). The degenerative process is rapid, so that by the second day of the period of bleeding the compact zone and the superficial part of the spongy zone have degenerated and a large proportion has been discharged into the cavity of the uterus (Fig. 39). It is certain that the whole of the compact zone of the functional layer is shed and probably most of the spongy zone of the endometrium. On the third day of the period of bleeding the surface of the endometrium is raw and the patulous glands of the functional layer open directly into the cavity of the uterus. Active degenera-

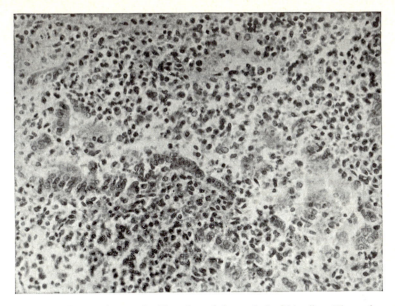

FIG. 40. Menstrual necrosis. First day of the period of bleeding. The endometrial gland is being broken up, and the stroma is infiltrated with round
cells and red blood corpuscles.

tion seems to be restricted to the first two days of menstruation; the subsequent bleeding is the result of oozing from the capillaries of the denuded
stroma. It is common to find relics of the glands and stroma of the endometrium in the shreds and clots passed on the first day of the period of bleeding,
which affords conclusive proof that a large part of the endometrium is shed
in normal menstruation. There is reason to believe, however, in cases of

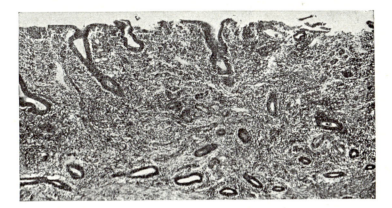

FIG. 41. Endometrium on the last day of the period of bleeding illustrating
the compact stroma and the method by which the denuded area is covered
by epithelium which grows over it from the glands.

abnormal uterine haemorrhage that the disintegration processes are not spread uniformly over the endometrium, but are localised to limited areas (see Figs. 38, 39 and 40).

Regeneration. Regeneration of the denuded epithelium is already in progress before menstrual bleeding has stopped and is complete forty-eight hours after the end of menstruation. Repair is brought about by the glandular epithelium growing over the bare stroma (see Fig. 41). It is not uncommon for relics of crenated glands to be found in the endometrium during the first two days following menstruation, and one of the great characteristics of the endometrium at this time is the presence of a large number of lymphocytes in the stroma. The relation between the cyclical alterations in the ovaries and in the endometrium will be discussed in Chapter 3.

The Decidua of Pregnancy. In the early weeks of pregnancy the structure of the endometrium is very similar to that found late in the secretory phase. The division into compact and spongy zones of the functional layer is more clearly defined. The basal layer can still be identified, but its glands, although staining more deeply than the hypertrophied glands of the spongy layer, show some degree of crenation and contain secretion. The lymphoid islands of the basal layer are not easily identified, for in the early weeks of pregnancy lymphocytes are disseminated extensively into the stroma of the spongy layer. The glands of the spongy layer retain the general form found late in the secretory phase, but they are much more crenated, so much so that the impression is given that they have increased in number. The cells lining the glands are irregular in shape and tend to be elongated with irregular processes projecting into the lumina of the glands and discharging secretion. It is not uncommon for small papillae to be formed which project into the glands, but in spite of the activity of the epithelium the basement membrane remains well defined. Activity is not restricted to the immediate vicinity of the implanted ovum, but is distributed uniformly through the endometrium of the body of the uterus. The compact layer shows the typical decidual reaction of pregnancy. The decidual cells are derived from stroma cells; they are stellate in shape, contain glycogen, and are surrounded by an intercellular fibrillary ground substance and by lymphocytes (see Fig. 42).

Ectopic Decidual Cells. Decidual cells are not restricted to the endometrium of the body of the uterus. Decidual reaction, in which decidual cells are surrounded by a fibrillary matrix and lymphocytes, has been demonstrated in various ectopic situations in the pelvis. The best example of ectopic decidual reaction is found on the surface of the ovaries during pregnancy, when small irregular reddish areas are easily recognised with the naked eye and show typical decidual reaction on histological examination. In the ovaries the decidual reaction is limited to the surface with very little invasion of the cortex. Ectopic decidual reaction is always very well marked beneath the peritoneum of the back of the uterus in the pouch of Douglas. It has been demonstrated in adenomyomata, in the walls of chocolate cysts, on the uterovesical fold of peritoneum and in the omentum. Decidual reaction can invariably be demonstrated in the isthmus region of the endometrium during pregnancy, but only rarely is the typical reaction found in the glands of the

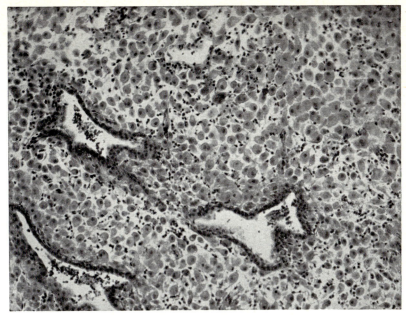

FIG. 42. Decidua of early pregnancy. The large decidual cells have a faintly staining cytoplasm which is eosinophilic. They are always surrounded by lymphocytes and the cells fuse with an intercellular matrix. (×110.)

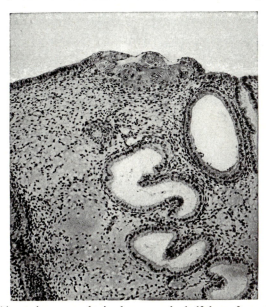

FIG. 43. This specimen was obtained seven and a half days after coitus (Rock and Hertig). It was computed that implantation had occurred forty-eight hours previously. The relation of the ovum to the surface epithelium and decidual glands can be seen.

cervical canal. A similar ectopic decidual reaction can be demonstrated during the latter part of the secretory phase of the menstrual cycle. The significance of ectopic decidual cells is unknown. It will be shown later that decidual reaction is controlled by the corpus luteum, but it is unknown why only cells with this curious distribution respond to the stimulus.

Transport of the Ovum

After ovulation, the ovum, surrounded by the corona radiata of granulosa cells, is transported into the Fallopian tube. The factors which control this migration are not known with certainty. Particulate matter, after injection

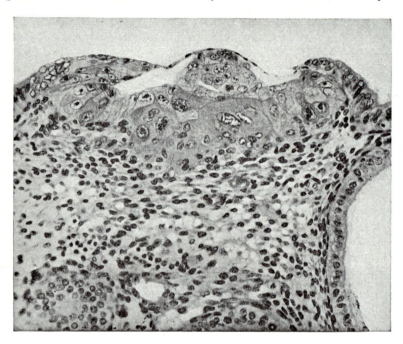

FIG. 44. The same specimen—higher magnification (Rock and Hertig). The trophoblast is represented by a syncytiotrophoblast which is well developed adjacent to the stroma, while the cytotrophoblast has developed irregularly and is less well defined. At the abembryonic pole there is only a thin layer of mesothelial cells. The opening in the surface epithelium is well shown. The embryoblast already shows an entoderm and ectoderm with an amniotic space and a suggestion of a yolk sac.

into the peritoneal cavity, is carried into the Fallopian tube, and it is generally believed that this motion is determined by currents induced by the ciliary movement of the tubal epithelium. It is possible that similar currents carry the ovum to the region of the abdominal ostium: otherwise it is very difficult to explain cases of abdominal migration of the ovum from the ovary of one side to the Fallopian tube of the other. Such cases are well authenticated in the human subject and have been induced experimentally in animals. Recent experimental work has indicated that ciliary movement is not the sole factor which controls the transport of the ovum. Corner and others have found that the spontaneous contractions of the Fallopian tube are increased during oestrus, and peculiar distortions and contractions of the Fallopian tube have been seen by endoscopic intraperitoneal examination of the pelvis of the Macaque monkey at the time of ovulation. Contractions of the human Fallopian tube are increased by oestrogen as well as by oxytocic agents and, more important, by prostaglandins E_1 and E_2 which are present in seminal

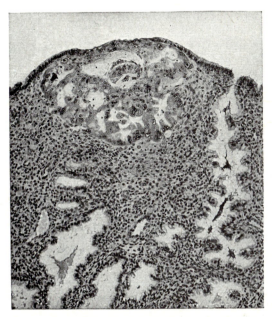

FIG. 45. Nine-and-a-half-day specimen (Rock and Hertig). Lacunae have developed in the syncytiotrophoblast while the cytotrophoblast at the embryonic pole is better developed than in the seven-and-a-half-day specimen. A few of the lacunae contain maternal blood. The embryo is bilaminar with ectoderm, entoderm, amniotic cavity and yolk sac.

fluid. The transport of the ovum from the surface of the ovary to the abdominal ostium seems to be determined by factors which approach rather to vitalism than to a simple mechanistic explanation. Similarly, it has been shown experimentally that the ciliary movement of the tubal epithelium is insufficient of itself to carry forward the large mammalian egg. Furthermore, it has been shown that premenstrual hypertrophy can be distinguished in the mucous membrane of the Fallopian tube which may have some bearing on the transport of the ovum. Fertilisation takes place in the outer part of the Fallopian tube. Corner has proved this to be the case with the sow, and the incidence of extrauterine gestation in the human subject shows that fertilisation can be extrauterine.

Rock and Hertig have shown that the interval between ovulation and nidation varies between five and eight days. Royal L. Brown showed, by placing the cervix of an extirpated uterus in a pool of semen, that the time taken for the sperms to migrate to the fimbriated end of the tube was about sixty-nine minutes. Allen, and subsequently other workers, have obtained specimens of ova in washings of the Fallopian tube. The ova obtained from tubal washings usually show signs of degeneration. Segmentation may occur *in vitro* and *in vitro* fertilisation has been seen by Rock and Hertig.

The Fertilised Human Ovum

Rock and Hertig obtained specimens of the early human ovum, one of the earliest of which was obtained seven and a half days after coitus (Figs. 43 and 44), and the ovum had already implanted. It consists of a flattened

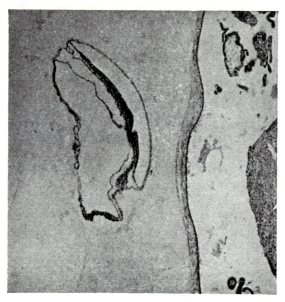

Fig. 46. Early human embryo dated as thirty-eight days from the first day of the last menstrual period. To the right lie chorionic villi and decidua. The embryo, which consists of two vesicles, lies in the extra-embryonic mesoderm. The amniotic sac which lies above and to the right is separated from the yolk sac lying below and to the left by the embryonic plate. The primitive streak is shown as a cup-shaped depression in the embryonic plate. The entoderm of the yolk sac has separated from the mesoderm which is burrowing laterally from the primitive streak.

blastocyst. Already a peripheral group of cells called the **trophoblast** has been differentiated, while an inner group of smaller cells forms the **embryoblast** of the embryo. The embryoblast lies in contact with that part of the trophoblast which lies adjacent to the stroma of the endometrium. At the abembryonic pole the trophoblast consists only of flattened cells, while at the embryonic pole it is actively proliferating. Already a peripheral group of massive deeply

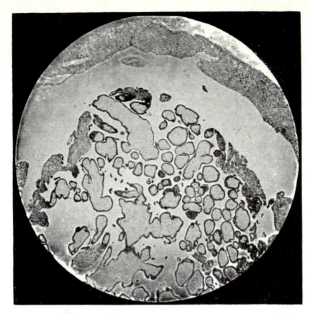

FIG. 47. Chorionic villi from an ovum which is calculated as thirty-eight days from the first day of the last period. Above lies the decidua capsularis, while below are primitive chorionic villi surrounded by cytotrophoblast.

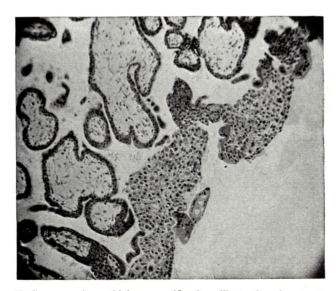

FIG. 48. Same specimen, higher magnification, illustrating the structure of primitive chorionic villi and the appearance of the cytotrophoblast. A few pieces of syncytium can be seen around the cytotrophoblast.

staining cells called the **syncytiotrophoblast** can be differentiated in the trophoblast, while a less prominent layer of **cytotrophoblast** consisting of large cells,
polyhedral in shape, with pale protoplasm, lines the inner part of the trophoblast layer. The embryo is a globular mass which already shows the two layers
of entoderm and ectoderm and within the ectoderm is a clear space—the
primitive amniotic cavity. The illustration shows that a yolk sac cleft can
already be distinguished in the entoderm. A slightly older specimen, obtained
nine and a half days after coitus (Fig. 45), shows that the defect in the endometrium through which the ovum has become implanted has been partially
repaired. There is no abembryonic wall and the original blastocyst structure
has disappeared. The embryo is bilaminar with a more pronounced amniotic
cavity. Vascular sinusoids are developing in the endometrium from branches

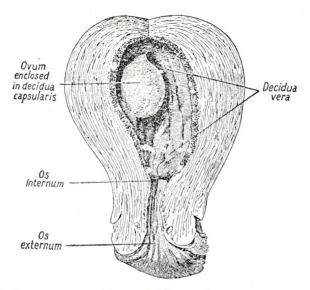

Ovum
enclosed
in decidua
capsularis

Decidua
vera

Os
Internum

Os
externum

FIG. 49. Pregnant uterus with ovum of four weeks' gestation. Natural size.
(Eden and Holland's "Manual of Obstetrics".)

of the spiral arterioles. Lacunae are appearing in the syncytiotrophoblast
which are designed to receive maternal blood and to constitute the future
intervillous space. The space within the cytotrophoblast is referred to as the
chorionic cavity, and the loose cells which it contains are called the cells of
the chorionic mesoderm. Thirteen and a half days after coitus, primitive
chorionic villi can be distinguished. They are formed from the cytotrophoblast. At this stage there is well-marked decidual reaction in the adjacent
endometrium (see Figs. 44 and 45).

The **allantois** develops early as a diverticulum from the yolk sac in the
region of the cloacal membrane. Blood islands can be distinguished in the
wall of the yolk sac very early in development and blood vessels pass along
the course of the allantois to reach the trophoblast. The **mesoderm** of the

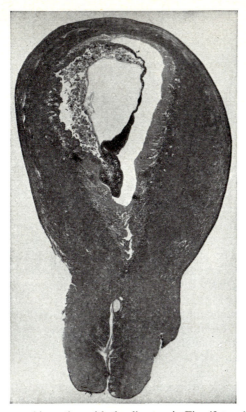

FIG. 50. Compare this section with the diagram in Fig. 49 to which it forms
an exact counterpart.

embryo arises by the division of cells at the base of the primitive streak and
the mesodermal layer stretches laterally between the ectoderm and the
endoderm of the yolk sac. The connecting stalk contains the allantois and its
blood vessels, together with primitive cells which resemble the cells of the
chorionic mesoderm. Subsequently the connecting stalk becomes the umbilical
cord (see Figs. 46, 47, 48, 49 and 50).

3 Physiology

In order to understand the normal and abnormal behaviour of the end organ of menstruation, the uterus, it is necessary to study the various components of the endocrine system which influence menstrual function.

THE PITUITARY

The anterior pituitary contains three histologically distinguishable cells, the chromophobe or parent cell, the eosinophil or alpha cell, and the basophil or beta cell. The alpha and beta cells are the functional units which secrete the active hormones. The total number of anterior pituitary hormones is unknown and only those of interest to the gynaecologist need be mentioned here. The suffix tropin*—the noun, or tropic*—the adjective, signifies a stimulant or influential action on the target organ—thus thyrotropic hormone of the anterior pituitary stimulates the specific release of thyroxin from the thyroid gland.

There are three gonadotropic hormones, the first two of which are secreted by the beta cells:

(1) **Follicle-stimulating Hormone** (FSH). This controls the ripening of the Graafian follicle and, in conjunction with luteinising hormone, causes ovulation. Its activity starts as menstruation is ceasing, reaches a peak at the seventh day of the cycle and then declines to disappear at about the eighteenth day. It is a watersoluble glyco-protein of high molecular weight. The carbohydrate fraction is mannose.

(2) **Luteinising Hormone** (LH) in conjunction with FSH, activates the secretion of oestrogen from the theca cells and also, in conjunction with oestrogen, causes ovulation. In the granulosa cells it initiates the earlier stages of progesterone production. It reaches peak secretion at the time of ovulation when FSH is declining. It is a water-soluble glyco-protein of high molecular weight. The carbohydrate fraction is mannose.

(3) **Luteo-tropic Hormone** (LTH) stimulates the actual secretion of progesterone, the precursor of which has been already stimulated by LH. It is probably the same substance as the mammogenic hormone prolactin and, if so, is secreted by the alpha cells of the anterior pituitary. It is chemically

---

* Gonadotropin versus gonadotrophin. It is debatable which is correct, although by strict Greek derivation tropin should be preferred. Common usage of trophin justifies its modern adoption and only classical purists will defend tropin. The reader may use whichever he pleases provided he has first read this footnote.

different from FSH and LH in that it is alcohol rather than water soluble nor is it a glycoprotein, but a protein. Its peak secretion occurs on the twenty-first day of the menstrual cycle. If pregnancy occurs, its secretion continues until the chorionic gonadotropins of the placenta assume its function, whereas, in the absence of pregnancy, its activity declines just before menstruation.

In the United Kingdom gonadotropin urinary levels are measured by the human menopausal gonadotropin unit (HMG) assayed on a 24-hour urine specimen. In the non-pregnant woman at the beginning of the menstrual cycle the HMG level is 10 units rising to 40 at the time of ovulation and then rapidly declining in a sharp curve to the basal level of 10 or under. This is of course a measure of pituitary gonadotropin excretion.

Extra-pituitary Gonadotropin. The human cytotrophoblast cells of the chorionic villi produce human chorionic gonadotropin (HCG) which resembles FSH and LH in being a glyco-protein except that the carbo-hydrate fraction is galactose. The presence of HCG in the urine of pregnant women and its biologically luteinising action is the basis of all pregnancy tests. If conception occurs HCG is recoverable fourteen days after ovulation and the tests should be positive seven days after the first missed period. Chorionic gonadotropin as opposed to pituitary gonadotropin is the urinary excretion production of trophoblastic activity and is measured in international units (1 I.U. = the activity of 0.1 mg. of a standard powder). The highest level is reached between the 7th and 10th week of pregnancy and may attain a level of 100,000 I.U. This level falls rapidly at the 12th week to reach a steady level at 5—10,000 units up to term. In twin pregnancy the titre is higher and with hydatidiform mole and chorion epithelioma the titre is such as to make possible a quantitative test for these conditions.

Adrenocorticotropic hormone (ACTH) stimulates the production of corticosteroids in the adrenal cortex and is produced by the beta cells. ACTH is closely linked with the melanocyte stimulating hormone (MSH). This hormone is increased at puberty when clinical pigmentation may be detectable and in pregnancy when it is obvious in the areola, cloasma (pigmentation of face and forehead, the so-called gypsy mark of pregnancy) and linea nigra of the abdomen.

Thyrotropic hormone acts on the thyroid and regulates the production of thyroxin. It is also produced by the beta cells.

Somatotropic or growth-promoting hormone acts directly on the skeletal system. It is a secretion of the alpha cells of the pituitary.

THE ADRENAL CORTICAL AND OVARIAN STEROIDS

The active hormones of the ovary and the adrenal cortex are steroids and in the adrenal cortex alone over thirty different steroids have been identified including oestrogenic steroids and progesterone. In fact, it is recognised that the adrenal cortex is an important source of extra-ovarian oestrogen. All steroids are derived from the cyclopentenophenanthrene nucleus in which the rings are distinguished by the letters A B C D and of which the carbon atoms are numbered 1 to 17.

To these 17 basic atoms of the cyclopentenophenanthrene nucleus additional atoms or groups of atoms may be added. Thus the pregnane nucleus is formed by the addition of side chains at C_{10}, C_{13} and C_{17}.

The presence of hydroxyl groups is indicated by the suffix—ol, and that of ketone groups by the suffix—one. Thus oestradiol signifies the presence of 2 hydroxyl groups and oestriol of 3.

By the addition of ketone groups at C_3 and C_{20} in the pregnane nucleus, the physiologically active steroid progesterone is produced.

The oestrogenic hormones are C_{18} compounds (with one side chain attached at C_{13}.)

Oestradiol (+2 hydroxyl groups)   Oestriol (+3 hydroxyl groups)

Oestrone,

The three main corticosteroid hormones of the adrenal cortex are aldosterone-corticosterone and hydrocortisone. These are C_{21} compounds with a hydroxyl group at C_{21}. They are all derivatives of cholesterol, a C_{27} compound, which as a result of ACTH action, loses its cholesterol side chain to become a C_{21} compound.

Cholesterol (C_{27} compound)

Under the influence of ACTH loses its side chain and forms $\triangle^5$—Pregnenolone (C_{21} compound)

Oxidation of the hydroxyl group produces Progesterone

Subsequent hydroxylation results in 17α-hydroxyprogesterone

and 17α, 21-hydroxyprogesterone

From this hydrocortisone results.

The biosynthesis of the corticosteroids, apart from the initial step of separation of the cholesterol side chain by ACTH, is effected by a series of adrenal enzymes.

The adreno-cortical steroids of interest to the gynaecologist are the following:

(1) Aldosterone is mineralo-corticoid in its action and influence on salt and water metabolism.

(2) Hydrocortisone is glucocorticoid and probably the principal corticosteroid, being found in the highest concentration in the adrenal vein. Its gluco-corticoid activity influences glycogen deposition and accounts for the hyperglycaemia and plethoric obesity of Cushings syndrome where gluco-corticoids are produced in excess.

(3) Dehydroepiandrosterone—a C_{19} compound—is entirely androgenic and, when produced in excess, may be one of the androgenic steroids responsible for the virilism of the androgenital syndrome.

(4) Adreno-cortical oestrogens have already been mentioned.

The Thyroid Gland

Disorders of the thyroid are at least five times as frequent in females as in males, and simple goitres and adenomas are known to undergo well-marked enlargement during pregnancy. In some women the thyroid enlarges at puberty and at the menopause, and the general belief is that the thyroid increases in size during pregnancy. This is possibly explained as the result of excessive output of anterior pituitary thyrotropic hormone. In *cretinism* the menstrual functions may not develop, or if they do develop, puberty is delayed and menstruation is irregular. In *adult myxoedema* menstruation may become irregular and scanty or it may cease, but occasionally the patients suffer from excessive menstruation or irregular menstrual periods. In hyper-thyroidism, the menstrual functions may not be disturbed although in advanced disease patients suffer from amenorrhoea or oligomenorrhoea.

APPLIED PHYSIOLOGY

Ovarian Hormones

Oestrogen. Natural oestrogens are C_{18} steroids, the main sources of which are the theca and granulosa cells of the Graafian follicles and corpus luteum, though the adrenal cortex is a secondary source of supply. Oestrogen is secreted as oestradiol, inactivated by the liver and excreted as conjugates of oestrone, oestradiol and oestriol in the urine whence they may be removed and assayed.

The excretion levels of the total end products of oestrogen rise from 10 mg. in 24 hours to 50 mg. at the time of ovulation, then decline to 25 mg. on the 16th day and fall steeply after the 24th day to 10 mg. at the onset of menstruation.

FUNCTIONS OF OESTROGEN:

(1) Feminisation and secondary sex characteristics. The texture of the female skin and hair, and the shape of the female form are considerably influenced by oestrogen.

(2) Specific action on the genital tract:

Vulva and vagina:

(a)   Development of vulva.
(b)   Vascular stimulation of vulva and vagina.
(c)   Epithelial stimulation of vulva and vagina.
(d)   Cornification of superficial layers of vagina, which appear as acidophilic polyhedral cells with a small pyknotic nucleus.
(e)   Deposition and metabolism of intracellular glycogen in vaginal epithelium. Characteristic changes in vaginal cytology.

Uterus:

(a)   Causes myohyperplasia of the myometrium and cervix.
(b)   Increases uterine vascularity.
(c)   Regenerates the endometrium after menstruation and is responsible for the proliferative pre-ovulatory hyperplasia of the endometrium.
(e)   Stimulant effect on the glands of the endocervix and their mucus secretion.

Fallopian Tubes:

Oestrogen stimulates the tubal musculature which is, in fact, morphologically specialised myometrium.

Ovary:

No action.

(3) Breast: Hypertrophy of the parenchyma of the breast increased vascularity, areolar pigmentation, but no galactogenic effect.

(4) Action on other endocrine glands: Oestrogen is depressant to FSH, luteotropic and thyrotropic hormones. It can be used to inhibit ovulation and the production of milk in the puerperal patient. It is stimulant to the luteinising hormone (LH) and thereby corpus luteum formation and, to a lesser extent, to ACTH.

(5) Skeletal system: It influences calcification of bone and the closure of epiphyses in the adolescent and is thus antagonistic to somatotropin. In the post-menopausal, decalcification of bone (osteoporosis leading to kyphosis) may be, in fact, due to oestrogen deficiency.

(6) Water and sodium metabolism: Oestrogen tends to cause water and sodium retention. An example is premenstrual tension which is caused by congestion secondary to water retention.

(7) Blood cholesterol levels are to a small extent controlled by oestrogen, hence the importance of ovarian conservation when performing a hysterectomy in a woman who gives a history of thrombo-embolic disease.

(8) Urinary oestriol estimations during pregnancy give a very good indication of placental function. The total may rise to 50 mgm. per day. Very low levels, below 10, are indicative of placental insufficiency.

Progesterone. The corpus luteum is the main source of progesterone. Although progesterone is an important intermediary product of synthesis of adrenal corticosteroids, it has little, if any, biological action from this extra-ovarian source. It is excreted in the urine as sodium pregnanediol glycuronide and recoverable as such for assay in the secretory phase of the menstrual cycle when it reaches as level of 3–4 mg. in the total twenty-four-hour urine. This figure presents only one tenth of the total progesterone production. During pregnancy the progesterone excretion level for 24 hours reaches 50–100 mg. in the middle trimester and rises to 100 or even 300 mg. at term. This very considerable output is entirely produced by the placenta as the corpus luteum is atrophic after the 14th week of gestation. Unfortunately, this assay is so complicated and expensive that very few laboratories in this country are prepared to undertake it and the clinician is thereby deprived of one useful means of assessing corpus luteum adequacy.

Like oestrogen, progesterone is inactivated in the liver.

ACTIONS OF PROGESTERONE

(1) Genital Tract:

Endometrium. Progesterone causes secretory hypertrophy and decidua formation in the endometrium if it has already been primed by oestrogen. This decidual reaction is, in reality, a water retention on the part of the stromal cell cytoplasm.

If pregnancy occurs, progesterone maintains this decidual state and is responsible for the early placentation of the ovum up to the twelfth week, after which the placenta itself manufactures progesterone as well as oestrogen and chorionic gonadotropin. The corpus luteum thereafter progressively degenerates.

If pregnancy does not occur, progesterone secretion ceases and progesterone withdrawal bleeding occurs. It is tempting to suggest that it is the withdrawal of progesterone which causes the bleeding of menstruation and this theory finds some support in the demonstration of progesterone withdrawal bleeding when the hormone is given therapeutically. It must, however, be remembered that women who have anovular cycles menstruate regularly and that the vascular changes characteristic of the endometrium about to menstruate can be produced experimentally and therapeutically by oestrogen alone without the presence of progesterone.

Myometrium

(a) Like oestrogen, progesterone causes myohyperplasia of the uterus and tubes.

(b) It increases the tone and strength of the rhythmic contractions of the uterus.

(c) It may be responsible for the pain of dysmenorrhoea by causing a hypertonus of the myometrium. (N.B. Anovular cycles are painless.)

(d) Progesterone increases the tone of the circular or sphincter muscle of the cervix and thus enhances its competence. It thus performs a physiological Shirodkar operation (see Chap. 20). In addition it increases the amount and viscosity of the cervical mucous glands and so produces a more tenacious mucous plug in the cervix.

(2) Under the influence of progesterone the vaginal smear shows characteristic changes. The cell pattern becomes one in which the cells are predominantly of the basophilic intermediate type with vesicular nuclei. These cells are clustered together with their edges curling or infolding—the so-called envelope effect.

(3) Breasts: Progesterone enhances the action of oestrogen and causes acinar epithelial growth. It is not lactogenic.

(4) Pituitary: It is possibly inhibitory to luteinising hormone.

(5) Like other steroids, it causes water and sodium retention and may be a contributory factor in premenstrual tension.

(6) Progesterone can be regarded a as weak pyrogenic agent in that it raises the body temperature by 0.5°C to 1.0°C. This is the basis of the interpretation of morning temperature charts in the investigation of infertility. If the temperature rises after ovulation by 0.5° C to 1°C this is stated to be a biphasic chart and is indirect evidence that ovulation has occurred.

(7) Action of progesterone on smooth muscle: It has a selective relaxant effect on all smooth muscle and this is most noticeable in pregnancy. The gastro-intestinal tract becomes hypotonic with delayed stomach emptying and colon stasis causing heartburn and constipation. The media of veins is hypotonic and this may well explain varicose veins and piles in the pregnant. The ureter becomes grossly dilated and tortuous.

Relaxin. Relaxin is a hormone which relaxes connective tissue and is probably produced by the ovary. It is a protein, water soluble and non-steroid. It has been prepared and marketed commercially but its therapeutic action is yet to be established. Relaxation of the fascial supports of the intervertebral joints may explain the liability of pregnant women to low back strain and backache whilst relaxation of the supports of the joints of the pelvis improves pelvic capacity.

Human Chorionic Gonadotropin (HCG)

Human chorionic gonadotropin is produced by the placenta (together with progesterone and oestrogens). It is assessed by an immunological method which has replaced the bio-assay used previously and the results are expressed as international units (I.U.).

The concentrations of HCG in both the serum and the urine follow a parallel course throughout pregnancy. HCG can be detected in the serum as early as the time of the first suppressed period, that is the 28th day. A rapid increase commences at about the 38th day, reaching a peak at about the 60th day and then falls abruptly from the 80th day to a level which remains fairly constant throughout the rest of pregnancy.

The actual peak values of HCG present in the urine per 24 hours varies between 20,000 to 500,000 I.U. These peak levels probably last for only three to four weeks, following which the daily excretion rate in the urine remains fairly constant at a level of between 5,000 to 10,000 I.U.

The exact role of HCG is obscure. It is definitely luteotropic. When the level of HCG falls at about the 80th day of pregnancy it is considered that the corpus luteum is no longer essential for the maintenance of the pregnancy.

Nearly all the diagnostic tests for pregnancy are based on the action of HCG and are either immunological or biological tests. Excessive growth of trophoblast, as seen in hydatidiform mole and chorion epithelioma produces large quantities of HCG, so that the pregnancy test may become positive when the urine is diluted (see page 141).

The Pituitary Gonadotropins

Three gonadotropic hormones are secreted by the anterior pituitary:
(1) Follicle stimulating hormone (FSH).
(2) Luteinising Hormone or the interstitial cell stimulating hormone (LH or ICSH).
(3) Luteotropin hormone (LTH). It is possible that LTH and prolactin are the same substance.

Pituitary gonadotropic hormones have not yet been chemically synthesised and until this has been done treatment must remain largely experimental. Owing to immense difficulties in assay techniques commercial pituitary gonadotropin does not necessarily contain biologically active and identical human hormones. The pituitary gonadotropins are chemically unstable proteins.

These hormones should be the logical therapy for certain pituitary ovarian dysfunctions such as in those instances where amenorrhoea occurs in the presence of normal reproductive organs, or when infertility is due to anovulatory cycles.

The position has been dramatically altered recently by Gemzell, who isolated from the pituitary of human cadavers at autopsy the active principle of the human pituitary follicle stimulating hormone (HPFSH). This had the advantage of not being inactivated by antibody formation and proved effective in producing ovulation in patients with both primary and secondary amenorrhoea, together with the production of polycystic ovaries. Unfortunately it requires ten human pituitaries to produce sufficient FSH to produce one ovulation, so that the difficulty of obtaining material and reasonable commercial marketing seems insuperable at present. The potency of the preparation is unquestionable since multiple pregnancies are common, quintuplets and even septuplets having been reported. Ovulation was successfully induced by Gemzell in 29 out of 40 patients with amenorrhoea.

In 1961 Greenblatt reported his results with clomiphene, a synthetic analogue of the non-steroidal oestrogen chlorotrianisene. In 96 patients 75 ovulated with 11 conceptions. Clomiphene is ineffective in primary amenorrhoea and most useful in secondary amenorrhoea. Its method of action is not yet fully understood.

A pituitary gonadotropin is also obtained from the urine of menopausal women (HMG). This preparation contains both follicle stimulating hormone (FSH) and luteinising hormone (LH). The individual assay of these two separate hormones is difficult to fractionate and potency varies widely with different preparations. The preparations are expensive, unstable and inactive by mouth.

CLINICAL APPLICATION OF HORMONE THERAPY

Oestrogen. In therapy oestrogen is effectively used both in the natural and synthetic form. It has been accurately standardised and the potency and dosage is known.

It is used as follows:

(1) To suppress anterior pituitary FSH, i.e. to convert painful ovular into painless anovular cycles in spasmodic dysmenorrhoea.

(2) To suppress anterior pituitary luteotropic hormone in the puerperal woman in order to suppress lactation.

(3) To stimulate the growth and vascularity of the Mullerian system. This obviously only works if the target organ is receptive.

(4) To test the sensitivity of the endometrium to oestrogen. This is a corollary of (3).

(5) To proliferate the epithelium of the endometrium, vagina and vulva.

(6) To develop the breast in patients with mammary hypoplasia.

(7) To control menopausal flushes by suppressing FSH production.

Less well defined indications for oestrogen therapy than the above are:

(8) To produce artificial cycles with oestrogen and progesterone withdrawal

bleeding at regular intervals in the hope of re-establishing normal menstrual rhythm in a woman with secondary amenorrhoea.

(9) To raise the blood oestrogen level above that of the threshold for bleeding and so arrest the uterine haemorrhage of metropathia. Very large doses are needed initially and as soon as treatment is stopped severe bleeding may recur.

Oestrogen therapy is largely substitutional and most of its results last only as long as it is continued.

The above are the more genuine indications for oestrogen but there are innumerable conditions for which it is given, many with little or no scientific basis.

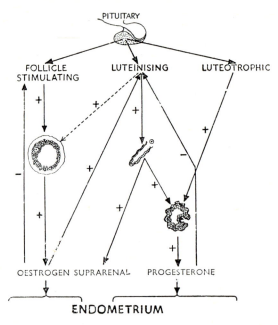

Fig. 51. A scheme illustrating the interrelation of the pituitary gonado-tropic hormones. + indicates stimulation and − indicates inhibition.

Progestogens. The natural product progesterone has been superseded in clinical therapy by the orally active synthetic progestogens, whose dosage and potency are accurate and reliable. The action of these drugs is somewhat selective, as the following examples will show.

(1) **Alkyl derivatives of 19-Norsteroids** (norethisterone, norethynodrel, norethisterone acetate—trade names Primolut N, Enavid and Anovlar respectively). This group is mildly oestrogenic, definitely progestational, ovulation inhibitory and somewhat haemostatic in dysfunctional uterine bleeding. Most are contraceptive. Some are certainly androgenic and can cause virilism in the female foetus of a pregnant woman.

(2) **Derivatives of progesterone** (dihydroprogesterone, duphaston and megestrol acetate which with added oestrogen is Volidan). These drugs have no oestrogenic but a marked progestational effect on the endometrium. They are used in the treatment of dysmenorrhoea and recurrent abortion. Effective by mouth.

(3) **Alkyl derivatives of testosterone.** 17 α ethinyl-testosterone (Ethisterone B.P., Progestoral) and dimethisterone (Secrosteron). The less potent of the progestogens but undoubtedly the most virilising.

(4) **Esters of 17 α hydroxyprogesterone.** 17 α hydroxyprogesterone 17n caproate (Primolut depot). This is given by intramuscular injection in doses of up to 250 mg. Its action continues for approximately one week.

The 17 α hydroxyprogesterone acetate is active by mouth. It has no oestrogenic effect and is weak or non-inhibitory to ovulation. Its main effect is progestational. The caproate is the safest of all progestogens as far as virilism is concerned.

Efficiency. All the progestogens except the 17 α hydroxyprogesterone caproate are effective by mouth. They take a few days to produce the maximum result on the target organ and this effect is short lived, i.e. progestogen withdrawal bleeding occurs within 48 hours of cessation of therapy. To be effective on the endometrium some priming with oestrogen is needed.

Side Effects. If given in large doses they can cause gastro-intestinal symptoms, nausea and vomiting. Headache and mild elevation of temperature are also seen. In fact all the symptoms of a pseudo pregnancy state may be observed—water retention, breast engorgement and tenderness and moderate uterine enlargement. Virilism has already been mentioned. Thrombosis of deep veins, pulmonary embolism and even arterial thrombosis are much publicised, if somewhat exaggerated, risks.

Therapeutic indications
  (a) In conjunction with oestrogen to produce secretory changes in the endometrium.
  (b) In conjunction with oestrogen to inhibit ovulation—the contraceptive pill.
  (c) In the treatment of dysfunctional bleeding.
  (d) In the treatment of dysmenorrhoea by producing anovular and therefore painless cycles—the same as (b) above.
  (e) To prevent abortion. To minimise the risk of foetal virilisation 17 α hydroxyprogesterone caproate should be used. It is especially indicated in habitual abortion, although some authorities doubt if it has any effect in preventing abortion.
  (f) In the non-surgical treatment of endometriosis. Here large doses up to 30 to 40 mgms. daily can be given for 9–24 months to induce a state of pseudo-pregnancy.
  (g) In the palliation and control of endometrial cancer. Progestogen in very large doses (up to 2 or even 5 gms. weekly) is not curative but can

cause temporary disappearance of metastases and certainly may prolong life for several months.

The indications for endocrine therapy and the treatment and dosage will be further considered under their respective headings in subsequent chapters. The above is a brief outline only.

THE PHYSIOLOGY OF MENSTRUATION

The proliferative phase of the endometrium represents the oestrogenic part of the menstrual cycle and is homologous with the pro-oestrous phase of lower animals. It is initiated and controlled by the hormone oestrogen which is almost certainly derived from the secretion of theca cells of the Graafian follicle. The secretory phase of the endometrium is controlled by the hormone progesterone, although the effect of progesterone is obtained only after the endometrium has been sensitised with oestrogen.

Although the activity of the endometrium is directly controlled by ovarian function and by the two hormones secreted by the ovary, the ovary itself is activated by the pituitary gland, the secretions of which are probably under the nervous control of the hypothalamus.

Oestrogen is liberated by the Graafian follicle and progesterone is secreted by the corpus luteum. The mechanism of ovarian stimulation by means of the gonadotropic hormones is complex and has already been referred to on p. 76. The follicle stimulating hormone (FSH) causes the development of a Graafian follicle in the ovary. The Graafian follicle under the influence of FSH together with only a minimal amount of the luteinising hormone (LH) secretes 17β-oestradiol. 17β-oestradiol has three functions. In the first place, it produces proliferative changes in the endometrium. Secondly, it inhibits further secretion of the follicle stimulating hormone by the anterior pituitary, and thirdly, it stimulates the anterior pituitary to secrete the luteinising hormone. The luteinising hormone has two functions. In the first place, it stimulates a Graafian follicle to secrete 17β-oestradiol, and secondly, it causes the follicle to rupture at ovulation and to form a corpus luteum. The luteotropic hormone may stimulate the corpus luteum to secrete progesterone. The hormone progesterone has two functions. In the first place, it stimulates the endometrium to undergo secretory hypertrophy, and secondly, it inhibits further production of the luteinising hormone by the anterior pituitary. It should be remembered that there is no evidence that any gonadotropic hormone has a direct effect upon the endometrium of the uterus.

The cause of menstrual bleeding is obscure. A popular hypothesis is that withdrawal of progesterone secretion is followed by menstrual haemorrhage, for uterine bleeding of this type can be induced experimentally. The hypothesis is almost certainly too simple and it is debatable whether menstruation is due to progesterone or oestrogen withdrawal or both. The point can only be of academic interest.

The urinary excretion levels of oestrogen in the menstrual cycle rise from a basal 10 mgm. in the 24 hours to 50 or even more at ovulation and then fall to 30 mgm. at the 22nd day and thereafter steeply to the basal 10 mgm. just before the next menstruation. A study of the coiled arteries of the endometrium shows that there is a slight regression shortly after ovulation and that a rapid decrease in thickness can be demonstrated even before menstruation starts. In the regression which starts during the few days prior to menstruation there is a decreased blood flow which may cause shrinkage of the endometrium from dehydration. During menstruation itself the reduction in the thickness of the endometrium is determined both by desquamation and by resorption. The coiled arteries become buckled with subsequent stasis of blood flow. The necrosis of the superficial layers of the endometrium is produced either by local stasis or by the clearly demonstrated vasoconstriction of the coiled arteries. Menstrual bleeding occurs when the open arteries damaged by necrosis relax and discharge blood into the uterine cavity. Some degree of venous haemorrhage also occurs. Fragments become detached from the superficial layer of the endometrium at the end of the first day.

The important features of the menstrual changes are the contraction and constriction of the coiled arteries. The ischaemia causes necrosis and disintegration of the superficial zone. The regeneration of the vascular system is probably brought about by the development of anastomosing arteries. The re-epithelialisation is brought about by cells growing from the mouths of the base of the glands that remain in the unshed basal layer of the endometrium.

In anovulatory menstruation there is the same shedding of a thin necrotic superficial layer of the endometrium, and it is to be presumed that exactly the same factor is at work to cause the vascular changes with resultant ischaemia. The cyclical bleeding of anovulatory cycles in which progesterone withdrawal can play no part emphasises the importance of oestrogen withdrawal in the normal ovulatory cycle as already stated.

THE HYPOTHESIS OF OESTROGEN WITHDRAWAL BLEEDING

The theory has been postulated that there is a certain intermediate level of oestrogen in the blood at which bleeding occurs from the uterus:

(1) If the level of oestrogen rises above this level—so-called super-threshold oestrogen level—no bleeding occurs. This super-threshold level can be obtained by giving a woman with dysfunctional bleeding very large doses of oestrogen and raising the blood level so that haemorrhage ceases and therapeutic amenorrhoea results as long as the oestrogen level is held at this height.

(2) Sub-threshold oestrogen level also results in amenorrhoea. This is again seen when both ovaries are removed surgically or destroyed by radiation, and in amenorrhoea due to ovarian failure.

(3) If the ovary is absent or destroyed but the uterus present, bleeding can be produced by giving oestrogen to raise the blood oestrogen to threshold level. This is exemplified by the post-menopausal bleeding due to excessive and uncontrolled oestrogen therapy usually in an effort to control hot flushes.

(4) If oestrogen therapy is being given in sufficient dosage to raise the blood level to super-threshold, as soon as it is suddenly withdrawn, in from

two to seven days the oestrogen level falls from super-threshold to threshold level and bleeding results.

(5) Normal menstrual cycles can be explained as follows: In the oestrogenic phase, blood oestrogen is at super-threshold level and gradually falls to threshold level at the end of the secretory phase, when bleeding results, i.e. menstruation.

(6) Ovulation spotting may be due to a temporary fall in oestrogen to threshold level.

Progesterone may act in a similar way and this would explain the phenomenon of progesterone withdrawal bleeding. In other words, in the secretory phase progesterone is at super-threshold level and acts as a substitute for oestrogen, which is now falling to threshold level. If conception does not occur, the combined effect of oestrogen and progesterone withdrawal causes a drop in these combined steroids to threshold level and so bleeding results.

Some support for the above theories is obtained by the fact that it is possible to postpone normal menstrual bleeding by giving large doses of oestrogen or progesterone, sufficient to maintain the oestrogen or progesterone above the threshold level after the normally produced ovarian hormones have fallen to threshold level. Though rarely indicated or advisable, this therapeutic feat is used clinically to suppress menstruation for a few days in athletes, entertainers and during the honeymoon.

MENSTRUATION

The Menstrual Rhythm. The menstrual cycle is usually one of twenty-eight days, measured by the time between the first day of one period and the first day of the next. The duration of the haemorrhage varies between three and five days, and the amount of blood lost has been estimated to be between 50 and 200 ml. An exact cycle of twenty-eight days is present only in a small

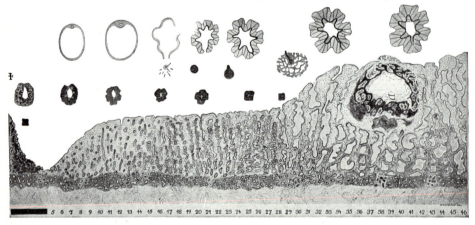

FIG. 52. Schröder's illustration of the relation between ovarian function and the changes in the endometrium during early pregnancy. (Veit-Stoeckel.)

proportion of healthy women. Frequently there is a departure of two or three days from the twenty-eight-day rhythm, while in others the cycle is one of twenty-one days. In some women the menstrual cycle is irregular, varying between three weeks and six weeks, and such irregularity may be present without any sign of anatomical defect of the genitalia. The cause of the normal menstrual rhythm of twenty-eight days is unknown. The rhythm may conveniently be regarded as one of the biological constants of adult women. Variations are found in different races, a shorter cycle being more prevalent amongst the women of tropical climates, while at the other extreme are the Esquimaux women who menstruate only during the time of the midnight sun.

Whatever its origin, it is now established that the rhythm is altered in gynaecological complaints only by disorders of the ovaries or of those ductless glands which influence the ovaries through their internal secretions. The menstrual rhythm cannot be influenced by disease of the uterus or the Fallopian tubes, but the amount of blood lost and the duration of the haemorrhage at a menstrual period are commonly affected by local abnormalities of the uterus and Fallopian tubes.

Characters of the Menstrual Discharge. The menstrual discharge consists of dark altered blood mixed with mucous secretion from the cervical canal and with the normal vaginal secretion. The dark fluid blood has a characteristic appearance. It is different from the uterine haemorrhage of carcinoma of the body of the uterus or from the haemorrhage of polypi or of abortion, but the same type of dark fluid blood is seen in cases of metropathia haemorrhagica. The normal menstrual discharge is peculiar in that it does not clot and contains no prothrombin though rich in calcium. Its fibrinogen content is low and it is presumed that the prothrombin is inactivated in the endometrium. The fluid contains, apart from red blood corpuscles, a preponderance of leucocytes. It also contains epithelial cells and cell debris. Small shreds of necrotic tissue can sometimes be identified. It is suggested that the blood discharged from the endometrium during menstruation may clot inside the uterus. Subsequently the clots are dissolved by an enzyme capable of proteolysis. This theory is not supported by the evidence of hysterectomy performed at the time of menstruation where the menstrual history is one of a normal loss. In such circumstances, few surgeons have ever found a clot in the uterus. Clots are passed if menstrual bleeding is excessive, and the passage of clots is a symptom met with in myomata and excessive haemorrhage, but the clots form in the upper vagina. If the menstrual discharge is examined on the first day of the period of bleeding, relics of the functional layer of the endometrium can be detected.

Symptoms

During menstruation a minority of women have no symptoms whatever. The majority notice minor symptoms varying from trifling to moderate but not ever incapacitating. The commonest of these is a heavy feeling in the lower abdomen and back probably due to pelvic congestion or increased vascularity of the uterus and rapidly relieved by the establishment of the flow. As a result of the pelvic hyperaemia, frequency of micturition and a feeling of fullness in the pelvis are often noticed, and it is not uncommon for any haemorrhoids which may be present to become more painful. Moreover, headaches, sleeplessness, palpitations and even migraine are common, and such physical disturbances as depression and irritability frequently develop. The female crime and suicide rate reaches its peak in the premenstrual phase. There is slight enlargement of the thyroid gland, and often the nasal mucosa becomes congested. Sometimes skin eruptions, such as acne, develop before menstruation. The mechanism of the causation of acne is not understood— it may be caused by giving progesterone whilst in others it may be cured by progesterone. Immediately before menstruation the blood pressure rises, together with the basal metabolic rate, the serum calcium and also the number of circulating red blood corpuscles. The body temperature falls half a degree or a little more as the result of progesterone withdrawal and this is one sign that conception has not occurred in those women who keep careful, regular temperature charts during treatment for infertility.

Two noticeable symptoms are fairly constant in most women at or just before menstruation. One is a tendency to disturbance of bowel habit, usually resulting in constipation though the other extreme is more rarely seen, and the other is a feeling of fullness or heaviness in the breasts even amounting to pain. Some of these premonitory symptoms when observed by an intelligent woman invariably give her warning of an impending menstrual period and serve the useful purpose of giving her time to adjust her social activities accordingly. They also warn her to take the necessary hygienic precautions against the menstrual flow. This premenstrual tension is probably due to an increased water and sodium retention and may cause a slight weight gain of 1–2 Kg. (2–4 lb.).

Menstrual Hygiene. Old superstitions and traditions die hard and slow, and the physiological process of menstruation is still regarded by many women as an unclean state which segregates them from the activities of normal life. The popular but sinister appellation of "the curse" recalls the original sin of Eve and suggests a period of mental and physical discomfort which darkens the calendar at regular intervals. Mother, relatives and friends may promote this idea of discomfort and pain by well documented accounts of their own suffering. Thus, early in her menstrual life a young girl is conditioned to the idea of dysmenorrhoea. She may be discouraged from the ordinary social intercourse of adolescence, games and parties being strictly interdicted, all domestic and outdoor bathing stopped, and she may be encouraged to stay at home, to be fussed over by an over-indulgent parent. To a suggestible girl in her teens, these psychosomatic factors are of profound importance and can soon be exploited to avoid every sort of unpleasant routine. A day off from school or the office and, later on, from household duties is a tempting avenue of escapism and, if spent in bed with a hot water bottle and meals brought up by mother or husband, can provide certain compensation for inactivity. It is surprising how many girls with dysmenorrhoea have dysmenorrhoeic mothers.

This attitude in parents towards menstruation is strongly to be deprecated. A sensible and frank explanation that menstruation is a normal physiological process, that stories of pain and illness can be largely discounted, instruction in the necessary hygiene and a firm but kindly under-emphasis of any symptoms that do arise will largely dispel most of the wrong ideas in the young adolescent mind. There is no necessity for any curtailment of social or school activities, games should continue to be played and life should continue in spite of this slightly inconvenient contretemps. There should, in fact, be no interruption of daily routine.

For the adolescent just starting to menstruate, it is wise to use an ordinary external sanitary pad which should be changed two to three times by day and once at night. For the ordinary loss this number will suffice and the average number used during a period will be twelve to eighteen pads. Later on, as adolescence advances into womanhood, some internal tampon will no doubt be preferred for its convenience, unobtrusiveness and ease of disposal. These intra-vaginal tampons are satisfactory and harmless but they are inadequate if the loss is heavier than average. They may be purchased in varying sizes, the smallest of which are suitable for the young woman with an unruptured hymen and although their use does involve a certain amount of intra-vaginal manipulation the advantages of internal protection are enormous. They have one surprising disadvantage: their liability to be overlooked and left in situ when they give rise to a profuse and evil-smelling discharge. Every gynaecologist has had the unpleasant experience of removing at least a few of these missing foreign bodies. For all women, the tampon has much to recommend it over the sanitary towel.

Premenstrual tension. The syndrome of premenstrual tension or congestion is well recognised and is caused by water retention. It may be for only a few hours but can last for up to ten days before the period and is usually dramatically relieved by the onset of the menstrual flow. It is well recognised that a rise of oestrogen and progestogen can cause a disturbance of water balance in the tissues. A good example of this is seen in the tissue oedema encountered in some cases of carcinoma of the prostate treated by massive dosage of oestrogen. Clinically, patients who suffer from premenstrual tension complain of feeling bloated and uncomfortable, a fullness in the head and congestion of the sinuses, pain and swelling in the breasts and abdominal distension and discomfort. Various treatments have been tried of which the most effective is restriction of salt intake with the addition, if required, of a diuretic such as chlorothiazide G. 0.5 morning and midday for the required number of premenstrual days.

This simple physical explanation is valid for those patients who have a demonstrable weight gain of sudden onset up to 4–5 lb. in the premenstrual phase. In a few the gain may be even more dramatic and reach 10 lb., but many patients show no weight gain and still suffer from premenstrual tension. In these there is a marked functional overlay and the condition must be regarded as largely, but not entirely, psycho-somatic.

Intermenstrual Pain. Mittelschmerz. Ovulation Pain. This intermenstrual pain has been attributed to the rupture of a Graafian follicle during ovulation. Usually the pain is restricted to about the fourteenth day; frequently the vaginal discharge is increased at the time, and in some instances there is a little bleeding as well. Intermenstrual pain is probably caused by tension within ovaries which have a thick tunica albuginea, for at about the time of ovulation the ovary contains a large ripe follicle. Another possible explanation of the pain is a local peritoneal reaction to the discharge of follicular contents and possible slight blood loss at the time of follicular rupture. Occasionally the intermenstrual pain is so severe that sedatives have to be given. The regular cyclical incidence of the pain and its timing usually give the correct clue to the diagnosis. No treatment, apart from reassurance and explanation, is necessary. Ovulation normally occurs 14 days before the next menstrual period, these two events being linked by the formation and decline of the corpus luteum. Thus ovulation occurs on the 14th day of a 28-day cycle and on the 21st day of a 35-day cycle. Mild or even severe pain is sometimes felt in the lower abdomen at the time of ovulation. It is frequently localised to the side on which ovulation has occurred.

On rare occasions ovulation is accompanied by intraperitoneal haemorrhage in sufficient quantity to cause quite severe abdominal pain similar to that of an extrauterine gestation. The clinical picture is one of acute local tenderness usually in one or other lower quadrant. If the condition is not recognised the abdomen will be opened, with a diagnosis of extrauterine gestation or appendicitis. The treatment should be conservative if these two serious possibilities can be excluded and as a rule the patient recovers in twenty-four hours, but the diagnosis can be proved subsequently by suspension of ovulation with hormones which will, of course, prevent the pain occurring.

PUBERTY

Like the climacteric, puberty has vague boundaries in time, whereas the menarche is a relatively sudden event. Puberty is a slow process involving several years during which the secondary sexual characteristics develop to maturity and menstruation is established. The menarche, or time of onset of menstruation, varies with race and, to some extent, family but the average for most girls is from twelve to thirteen years of age. The process of puberty can be largely explained by activity of the anterior pituitary which stimulates, by its various tropins, the various endocrine glands under its control. Somatotropin causes a fairly sudden increase in skeletal growth, gonadotropin stimulates ovarian activity which, in turn, produces the secondary sexual characteristics, increase in breast size, development of external genitalia, axillary and pubic hair, and enlargement of the internal genitalia resulting in menstruation. ACTH stimulates the adrenal which is in part responsible for some of the phenomena and an increase in gluco-corticoids may explain the tendency to a transient, mild adolescent obesity. The adrenal activity possibly explains the liability to acneiform eruptions on the face and trunk. Thyrotropic hormone activity accounts for the slight noticeable enlargement of the thyroid. It is, however, the rising surge of oestrogen which dominates the changing picture of adolescence.

Puberty may be precocious, occurring two or three years before the expected and recognised average, or delayed perhaps five years after. If anatomically and clinically normal, most girls menstruate spontaneously by the age of eighteen or nineteen and these aberrations from the normal need cause no anxiety nor indicate any treatment, in spite of parental anxiety or attempted coercion.

THE MENOPAUSE

Strictly speaking, the menopause should be defined as the time at which menstruation ceases and not used synonymously with the climacteric, which is the phase of waning ovarian activity and may start two or three years before the menopause and continue for two to five years after it. The climacteric is thus a phase of adjustment between active and inactive ovarian function and may occupy several years of a woman's life. In deference to common though incorrect usage the word menopause has been retained in the text.

The menopause occurs between the ages of 45 and 50; the average age of onset is 47, so that the child-bearing period of life covers a period between thirty and thirty-five years. It is the authors' opinion that the onset of the menopause is later than it was thirty years ago and patients are occasionally seen menstruating quite regularly at 55. This prolongation of menstrual activity is probably due to an improvement in the general health and environmental conditions of women. It has certainly nothing to do with parity or the age at which the menarche occurs. There are variations in the time of onset amongst individual races. A late onset of the menopause is frequently associated with the presence of uterine myomata or of some degree of myohyperplasia. In some women menstruation ceases abruptly during the third decade of life without producing any severe disturbances of the general health. After the menopause ovarian activity ceases, and ripening follicles and corpora lutea no longer develop in the ovaries. The interstitial cells remain for a few months, but within a year of the completion of the menopause ovarian activity has ceased and even primordial follicles have disappeared. As the result of cessation of ovarian activity, reactions develop in the other ductless glands which are responsible for many of the menopausal symptoms which arise. The FSH of the anterior pituitary rises as a result of the fall in oestrogen level, and the urinary gonadotropin may even reach a level sufficient to give a false positive to biological pregnancy tests. Menopausal urine is thus one commercial source of gonadotropin (HMG). The figures reach a peak of 1,000 HMG units which is fifty times greater than in the menstruating adult. Sclerotic degenerative changes can be demonstrated in the ovarian vessels and thickening of the intima is particularly noticeable. It is of interest that a menopause develops in the human female, whereas lower animals retain normal follicles and ova in their ovaries with the result that fertility continues into old age.

Anatomical Changes. The genitalia undergo atrophy and retrogression. The ovaries become shrunken and their surfaces grooved and furrowed. The plain muscle of the Fallopian tube undergoes atrophy, cilia disappear from the tubal epithelium, and the tubal plicae are not so prominent. The uterus becomes smaller through atrophy of its plain muscle, so that the connective tissues are relatively more conspicuous when sections are made through the myometrium. The endometrium is represented only by the basal layer with its compact, deeply staining stroma, and by a few simple tubular glands. The functional layer can no longer be demonstrated, premenstrual hypertrophy is never seen, and the lymphoid tissue also disappears. It is common for some of the glands of the endometrium of the body of the uterus to become cystically dilated even before menstruation has ceased, and such cystic glands are often to be demonstrated in the endometrium after the menopause. The cervix becomes smaller and its vaginal portion is represented in old women by a small prominence in the upper part of the vagina. The vagina becomes smaller and tends to be conical with the apex of the cone in the situation of the cervix. The action of oestrogen causes the growth of the cervix into the upper vagina at puberty producing the four vaginal fornices. The fornices gradually disappear as the cervix regresses after the menopause. The vaginal epithelium becomes pale, thin and dry, and during its involution is readily infected, so that senile vaginitis results. The vulva atrophies and the vaginal orifice becomes smaller, so that dyspareunia is a common symptom. The skin of the labia minora and of the vestibule becomes pale and dry, and there is a reduction in the amount of fat contained by the labia majora. The pubic hair is reduced in amount and becomes grey. The skin around the vaginal orifice and urethra loses some of its resistance to infection as the epithelium becomes thin so that red patchy areas are often seen in patients past menopausal age. The pelvic cellular tissues become lax and the ligaments and tissues which support the uterus and vagina lose their tone, so that there is a tendency for prolapse to become more marked. It is well known clinically that patients quite often seek treatment for prolapse shortly after the menopause.

In addition to local atrophy of the generative organs, general disturbances develop which are almost certainly caused by alteration of the endocrine balance, which was maintained during the child-bearing period of life. Fat is deposited around the breasts, hips, nates, and abdomen. Although the mammary glandular tissue atrophies, the deposition of fat frequently makes the breasts more pendulous. The skin becomes wrinkled and quite commonly hair grows round the lips and chin. In most cases the blood pressure rises, and cardiac irregularity and tachycardia sometimes occur. Arthritic changes often develop in the joints, and in some women a well-marked osteoporosis may be seen, particularly in the spine and pelvic girdle, which renders these bones more liable to fracture.

The oestrogenic hormones are secreted in a very small amount by postmenopausal women and the most likely source of this oestrogen is the adrenal cortex. The gonadotropic hormones appear in high concentration at the menopause because they are not inhibited by oestrogen.

Menopausal Symptoms

(1) Menstrual. The three classical ways in which the periods cease are:
  i. Sudden cessation.
  ii. Gradual diminution in the amount of loss with each regular period until
      they disappear.

iii. Gradual increase in the spacing of the periods until they cease for an interval of six months.

Any patient who bleeds after a gap of six months must be considered to be suffering from post-menopausal bleeding and treated as such (p. 104). Continuous bleeding, menorrhagia, irregular bleeding or other menstrual abnormalities are not normal. They must be investigated despite the common belief that they are "signs of the change".

(2) *Cardiovascular:* The commonest and most noticeable symptoms are hot flushings and sweatings. The flushings are waves of vasodilatation affecting the face and neck which last for about two minutes and are frequently followed by severe sweating. Several of these flushes may occur in a day and they may be induced by trivial incidents in nervous women. They are often worse at night in bed and the profuse night sweats disturb the patient's rest. Some patients become acutely conscious of their presence and shrink as a result from the ordinary contacts of social intercourse. This increases their introspective tendencies and makes a trivial symptom one of all absorbing importance. Functional derangements of cardiac action with palpitations are common and anginal pains of effort are complained of at this time.

(3) *Neurological and Emotional:* Paraesthesiae, which take the form of sensations of pins and needles in the extremities, are again extremely common. Headaches and noises in the ears are often complained of, while psychical disturbances which take the form of irritability, depression and even melancholia are frequent. Sexual feeling is quite often increased when the menopause is in progress, and is probably induced by a raised androgen secretion from the adrenal cortex.

The condition of **pseudocyesis** is infrequent. Patients who are probably disturbed psychically attribute the amenorrhoea to pregnancy, a view which is supported by the increase in the abdominal girth caused by the deposition of fat. It is often difficult to convince such a woman that her symptoms are menopausal.

In a severe case of pseudocyesis the patient will produce most convincing physical signs. She will point out the enlargement of the breasts, due in reality to localised obesity, and by aerophagy and flatulent distension will produce a sizeable abdominal swelling. As constipation is frequently troublesome at the menopause, this associated with borborygmi will be interpreted by her as foetal movements. Some patients are almost impossible to convince that they are not pregnant and only prolonged observation and repeated negative tests will eventually disillusion them.

(4) *Gastro-intestinal Symptoms:* The most noticeable of these is an almost universal tendency to flatulent distension of the colon which is often so marked that the patient suspects that she may have some abdominal tumour. This distension is associated with a tendency to constipation. Barium enema may show colon spasm and, in the more obese patient, diverticulosis. It is naturally important with any alteration of bowel habit to exclude a carcinoma. Flatulent and functional dyspepsias are also common and these are often associated

4*

with an increase in appetite for carbohydrates with resulting obesity and abdominal discomfort.

(5) *Locomotor System:* Menopausal arthropathy, osteoarthritis, fibrositis, backache, and intervertebral disc lesions are all common complaints at the menopause. Whether the basis of these conditions is vascular or endocrine is questionable as is the role of the menopause in their causation.

(6) *Endocrine System:* Slight virilisation as seen in the increased hirsutism is probably adrenal in origin as is, perhaps, the obesity. Slight degrees of hypothyroidism are also noticed with lowered B.M.R., raised cholesterol, brittleness of hair, dryness of skin, lassitude and reduction of mental power and concentration.

(7) *Genital Tract:*

   (a)   Vulva: There is a progressive atrophy over the years. The vulval skin becomes pale, thin and almost translucent.
   (b)   Vagina: This becomes dry, the epithelium atrophic, glycogen is low or absent in the cells, the pH rises and senile vaginitis is a likely sequel.
   (c)   Cervix: The cervix atrophies, the glands cease their activity and mucous secretion is diminished. An obliterative stenosis may result in a senile pyometra.
   (d)   Uterus: This diminishes in size, the myometrium and endometrium atrophy and fibroids, if present, shrink in size but do not disappear. They are liable to undergo hyaline and calcareous degeneration.
   (e)   Ovaries: These show an increased refractory state to gonadotropins and ovulation finally ceases after which the ovary atrophies with gradual decrease in oestrogen production. It must not be thought that all menopausal menstruation is anovular and that these patients are, therefore, infertile. Many a child has been conceived in the very late forties largely because women consider themselves beyond the possibility of conception and become slack in their contraceptive drill.

There is much variation in the manner in which the menstrual periods cease at the time of the menopause. Only three variations should be regarded as physiological. These are described on p. 96. Any departure from these three forms should be regarded as pathological. It is a common misconception that irregular and excessive uterine haemorrhage is a characteristic symptom of the menopause. Even to this day cases of carcinoma of the uterus are missed in their early stages because the irregular haemorrhage caused by the carcinoma is regarded as menopausal. Any form of irregular haemorrhage arising in women of menopausal age should be investigated with the utmost care. Vaginal speculum and cytological examination must be insisted upon. The uterus should be curetted and the curettings must be examined histologically. One of the worst mistakes ever made in gynaecology is to fail to diagnose carcinoma of the uterus when the growth is at an early stage of development.

Apart from carcinoma of the uterus, other gynaecological conditions, such as myomata, polypi, etc., give rise to irregular haemorrhage which very often can be easily treated and cured. All patients who suffer from irregular haemorrhage at the time of the menopause should therefore be carefully examined to determine the cause of this irregularity. Acute menopausal symptoms may develop as the result of the surgical removal of both ovaries, and they may also be induced by the use of X-rays or radium to produce an artificial menopause. The menopausal symptoms are not usually severe in women younger than 30, and there is no knowledge of the factors which determine whether any particular patient will develop severe symptoms.

Treatment of Menopausal Symptoms. Like dysmenorrhoea, the menopause is largely bedevilled with old wives' tales and the patient is psychologically conditioned into a state of anxiety neurosis by the case histories, told with painstaking detail, of her friends and relations. Many women are obsessed with the conviction that their physical, mental and sexual lives will now rapidly decline into a state of uselessness and senescence. More sinister than this is the firm conviction, often at a subconscious level, that malignant disease is a likely event at the menopause.

The first duty of a doctor, when handling the menopausal patient, is to spend plenty of time in explaining the exact physiological state in simple language that is intelligible to his patient, discovering her fears and reassuring her, and answering patiently but convincingly all the little questions that are on her mind. He should then make a thorough examination of the whole patient and, finally, a careful bimanual pelvic examination with vaginal speculum examination, always including cytological screening. He is then in a position to pronounce his patient a fit woman with a normal pelvis and assure her that there is no evidence of cancer, if that is her fear. He should arrange to see her at regular intervals until she has reached the calm waters of the completed climacteric. This means a final and happy adjustment to her new hormonal state of lessening ovarian activity. This supervision will involve careful attention to a low carbohydrate, average protein diet and strict control of incipient obesity; regular exercise to maintain muscular and general physical fitness; encouragement of external interests to boost her psychological outlook and combat any tendency to introspection and depression. Attention to minor ailments like constipation and piles, varicose veins and the arthropathies by physiotherapy are important. Finally, a regular pelvic examination is essential at least once a year and preferably at half-yearly intervals, this to include cytological screening.

Small doses of phenobarbitone with or without a mild tranquilliser may relieve moderate symptoms, and only in the more severe cases resort to oestrogen should be necessary—for example, where flushes are frequent and severe and have become an interference to her normal life. The flushes and sweats are caused by excessive FSH production which can be suppressed by oestrogen. The results of the treatment are excellent and most patients respond within one or two days.

The efficacy of oestrogen can be gauged by the reduction in the number and severity of the flushes occurring in twenty-four hours, the aim being to reduce the number of flushes to a reasonable level rather than their complete suppression. The exact dose must be determined by trial, and it is best to start with a small dose such as 0.01 mgm. ethinyl oestradiol daily which may later be adjusted to the patient's requirements. It is best only to prescribe enough pills for a short course of one month and then assess the effect. Thereafter, the dose should be reduced for the next month and the patient then gradually weaned from the oestrogen by tapering the dosage further. For the next month or two no treatment is given and then only resumed if the flushes again become intolerable, when a further course of similar dosage is given.

If one oral preparation of oestrogen causes headache or nausea, it is often possible by changing to another preparation to find one in which the side-effects are avoided. Comparatively small doses must be used when changing the preparation. In terms of stilboestrol, the daily dose should not exceed 0.50 mgm., remembering that ethinyl oestradiol is twenty times more potent than stilboestrol.

A word of warning must be given in the abuse of oestrogen at the menopause. Many women are given oestrogen in large doses over a long period with the inevitable outcome that either oestrogen withdrawal bleeding results or that bleeding occurs from oestrogen hyperplasia of the endometrium. This gravely confuses the picture in that it is difficult to know whether this post-menopausal bleeding is due to the abuse of oestrogen or to malignant disease of the corpus uteri. The safest course to take will be to admit the patient for a diagnostic curettage even if it is fully realised that the result will most certainly be negative. Many hospital beds are blocked and much public money is wasted as a result of oestrogen overdosage, which now provides the commonest cause of post-menopausal bleeding.

The action of oestrogens in suppressing menopausal symptoms can be enhanced or potentiated by the addition of testosterone. Nevertheless the administration of androgen for this purpose to the menopausal female is to be deplored owing to the risk of producing masculinisation symptoms.

The modern cult of "Feminine Forever" has received a lot of publicity. Many women have been led to fear the imagined tragedy of the menopause with its supposed ageing, grey hair, wrinkles, dry skin, loss of vaginal secretion, loss of libido and sexual satisfaction as well as mental acuity. In order to avoid these changes and to "stay young" in body and spirit they take cyclical oestrogen or oestrogen/progesterone mixtures for many years in a dose of 1 tablet daily for 24 days each month. Withdrawal bleeding occurs two or three days after completing each course. Continued uncontrolled oestrogen administration is not recommended partly because continued stimulus of the endometrium may be carcinogenic and partly because prolonged bleeding may eventually occur necessitating diagnostic curettage.

There is no need for any woman to suffer symptoms of post-menopausal atrophy. Annual gynaecological examinations should be undertaken at which the early signs of change are noticed and corrected by the administration of mgm. 0.01 ethinyl oestradiol for seven days a month for four months.

4 Gynaecological Diagnosis

It is often difficult in gynaecological practice to obtain an accurate history from the patient. Some women dislike discussing even normal menstruation with their medical attendant, and diplomacy may be necessary to discover the exact nature of the patient's complaint. Abstruse technical terms must be avoided and plain, basic English used when obtaining a menstrual history, so that the patient understands exactly the significance of the question and answer. The question "What is your menstrual cycle?" may be meaningless to a simple citizen, but every woman knows the answer to "How often do you have a monthly period?" Some women have a curious reluctance to admit such symptoms as excessive haemorrhage, continuous bleeding or discharge, and are easily distressed when leading questions are put with too much frankness. In some cases of dyspareunia and sterility it may be almost impossible to determine exactly what complaint the patient has, unless the question is approached very tactfully by roundabout means. First endeavours should therefore be directed towards gaining the patient's confidence; details in the history can conveniently be left until later.

The best way for a doctor to obtain a patient's confidence is to convince her that he is applying to her particular problem his whole concentrated scientific training and to present an impersonal but sympathetic attitude. It is not always possible in a single session to overcome the inhibitions of the nervous or the evasions of the deceitful. Subterfuges frequently cover some point in the history of which the patient is ashamed, such as venereal disease or self-induced abortion. When the examiner feels that he has reached an impasse, it is good practice to see the patient again at an early date, briefly recapitulate the history and repeat the physical examination. Such a second interview lessens the embarrassment of the patient and frequently results in a frank discussion that is most profitable to accurate diagnosis.

Probably in no other branch of medicine is an accurate history more essential for diagnosis than in gynaecology. When there is any disturbance of menstruation it is necessary to obtain the exact dates of the menstrual irregularities and much time has to be spent in obtaining such accurate records. It is essential to have a calendar available when the history is being taken. It is impossible to be exact in gynaecological diagnosis unless accurate histories of this kind have been carefully elicited. When an accurate gynaecological history is available, a large number of gynaecological affections can be suspected and often diagnosed from the history alone. Time spent on the patient's history is never wasted. Mistakes in diagnosis are as often due to inaccuracy and inadequacy of history as to omission to elicit physical signs. The history should be taken systematically and questions should be asked according to a strict routine. Unless every point in the history is investigated, errors in diagnosis will be made and concomitant abnormalities may be missed. In hospital practice a printed case sheet is helpful in teaching students and house officers thoroughness and accuracy.

It is well to start the questions by asking the patient to describe what she is complaining of and to allow her to state in her own words what type of pain and what irregularity of menstruation may be present. If menstrual irregularities are complained of, it will usually be found that patients become confused in recalling dates, the establishment of which may require much patience and firmness on the part of the history taker.

General History

There is a tendency amongst students when seeing gynaecological patients to concentrate on the pelvis to the exclusion of the other systems and it is a sad but sobering thought that this misdemeanour can also apply to their tutors. A brief survey of the whole patient must be made since the primary cause of her trouble may well be extragenital. A history of pulmonary tuberculosis in the infertile suggests the possibility of genital extension of the primary pulmonary disease.

Menstrual History

(1) The patient should be asked at what age the menstrual periods began. A late onset of puberty is not usually significant though it may suggest pituitary-ovarian dysfunction. Many girls do not menstruate according to an exact calendar and late starters at 16 or even 18 years of age rapidly develop a normal regular cycle and have a normal fertility. An early onset of puberty suggests undue activity of the ovaries which may be constitutional and unaccompanied by any local disease such as a granulosa cell tumour of the ovary, though this must naturally be excluded in the physical examination.

(2) The normal menstrual rhythm. The menstrual cycle is often irregular during the few years subsequent to puberty, but at about the age of 17 or 18 the normal cycle for the individual has become established. It should be borne in mind that the menstrual cycle is the time intervening between the first day of one period and the first day of the next. When a patient states that she menstruates every month she does not necessarily mean that the menstrual cycle is twenty-eight days; she may mean that the interval between the last day of one period and the first day of the next is twenty-eight days. Unless the normal menstrual cycle, as distinct from the interval between periods, is taken as the basis, confusion is certain to follow. For example, with myomata the duration of menstrual loss is prolonged so that the interval between periods is reduced and the patient may complain that she menstruates more frequently than before, when actually the menstrual cycle itself is unaltered. Similarly, it will often be found, if patients are questioned closely, that there has been a variation of a few days from the cycle of twenty-eight days, and even a difference of as little as one or two days may be of importance in the history when such conditions as ectopic gestation are being considered. The term **menorrhagia** is used when the menstrual cycle is unaltered but in which

the duration of the menstrual bleeding is prolonged or its quantity increased. **Polymenorrhoea** or **epimenorrhoea** refers to those cases in which a previous cycle of twenty-eight days is shortened to one of about twenty-one days or less and subsequently remains constant at that rhythm. If the problem is not urgent and an accurate menstrual history not readily obtainable, it is reasonable to give the patient a menstrual chart and ask her to fill it in carefully and produce it at a subsequent visit. This graphic evidence is always more convincing to both observer and patient than the verbal recital which is often exaggerated.

(3) The amount of blood lost during each period is difficult to assess. A loss which one woman would call excessive is regarded by others as normal, and the number of diapers used may be misleading, for obviously there are variations in individual cleanliness. The passage of large clots always means that the menstrual haemorrhage is excessive. An excessive menstrual period leaves the patient tired and listless, so that when severe bleeding is suspected, enquiries should be made as to the patient's general condition at the end of the menstrual period. She may in addition complain of symptoms of anaemia such as breathlessness on exertion, faintness, dizziness and palpitation. Inspection of conjunctivae and palate will confirm the significance of these symptoms but the haemoglobin estimation is the final arbiter. Simple menorrhagia is characteristic of myomata, myohyperplasia and inflammatory lesions of the Fallopian tubes.

(4) The date of the last normal period should always be recorded, that is, the period preceding the menstrual abnormality under investigation. The onset, frequency, duration and amount of any subsequent bleeding is now noted with particular reference to the date of this abnormal bleeding in relation to the date of the last normal period.

For example, if the last normal period in an otherwise healthy young girl with a regular twenty-eight-day cycle occurred six weeks ago and she missed her next period but started bleeding yesterday, this history is very suggestive of an extrauterine gestation or a threatened abortion. The diagnosis should largely be made on the accurate correlation of the normal and abnormal bleeding.

Menstrual Abnormalities: Haemorrhages

Menorrhagia has already been mentioned and defined as excessive menstrual loss with preservation of the normal cycle, i.e. 4/28 becomes 7-10/28. It is caused by any condition which increases the surface area of the menstruating endometrium, e.g. fibroids, polypi or any increase in uterine vascularity, e.g. the congestion of pelvic inflammatory disease.

Polymenorrhoea (Epimenorrhoea) has also been mentioned and defined. It is sometimes associated with menorrhagia, when the term epimenorrhagia is used. The cause of epimenorrhoea is usually ovarian rather than uterine. A good example is the ovarian congestion of pelvic inflammatory disease. Another cause is disturbance of ovarian function due to pituitary ovarian disharmony.

Metrorrhagia. In metrorrhagia the menstrual cycle remains unaltered but superimposed upon the normal menstrual bleeding is an irregular haemorrhage which is intermenstrual in type. Metrorrhagia is a symptom of uterine polypi and of carcinoma of the cervix or body of the uterus. The cause of metrorrhagia always lies locally in the pelvis. Since metrorrhagia should always suggest a uterine cancer, any patient with this presenting symptom must be immediately and carefully examined by every means available to exclude this serious diagnosis. Such examination will almost certainly demand admission to hospital for biopsy and curettage.

Continuous Bleeding. Some patients suffer from continuous uterine haemorrhage so that the normal cyclical bleeding can no longer be distinguished. Continuous bleeding of this kind is met in abortion, ectopic gestation, carcinoma of the cervix or endometrium, metropathia haemorrhagica and with some uterine polypi. In abortion there is a history of missed periods followed by excessive bleeding: in ectopic gestation the vaginal bleeding is small in amount and usually consists of dark altered blood. In most ectopic gestations the haemorrhage starts about six weeks after the last normal period and almost invariably the patients give a history of severe abdominal pain. With metropathia haemorrhagica there is usually a history of a missed period; the haemorrhage is small in amount, although, if continuing for a long time, it may lead to a severe degree of anaemia. There is, however, no history of abdominal pain in metropathia. With carcinoma of the cervix the continuous haemorrhage is often accompanied by an offensive discharge.

Pregnancy Haemorrhages. It is important to distinguish between the haemorrhages associated with pregnancy and the haemorrhages caused by purely local gynaecological abnormalities. The haemorrhages of early pregnancy should always be borne in mind when patients with irregular haemorrhage are being investigated. The haemorrhages of early pregnancy are as follows:

(a) It is not uncommon for patients to have slight vaginal bleeding in the first few months of pregnancy at times corresponding to the suppressed periods.

(b) All types of abortion may lead to irregular uterine bleeding.

(c) In ectopic gestation uterine bleeding is almost invariable.

(d) Irregular haemorrhage is also a symptom of hydatidiform mole.

Later in pregnancy the different types of antepartum haemorrhage have to be considered. It should also be borne in mind that such conditions as mucous polypi, vascular erosions and carcinoma of the cervix may be coincident with pregnancy and cause irregular haemorrhage.

Postmenopausal Haemorrhage. Postmenopausal haemorrhage is, by definition, any bleeding from the genital tract in a woman of menopausal age who has not had a period during the preceding six months or longer. This symptom is of very great clinical importance since all patients suffering from postmenopausal haemorrhage must be investigated to exclude a genital tract cancer. Postmenopausal haemorrhage occurs particularly in carcinoma of the cervix and carcinoma of the body. It may arise from carcinoma of the vagina and rarely with carcinoma of the ovaries. Local conditions at the vulva such as a urethral caruncle may cause bleeding, while senile vaginitis often produces a bloodstained discharge. Pressure ulcers from retained ring pessaries may also bleed. Innocent conditions of the cervix which cause bleeding are polypi and erosions. More rarely a myoma produces postmenopausal haemorrhage, and senile endometritis and intermittent pyometra also cause haemorrhage. The rare sarcomata of the uterus may ulcerate and cause bleeding. Some functioning ovarian tumours, such as the granulosa cell tumour and theca cell tumour also cause postmenopausal haemorrhage. Haemorrhage can occur after the administration of such oestrogens as stilboestrol. The popularity of oestrogens in the treatment of menopausal complaints has greatly increased this type of postmenopausal bleeding. The fact that the patient may give a history of having taken oestrogens does not exclude the possibility of uterine cancer. This danger must be strongly emphasised and, if the slightest doubt arises in the mind of the gynaecologist, a diagnostic curettage must be performed in order to exclude a cancer. In patients who give a history of bleeding after taking oestrogens, cytological screening provides helpful but not entirely exclusive evidence.

Vaginal Discharge

(1) **Physiological.** In healthy women the vagina contains a small quantity of watery secretion: it contains mucus, desquamated epithelial cells, Döderlein's bacilli and lactic acid. The Döderlein's bacilli ferment the glycogen in the desquamated epithelial cells to form lactic acid which is essential to the defence mechanism of the healthy vagina. Under certain circumstances a healthy woman may become aware of this vaginal moisture to such an extent that it is discharged from the introitus as a vaginal discharge. The normal secretion of the vagina is composed of vaginal transudate, mucus from the endocervical glands, mucus from the endometrial glands (especially during the secretory part of the cycle) and secretion of Bartholin's glands.

1. A physiological discharge may become apparent at the time of ovulation when the high peak of oestrogen provokes the endocervical glands into excessive secretion.

2. As a result of sexual stimulation, when the main increasing component comes from Bartholin's gland.

3. As a result of premenstrual congestion where there may be an increase of discharge for two or three days before the period.

4. During pregnancy, when general pelvic congestion and vaginal transudate are responsible for the increase.

The vulval sebaceous apocrine and sweat glands are also important, especially the apocrine glands since they furnish a special odour which may be appreciated by the patient who as a result complains that the discharge has an offensive smell.

Leucorrhoea. The term leucorrhoea should be restricted to a simple increase in the normal vaginal secretion as described above, but nowadays it is used incorrectly to describe any white vaginal discharge of a non-purulent nature.

(2) **Pathological.** A white vaginal discharge. Since few women complain

directly of vaginal discharge it is usually necessary to ask a direct question. If a patient has vaginal discharge it is necessary to know the colour, the quantity, the duration of time that it has been present, whether or not it is malodorous or irritating and if it contains blood.

A white vaginal discharge is a very common complaint and whilst it may well be the result of some local pathological lesion, very frequently no cause can be found. Such a discharge is non-irritating and non-odorous and never contains blood. It may commence at or shortly after puberty, when it is usually caused by a cervical erosion of the so-called congenital type. It may commence during pregnancy and continue after the termination of pregnancy, when it may also be caused by a cervical erosion. Other causes such as cervical polypi, mild endocervical infection, cervical lacerations may also be responsible. A very low grade vaginal infection may also lead to excessive vaginal or cervical secretion with the production of a white vaginal discharge.

It is always difficult to assess the margin between a physiological secretion and a pathological discharge, and the subjective interpretation of the patient is important, for example a sensitive introspective patient of fastidious habits will readily translate a minimal physiological discharge into a copious malodorous discharge with a self-diagnosis of malignant disease.

Too much enthusiastic douching with antiseptics is irritant to the vagina and cervix and promotes the very condition it is designed to control. Some patients are sensitive to these various douche solutions and develop an idiosyncrasy or allergic reaction to them. They may even develop a generalised skin reaction on other parts of the body. An example of this vaginitis medicamentosa is seen in arsenic sensitivity from the use of arsenical pessaries.

An irritating discharge. The two classic causes of an irritating discharge are infection by the trichomonas vaginalis and candida albicans giving rise to acute or chronic trichomonas or monilial vaginitis.

A yellow discharge. Almost any vaginal or uterine infection may cause yellow discharge. Bacterial infections of the vagina, infected cervical polypi or erosions together with endocervical infection may give rise to a yellow discharge. In acute gonorrhoea the discharge is often yellowish or greenish in colour and causes extreme soreness, pain and tenderness of the vulva. Purulent discharge may also be present in association with septic abortion, puerperal sepsis, pyometra. Any infected discharge may be associated with vulval discomfort or soreness.

Offensive vaginal discharge is characteristic of necrotic lesions in the genital tract, such as carcinoma of the cervix, septic myomatous polypi, septic abortion and of the rarer growths such as sarcoma of the uterus and carcinoma of the vagina. It is also present when foreign bodies such as pessaries and tampons have been forgotten and retained in the vagina. The discharge caused by the trichomonas also has a characteristic odour.

Bloodstained discharges occur with oestrogen deficiency (so-called senile vaginitis), carcinoma of the cervix and body of the uterus, cervical polypi, infected and degenerate submucous fibroid polypi. Any ulcerated lesion of the genital tract whether inflammatory or malignant will produce a bloodstained discharge, e.g. ulceration of the posterior fornix from a retained pessary.

When bloodstained discharge occurs before the menopause the possibility of intrauterine pregnancy must always be considered. A bloodstained discharge may be caused by retained products of conception or by a placental polyp.

A watery vaginal discharge is uncommon, apart from obvious causes such as urinary fistulae where the high urea contents of the discharged fluid is diagnostic. Discharges of this kind have been described in the condition known as hydrops tubae profluens when a hydrosalpinx has been supposed to discharge its contents through the interstitial portion of the tube into the cavity of the uterus. In carcinoma of the Fallopian tube the discharge has been aptly described as amber coloured. During pregnancy a watery discharge is more frequent. In hydrorrhoea gravidarum the watery discharge is probably due to leakage of the liquor amnii through rupture of the membranes above the level of the internal os.

Faecal discharges, when proved to be of vaginal origin and not contaminant from the adjacent bowel, are self-evident proof of a recto-vaginal fistula.

PAIN

Menstrual Pain. During normal menstruation some degree of abdominal discomfort is usual, but the pain of **spasmodic dysmenorrhoea** may be so severe that the patient is incapacitated. When enquiries are made as to menstrual pain it is important to determine its time of onset. In spasmodic dysmenorrhoea the pain develops typically on the first day of the period of bleeding when, in addition to the usual abdominal discomfort, there is violently severe pain felt in the lower abdomen which may cause fainting and vomiting and be of such intensity that the patient is forced to lie down. This type of pain rarely lasts for more than twelve hours when it is followed by the usual abdominal discomfort which persists but decreases throughout the period of bleeding. In some cases of spasmodic dysmenorrhoea, the severe pain develops on the day before the period begins. In **congestive dysmenorrhoea,** the patients complain of a dull pain in the back and in the lower abdomen which arises two or three days or even longer before the onset of the menstrual flow and which is relieved by the bleeding though a feeling of heaviness in the pelvis may continue throughout the first days of the loss or even for its whole duration. When myomata are present, painful uterine contractions during menstruation may develop if the tumour becomes submucous or polypoidal. With chocolate cysts of the ovaries severe pain is complained of during the three or four days before the onset of menstruation, although frequently severe abdominal pain may be present during the period of bleeding.

The severity of all types of menstrual pain must be judged by its effect upon the individual patient. Pain which causes incapacitation of working women is obviously severe whereas pain in the affluent may be suspect as a plausible excuse for evading unwelcome or unattractive duties.

Abdominal Pain. Severe abdominal pain, not in any way related to menstruation, is present in ectopic gestation, acute salpingo-oöphoritis, twisted ovarian cysts and torsion of subperitoneal myomata. In these four conditions the pain is extremely severe, and in tubal rupture with diffuse intraperitoneal bleeding the pain is comparable in severity to that of perforated peptic ulcer and is associated with shock and collapse. In tubal abortion, the pain is intermittent and colicky, and though severe, less so than that caused by a massive intraperitoneal haemorrhage. In pelvic peritonitis caused by inflammation of the uterine appendages or septic abortion, the pain is acute in onset but less dramatic than that of ectopic gestation. It is severe and frequently causes nausea and vomiting. Uterine myomata do not cause abdominal pain except when they undergo degeneration, apart from which condition they are almost symptomless, although they may cause a feeling of heaviness in the lower abdomen and pelvis.

Almost all benign and malignant tumours of the ovary, whether cystic or solid, are initially symptomless. It is only the dramatic event of torsion which draws attention to their presence. An obviously malignant tumour, hard, irregular and fixed, if associated with localised pain suggests widespread and inoperable local infiltration and carries a depressing prognosis. Cancer when operable is painless and once painful it is usually inoperable.

Pain in the Back. This is a common symptom in gynaecological practice though it is rarely due to a strictly gynaecological cause, being far more frequently of orthopaedic origin. Backache arising after childbirth may sometimes be due to sacro-iliac or lumbo-sacral strain or even a prolapsed intervertebral disc. Backache is also encountered when there has been previous parametritis with resultant fibrosis in Mackenrodt's and the utero-sacral ligaments. It should be suspected that any backache higher than the first sacral vertebra is unlikely to be of gynaecological origin.

Dyspareunia is defined as pain or difficulty with intercourse. It will be discussed in greater detail later. Its causes may be briefly summarised as any painful obstructive lesion at the vaginal introitus or in the vaginal canal, painful inflammatory conditions in these two situations and deeper-seated lesions such as endometriosis of the uterosacral ligaments and retroversion of the uterus with tender prolapsed ovaries.

When the history of pain is being taken, these points must all be borne in mind. The patient must first be asked if she has any pain and, if so, the relation of the pain to menstruation must be investigated, as must also be the situation, severity and date of development of the pain. It is always instructive to request the patient to point out with her finger the exact situation of the spot of maximum pain. Quite often she is able to do this with anatomical exactitude, e.g. in ovarian pain, she will indicate a spot one inch above the mid-point of Poupart's ligament. A vague gesture which encompasses the upper abdomen usually indicates an extra-genital origin and suggests the possibility of functional overlay.

Previous Pregnancies. It is a common experience in gynaecological practice to find that many gynaecological affections date from an earlier confinement or miscarriage. The history of previous pregnancies, confinements miscarriages should therefore be taken most carefully. Enquiries should be made as to the dates of these confinements. If it is found that a patient has not conceived for a long time, and if it is discovered that during the last puerperium the patient had puerperal sepsis, occlusion of the Fallopian tubes as the result of salpingitis will be suspected. Questions should be asked to determine whether the confinements were difficult, whether instruments were used, and whether the perineum was lacerated. Positive answers suggest the likelihood of genital tract injuries. A history of persistent lochia or of a persistent blood-stained discharge from the uterus is suggestive of an infection of the uterus. Similarly, a history of backache which exactly dates its onset from the time of the confinement and not before it, suggests the possibility of subinvolution but by no means conclusively since minor orthopaedic lesions such as sacro-iliac strain may have been caused by the lithotomy position during a forceps delivery.

Urinary Symptoms

Affections of the urinary tract are common complications of gynaecological abnormalities and the following symptoms should be enquired about as a routine.

Pain on Micturition. Cystitis causes painful micturition and patients complain of severe discomfort at the end of the act of micturition. Scalding micturition is characteristic of the urethritis of gonorrhoea and of coliform infections.

Retention of urine occurs with retroverted gravid uterus, myomata incarcerated in the pelvis, and more rarely in cases of haematocolpos, pelvic haematocele and ovarian cyst impacted in the pelvis. The commonest cause of retention of urine in gynaecological practice, however, is postoperative retention following operations upon the vagina, perineum and rectum.

Difficulty in micturition is a symptom of severe cystocele or complete procidentia. When the patient strains to micturate the cystocele protrudes from the vagina and it may be necessary for the patient to press back the cystocele before she is able to pass urine.

True incontinence of urine is a symptom of urinary fistulae. It is marked by the continuous dribbling of urine from the vagina. If the fistula is small the leak may only be noticeable when the bladder is full, and it may be less at night when the patient is in bed.

False or stress incontinence is a common symptom in prolapse. The patient complains that she has imperfect control over micturition so that the urine dribbles away if the intra-abdominal pressure is raised when the patient laughs or coughs, sneezes, lifts a weight or even mildly exerts herself as when walking rapidly. In the severest examples of stress incontinence, not even these simple tests are required to demonstrate the lack of control.

Frequency of micturition is present during the early weeks of pregnancy, as it is later in pregnancy when the patient is approaching term. Frequency of micturition develops with urinary infections, in prolapse and when pelvic tumours press on the bladder, in addition to the usual diseases of the urinary tract which cause frequency.

Rectal Symptoms

Certain diseases of the rectum and sigmoid colon frequently cause difficulty in gynaecological diagnosis. Diverticulitis and carcinoma of the sigmoid colon may be difficult to distinguish from malignant disease of the ovaries; proctitis is sometimes a complication of the radium treatment of carcinoma of the cervix, and haemorrhoids are commonly found complicating gynaecological diseases. Patients should therefore be asked if there is any pain or difficulty on defaecation and also whether there has been any discharge of blood, pus or mucus from the rectum. If a rectovaginal fistula is present, the patients suffer from incontinence of faeces.

Past Illness

Patients should be asked whether they have had any serious illness in the past and whether they have undergone any surgical operation. Many women have short and inaccurate memories and abdominal examination frequently discloses a scar about which they have failed to make any mention in the history. However trivial the illness or operation and however distant its date in the past, it may have a profound influence on the present complaint. For example, pelvic peritonitis resulting from either appendicitis or tuberculous peritonitis may cause subsequent sterility. Moreover, past illness such as phthisis and morbus cordis may contraindicate operative treatment and will certainly call for an expert assessment of the patient before the administration of an anaesthetic.

EXAMINATION

The examination of all gynaecological patients should be complete. No system should be neglected since a thorough examination of the patient may elucidate diseases of the cardiovascular and respiratory systems which may modify subsequent operative procedures. During examination of the chest the blood pressure should invariably be recorded and the breasts carefully examined. Many an early carcinoma of the breast has been first diagnosed in gynaecological out-patients. The characteristic changes of pregnancy may be noted and valuable information of ovarian function can be deduced from the state of the breast. Activity of the breasts is manifested by hypertrophy, by the presence of dilated veins on the surface, by the development of Montgomery's tubercles, and by the production of a secondary areola. During pregnancy the breast tissue becomes more granular, and a clear secretion can be expressed from the nipple. Well-marked activity of the breasts is restricted to pregnancy, but some hypertrophy is common in the new-born and at puberty, and can also be detected after taking the contraceptive pill containing progestogen. It is extremely important to be able to recognise the early signs of activity in the breasts, as such activity can be detected in cases of ectopic gestation. It will be convenient to examine the thyroid at this time, and an assessment of any thyroid dysfunction should be made. The central nervous system should not be neglected, and this especially applies to obscure cases of urinary incontinence in which a urethrocele has been wrongly blamed as the cause, whereas the patient is really suffering from disseminated sclerosis. The abdomen is next examined, the gastro-intestinal tract and the kidneys being palpated. Gall-bladder disease is not uncommon in gynaecological patients, and in malignant ovarian tumours the primary growth may be in the stomach. Tumours in the pelvis are by no means the exclusive property of the genital tract; appendicitis, regional ileitis, diverticulitis and carcinoma of the caecum and colon may all present them-selves as gynaecological tumours. Ureteric obstruction is common with large pelvic tumours and cancer of the cervix, and the resulting hydronephrosis may be easily felt if its possibility is remembered. The urine is always tested and diabetes is often found in cases of severe and intractable vulvitis.

Finally, a bimanual pelvic examination is made of the uterus and its appendages, after which the rectum should be examined digitally and, if necessary, by proctoscope. Apart from the gynaecological information obtainable by rectal examination this important step will exclude a carcinoma of the large bowel in the pelvis.

Abdominal Examination

Abdominal examination must be performed systematically by inspection, palpation, percussion and auscultation. The examination should be made from the right side of the patient and the abdomen should be completely exposed. The obligatory stance of the examining clinician on one or other side of the patient is of course nonsense, as is the use of either the right or left hand for certain manoeuvres. A doctor should stand in the place which is most useful for what he is doing at that moment and he should use the hand which gives him the maximum information and which is most comfortably suited for that particular purpose.

Inspection. Many gynaecological tumours produce large abdominal swellings which arise from the pelvis and of which the upper and lateral limits are apparent. In such cases the abdomen is more prominent below the level of the umbilicus. In the presence of ascites the abdomen, though protuberant, is flattened in the region of the flanks; moreover, in ascites dilated veins can usually be seen beneath the skin running longitudinally in the flanks. Eversion of the umbilicus is a physical sign of intra-abdominal pressure, and is seen with large ovarian tumours, ascites and pregnancy. The mobility of the abdominal wall on respiration should be investigated. With pelvic tumours which extend into the abdomen, the abdominal wall moves over the tumour during inspiration so that the situation of the upper limit of the tumour is apparently altered. In pelvic peritonitis the abdomen is distended and its movements below the level of the umbilicus are restricted. Striae gravidarum develop during pregnancy but are not uncommon with large abdominal tumours in young women.

Palpation. The examining hands should be warm and the hand and fingers flattened in extension. It will be found that the abdomen can be best examined with the left hand, if the examination is made from the right side of the patient. Gynaecological swellings extend upwards from the pelvis, and it is easier for the left hand to palpate the upper border of the swelling than the right, for the sensitive ulnar border is more likely to detect small swellings arising from the pelvis. Most gynaecological swellings are easily felt, and it is unnecessary to exert much pressure upon the abdominal wall. Myomata have a peculiar solid consistence except when they have undergone cystic degeneration; their surfaces are smooth except when the tumour is bossed through the presence of multiple myomata. Ovarian cysts have smooth surfaces and fluctuate; they can be demarcated above, but large cysts are not always defined laterally. The typical ovarian cyst has a peculiar tense consistence which is very characteristic. The pregnant uterus is soft, and if patience is exercised, may be found to contract under the hand. The foetus can be outlined after about the twenty-fourth week, and before then external ballottement can be elicited. The pyriform shape and the peculiar consistence are characteristic of the pregnant uterus. The full bladder projects anteriorly more than any other abdominal swelling: it is not movable, and is usually extremely tender. In all abdominal swellings the possibility that the tumour is either the full bladder or the pregnant uterus must be borne in mind. It is easy to diagnose a full bladder or a pregnant uterus if either condition is suspected: mistakes are made when these possibilities are neglected. The passage of a catheter will always eliminate one of these two.

It may be extremely difficult to determine whether abdominal swelling in a fat woman is due solely to the presence of fat or whether there is an accompanying intra-abdominal swelling. In such a situation more reliance should be placed upon the physical signs elicited by percussion than those found by palpation.

Extreme tenderness on palpation below the level of the umbilicus is characteristic of peritoneal irritation. Tenderness of a well-marked degree is present in ectopic gestation and twisted ovarian cyst. A red degenerate myoma is also tender but less so than a twisted ovarian cyst.

Percussion. Uterine myomata and ovarian cysts are dull to percussion, but the flanks are resonant. Dullness in the flanks and shifting dullness indicate the presence of free fluid within the abdominal cavity. Ascites of this kind is present with most malignant ovarian tumours. With tuberculous peritonitis, encysted ascites, and rarely with large pelvic haematoceles, abdominal tumours may be palpated which are tympanitic on percussion as the result of adherent bowel.

Auscultation. Auscultation of an abdominal tumour may lead to the detection of the foetal heart sounds or of foetal movements. A uterine souffle may be detected not only over the pregnant uterus, but also with large myomata.

The importance of auscultation for bowel sounds in the diagnosis of paralytic ileus, peritonitis and intestinal obstruction cannot be over-estimated. The return of bowel sounds in paralytic and peritonitic ileus is a sign of effective treatment and marks the turning point in this serious post-operative complication. This sign should never be neglected.

Routine examination of the abdomen should include not only the details which have just been mentioned, but also the examination of the kidneys, liver and gall bladder, stomach and large intestine. Unless these organs are examined mistakes will be made. For example, in cases of pelvic tumour an examination of the upper abdomen may lead to the identification of a carcinoma of the stomach or of large metastases in the omentum and liver. Such findings influence not only the diagnosis but also the subsequent treatment.

Vaginal Examination

No vaginal examination should be made without certain formalities.

(1) The patient should be instructed to empty the bladder immediately before the examination. She has no doubt already done this on leaving home and may consider this good enough. The gynaecologist must take into consideration the intervening period of waiting during which considerable urinary output occurs. Every student knows that the ordeal of examination causes diuresis. As a reservation it should be stated that stress incontinence is best demonstrated on the unemptied bladder.

(2) A heavily loaded colon is notoriously responsible for the production of a false pelvic tumour. When it obstructs exact diagnosis, especially in the left fornix, it should be emptied by an aperient and the patient re-examined at the next available opportunity.

(3) A chaperone should always be present. In hospital this presents no problem but in domiciliary practice the district nurse or some sensible relative or female friend should be available.

(4) The doctor making the examination should explain simply and clearly that he is going to make an internal vaginal examination, and should obtain the patient's consent thereto. In the case of a girl under eighteen, the mother's consent should be obtained and her presence at the examination insisted upon.

(5) The necessary equipment must be available: gloves, sterile lubricant, specula, sponge-holder, swabs and a powerful and easily adjusted light.

In most clinics in the U.K. it is customary to make vaginal examinations with the patient lying in the left lateral position. The patient lies on her left side with the buttocks well over to the edge of the couch, with the right knee drawn up towards the chin and with the right shoulder thrown over to the opposite side of the couch. This position can easily be assumed from the dorsal position in which the patient has been lying during the abdominal examination. The left lateral position gives a good exposure of the external genitalia, and specula can be easily inserted with the patient in this position. Quite often the left appendages can be more easily felt when the patient is lying on her left side than when lying in the lithotomy position. Women naturally prefer being examined in the left lateral position than in the lithotomy position because it is more comfortable and certainly less undignified. Since she cannot see the manipulations and the instruments of the examiner she is not frightened so easily in the lateral position. The lithotomy position is, however, more convenient for examining the external genitalia and the cervix. One further advantage of the left lateral position is that it enables the gynaecologist to instruct his pupils without undue embarrassment to the patient. He can, for instance, demonstrate a cervical erosion to one or two students without her being fully conscious of their presence, though her consent to such a demonstration should be tactfully secured beforehand.

A disposable glove should always be worn on the right hand during vaginal examination, but it will be found that bimanual examinations can be carried out more accurately if the left hand is bare.

Vaginal examinations should be made systematically and a strict routine should be followed if the examination is to be complete, Students should remember that an accurate vaginal examination depends upon a knowledge of anatomy and upon experience, and the more important factor of the two is experience. Students should never lose an opportunity of making a vaginal examination even in normal patients. It is impossible to acquire the technique of bimanual examination without practice, and much experience is required before gynaecological abnormalities can be detected with any accuracy. Failures to find physical signs in gynaecology mostly depend upon incomplete examinations; the average student does not follow a strict routine in his examination, and tends to be satisfied if he has succeeded in locating the uterus. The more examinations a student makes the more confidence will he acquire as to his ability to elicit physical signs.

External Genitalia. The vulva is first examined, the labia, clitoris, urethral meatus and vaginal orifice being inspected in turn. Most abnormalities of the vulva are easily recognised by inspection. It will sometimes be found helpful in order to expose the anterior aspect of the vulva to ask the patient to raise her right knee. The correct position of the patient in the left lateral position is essential, the most important point being the position of the patient's left buttock on the very edge of the examining couch (see Fig. 53). Shy and nervous patients tend to revert to the opisthotonic posture of defence and to withdraw from inspection the very part under examination. The urethra should be inspected for evidence of urethritis, caruncle, prolapse of the mucous membrane and carcinoma. In acute gonorrhoea the meatus is reddened and pus can be seen coming from the urethra; the orifices of Skene's tubules, which lie immediately within the meatus, are reddened and inflamed, and the ducts of the periurethral glands are also conspicuous by their red colour.

The hymen should be examined and if intact usually contraindicates vaginal examination, which is best deferred until it can be performed under an anaesthetic. Abnormalities of the hymen, such as hymen rigidus, should be recorded. In patients of postmenopausal age, reddening of the epithelium around the hymen and vaginal orifice is seen in kraurosis vulvae and is associated with the development of white opaque areas on the adjacent epithelium. The ducts of Bartholin's glands should be inspected. The mouths of the ducts lie external to the hymen at the junction of the anterior two-thirds and posterior one-third of the vaginal orifice. In gonorrhoea the mouths of the ducts are reddened, and quite frequently pus can be seen exuding from the ducts. Bartholin's gland cannot be palpated except when it is enlarged, but in acute gonorrhoea the gland can be felt quite easily, deep to the tissues of the labia at the level of the posterior third of the vaginal orifice. In Bartholin's abscess, a fluctuating swelling is found in the situation of the gland, which extends anteriorly and may discharge itself on the inner surface of the labium minus. Bartholin's cysts lie deep to the tissues of the labium minus and extend anteriorly along the course of the labium minus so that it is stretched over the swelling. Herniae, cysts of the canal of Nuck, lipomata and adeno-myomata are found more laterally in the tissues of the labium majus. The perineum should be inspected for scars and old lacerations: complete tears of the perineum are easily recognised because the red mucous membrane of the rectum fuses with the posterior vaginal wall without the intervention of the tissues of the perineal body.

The patient should now be asked to cough or strain down to enable any prolapse which may be present to be detected. If there is any prolapse it is important to know exactly which structures are affected: whether the prolapse

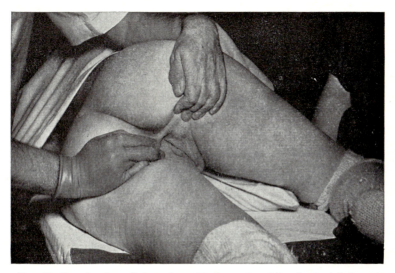

FIG. 53. Examination of the vulva with the patient lying in the left lateral position. Note the importance of upward traction on the right buttock in order to expose the vaginal introitus.

consists of the anterior vaginal wall, the cervix or the posterior vaginal wall or all three together. In all cases of prolapse of the posterior vaginal wall a rectal examination must subsequently be made to determine whether there is an associated rectocele.

Internal Examination. One or two fingers of the right hand, lubricated with sterile liquid paraffin, are now inserted into the vagina. The use of antiseptic creams is not recommended. If a culture of the vaginal discharge is required the antiseptic interferes with the growth of organisms, and some women are sensitive to the commonly used antiseptics. If liquid paraffin is used, being clear and colourless, it does not obscure a true picture of any vaginal discharge present. Even liquid paraffin, however, interferes with the microscopical picture, and when investigating a vaginal discharge it is best to use plain clean water as a finger lubricant until all smears have been taken.

The most sensitive part of the vulva lies anteriorly in the region of the clitoris and urethral meatus; if, therefore, there is difficulty in inserting two fingers, the perineal body should be pressed posteriorly. The next step in the examination is palpation of the perineal body and of the levator ani muscles. The perineal body is examined by placing two fingers in the vagina, flexing them posteriorly and palpating the perineal body between these fingers and the thumb which is placed externally. In this way the thickness of tissue contained in the perineal body and the tone of the contained muscles can be judged. The fingers are now turned and flexed laterally above the level of the levator ani muscles. The levator muscles can easily be palpated between the vaginal

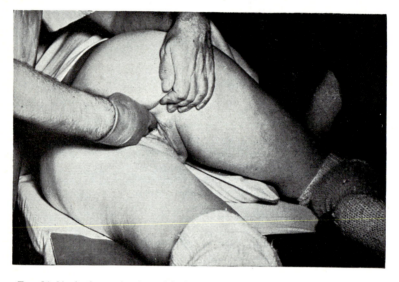

Fig. 54. Vaginal examination with the patient in the left lateral position. Two fingers of the right hand have been introduced into the vagina.

fingers and the thumb placed externally over the labium majus. The tone of the levator muscles can then be judged and in cases of prolapse the degree to which the muscles have separated can be estimated very accurately. The next step is to examine for evidence of vaginal discharge. The discharge may be seen during inspection of the vulva, but quite often the discharge first appears after the fingers have been placed in the vagina. The characters of the discharge should be noted. In gonorrhoea the discharge is purulent, profuse and greenish in colour; in trichomonas infections the discharge is thin and fluid, yellowish in colour, and associated with reddening of the vaginal walls. Small bubbles of gas can be seen in the discharge and this characteristic frothy appearance is strongly suggestive of the presence of trichomonas. Fig. 54.

The vagina is now examined by palpation and such gross abnormalities as septate vagina and carcinoma of the vagina are easily detected. Vaginal scars caused by old lacerations are most prominent near the cervix where they are often found to be continuous with lacerations of the cervix itself. During pregnancy, in addition to its mauve discoloration, the vagina is softened, particularly in the upper part. In prolapse the vaginal walls are lax with little sense of resistance of the perivaginal tissues.

The Cervix

When the uterus is in its normal position of anteflexion and anterversion, the first part of the cervix felt by the examining fingers is the anterior lip. In retroversion the cervix is directed downwards and forwards, so that its lowest part is either the external os or the posterior lip. A slender conical cervix is often seen in adolescents, while with chronic cervicitis it is common to find the cervix enlarged. Congenital vaginal elongation of the cervix is easily recognised by the depth of the vaginal fornices, and quite often the cervix projects almost half-way down the vagina. In nulliparae the external os is circular, while after childbirth an anterior and posterior lip can be distinguished. Lateral laceration of the cervix is frequent in multiparous women and in most cases the cervix is torn on the left side. Severe lacerations of the cervix are usually the result of the application of forceps before full dilatation of the os, and they may be found both in the anterior lip and in the posterior lip when scar tissue can often be traced backwards to the posterior vaginal wall. The normal cervix is smooth and its texture is firm. A carcinoma of the cervix bleeds vigorously on examination. It is friable, and usually there is well-marked induration at the periphery of the carcinoma. Such abnormalities as polypi may be detected. Erosions are difficult to distinguish with a gloved finger, although a difference in texture giving a feeling like velvet around the external os is suggestive of the presence of an erosion. Speculum examination, however, is necessary before the presence of an erosion of the cervix can be established. Dilatation of the external os is present when polypi lie within the cervical canal and with retained products of conception following abortion. While the cervix is being examined the patient should again be asked to strain down, and in this way any prolapse of the uterus which may be present can be recognised and its extent assessed by slightly withdrawing the examining fingers and asking the patient to cough when the prolapsed cervix descends down the vagina.

Examination of the cervix should be systematic, and the following points should be investigated as a routine.

(a) The direction in which the cervix is pointing.
(b) Whether the cervix descends upon straining.
(c) The texture of the cervix.
(d) The degree of dilatation of the external os.
(e) Whether the cervix bleeds on examination.

Bimanual Examination

The uterus and its appendages should now be examined bimanually. Two fingers of the right hand are placed in the anterior fornix of the vagina against the front of the vaginal portion of the cervix. These fingers press up the uterus while the external hand placed on the lower abdomen is brought

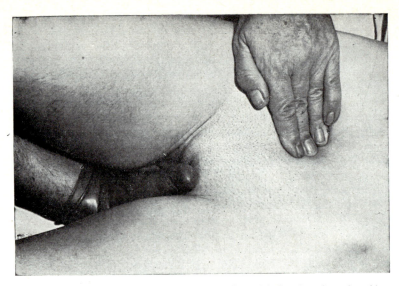

FIG. 55. Bimanual examination. Two fingers of the right hand are introduced into the vagina and the left hand is placed well above the symphysis pubis.

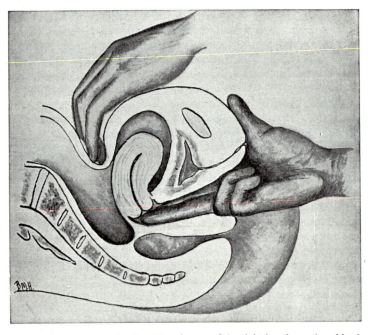

FIG. 56. Bimanual examination. Two fingers of the right hand are placed in the vagina and press the cervix upwards and backwards. The external hand is placed on the lower abdomen and is insinuated behind the uterus. The uterus is then felt between the fingers of the two hands

to lie behind the uterus. The uterus is then palpated between the fingers of the two hands. Beginners are apt to forget that most of the physical signs elicited by bimanual examination are detected with the external hand. A common error is for the fingers of the right hand to push upwards in the direction of the symphysis pubis rather than towards the lumbar vertebrae. The pressure exerted by the left hand should be not only downwards but from behind forwards. A mistake which is frequently made is to place the left hand immediately above the symphysis pubis and simply to press downwards.

The left hand should be placed on the abdomen well above the level of the symphysis pubis and the fingers of the left hand should reach as far back as possible before being drawn downwards and forwards to meet the uterus. The technique of bimanual examination is difficult to describe in words; experience alone teaches the method to be followed (see Figs. 55 and 56).

A carefully and skilfully performed bimanual examination in the hands of an experienced clinician will, in most cases, provide enough evidence to reach an accurate diagnosis. There are, however, some patients in whom the findings are inadequate or equivocal:

(1) The obese patient, whose abdominal wall is impermeable to the fingers of the external hand so that the boundaries of the fundus cannot be defined.

(2) The extremely nervous patient, on whom tact and patience makes no impression in the promotion of abdominal relaxation.

(3) The intact virgin, who normally belongs to the above class and in whom only an abdomino-rectal examination is possible.

(4) Certain doubtful cases—such as suspected extrauterine gestation in which the findings are suspicious but not conclusive, and in which further evidence is required before laparotomy.

In all these patients examination under an anaesthetic with bowel and bladder completely empty is strongly recommended. The anaesthetic must give genuine abdominal relaxation and not merely render the patient unconscious but with the abdomen tense, as so often happens.

The Uterus

During the bimanual examination of the uterus the following points are investigated in turn.

The Position of the Uterus. Normally the uterus lies in the midline. It may be congenitally displaced to one side when it usually lies to the left, or it may be laterally displaced by such swellings as myomata of the broad ligament, ovarian cysts, adnexal inflammatory swellings, tubal gestation and the effusion of parametritis. In some cases the uterus is drawn over to one side as the result of contraction of scar tissue in the parametrium resulting from previous parametritis or obstetric injuries.

The retroverted uterus is not easily palpated bimanually, but the fundus of the retroverted uterus can readily be detected through the posterior fornix. After bimanual examination it will be possible to say whether the uterus is anteflexed or retroflexed, anteverted or retroverted.

The Size of the Uterus. Experience is necessary before an opinion can be given as to whether the uterus is of normal size when the patient is fat. Owing to the thickness of the abdominal wall the impression is often given on bimanual examination that the uterus is enlarged. In ovarian deficiency conditions the uterus is hypoplastic.

The Surface of the Uterus. Bosses on the surfaces of the uterus indicate the presence of myomata (see Fig. 57).

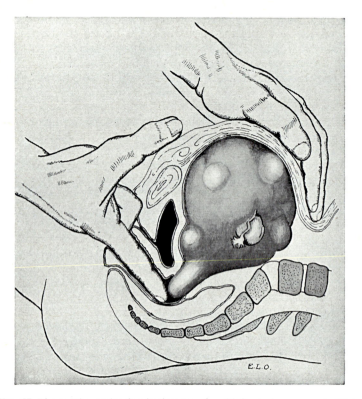

FIG. 57. Bimanual examination in the case of multiple uterine myomata. Note how the external hand is placed high in the abdomen, well above the level of the tumour. Movements are transmitted between the two hands directly through the tumour. (After Halban Seitz.)

Mobility of the Uterus. The normal uterus is movable to some degree in all directions. This mobility is restricted (i) in carcinoma of the cervix when the parametrium has become infiltrated with growth; (ii) when fibrous tissue has formed in the parametrium either as the result of parametritis or following upon extensive lacerations of the cervix and vaginal vault; (iii) with peritoneal adhesions resulting from salpingo-oöphoritis; (iv) in the presence of external endometriosis of the ovaries. (v) If the uterus contains fibroids, one of which accurately fits the pelvis, uterine mobility is obviously limited.

The Uterine Appendages. Before an attempt is made to palpate the uterine appendages the position of the uterus must be established. With some pelvic tumours there may be difficulty in deciding whether the tumour is the enlarged uterus or whether it is a swelling of the appendages. When the uterus cannot be outlined with certainty the following investigations should be made. Try to follow up the cervix with the fingers in the vagina to discover with which swelling the cervix is continuous. Next, press down upon the

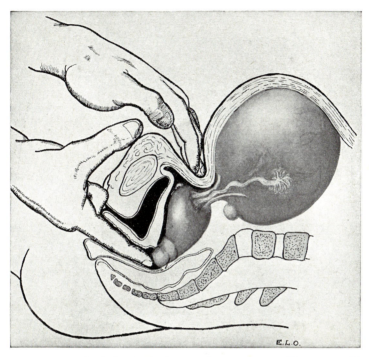

Fig. 58. Bimanual examination in the case of an ovarian cyst. The nature of the tumour is determined on bimanual examination because the uterus can be identified apart from the abdominal tumour. Compare Fig. 57. In some cases the pedicle can be distinguished if the fingers in the vagina are placed high up in the posterior fornix. Movements of the abdominal tumour are clearly not transmitted to the cervix. (After Halban Seitz.)

abdominal swelling and determine whether the cervix itself is pushed down (Fig. 57). Movements of the body of the uterus are always transmitted to the cervix; on the other hand, movements of an ovarian cyst are usually not transmitted. Similarly, move the cervix in the vagina and determine whether such movements are transmitted to the abdominal swelling: if so, the abdominal swelling is almost certainly the uterus. The fundamental sign of an adnexal swelling is that it can be identified separate from the uterus (Fig. 58). Conversely, unless a swelling can be distinguished separate from the uterus the diagnosis of an adnexal swelling should never be made with certainty.

In the identification of the uterine appendages the two fingers are placed in the lateral fornix of the vagina: the left hand is placed to one side of the uterus and efforts are made to outline the adnexa between the fingers of the

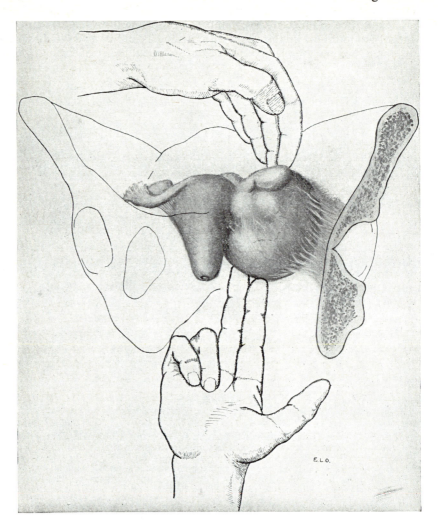

Fig. 59. Bimanual examination in the case of a pyosalpinx. Note that the uterus is displaced over to the opposite side. The fingers in the vagina are moved to one side of the cervix, and they feel the lower pole of the swelling. (After Halban Seitz.)

two hands (Fig. 59). A similar technique is used to that employed in palpating the uterus. Sometimes, however, it will be found that the ovaries can best be palpated by pressing them against the lateral wall of the pelvis; this is particularly so in the case of the right ovary. It should be clearly stated that even in the hands of the most experienced, the normal tube is never palpable and that only the ovary is felt. If the tube is palpable it is diseased.

Some patients are extremely easy to examine so that the ovaries can easily be felt. Swellings of the uterine adnexa tend to prolapse behind the uterus into the pouch of Douglas rather than to extend upwards. For this reason the pouch of Douglas should be examined through the posterior fornix in an endeavour to detect the lower pole of an adnexal swelling.

Inflammatory swellings of the uterine appendages are tender and fixed, while ovarian tumours have smooth surfaces, are not tender, and can usually be moved easily. Tubal gestations have a characteristic consistence because most of the swelling is composed of blood clot. With hydrosalpinx and pyosalpinx it is often possible to distinguish their retort-like shape with the dilated ampullary part of the tube prolapsed behind the uterus into the pouch of Douglas. In parametritis a dense induration is felt to one side of the uterus, which may extend laterally to the pelvic wall, from which the uterus can be distinguished with difficulty.

The Pouch of Douglas. The pouch of Douglas can be examined very easily through the posterior fornix, because only the peritoneum and the posterior vaginal wall intervene between the posterior fornix of the vagina and the peritoneal cavity. The commonest swelling felt through the posterior fornix is a collection of faeces in the rectosigmoid. Next in order of frequency comes the retroverted body of the uterus. Pelvic abscesses in the pouch of Douglas produce dense indurated swellings in which areas of softening can be detected. Pelvic haematoceles have the characteristic consistence of blood clot and produce fixity of the surrounding structures. The lower poles of ovarian tumours and adnexal inflammatory swellings can also be felt in the pouch of Douglas, while the presence of discrete hard fixed nodules is a characteristic finding in cases of malignant ovarian tumours. Pelvic endometriosis gives somewhat similar signs to an ovarian carcinoma in that small nodules may be palpable in the posterior fornix. In endometriosis the uterus is fixed and the ovaries may contain palpable chocolate cysts. Bimanual examination is usually tender and the history of pain and the age of the patient are also helpful in diagnosis. Ovarian cancer on the contrary is painless and its palpation elicits no local tenderness. The swelling of diverticulitis can be felt in the pouch of Douglas on the left side, and it is usually possible to establish that such swellings are separate both from the uterus and from the left appendage. The swelling of diverticulitis is tender and fixed. Such swellings may give rise to difficulty in diagnosis, but if the possibility of diverticulitis is borne in mind the diagnosis should be established by a barium enema. Carcinoma of the sigmoid colon gives similar signs.

Speculum Examination

The next step in the pelvic examination is to pass a speculum in order to examine the vagina and cervix visually. It is argued by some schools that inspection should precede palpation and that the speculum should be passed before the digital vaginal examination. The best form of speculum to use is the self-retaining bivalve speculum of Cusco or some modification of it. It can be

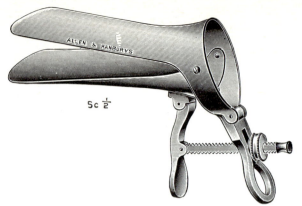

FIG. 60. Cusco's speculum.

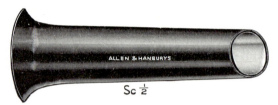

FIG. 61. Ferguson's speculum

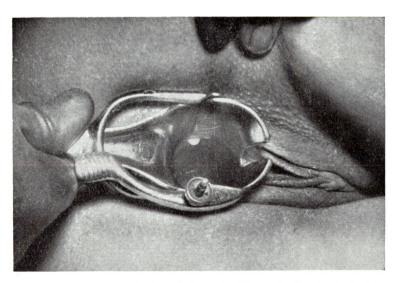

FIG. 62. Speculum examination of the cervix. The patient is lying in the left
lateral position and a Cusco speculum (Brewer's modification) has been inserted into the vagina.

inserted without causing discomfort, be opened out and adjusted to the size of the vagina, and above all it is self-retaining. For routine examination with the patient lying in the left lateral position, Cusco's speculum is strongly recommended (see Figs. 60 and 62).

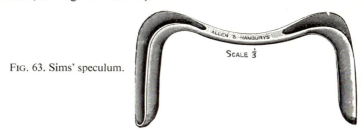

FIG. 63. Sims' speculum.

For clinical examination, the authors have now abandoned all other specula and use only three sizes of Cusco's speculum. The smallest for nulliparae, the medium for most routine work and the large size for the patulous, prolapsed vagina of the multipara. They reserve Ferguson's speculum for out-patient cauterisation of the cervix or of the vaginal vault granulations often seen after total hysterectomy since it provides maximum protection to the vaginal walls against accidental burns (see Fig. 61).

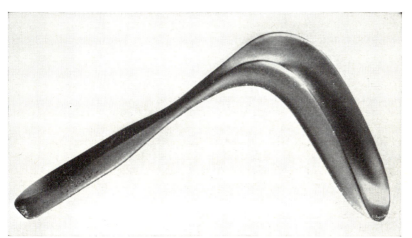

FIG. 64. Single-bladed modification of Sims' speculum as used by the authors. This is more simple to use than the Sims' speculum.

Sims' speculum was devised by Marion Sims for exposing vesico-vaginal fistulae and was intended for use with the patient lying in the left lateral position (see Fig. 63). Sims' speculum is an extremely useful instrument to use when the patient is lying in the lithotomy position, but assistance is required if it is employed to expose the cervix when the patient is lying in the left lateral position. If Sims' speculum is used, it should be modified as a single-bladed speculum similar to that of Milligan (Fig. 64). The single-bladed modification is much handier to use in the lithotomy position as the second blade of the double-bladed variety frequently gets in the way.

During the insertion of the speculum the vaginal wall can be examined for such abnormalities as colpitis senilis and colpitis granulosa. The cervix can be examined by inspection for such abnormalities as erosions, lacerations, polypi and carcinoma. Illumination of the vagina can be obtained by the use of an electric torch or by an adjustable lamp or with an illuminated plastic speculum of the Coldlite type. Speculum examination of the cervix should be employed as a routine and it is essential in all cases in which vaginal haemorrhage has followed bimanual examination. Early carcinoma of the cervix cannot be detected by palpation.

While the cervix is exposed by a speculum, further investigations can be carried out. It may be necessary to make bacteriological examinations of the discharge from the cervical canal. The discharge from the cervical canal is then collected either with a platinum loop or with a throat swab. In other cases, small mucous polypi can be twisted off the cervix, while in cases of suspected carcinoma a small piece can be excised from the suspicious area with long pointed scissors or a small conchotome. Similarly, in cases of retroversion it may be decided to attempt to replace the uterus by fixing a pair of volsellum forceps on the anterior lip. It is often stated that the cervix is insensitive: this is not strictly true, but there is usually very little discomfort either in twisting off polypi from the cervix or in attaching single-bite fine-toothed volsellum forceps to the anterior lip. It is now our routine practice to take cervical and vaginal smears for cytological examination in all patients.

Rectal Examination

Rectal examination should be performed more often during gynaecological investigations. In virgins bimanual examination of the pelvis is carried out with one finger inserted into the rectum. The method is not so exact as bimanual vaginal examination, but it often allows the ovaries to be more easily identified. In parametritis and carcinoma of the cervix, rectal examination is performed as a routine, for the uterosacral ligaments are easily felt by rectal examination and any induration present can be recognised. The uterosacral ligaments are sometimes thickened and tender in patients suffering from endometriosis. A rectal examination should be made whenever swellings or indurations either of the posterior vaginal wall or of the pouch of Douglas have been detected. In this way it will be established whether the swellings lie in front of the rectum. Unless rectal examinations are performed as a routine in such cases, tumours such as carcinoma of the rectum will be missed. A rectal examination should always be made when the patient has complained of rectal symptoms which may be caused by such conditions as haemorrhoids, anal fissures and polypi. The passage of a small well-lubricated proctoscope is an essential part of all rectal examinations.

A useful refinement of the rectal examination and one which is not used often enough and which should be better known, is the bi-digital examination. The index finger of the right hand is placed in the vagina and the middle finger in the rectum. A bimanual pelvic examination is then performed. The rectal and vaginal fingers can then more accurately assess the position of an obscure pelvic tumour and can usually confirm its relationship to the large bowel and ovary. By this means it is, therefore, often possible to say that a given pelvic tumour is either ovarian in origin or primarily situated in the bowel, e.g. carcinoma of the recto-sigmoid.

Examination of Vaginal Discharge

A bacteriological examination must never be omitted when investigating a patient complaining of a vaginal discharge. In suspected gonorrhoea, material for examination must be collected from the urethra, the ducts of Bartholin's glands, from the cervix and from the anal canal. A finger should be inserted into the vagina and the urethra massaged against the posterior surface of the symphysis pubis so that the discharge is expressed from the urethral meatus. This discharge is collected with a platinum loop. Similarly, on compression of Bartholin's glands, pus may be expressed from the ducts; if so it should be examined bacteriologically. The technique of collecting the discharge from the cervix has already been described in the paragraph dealing with speculum examination. The positive demonstration of the intracellular gonococcus in the pus cells of the vaginal discharge is rendered difficult by the presence of other organisms in considerable numbers.

With trichomonas infections the vaginal discharge should be collected in a platinum loop from the posterior fornix, using a Cusco's speculum. When diluted in warm normal saline the characteristic features and movements of the organism when seen under the microscope are diagnostic. It can also be demonstrated in stained films if special stains are used. A solution of 1% brilliant cresyl violet is a most valuable method for trichomonas staining, for leucocytes and bacteria do not take up the dye. Giemsa's stain also allows the trichomonas to be seen easily. Failure to visualise the trichomonas when there is strong clinical suspicion of its presence, calls for a selective culture using a special medium containing antibiotics to inhibit all contaminant organisms. Using this selective mechanism many suspect cases of trichomoniasis will be positively diagnosed when negative to the simple microscopic examination.

Vaginal moniliasis has become increasingly common due to the use of antibiotics often for some extragenital infection. The discharge is characteristic: thick, white cheesy plaques are seen lightly adhering to the vaginal and sometimes to the vulval epithelium. When these are removed a petechial haemorrhagic patch is left which tends to bleed. These plaques are often accompanied by a profuse, thin, watery discharge which is highly irritant to the vulva which presents a glazed or oedematous, inflamed appearance. A throat swab should be rotated in the white discharge and transferred to a test-tube containing warm normal saline; this can be examined under the microscope immediately or is sent at once to the laboratory where a direct smear examination will demonstrate the characteristic appearance of the fungus with mycelial threads and spores. The fungus can be cultured in Sabouraud's medium as confirmatory evidence. The clinical appearance is usually sufficient for diagnosis but cultural methods will double the number

of positive diagnoses. It must be remembered that moniliasis and trichomoniasis may co-exist.

Examination of the Urinary Tract

In every gynaecological out-patient consultation the urine should be
examined chemically for albumen and sugar and a microscopical examination
should also be made when urinary infections are suspected.

Patients with urinary symptoms are best investigated by a urologist who
will make a full examination including cystoscopy. This is particularly
important where a recurrent urinary tract infection has been wrongly attributed to some gynaecological cause such as a cystocele when it is in fact due
to a purely urological lesion. A history of evident or suspected haematuria
is always most significant since carcinoma of the urinary tract quite commonly
presents as a gynaecological problem in the first instance. It is the authors'
strong conviction that all patients with stress incontinence should have a full
urological investigation including cysto-urethroscopy before being subjected
to a gynaecological repair operation. In carcinoma of the cervix infiltration
of the bladder is best recognised by cystoscopic examination. In the earliest
stage of involvement of the bladder there is a bullous oedema of the bladder
wall; later, retraction of the bladder wall develops, while in advanced carcinoma the growth ulcerates into the cavity of the bladder. In patients
with carcinoma of the cervix an intravenous pyelogram is an essential part of
the treatment and should never be omitted. Early ureteric obstruction will,
if present, be detected and retrograde pyelography can be performed if
necessary.

Cervical Biopsy

The scope of consulting room or out-patient biopsy in the unanaesthetised
patient is steadily diminishing in favour of a full-scale cold cone biopsy
which removes all actually or potentially malignant areas and for which an
anaesthetic is needed. This examination naturally includes a full and thorough
diagnostic curettage. The reason for the above statement are as follows:

1. A random biopsy with punch forceps may easily miss the actual area
    of malignant infiltration.
2. A surface lesion which is evident to inspection or speculum examina-
    tion may be superimposed upon a deeper seated infiltrated carcinoma
    of the endocervix.
3. No out-patient biopsy however enthusiastically performed can ever
    compete for thoroughness with that performed in the operating theatre
    under an anaesthetic.
4. Control of haemorrhage by packing or suture is always more efficient
    in the anaesthetised patient.

It is our present practice to limit out-patient biopsy of the cervix to those
patients whose lesion is obviously malignant and in whom it is easy to obtain
a suitable piece of growth without causing heavy bleeding, i.e. the friable
exophytic type of growth. If bleeding should occur it is best controlled by

packing and not cautery since the latter spoils the specimen for histological examination if hysterectomy should subsequently be indicated.

Endometrial Biopsy

This method of investigation is useful to establish the presence of ovulation but it should not be employed for the diagnosis of endometrial cancer. The patient must be placed in the lithotomy position and the cervix exposed and pulled down with fine, single-bite volsellum forceps. Strict asepsis is necessary. The practical object of the investigation is to remove strips of endometrium from the body of the uterus. The dangers of the operation are sepsis, perforation of the uterine wall and abortion if the patient should have an undiagnosed pregnancy. Under no circumstances should the investigation be made if there is latent or active sepsis in any of the pelvic organs. If carcinoma of the body of the uterus is suspected, it is essential to anaesthetise the patient, to perform a curettage and to explore every part of the cavity of the uterus.

The theoretical object of endometrial biopsy is to determine the degree of secretory hypertrophy from examination of the endometrium removed. In this way the cycle can be classed as ovulatory or anovulatory and as a method of study of ovarian function endometrial biopsy is of great value. An expert gynaecological histologist will be able to determine from an examination of the material removed the degree of ovarian insufficiency, from complete absence of oestrogen effects on the endometrium to those which show proliferative and hyperplastic endometrium as the result of prolonged oestrogenic stimulation without the influence of progesterone, as in the eondition of metropathia haemorrhagica.

Out-patient endometrial biopsy has a limited usefulness. If the specimen obtained gives a clear-cut histological picture in conformity with the clinical findings it is valuable, but it must be remembered that a random sample of endometrium obtained with difficulty in a nervous patient may not be representative of the true overall endometrial picture and for this a full-scale diagnostic curettage is essential. The instrument used may be either a thin delicate curette or a hollow curette with an aspiration syringe attached through which pieces of tissue can be drawn. The operation is simple. The difficulty lies in the interpretation of the material examined.

Aspiration of Douglas' Pouch

This operation is extremely simple to perform. The patient is placed in the lithotomy position and the posterior lip of the cervix drawn forwards and downwards with volsellum forceps while a speculum retracts back the posterior vaginal wall. The vaginal wall behind the cervix is disinfected and a long needle attached to an aspiration syringe by a bayonet attachment is introduced into Douglas' pouch. The aspiration of pus confirms the diagnosis of a pelvic abscess while the presence of blood indicates a pelvic haematocele from an extrauterine gestation. This examination is best performed in an operating theatre under full asepsis and where everything is in readiness to proceed to laparotomy if indicated.

Culdoscopy*

An elaboration of the last method was introduced in America by Decker and Cherry in 1944 and has since then been favourably reported on in this country by Jeffcoate. A previous bimanual examination should exclude gross pelvic pathology such as advanced endometriosis or the fixed retroversion of chronic pelvic inflammatory disease. The bladder is emptied by a catheter and the patient is intubated to secure a clear airway for the anaesthetic.

TECHNIQUE. The apparatus consists of a special trocar with a guard on the sheath 3 cm. from the tip to control the depth of introduction. Carbon dioxide is used to displace the viscera. The actual culdoscope resembles a cystoscope. Illumination is by dry battery. See Fig. 66.

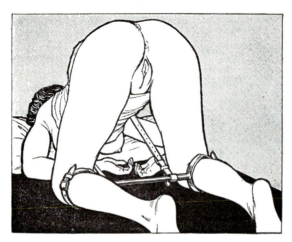

FIG. 65. Anaesthetised patient in knee-chest position. Clover's crutch used to control the position of the patient as advocated by Jeffcoate. (From Shaw's *Operative Gynaecology*, E. & S. Livingstone.)

The patient is placed in the knee-chest position, the vagina sterilised and the posterior lip of the cervix grasped with a volsellum. The puncture is made about 25 mm. behind the cervix and in the midline. Before the trocar is withdrawn carbon dioxide is introduced by the side tap on the cannula. The introduction of the gas and the force of gravity allow the bowel to fall away from the pouch of Douglas. The culdoscope is now introduced. Fig. 65.

All the normal contents of the pelvis should be visible for inspection and the usual cystoscopic manoeuvres are used to bring different aspects under scrutiny. Abdominal manipulation, traction on the cervix and gentle pressure by the lip of the instrument will help to display the various structures. Culdoscopy can be combined with tubal patency testing, using a dye in saline introduced into the cervical canal as in the operation of hysterosalpingography (p. 344).

* The sections on TECHNIQUE and COMPLICATIONS together with Figs. 65 and 66 are taken verbatim from Shaw's *Operative Gynaecology*, 2nd ed., revised by John Howkins, by permission of the publishers, E. & S. Livingstone Ltd., Edinburgh.

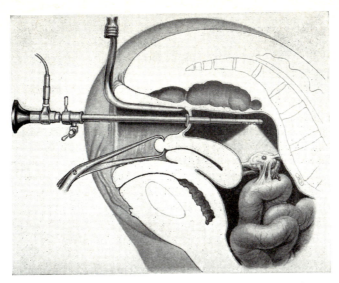

Fig. 66. Culdoscope in position showing typical view of the pelvic contents with small gut adherent to the appendage.

When the examination is finished the culdoscope is removed but the sheath is left in position. The patient is placed on her back or side and pressure is exerted on the abdomen to expel as much gas as possible. The carbon dioxide gas should be completely absorbed in 24 hours and until this absorption is complete the patient will experience shoulder pain. The small vaginal wound is sutured by one stitch but can be left unclosed.

SOME POSSIBLE INDICATIONS FOR CULDOSCOPY:

1. Diagnosis of extrauterine gestation.
2. Diagnosis of endometriosis in its early and clinically undemonstrable state.
3. In the investigation of obscure pelvic pain.
4. In the exact diagnosis of a pelvic mass.
5. In the investigation of infertility.
6. In patients with suspected Stein-Leventhal syndrome and virilism.
7. In the investigation of certain menstrual disorders.

COMPLICATIONS: (1) Pneumoperitoneum causing discomfort and shoulder pain. This can be minimal if the abdomen is emptied of gas after the operation and should only last for 24 hours.

(2) Emphysema due to entering the cellular tissues behind the cervix.

(3) Puncture of an adherent bowel, usually the rectum. Observation and antibiotics should be sufficient in the treatment of this accident.

CONTRAINDICATIONS. Chronic pelvic inflammatory disease or advanced endometriosis with obliteration of the pouch of Douglas.

In summary, culdoscopy is a useful accessory to exact pelvic diagnosis and its employment may well save the patient and the hospital the expense and wastage of a bed after an unnecessary laparotomy. The fact that it has not achieved any popularity in the United Kingdom does not condemn it and it will probably find an occasional place in our future practice. It is simple, safe and, within its limits, effective.

Peritoneoscopy

During the past fifty years sporadic efforts have been made to popularise peritoneoscopy. Recently (1965) Steptoe has introduced certain refinements of technique that should establish this simple, cheap and time saving alternative to laparotomy. By using an extra abdominal source of light transmitted by means of fibre lighting it is now possible to provide a powerful illumination for the telescope and for photography.

Briefly, the technique is as follows:

1. The patient is admitted for 36 hours to hospital.
2. Full pre-operative preparations as for laparotomy are essential.
3. The bladder is emptied by catheter.
4. The patient is placed in the lithotomy-Trendelenburg position.
5. A pneumoperitoneum of 4 litres of carbon dioxide is introduced and the volume measured on the anaesthetic flow meter. A special needle is introduced just lateral to the rectus muscle for the pneumoperitoneum.
6. A separate midline stab 3–4 cm. below the umbilicus is made for the introduction of the trocar and cannula of the telescope. On entering the peritoneal cavity the trocar is withdrawn and the telescope inserted.
7. By manoeuvring the telescope, altering the position of the uterus by a sound previously placed within the uterus or by an insufflation cannula manipulated from the vagina and changing the position of the patient, it should be possible to obtain a good view of the pelvis and its contents.
8. The examination concluded the telescope is withdrawn and the gas encouraged to escape through the cannula by flattening the patient's position to horizontal and gently compressing the abdomen.
9. The cannula is then withdrawn and one skin clip is inserted.

Although this examination is quite feasible under a local anaesthetic, a general is preferred to minimise the discomfort of the pneumoperitoneum.

The advantages of peritoneoscopy over culdoscopy are:

1. The field of vision is far wider and with experience as informative as laparotomy.
2. Peritoneoscopy is applicable in just those patients where culdoscopy is impossible, e.g. pouch of Douglas obliterated by endometriosis or pelvic peritonitis and dense adhesions.
3. The indications for its use are all those covered by culdoscopy.
4. Its dangers are the same as for culdoscopy and are negligible.
5. Its contraindications are very few apart from a history of general peritonitis, adhesive tuberculous peritonitis and a heavily scarred abdomen.

Cytology. The diagnostic reliability of vaginal and cervical cytology is now established not only for malignant disease but also in the assessment of sex hormone activity. It is a quick, convenient, inexpensive out-patient method of hormone assay comparing favourably with the more complicated and expensive biochemical investigations.

Technique. All surface cells of the genital tract possess the property of exfoliation and this exfoliative material is readily obtainable for cytological examination.

(a) **Aspiration of the posterior fornix** will contain exfoliated cells from any part of the genital tract and if malignant cells are present does not tell us the situation of the growth. A glass pipette with a suction bulb is used and the aspirated material spread evenly on a slide and fixed in equal parts of 95% alcohol and ether.

(b) **Cervical scrape** using Ayre's spatula revolved over the whole 360 degrees of the portio vaginalis of the cervix, after it has been well exposed with a Cusco's speculum. This smear is specifically designed to confirm or exclude a carcinoma of the cervix.

(c) To exclude an **endocervical** growth the endocervical canal should be scraped with a small spoon or aspirated and a separate slide made.

(d) If **carcinoma of the endometrium** is suspected and requires exclusion a further smear from the cavity of the uterus should be obtained by suction cannula.

(e) For **hormonal assay** the lateral wall of the upper third of the vagina is lightly scraped. This is the part of the vagina most sensitive to hormonal influence.

The Cytological Diagnosis of Uterine Cancer

This method was introduced by Papanicolaou and Traut in 1943. The material for cytological examination may be obtained in two ways. The first method is to make a vaginal smear from the posterior fornix in the manner already described. This will contain the normal vaginal squames and also cells exfoliated from the cervix and a few from the endocervix and endo-

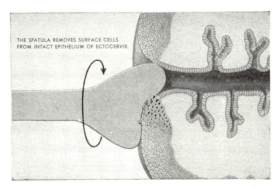

THE SPATULA REMOVES SURFACE CELLS
FROM INTACT EPITHELIUM OF ECTOCERVIX.

FIG. 67. Surface biopsy of cervix. (Ayre, "Cancer Cytology of the Uterus," Grune & Stratton Inc.)

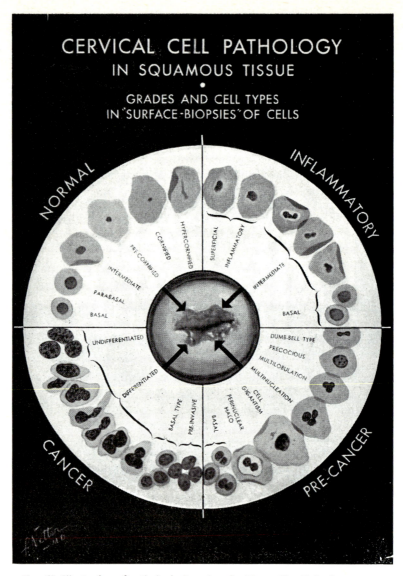

F1G. 68. Illustration of pathological grades of epidermoid cells in the squamo-columnar junction of the cervix. Cells arising in this location were procured by a uniform cell-scraping technique. Classification of cell types is based upon thorough study, evaluation of cell characteristics and pathological features, and is finally correlated with corresponding histological studies of the tissues. No attempt is made to classify cells exfoliated from other tissue areas, such as the endometrium. The squamo-columnar junction is a vital zone to the female, since this is the focal point where cancer arises. Grading of cells depends upon knowledge of origin of cell sample, on securing a rich concentration of cells, and, of greatest importance, on correct correlation with histological findings.

metrium. In common with all cancers of Müllerian tissue, carcinoma of the cervix exfoliates its superficial cells, and these will, therefore, be picked up from the vaginal pool. The second method is to make a smear directly from the cervix, the so-called "surface biopsy" described by Ayre. A wooden spatula, shaped so that a portion of one end will fit into the external os, is applied with light pressure to the cervix and is rotated through 360 degrees (Fig. 67). The material obtained is smeared on a glass slide and fixed immediately as previously described. If carcinoma cells are subsequently found in one smear, the area of the cervix to be submitted to biopsy may be defined

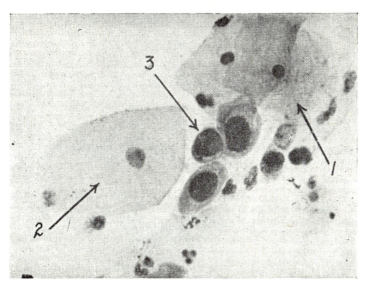

FIG. 69. Cornified Cells and Cancer Cells. Cervical smear from edge of clinical carcinoma showing normal, mature cornified cell (1), an intermediate cell (2), in close association with malignant cells (3). (From Ayre's "Cancer Cytology of the Uterus", Grune & Stratton Inc.)

more accurately by means of colposcopy. To improve the diagnostic accuracy in carcinoma of the endometrium, an intrauterine cannula attached to a strong suction bulb should be inserted into the cavity of the uterus. As this cannula is slowly withdrawn, negative pressure is exerted and thus a fairly representative sample of the endometrial cytology is obtained. The aspirated material is expelled onto a slide and fixed for staining in the usual manner. It will be remembered that there are three types of normal cell found in vaginal smears. The basal cells are small, rounded and basophilic, the cells from the middle layer are transparent and basophilic, while the cells from the superficial layer are acidophilic with characteristic pyknotic nuclei. In addition, endometrial cells, histiocytes, blood cells and bacteria can often be seen. Malignant cells are hyperchromatic with a great increase in chromatin content. The nuclei vary in size and there is usually only a small amount of cytoplasm in the undifferentiated malignant cell (see Figs. 68 and 69).

Papanicolaou Classification.

Group I.—Normal: no evidence of malignant or atypical cells.

Group II.—Atypical cells probably resulting from infection or lesions such as erosions. No evidence of malignancy.

Group III.—Cells present that are suspicious of malignancy.

Group IV.—Few malignant cells present.

Group V.—Large numbers of malignant cells present.

SIGNIFICANCE OF PAPANICOLAOU CLASSIFICATION

Group I.—Normal

Group II.—Vaginal or cervical infection which should be investigated and treated.

Group III.—Suspicious: merits repeat smear and, if repeatedly positive, further investigation, diagnostic curettage and cold cone biopsy of the cervix as in IV and V.

Groups IV and V.—Positive: further investigation must be undertaken (e.g., biopsy and curettage) until the source of the cells is found and the diagnosis confirmed.

Reliability of Vaginal Smears. The reliability of vaginal smears depends upon the efficient preparation and preservation of the specimen, its processing and the efficiency and skill of the cytologist. The accuracy of smear reports for carcinoma of the cervix varies from 95% to 100%. The accuracy of Group V smears is almost 100%, especially if they are combined with subsequent adequate biopsy, and in a significant number of those cases where the biopsy has been negative the final result has proved the smear to be correct. The cytological false negatives may be as high as 10% for a single examination, but if repeat examinations are employed as part of a screening programme the false negatives are less than 1%.

The accuracy of vaginal smears in the diagnosis of endometrial carcinoma is low (about 70%) but if endometrial smears are used the accuracy is over 90%.

Value of Vaginal Smears. It must be stressed that, in the diagnosis of cancer, vaginal smears are no more than an aid to a diagnosis that must be proved by biopsy and standard histological examination. The main value of vaginal smears lies in the use of the technique for screening large numbers of people in order that carcinoma of the uterus may be diagnosed earlier. In this respect the value of screening large numbers of women in order to diagnose carcinoma *in situ* (pre-invasive carcinoma) is of paramount importance, since by this method the precursor of invasive cancer can be diagnosed before a clinical lesion appears or whilst any visible lesion is apparently benign. There is much evidence to show that carcinoma *in situ* exists for a period of up to ten years before the lesion becomes invasive and cytological screening of patients during this period could do much to eliminate invasive carcinoma of the cervix.

It is reasonable to enquire what percentage of unsuspected cancers, including carcinoma *in situ*, can be expected to be diagnosed by cytology.

When screening the female population over the age of 30 it is found that five abnormal smears are obtained per 1,000 women examined.

Cytological screening can therefore be expected to discover unsuspected, mostly *in situ* carcinoma in four to ten of every 1,000 women screened. A trained cytologist cannot be expected to read more than a maximum of thirty slides a day owing to eye fatigue, and he requires ten months' training, before he acquires efficiency and reliability. His total annual output is therefore about 6,000 slides when trained and his training is expensive. From an economic point of view, it is estimated that the discovery of one unsuspected cancer costs £500. Such financial objections are likely to limit the scope of cytology, at any rate in this country, to large specialist centres. In these it is likely to be of most use when applied to the gynaecological out-patient whose cervix discloses on clinical examination a supposedly benign lesion such as erosion. Finally, this useful and fairly reliable method of investigation is not infallible and it must never become an alternative to a proper clinical examination.

Hormonal Assay for Vaginal Cytology. This is the second main use of vaginal cytology and one of steadily increasing importance owing to its speed, cheapness, availability and accuracy.

(a) **Assessment of oestrogens.** Oestrogens produce a cytological picture where mature epithelial cells are large eosinophilic cells with pyknotic nuclei. The background is clear, containing a few bacteria and leucocytes. The number of mature eosinophilic cells per 100 cells counted is expressed as the Karyopyknotic index. This index is high in the early part of the menstrual cycle and falls after ovulation. It is also low during pregnancy.

(b) **Progesterone Assessment.** The cell pattern is predominantly basophilic with intermediate cells having vesicular nuclei. In pregnancy the cells tend to show curling and folding—the envelope effect—and they tend to form clusters.

The cytologist must be given details of the patient's age, date of last menstrual period, the details of her normal menstrual pattern, if any hormone therapy has been used, e.g. the contraceptive pill, and the date of the last dose.

Colposcopic Examination of the Cervix

The purpose of this examination is to enable the clinician to make a detailed study of the portio vaginalis and its epithelial coverings. The method is now widely used and its value recognised. In principle, the colposcope enables a binocular examination of the cervix to be made at magnifications of from 6 to 40 diameters. Different types of illumination can be used to help differentiate the vascular and other changes in the epithelia.

The method was introduced by Hinselmann in 1927. His original apparatus was of low magnifying power. The modern instruments have been much elaborated and improved. The illustration (Fig. 70) shows one of the more recent colposcopes which has an adaptation for photography.

The lithotomy position is used for this examination and the cervix is exposed with a speculum. The cervix is swabbed clear of excess mucus and it can then be examined in detail.

The portio of the normal cervix is covered with squamous epithelium which takes on a mahogany brown colour when stained with iodine in Schiller's test. The staining ceases at the mucocutaneous junction of the external os as the mucosa of the endocervix contains no glycogen.

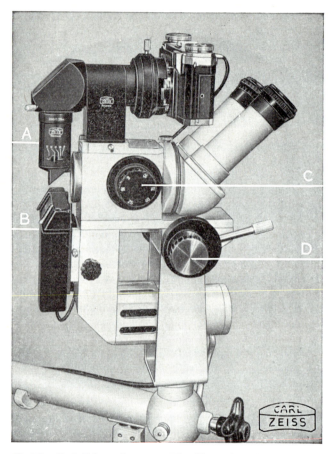

Fig. 70. The Carl Zeiss colposcope. The illustration shows the binocular viewing unit. Note the camera attachment (A) and electronic flash unit (B) for making photographic records. The magnification (C) and focusing (D) controls are also shown. (Courtesy of Rayner & Keeler Ltd.)

Where an erosion is present, the squamous epithelium is replaced by the red glistening columnar epithelium which is bathed in mucus and has a papillary structure. If this is swabbed with 2% acetic acid or 5% silver nitrate, the mucus is precipitated as a white substance demarcating the edges of the papillae. The colposcope enables the openings of the glands to be seen, and this appearance enables a clear distinction to be made between a true erosion and a carcinoma.

When regeneration of the squamous epithelium has begun, there is regression of the eroded area and flame-shaped areas of young squamous tissue cut into the regular papillary pattern of the erosion. This young tissue does not take up the iodine stain well as its glycogen content is low.

Leukoplakia is another condition occurring on the cervix in circumscribed areas which can be distinguished by the colposcope and which are also iodine negative. The characteristic pattern is a mosaic of enclosed fields as seen by an aviator, the size and shape of the fields being remarkably uniform.

Carcinoma of squamous-cell or adenomatous type shows none of the regularity of the foregoing tissues and, in addition, there is marked disorder in the arrangement of the superficial blood vessels which have lost their normal arborescence and become distorted into corkscrew and comma shaped patterns. Telangiectatic areas are also seen in which the calibre of the capillary lumen is greatly widened. The epithelium shows irregular yellow glossy areas with ulceration. These areas are iodine negative.

In summary, the great value of colposcopy lies in its ability to differentiate the benign from the malignant lesion and to pinpoint the exact position from which a biopsy should be made. In the exact localisation of the site of malignant process lies the greatest justification for this special investigation without which a random biopsy may well miss the very spot which contains the early cancer.

Investigations

Radiological investigation should be more widely employed in gynaecological practice. Apart from the genital tract the chest must be X-rayed in all cases of suspected genital tuberculosis and to exclude metastases from malignant pelvic disease. The gastro-intestinal tract may harbour a small primary carcinoma in stomach or colon in cases of malignant ovarian tumour. A barium meal or enema is essential in elucidating obscure tumours in the right or left lower quadrant, such as regional ileitis on the right and diverticulitis and carcinoma of the sigmoid on the left side. In all cases of backache in which prolapse or retroversion has been incriminated as the possible cause the spine and sacro-iliac joints should be X-rayed, and the old adage remembered that if a woman complains of backache there is usually something wrong with her back.

An intravenous pyelogram will often provide vital information of ureteric abnormality or obstruction and may show the presence of an ectopic or supernumerary ureter opening in the vagina, the absence of one kidney, an ectopic pelvic kidney, obstructions due to fibroids, pyosalpinx or pelvic carcinoma (see Fig. 71). Lateral cystograms are useful in the investigation and treatment of stress incontinence. In endocrinopathies the pituitary fossa should be X-rayed.

Radiological investigation of the pelvis may be useful in diagnosing pregnancy after the fourteenth week. The possible risks of foetal damage have, however, limited its employment. Calcified fibroids show well and the teeth in a dermoid cyst can be demonstrated (see Figs. 72 and 73). The place of hysterosalpingography will be discussed later in the investigation of infertility. Rarer uses of X-rays include the demonstration of an advanced extrauterine pregnancy or the presence of a lithopaedion. Foreign bodies in the uterine cavity can be clearly demonstrated (Fig. 74).

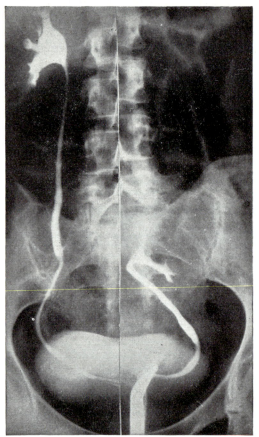

Fig. 71. Composite X-ray showing ectopic pelvic left kidney demonstrated by retrograde pyelography. (Clinically diagnosed as left ovarian tumour.)

A recently introduced refinement of radiological diagnosis has been named gynaecography. It is really the obverse of hysterosalpingography where the contrast medium introduced outlines the cavity of the uterus and Fallopian tubes, whereas gynaecography using a pneumoperitoneum of carbon dioxide gas outlines the peritoneal surface of the uterus and appendages. It is thus an external as opposed to an internal hysterosalpingography. Extremely clear and excellent pictures can be obtained and the method is of great value in confirming the presence of small ovarian swellings or Stein-Leventhal's

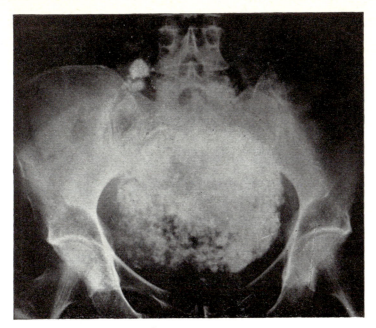

FIG. 72. X-ray of pelvis showing a calcified fibroid.

syndrome. The gas can be introduced through the cervix by the technique of tubal insufflation. If there is tubal spasm or obstruction a separate puncture must be made either transvaginally as in culdoscopy or transabdominally as in peritoneoscopy.

Biological Tests for Pregnancy

The Zondek-Aschheim test depends upon the excretion of chorionic gonadotropins in the urine and is positive only when living chorionic tissue is present in the body as in intrauterine pregnancy, extrauterine pregnancy, retained and living placental tissue, hydatidiform mole and chorionepithelioma. In the last two instances the test may be positive in high dilution of 1 in 200, or even 1 in 1,000. If hydatidiform mole or chorionepithelioma is suspected a quantitative test should be requested. It is preferable to use a morning specimen of urine to which a drop of xylol or toluol has been added. Immature female mice, less than three weeks old, are used as test animals, and the urine is injected subcutaneously. The animals are killed on the fifth day. The test is positive if the ovaries show haemorrhagic follicles or corpora lutea. This is the oldest and probably still the most reliable pregnancy test. It is still occasionally used where the more popular modern tests are equivocal.

In the Hogben test, the Xenopus toad is used as the test animal and urine is injected subcutaneously into the dorsal lymph sac. The test is speedy and eggs are voided if the test is positive at an average of eight hours afterwards. The test is not as reliable as the Zondek-Aschheim and may give a false negative of up to 10%.

An alternative to the Hogben test is the male toad test using the Bufo-Bufo which is an English native, readily obtainable and cheap (1s. 6d.). The toads are hardy and can be used indefinitely with rest intervals of ten days.

Immunological Tests for Pregnancy. The basis of this test is the inter-reaction of gonadotropin antibodies and the chorionic gonadotropin of pregnancy urine. The advantage of these tests is speed—results in two hours or less—cheapness and simplicity of performance. The immunological test has

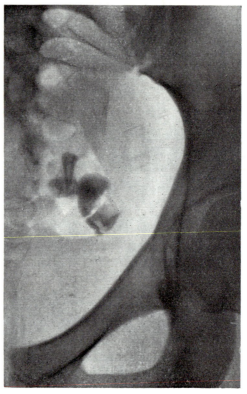

FIG. 73. X-ray of pelvis showing teeth in an ovarian dermoid cyst.

therefore become the standard laboratory procedure for pregnancy testing.

Practitioners are advised to use only the large pregnancy diagnosis laboratories, where a high degree of accuracy is maintained, and small laboratories doing a limited number of tests should be avoided. A wrong diagnosis of pregnancy is one of the most embarrassing experiences to practitioner and patient and is not readily forgiven by the offended party. The following advice will be helpful in avoiding mistakes:

(1) At least ten days should elapse after the first missed menstrual period before submitting urine to the laboratory.

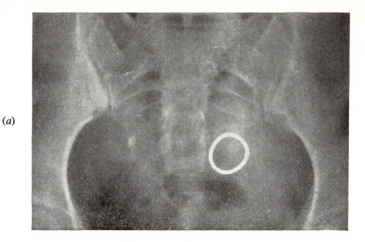

(a)

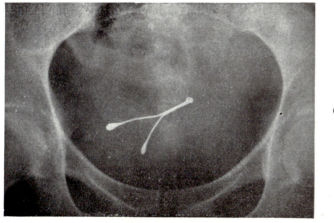

(b)

(c)

Fig. 74. Shows three
foreign bodies in
the uterine cavity.

(a) Grafenberg ring.
(b) Wishbone
            pessary.
(c) Hair grip.

(2) The first morning specimen which is richest in gonadotropin should be sent.

(3) The specimen should be collected in as clean and aseptic a manner as possible. The vessel must be thoroughly rinsed in warm clean tap water to remove every vestige of detergent.

(4) If the result is at variance with the clinical findings the test should be repeated.

Pregnancy tests should become negative forty-eight hours after parturition or after the death or abortion of the ovum, provided that no living chorionic tissue remains in the decidua.

The Operation of Curettage

The operation of curettage should be regarded as a most valuable method of diagnosis in gynaecology; in fact, the main indications for curettage are diagnostic. It is, therefore, used in investigating:

(1) All irregular or excessive uterine haemorrhages irrespective of the age of the patient; the commonest and most important age group includes the post-menopausal patient. The histological examination of the endometrium may provide exact proof of the diagnosis as in the cystic glandular hyperplasia of metropathia, and suggest a logical line of treatment.

(2) As a means of excluding or confirming a suspicion of endometrial cancer.

(3) To establish the fact of ovulation by the presence of secretory pro-gestational changes late in the cycle.

(4) It is sometimes helpful in disclosing the presence of some intrauterine cause of bleeding, e.g. endometrial polypus or a small submucous myoma or fibroid polypus.

(5) For persistent post-abortional bleeding where the cause is retention of the placenta or membranes.

(6) In the incidental diagnosis of uterine abnormality—usually a persistent septum, partial or complete.

A general anaesthetic is necessary and the operative procedures are similar to those described in the operation of dilatation of the cervix (see p. 447). Absolute asepsis is required and the operation must be performed in an operating theatre. The operation should not be performed in the presence of gross cervical infection until this has been treated or controlled, and the same principle applies to endometrial and acute adnexal inflammation. A possible exception is the removal of retained products of a septic abortion under antibiotic coverage. The whole of the endometrium should be scraped away and each wall and angle of the uterus must be curetted in turn. A blunt curette should be used in postpartum and postabortion cases because of the risk of damage to the soft friable myometrium. The dangers of the operation are perforation of the uterus, splitting of the cervix and extension of a pre-existing infection resulting in endosalpingitis and occasionally pelvic peritonitis.

Other Examinations

A haemoglobin estimation should be done on every gynaecological patient complaining of excessive uterine bleeding and it is sometimes advisable to perform a full blood count if there is any clinical suggestion of a primary blood disorder. In pelvic inflammatory disease, a white blood count and E.S.R. are essential.

It cannot be too strongly emphasised that failures and mistakes in diagnosis usually depend upon incomplete investigation. Before operation is performed upon any patient, a complete examination of the cardio-vascular, respiratory and urinary systems must be made.

PROGNOSIS

At the completion of the examination it is necessary to give an opinion both to the patient and to the nearest responsible relative. A truthful opinion both as to diagnosis and prognosis must always be given to the patient's relatives. As a general rule, it is a mistake to tell a patient that she is suffering from some grave disease, and it should be regarded as a principle not to tell a patient that she has cancer. The lay public is not yet sufficiently educated and conditioned to accept a diagnosis of cancer with equanimity and to most patients the very word spells inevitable doom. The fact that many genital tract cancers are curable does little to dispel the feeling of utter hopelessness which the diagnosis of cancer inspires. There are, however, exceptional circumstances in which this guiding principle must be disregarded, and of these a good doctor is the best judge. Fortunately, innocent growths of the female generative organs are frequent, and most women are aware that myomata are common. If a patient suffering from carcinoma asks a direct question as to whether a carcinoma is present or not, the answer should be that she has an ulcer which may very well become malignant unless it is treated appropriately. It is important always to be truthful to the relatives both as regards the diagnosis and prognosis. In cases of carcinoma of the cervix it should be pointed out to the relatives that the patient has a cancer of the womb, that they must realise the gravity of such a disease, but that if properly treated the average five-year survival rate is approximately 60% to 75%. A frank statement of the case in this way indicates to the relatives the gravity of the disease and gives hope in a way which is perfectly truthful.

5 Malformations of the Female Generative Organs

A brief summary of the development of the urogenital system in the female is necessary for the proper understanding of the congenital malformations that may be encountered in practice. Most of these abnormalities are extremely rare and many are of academic interest only, but failure to appreciate their possible presence will lead to perplexity and misdiagnosis.

Gonad. At an early stage of development every embryo is sexually undifferentiated in so far as its gonad is concerned and hence is potentially bisexual. It is after the sixth week that the genital ridge shows signs of masculinity, i.e. that it is destined to be a testis if the sex is male. It is believed that this early primitive testis provides the androgenic hormones which dictate the pattern of development in the Wolffian duct and urogenital sinus, with regression of the Müllerian ducts, by which a male is automatically recognised as such.

If an embryo is destined to be female, the gonad has assumed histologically recognisable ovarian characteristics by the tenth week. The role of oestrogen derived from the primitive ovary is, however, of less importance in developing the female characteristics, such as development of the Müllerian ducts and regression of the Wolffian system, than the comparable action of androgen in the male. It is suggested, in fact, that the basic sexual pattern is female in all embryos and that it is the androgen of the male which causes the male elements to predominate and the absence of androgen in the female which permits the development of the female pattern, rather than the influence of oestrogen which plays a less important part. A consideration of these hypotheses will help the student to understand some of the problems of intersexuality.

Thus, if the early embryonic state of bisexuality or non-differentiation persists into adult life, the result is that rare being—the true hermaphrodite. The gonad is an ovo-testis in which both testicular tubules and ova are histologically demonstrable. At laparotomy, recognisable structures derived from both Wolffian and Müllerian systems are present. The external genitalia are abnormal with, usually, a small phallus, hypospadias, absence of the lower part of the vagina and ectopic or mal-descended testes.

It is important to appreciate that, in the female embryo, the gonad is differentiated into a primitive ovary by the tenth week and, by the twelfth week, the Müllerian system is fully differentiated into its ultimate pattern of Fallopian tubes, uterus and upper three-quarters of vagina. The final differentiation of the urogenital sinus into female urethra and lower quarter of vagina is, however, delayed until the sixteenth to seventeenth weeks.

In the female pseudo-hermaphrodite, the gonad and Müllerian system is normal though, perhaps, under-developed as far as the level of the urogenital sinus. The Wolffian system does not, in any way, persist more than in the normal female, e.g., such vestigial structures as paroöphoron or epoöphoron and Gärtner's duct. But the phallus is hypertrophic, the labia majora may be fused in the midline like the scrotum, and the urogenital sinus opens at the base of the hypertrophied clitoris. Almost invariably, the adrenal glands are hyperplastic so that it is reasonably certain that the cause of female pseudo-hermaphroditism is abnormal cortical androgen produced in excess. This hormone operating on the not yet differentiated urogenital sinus between the twelfth and sixteenth weeks of embryonic life causes virilisation of the external genitalia. At birth the child may be regarded as a male with hypospadias. The vaginal orifice, although present, is concealed by the perineal membrane from fusion of the genital folds in the mid line. Adrenal hyperplasia may cause electrolyte imbalance with feeding difficulties or even death if the condition is not recognised. Nuclear sexing of such a child is essential.

Müllerian ducts. The paramesonephric (or Müllerian) duct appears in the upper lateral part of the intermediate cell mass close to the primitive gonad and in the region of the mesonephros at about the seventh week of intrauterine life. It is formed by an invagination of coelomic mesothelium and lies lateral to the dorsal mesentery of the gut. The caudal tip of this invagination consists of a solid band of cells which grows in a caudal direction lateral to the mesonephric duct (the Wolffian duct). In the female the mesonephric ducts and their associated mesonephric tubules degenerate and persist only as the vestigial Kobelt's tubules, epoöphoron, paroöphoron and Gärtner's duct. Cysts may arise from this residual mesonephric apparatus in the broad ligament and vagina.

As the paramesonephric ducts grow caudally they approach each other in the midline and cross the mesonephric ducts. Partial fusion occurs between the two paramesonephric ducts, which now continue to grow caudally. It must be remembered that the growing or advancing tip of the duct is a solid band of cells and that canalisation occurs later. The cranial part of the paramesonephric duct develops into the Fallopian tube, the middle part the uterus, and the lower part forms the upper three-quarters of the vagina.

The lower ends of the two fused paramesonephric ducts, at first separated from each other by a septum, become the single uterovaginal canal, the caudal end of which projects as the Müllerian tubercle into the urogenital sinus. Between the urogenital sinus and the caudal tip of the paramesonephric ducts there grow two solid bilateral proliferations of cells separating the sinus from the caudal end of the fused paramesonephric ducts. These proliferations are called the sinovaginal bulbs and will later become canalised to form the lower part of the vagina. The hymen is probably derived from the junction of the sinovaginal bulbs and the urogenital sinus. Failure of canalisation in the sinovaginal bulbs will lead to all types of vaginal atresia from a thin, imperforate hymeneal membrane to complete absence of the lower quarter of the vagina.

The development of the female genitalia consists, in the main, of the fusion of the two paramesonephric or Müllerian ducts with their subsequent canalisation and hypertrophy, and as this process may be arrested at any stage, a large number of different forms of mal-development have been recorded.

(1) **Aplasia** in which organs have failed to develop.

(2) **Hypoplasia** in which organs are rudimentary.

(3) **Atresia** in which there is either complete or partial failure of canalisation of the Müllerian ducts.

(4) **Müllerian duct** anomalies.

(5) **Hermaphroditism and pseudo-hermaphroditism,** in which there are abnormalities of development of the sex glands and external genitalia.

(6) Developmental defects of urogenital sinus.

Aplasia

(i) **Ovary.** Complete aplasia of the ovary is a most uncommon rarity but ovarian agenesis, in which there is complete absence of sex cells and the ovarian substance consists of an undifferentiated stroma, is well recognised. This ovarian abnormality is the basis of Turner's syndrome (vide p. 166) or gonadal dysgenesis, the gonads being white streaks of functionless stroma in the normal ovarian position on the back of the broad ligament. The chromosome complement is 45 XO.

(ii) **Fallopian Tube.** As the Müllerian duct system develops from above downwards, aplasia of the lower parts is commoner than that of the upper. Complete absence is occasionally seen but it is often found that the abdominal ostium is present even if the rest of Müller's duct is absent. (See Fig. 43.)

(iii) **Uterus.** A complete failure of development of both Müllerian ducts is only possible if there is a simultaneous non-development of the urinary system. Similarly unilateral aplasia is very rare and is represented by uterus unicornis. This anomaly is usually associated with some developmental defect of the urinary system. It should be noted also that the absence of the vagina may be associated with a single ectopic pelvic kidney, and in such patients an intravenous pyelogram is advisable before any attempt at surgical reconstruction.

(iv) **Vagina.** In some patients the vagina fails to develop along the whole of its length. Usually there is a depression in the situation of the hymen, and the uterus, if present, is either duplicated or rudimentary. In patients of this kind the ovaries may function normally although menstruation and sexual intercourse are impossible. Such patients may wish to marry and be willing to undergo operation for the construction of an artificial vagina. Patients have very rarely been reported in whom an artificial vagina was constructed in the presence of a normal uterus, and who subsequently conceived and were successfully delivered by Caesarean section. In these patients the vaginal atresia has usually been the result of scarring from chemical burns or operative injury and infection, and not as the result of congenital defect, where the uterus is so grossly malformed that conception is impossible. Several methods have been used in the construction of an artificial vagina.

TREATMENT: The modern method of fashioning an artificial vagina due,

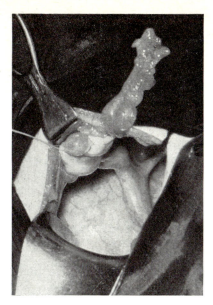

FIG. 75A. A patient with complete absence of the vagina in whom laparotomy disclosed entire aplasia of the genital tract with the exception of the upper half of both tubal ampulae.

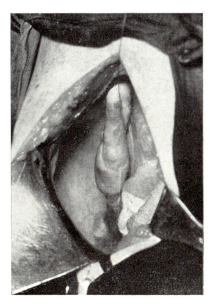

FIG. 75B. Ovary from same patient as Fig. A. The ovary occupied a position with its lower pole at the pelvic brim and its upper pole in the region of the kidney. This is the normal foetal position before pelvic migration.

in this country, to McIndoe is not only extremely simple but gives very good results. The patient is anaesthetised and placed in the lithotomy position. A transverse incision is made between the urethral orifice and the anus and the space between the urethra and the rectum is opened up. The separation is quite easy. A mould of polyvinyl sponge cut into the shape and size of the artificial tunnel created between the bladder and rectum is inserted into a Ferguson speculum of acceptable size and the speculum enclosed in a razor skin graft taken from the thigh. This graft is sewn down each side into the shape of a sack before being threaded over the speculum. The speculum covered with the graft and containing the sponge is inserted into the new vaginal cavity and gently pushed home. The speculum is now withdrawn leaving the graft in situ with the sponge mould exerting gentle, even, centrifugal pressure in all directions. Graft and mould are left in position by suturing the labia minora together over the base of the mould. The sponge is removed in 14 days and the patient is taught to insert by herself a plastic dilator which should be worn at night for four months. Thereafter natural coitus should be employed, though the dilator may be needed as an accessory for a few more months until all risk of contracture has passed. The artificial vagina is quite acceptable both psychologically and as a functional unit.

Williams' Operation. As an alternative to the skin grafting operation. This is a much simpler operative procedure in which an artificial vaginal tunnel is created by suturing together the labia minora. No attempt is made to open the space between the urethra and the rectum. The tunnel created between the labia minora by the Williams' operation provides an artificial vagina which is psychologically and functionally satisfactory.

Hypoplasia

This is more common than aplasia. One of the best-known examples is the foetal uterus or, as it may be more accurately called, the uterus bicornis rudimentarius solidus in which the uterus is not canalised and menstruation is impossible. Asymmetrical hypoplasia is seen typically in the uterus unicornis with rudimentary accessory cornu. An accessory cornu may be either solid or it may be canalised, in which case, unless it communicates with the main cavity of the uterus, its menstrual discharge is retained with a resulting haematometra in the mal-developed half of the uterus which presents clinically as a tender swelling attached to the uterus. In some cases of accessory cornu a fertilised ovum becomes implanted and gives rise to an ectopic gestation within a rudimentary cornu.

Symmetrical hypoplasia of the uterus, less severe in degree than that seen in uterus rudimentarius solidus, is seen in the infantile uterus and in the uterus which is termed the small adult uterus or the pubescent uterus. In the newborn, the body of the uterus is relatively ill-developed so that the cervix is longer than the body. All grades of development between a uterus of this type and a normal adult uterus are known. In the hypoplastic uterus of the adult, the cervix is long, slender and conical with a small external os, the so-called and misnamed congenital hypertrophy of the cervix. The body of the uterus is smaller than normal and quite frequently is acutely anteflexed.

The clinical condition termed **hypoplasia genitalis** is more often diagnosed than anatomically tenable and is recorded as being primarily due to a functional insufficiency of the ovaries. The uterus is of the small adult type with a slender conical cervix, a cavity of 5 cms. or less with poorly developed endometrium, and the vagina is short and narrow. The vulva itself is small, the labia contain only a small amount of fat and the perineum is depressed to produce what is termed a scaphoid perineum. Frequently the uterus is congenitally retroflexed: sometimes it is acutely anteflexed, producing a form called the cochleate uterus. The Fallopian tubes are relatively long, they show a well-marked tortuosity, and the plicae are ill-developed. The ovaries are elongated and often lie higher in the pelvis than normally.

The onset of puberty is usually delayed and menstruation is often irregular, so that the menstrual cycle is prolonged to between six and eight weeks. Severe dysmenorrhoea is a common symptom and there is a tendency for such patients to be sterile. The patients are usually of the "petite" type with small bones and the pelvis is of the generally contracted type.

The clinical syndrome is easily recognised, and such patients are frequently seen in gynaecological practice because of the attendant symptoms of dysmenorrhoea, sterility, dyspareunia and frigidity.

Atresia

The most important malformations are the result of failure of canalisation of the Müllerian ducts, which it should be recalled occurs progressively from above downwards.

Atresia of the Fallopian tubes may be partial or complete, when it gives rise to sterility. (See Fig. 75).

Complete atresia of the body of the uterus is a very rare malformation, but partial atresia in one half of the Müllerian duct system is seen in the rudimentary horn of a bicornuate uterus and on the deformed side there may also be an atresia of the cervix. When the patient menstruates this may give rise to a unilateral heamatometra in the rudimentary horn.

Congenital atresia of the vagina, in which the vagina is imperforate, is a rare malformation. In such cases the occlusion of the vagina is situated either in the upper third of the vagina or immediately above the level of the hymen. The commonest form of atresia that is seen is so called **imperforate hymen.** In this condition the membrane occluding the vaginal orifice consists of two layers, the lower of which represents the normal hymen, while above this and adherent to it lies an imperforate septum which is found on histological examination to be covered by transitional epithelium on its inner surface. Such cases are attributed to failure of the lowest part of the Müllerian ducts or the sinovaginal bulbs to canalise rather than to failure of that part of the cloacal membrane which forms the hymen to break down. Atresia of the vagina and of the hymen is not necessarily a congenital malformation. Such inflammatory conditions as gonococcal vulvovaginitis of children and the very rare diphtheritic infection of the genitalia can lead to the formation of adhesions which produce atresia. Douching with strong antiseptic solutions such as lysol or corrosive sublimate, usually in an attempt to procure abortion or avert venereal disease, may result in sloughing of the vagina. During healing the raw surfaces adhere with scarring and atresia. Similarly, the cervix may became occluded after such cervical operations as partial amputation and repair, in which technical errors have been made. It also occasionally results from cauterisation of the endocervix or the operation of diathermy conisation. Menstrual blood then collects in the uterus and produces haematometra.

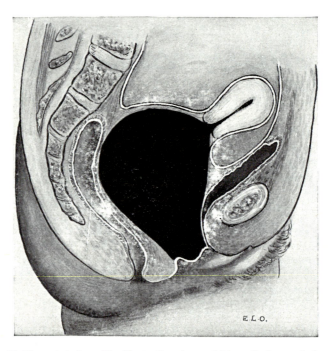

FIG. 76. Haematocolpos. The illustration shows: (*a*) how the hymen bulges externally; (*b*) how the distended vagina is easily palpable from the rectum; (*c*) how the uterus can be felt from the abdomen on the top of the swelling; (*d*) how retention of urine may result from elongation of the urethra. (After Stoeckel.)

Haematocolpos. The most important type of atresia is the congenital form in which the lower end of the vagina is imperforate either just above the hymen or at its level. The obstruction is not therefore necessarily the hymen which is present and normal below the atresia. The history obtained reveals that the expected onset of menstruation is delayed and that at monthly intervals the patient complains of pain in the lower abdomen and of such general disturbances as headaches, constipation and malaise. The patient or the patient's mother may seek medical advice either because the onset of menstruation has been delayed or because retention of urine has developed. The patients are usually about 16 years of age. In cases of imperforate hymen menstruation proceeds rhythmically, but the menstrual discharge becomes pent up in the vagina and causes the condition known as haematocolpos. By the time the patient seeks medical advice a large tumour has developed which fills the pelvis and which can be easily palpated in the lower abdomen and may be visible when the patient is examined from a lateral viewpoint. On vaginal examination the imperforate hymen bulges externally and the retained dark-coloured blood can be seen through the thin almost translucent septum. The retained menstrual discharge is fluid, consists of mucus and altered blood and contains a high percentage of calcium (see Figs. 76 to 79).

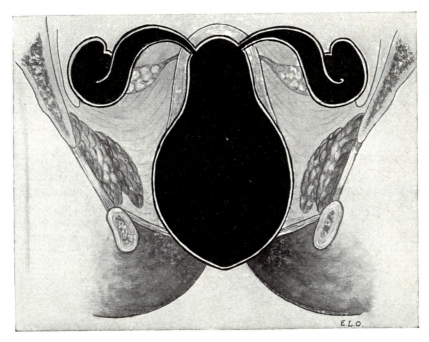

FIG. 77. Atresia hymenalis with haematocolpos, haematometra and haematosalpinx. (After Stoeckel.)

The vagina is capable of very great distension, so that in cases of haematocolpos it is not uncommon for a large tumour to be found which almost completely fills the pelvis, pushes the bladder forwards and upwards, almost occludes the rectum, and extends out of the pelvis into the abdominal cavity. The contents may amount to three or four pints. The uterus can be palpated on the upper surface of the tumour by abdominal examination. In late cases of haematocolpos the pent-up menstrual discharge not only fills the vagina but distends the uterus and produces a haematometra. The blood may extend upwards into the Fallopian tubes and pass into the peritoneal cavity where, by producing peritoneal irritation, adhesions are formed around the

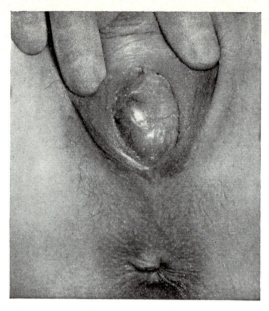

FIG. 78. Vaginal introitus of a girl aged 16 showing bulging membrane due to haematacolpos.

abdominal ostium of the Fallopian tube which close the lumen and lead to the production of a haematosalpinx. Such cases, however, are extremely rare, and in most instances of imperforate hymen the retention of blood is restricted to the vagina. Haematometra and haematosalpinx should be regarded as very exceptional complications of imperforate hymen. Very rarely

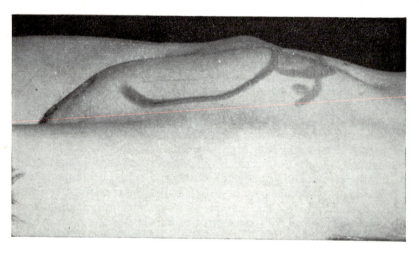

FIG. 79. The same case as Fig. 78 showing the surface markings of the uterus and vaginal tumour.

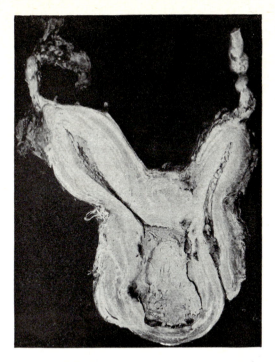

Fig. 80. Double uterus. The right cornu does not communicate with the vagina but the left cornu does. On the right side the cervical canal was distended with menstrual blood which subsequently became infected and led to salpingitis and pelvic peritonitis.

the haematosalpinx ruptures and discharges its contents suddenly into the peritoneal cavity, when severe pain is produced and the patient passes into a condition of shock and collapse very similar to that seen in a case of ruptured extrauterine gestation.

Diagnosis

The diagnosis of haematocolpos is made without difficulty, because the bulging septum at the vaginal orifice is obvious. Simple haematocolpos, in which the retention of the menstrual discharge is restricted to the vagina, should not be regarded as a dangerous condition. If, however, the uterus and Fallopian tubes have become distended with blood, the condition is potentially dangerous because of the risk of ascending infection. The retained menstrual fluid affords an excellent medium for the growth of micro-organisms, and pelvic peritonitis may follow evacuation of a haematocolpos if it is complicated by haematometra and haematosalpinx. For this reason the abdomen should be examined carefully in cases of haematocolpos, and if the uterus is enlarged or if there is tenderness in the region of the Fallopian tubes a graver prognosis must be given. In vaginal atresia and cervical atresia where the obstruction affects the upper vagina or cervix, distension of the uterus and Fallopian tubes with blood is much more frequent than with atresia at the lower end of the vagina.

A comparable form of atresia is that in which the uterus is bicornuate with one horn of the uterus shut off from the vagina, in which the menstrual discharge is retained. Such cases are met with clinically in patients who are usually over the age of 20, and there is a variety of types. Sometimes there is duplication both of the uterus and the vagina, when a large tumour, comparable in size to that found in cases of haematocolpos, may develop. The more common form is when the maldevelopment is restricted to the uterus and the menstrual discharge is retained in an accessory horn. Severe abdominal pain is then complained of, and on examination a tense, tender, fluctuating tumour is found to one side of the uterus. Not uncommonly the retained blood becomes infected and gives rise to salpingo-oöphoritis and pelvic peritonitis. The exact diagnosis is usually made at laparotomy, when it should be borne in mind that an accessory cornu is recognised by the position of attachment of the round ligament (see Fig. 80).

Treatment

The treatment of haematocolpos consists in excising the septum at the lower end of the vagina and of inserting, if necessary, a few haemostatic sutures in the cut edges. It is now known that the most important consideration is to determine whether the uterus and Fallopian tubes are distended with blood. After the evacuation of the haematocolpos, while the patient is still under the anaesthetic, the cervix should be exposed with specula. If the os is found to be closed it can be taken as certain that the menstrual discharge is not retained either in the uterus or in the Fallopian tubes and no further treatment is required. If, on the other hand, the cervix is dilated and a haematometra is present, no bimanual examination should be made for fear of disseminating any infection upwards and the patient must be given a full course of prophylactic antibiotics. As long as the response to conservative treatment is favourable it is unnecessary to do anything more than keep the patient under observation and, at the end of a month, perform a bimanual examination. It will then be found that uterus has involuted to normal and that all the abnexal swelling has subsided. The only untoward sequel may be tubal occlusion which can be treated later, if necessary, when the patient is married. It should be emphasised that haematometra and haematosalpinx are rare complications of haematocolpos because the patient will seek advice before the advent of this upward extension.

Müllerian Duct Anomalies

(Duplications and Malformations of the Uterus and Vagina)

If the two Müllerian ducts fail to fuse along the whole of their lengths, and if they develop normally and remain separate, a condition which is termed **uterus didelphys** results. In uterus didelphys, the two vaginas open at the vulva where a vaginal septum can be seen. A cervix lies at the top of each vagina and the two parts of the uterus above the level of the cervices

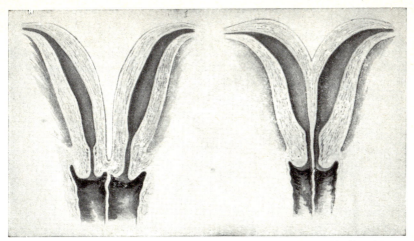

FIG. 81. Uterus didelphys.　　FIG. 82. Uterus bicornis bicollis with
septate vagina.

are completely separate since there is no fusion at any point between the two
halves of the uterine body (see Figs. 81 and 87).

From this complete degree of separation of the two Müllerian ducts
there are all sorts and varieties of imperfect and incomplete fusions. Very
few of these have any clinical importance, and most forms are extremely rare.
In **uterus duplex** and **vagina duplex** the two Müllerian ducts are partially
fused in the region of the body of the uterus, and one side is usually better
developed than the other (see Fig. 82).

In **uterus bicornis bicollis** the vagina is single, but the two cornua of the
uterus remain separate and two complete cervices project into the
vagina. Occasionally only a partial vaginal septum is present.

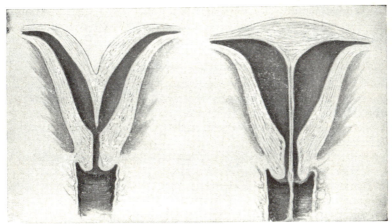

FIG. 83. A uterus bicornis unicollis.　　FIG. 84. A uterus septus.

In **uterus bicornis unicollis** the two cornua of the uterus are separate in the region of the body, but there is a single cervix and a single vagina (see Fig. 83).

In **uterus septus,** although the two Müllerian ducts have fused, a median septum passes from the fundus of the uterus through the cervix and may extend into the vagina (see Fig. 84).

In **uterus subseptus** this septum is restricted to the body of the uterus (see Fig. 85).

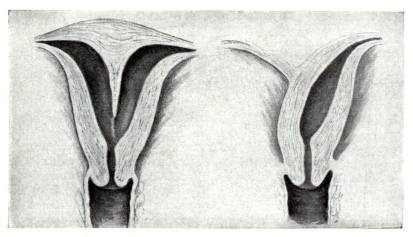

FIG. 85. A uterus subseptus.   FIG. 86. A uterus unicornis with a rudimentary horn.

Arcuate uterus. In this deformity, there is no actual septum in the region of the fundus but, instead of the usual dome-shaped convexity of the fundus, there is a shallow concave depression.

A **septate vagina** may be partial or complete as in uterus didelphys. If incomplete the septum, though it may occur only in the upper half, is usually situated in the lower end and represents an incomplete canalisation of the sino-vaginal bulbs.

Clinical Aspects of the Malformations of the Uterus

Such malformations as septate vagina may cause difficulties during coitus and during parturition. If the vaginal septum causes obstruction during childbirth it can easily be divided between clamps.

A partially or completely septate uterus may give rise to certain obstetric complications:

(1) Pregnancy in an accessory, rudimentary horn will be considered under extra-uterine gestation.

(2) These patients have a high incidence of abortion in the middle trimester and of premature labour.

(3) Malpresentations which resist correction may suggest a septate uterus, e.g. transverse lie is associated with an arcuate uterus.

(4) Obstructed labour can occur if one half of the uterus is impacted below the presenting part of the foetus in the other.

(5) Retained placenta is common and it is often when manual removal is being performed that the septate condition is first diagnosed.

The more complete the septum, the less the incidence of obstetric complications and, in fact, many patients with these anomalies have uneventful pregnancies and labours.

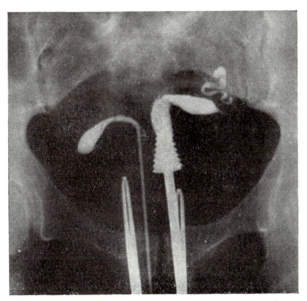

FIG. 87. Double hysterosalpingography of uterus didelphys. The screw cannula in the left cervix is radio-opaque; the right cannula does not show. Note that there is filling of the left Fallopian tube only.

Partial duplication of one or both Müllerian ducts is occasionally seen usually affecting the upper part of the tube where an accessory abdominal ostium may be found. Accessory Fallopian tubes have also been described.

Hermaphroditism and Pseudohermaphroditism

In true hermaphroditism the glands of both sexes must be present in the same individual. Such cases are very rare. In the museum of St. Bartholomew's Hospital there is a specimen obtained from an adult in whom the external genitalia were of the male type with normally developed penis and scrotum. Neither testis had descended into the scrotum and at post-mortem examination the uterus masculinus was represented by a uterus which was larger than the normal adult uterus, while on each side of the uterus was attached an ovary. Examples of this kind are extremely rare, and in most cases the accessory sex gland is atrophic and shows no evidence of functional activity.

In other cases the sex glands have been found to consist partly of ovarian and partly of testicular tissue. Berlinger has described an example of a combined gland (ovo-testis) in which follicles and corpora lutea as well as spermatogonia and spermatocytes were present.

In pseudo-hermaphroditism the sex glands are of one sex, while the external genitalia resemble those of the opposite sex. The ovaries may descend within the inguinal canal to lie in the labia majora, and if the clitoris is hypertrophied the external genitalia superficially resemble those of the male. This condition is best termed female pseudohermaphroditism (see Figs. 94 and 95). In the opposite type the testes fail to descend into the scrotum, the penis is ill-developed, and as a result of an extreme degree of hypospadias the external genitalia resemble those of the female (male pseudohermaphrodite).

Developmental Defects of Urogenital Sinus

(i) **Epispadias** is seen only rarely in women. There are different degrees of maldevelopment of the anterior wall of the urethra and bladder. In the mildest form the maldevelopment is restricted to the anterior parts of the labia minora and the clitoris; in some cases of this kind the symphysis pubis fails to develop, giving rise to the condition known as split pelvis. In such cases owing to the wide separation of the levator ani muscles the patients suffer from prolapse whether they have borne children or not.

Various plastic operations have been described to remedy the defect in the anterior wall of the urethra and to control the accompanying incontinence of urine.

(ii) **Ectopia Vesicae.** Ectopia vesicae is seen infrequently in the female. In this condition there is an absence both of the anterior wall of the bladder and of the lower part of the abdominal wall. The symphysis pubis also fails to develop, as does the anterior wall of the urethra. In ectopia vesicae the red mucous membrane of the bladder projects forwards in front of the anterior abdominal wall: the two ureteric orifices discharging urine are visible. Treatment consists in implanting the ureters into the sigmoid colon and subsequently closing the bladder and repairing the anterior abdominal wall.

(iii) **Hypospadias.** Hypospadias probably never occurs in the female.

Malformation of the Rectum and Anus

(i) **Imperforate Anus.** This condition is due to failure of the cloacal membrane to break down between the anal depression and the intestine.

(ii) **Atresia Recti.** The lower part of the rectum fails to develop, and such cases are much more unfavourable to treatment than the relatively simple atresia of the anus.

(iii) **Congenital Rectovaginal Fistulae.** Various types of malformations of the rectum and vagina are due to imperfect separation of the rectum from the urogenital sinus. In some cases the anus may be represented by a depression in the normal position, but the rectum opens on to the surface in the situation of the perineum, so called perineal anus. In other cases the lower part of the rectum ends partly by way of a normal anal canal and partly by way of a fistula opening on to the surface in the situation of the perineal body, or one opening into the posterior vaginal wall, termed the vaginal anus.

It is a surprising fact that patients who have an ectopic perineal or vaginal anus suffer little inconvenience and acquire quite good bowel control. During childbirth, however, there is a considerable risk of a severe and complicated third degree tear and for this reason these patients are best delivered by Caesarean section.

If surgical correction of a vaginal or perineal anus is contemplated the sphincter control of the normally situated transplanted anal canal may never be as good as the previously abnormal situation.

6 Sex and Intersexuality

The sex of an individual is the result of a number of different operative factors. It has been suggested that the basic sex is female and that masculinity of the male organs is the result of the influence of androgens on the developing Wolffian duct with a resultant atrophy of the Müllerian system. In other words, an early embryo is potentially bisexual up to the sixth week of intrauterine life.

In determining the sex of a patient, the following factors should be considered:

Denver System for Human Chromosomes

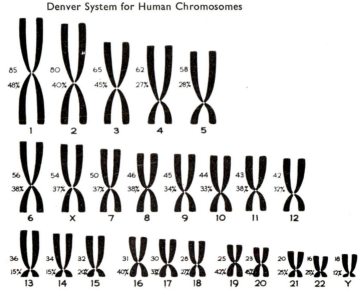

Fig. 88. An idealised chromosome set, numbered according to the internationally agreed Denver system. Note that only one of each pair is represented. The small figures beside each chromosome indicate approximately the relative length of the whole chromosome, and the proportion of the total length occupied by the short arm. (By permission of Dr. Bernard Lennox and *The Lancet*.)

Genetic Sex. The nuclei of humans contain a diploid number of chromosomes, 22 pairs of autosomes and 1 pair of sex chromosomes, making a total of 46. During maturation, a reduction division results in each ovum or spermatozoon containing only the haploid number of 22 unpaired autosomes and one sex chromosome. In the ovum, the sex chromosome is always X but, in the spermatozoon, it is either X or Y. The relative numbers of X and Y carrying spermatozoa is equal. As the spermatozoon carries either an X or a Y chromosome, fertilisation results in a 46 chromosome pattern carrying either an XX or XY—a genetic female or genetic male respectively. Thus the original diploid number of chromosomes is restored—22 pairs of autosomes plus the paired sex chromosome—46 in all. The chromosomal sex of an embryo is, therefore, determined at the very start of his or her career and every cell in the body is thereafter labelled by a chromosomal pattern either male or female. The fact that a very rare and select few may have abnormal chromosome arrangements such as is seen in Turner's and Klinefelter's syndrome need not invalidate this basic rule. Chromosomal sex can be determined by a study of the leucocytes or by simply taking a smear from the buccal mucosa. The nuclei of chromosomal females contain a small stainable body, the sex chromatin, and, therefore, female cells are termed chromatin positive. In epithelial cell nuclei this small peripherally situated, darkly staining nodule is called a Barr body. Male cell nuclei lack this body and are, therefore, chromatin negative. This chromatin nodule has been shown to consist of desoxyribonucleic acid. It measures 1μ in diameter and is present in approximately 75% of female cells. A distinctive and similar type of nuclear appendage, shaped like a drumstick, is seen attached to the nuclear substance of female neutrophils. It is also possible to sex eosinophils. The sex of the foetus can even be determined in utero by examining desquamated epithelium in the liquor amnii (see Fig. 89).

External Anatomical Sex. The shape of the body contours, the development of the musculature, the characteristics of the bones (notably the pelvis), the distribution of hair on face and body, and the external genitalia are strong presumptive evidence of either sex. The act of parturition is almost but not quite incontrovertible.

Internal Anatomical Sex. If, at laparotomy, a recognisable uterus, Fallopian tubes and ovaries are present, these female organs are strong presumptive evidence that the individual is a female. The rare exception is the true hermaphrodite.

Gonadal Sex. This depends on the histological appearance of the gonad from the study of a biopsy or from removal of the organ. It is not entirely diagnostic as in the case of an ovotestis in which both female and male elements are histologically demonstrated. Also, it is possible to have a rudimentary testis on one side and a rudimentary ovary on the other. Such findings are, however, so rare that the sex of the gonad is a reasonably reliable guide to the true sex of an individual.

Hormonal Influences. In the female pseudohermaphrodite, it has been seen that an excess production of androgenic hormone by adrenal cortical hyperplasia can modify the external genitalia of a genetic female. Hypertrophy of the phallus, fusion of the labia majora and hirsutism may cause the parents to consider their child to be a male. The virilising tumours of the ovary, such as arrhenoblastoma, can cause hirsutism, hypertrophy of the clitoris, deepening of the voice, masculine body contours and amenorrhoea. The exhibition

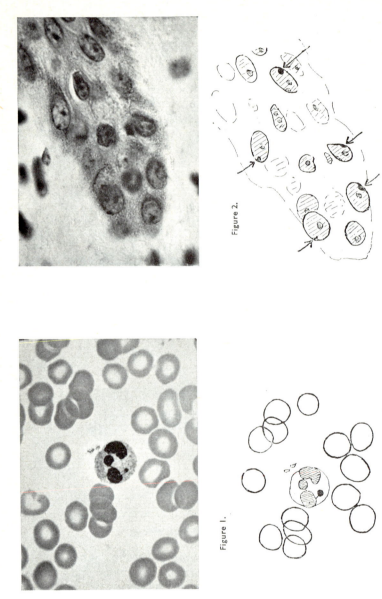

Figure 2.

Figure 1.

FIG. 89. (1) The typical chromatin nodule in a neutrophil leucocyte in the female. The nodule illustrated is $1 \cdot 4\mu$ in diameter, while neighbouring red blood cells measured on the average $7 \cdot 3\mu$. Coverslip preparation. Jenner Giemsa stain. × 1,200. (2) Typical nodules in the nuclei of the epithelial cells of the skin. An average nodule measures $1 \cdot 6 \times 0 \cdot 9\mu$, while red cells in a neighbouring blood vessel measured on the average $5 \cdot 6\mu$. × 1,200. (Davidson & Smith, 1956, *Postgrad. Med. J.*)

of oestrogen in the male can cause gynaecomastia. These are all examples of how hormones, natural or therapeutic, can modify but not alter the sexual organs and secondary sexual characteristics. Figs. 94 and 95.

Psychological Sex. Many men and women are psychologically dominated towards sexual inversion, a persistence of the childhood tendency. Effeminate behaviour, speech, dress and sexual inclination proclaim this fact. Transvestism is the most obvious and complete example where men dress in women's clothes and vice versa.

Environment and Upbringing. There are many examples of genetic males and females brought up by their parents in the mistaken sexual category who have acquired over the years the habits and mental inclinations of the opposite sex to a sufficient degree to pass as members of the wrong sex.

Clinical Diagnosis of Sex

External Appearance. Most men look like men and women like women because of the so-called secondary sexual characteristics. A man is broad-shouldered, more hirsute, especially about the face and chin, his scalp hair is coarser, his pubic hair grows in a triangular pattern with the apex towards the umbilicus; his nature is more aggressive and robust, his voice deep and his sexual instincts inclined to the heterosexual. A woman has narrow shoulders, broad hips, is rarely hirsute, has fine, abundant scalp hair, more delicately modelled features, and a typical pattern of pubic hair—a triangle, apex downwards with a flat base at the upper level of the mons; her voice is softer, her nature is supposed to be less self-assertive and aggressive than the male and her sexual instincts are heterosexual; a well developed breast is probably the strongest external evidence of femininity.

External Genitalia. In the male, the phallus is well developed, the urethra opens in the glans, the scrotum is rugose from the presence of the dartos muscle—an almost exclusively male possession—and the testicles are in the scrotum. In the female, the phallus is rudimentary, the urethra opens into the vestibule, the labia majora are smooth and bifid and do not possess a dartos muscle, and, as a rule, a vagina is present.

Internal Genitalia. Bimanual examination discloses a uterus and appendages in the female.

Signs of Feminism in the Male

External Appearance. Feminine figure, poor musculature, a tendency to obesity, high-pitched voice, absence of hirsutism and feminine personality and sexual inclinations. Gynaecomastia (Fig. 90).

External Genitalia. Hypospadias (urethra opening below phallus), underdevelopment of phallus, split scrotum and undescended testicles.

Clinical Examples

(A) Feminism: (i) *Male Pseudohermaphroditism*. There is often a strong familial tendency to this disorder and several examples may appear in the same family and in different generations. Apart from the external genitalia, male pseudo-hermaphrodites look like females and are brought up as such.

Their bodily conformity is male apart from scanty pubic and axillary hair. The phallus is usually under-developed with hypospadias and the testicles are undescended and mal-developed. A shallow vagina is sometimes present.

(ii) *Turner's Syndrome.* In this syndrome the genetic sex is usually male. The nucleus possesses only 45 chromosomes, i.e. 22 pairs of autosomes plus a sex chromosome XO. The absence of the Y chromosome resembles the female

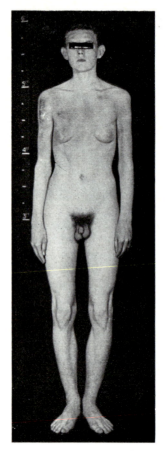

FIG. 90. Gynaecomastia in an otherwise obvious male.

but these patients are, like males, chromatin negative, i.e. their nuclei contain no nuclear satellite body and no drumsticks in the neutrophils. It should be explained here that the presence of a Barr body is dependent upon the presence of the second X chromosome and if the chromosome pattern is XXX or XXXY the extra X complement renders the eccentric chromatin nodule either larger in size or number.

The condition has been called ovarian **agenesis** or gonadal dysgenesis

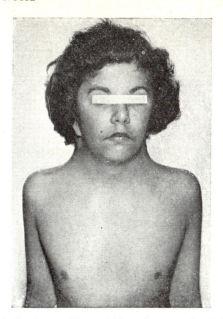

FIG. 91. Turner's Syndrome. Note webbing of neck and aplasia of breasts.

because, at laparotomy, the gonad is found to consist of undifferentiated stroma with absence of sex cells, a mere strip of fibrous tissue attached to the back of the broad ligament like a pale strip—the so-called "streak" gonad. The patients are clinically of short stature though not actual dwarfs, the trunk is muscular, the neck is short and webbed, cubitus valgus is notable, the breasts are not developed and pubic and axillary hair is scanty or absent (Figs. 91 and 92). Exaggerated epicanthic folds may be present, one of the obvious defects first noticeable on examining the patient. The vagina and

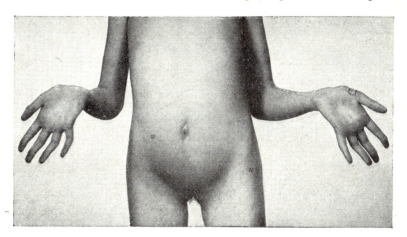

FIG. 92. Turner's Syndrome. Note marked cubitus valgus.

uterus, if present, are under- or mal-developed. Other gross congenital abnormalities are present such as coarctation of the aorta which is, incidentally, commoner in males than in females. Deformities of the digits are also seen.

The classical picture of Turner's Syndrome as described should have a chromosomal pattern of XO. There are, however, variants in which the mosaicism of XO/XX or even XO/XY produce less clear-cut syndromes, e.g. a normal appearing female apart from gonadal dysgenesis.

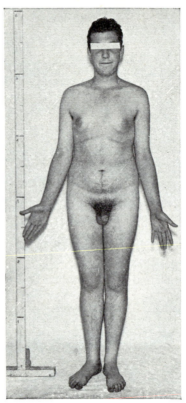

Fig. 93. Klinefelter's syndrome. Note the superficially normal male genitalia, gynaecomastia and tendency towards female distribution of pubic hair.

Superfemale (Triple X chromosome). The possession of an extra X is not excessively rare since it is quite compatible with complete feminine normality. There is, however, a well recognised triple X syndrome in which the patient, often mentally subnormal, suffers from scanty or irregular menstruation and infertility. Clinical examination may reveal hypoplasia of the genital tract. The importance of chromosomal studies in such a patient is obvious and will play an increasing role in our future investigations.

Klinefelter's Syndrome. The patient with this rare disorder externally resembles a male in general body conformity, the penis is small or normal in size, the testes are small but, as a rule, are normally placed although there is, on biopsy, hyaline degeneration of the seminiferous tubules as a result of which sterility may be the presenting symptom. Gynaecomastia is frequently present and the voice may be high-pitched and the appearance eunuchoid. The patient is often mentally defective or delinquent. Most of these patients are sex chromatin positive like females because of the extra X complement and chromosome analysis shows them to possess 47 chromosomes instead of the normal 46 due to the presence of an XXY chromosome. Fig. 93.

(B) Virilism. In patients exhibiting virilism, the chromosomal and gonadal sex is female and the accessory sex organs of the Müllerian origin are also female. The external genitalia, however, resemble the male.

Clinical Features. The body conformity is largely male with good muscular development and broad shoulders. The voice is deep and the thyroid cartilage prominent. Hirsutism is present to a remarkable degree, with a male distribution of hair. One patient of the author's shaves daily and, though only 23 years of age, shows signs of incipient baldness of masculine distribution. Legs and arms are also hirsute. The psychological sex is often, but not invariably, male.

The external genitalia show hypertrophy of the clitoris and fusion of the labia majora due to failure of the cloacal membrane to divide. The vagina is often absent if the cause is congenital. Figs. 94 and 95. The breasts are underdeveloped.

Clinical Varieties. (1) *Adreno-genital Syndrome*. This is due to a hyperplasia of the adrenal cortex and there are two types:

(*a*) **Congenital or intra-uterine adreno-genital syndrome** in which the primary defect is a block in the conversion of 17-hydroxyprogesterone into hydrocortisone due to an enzyme failure. The normal adrenal cortex produces three C_{21} compounds: hydrocortisone, corticosterone and aldosterone, and, in addition, certain androgens—C_{19} compounds. The production of 17-hydroxyprogesterone which is mildly androgenic in action is controlled by ACTH and this, in turn, is controlled by the reciprocal action of hydrocortisone. If, therefore, the hydrocortisone—ACTH inter-action is upset by a deficiency of hydrocortisone, the pituitary produces an excess of ACTH which leads to adrenal cortical hyperplasia and excess output of androgens, notably 17-hydroxyprogesterone. The main androgenic activity of 17-hydroxyprogesterone is due to its conversion into $\triangle^4$ androstenedione and hence to other orthodox androgens. These androgens are responsible for the virilising effects on the urogenital sinus and hypertrophy of the clitoris results with persistence of fusion of the labia majora to resemble a scrotum. The miniature vagina opens into the urogenital sinus and the external appearance is that of a male with hypospadias. The diagnostic feature is the very high value of 17-ketosteroids excreted. As expected the chromosomal pattern in these girls is invariably XX.

The treatment of this condition consists in the exhibition of cortisone or hydrocortisone or the newer synthetic corticosteroids such as prednisone or prednisolone (2.5 mgms. twice daily is an adequate maintenance dose in the

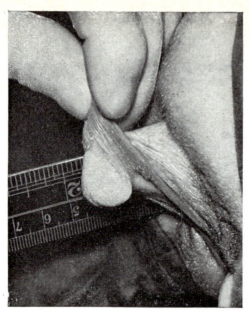

FIG. 94. Phallus of female pseudohermaphrodite showing hypertrophy and masculine appearance of glans.

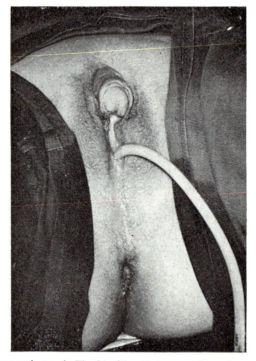

FIG. 95. Same patient as in Fig. 94 with catheter passed into immature vagina.

adult and will restore the output of 17-ketosteroids to normal). The continued use of these drugs carries certain dangers of adrenal deficiency due to suppression of ACTH and this especially operates at times of stress as, for example, if the patient needs an anaesthetic at which time cortisone coverage should be given during the period of stress (i.e. one day before, on the day of operation and for three days afterwards) (Fig. 96).

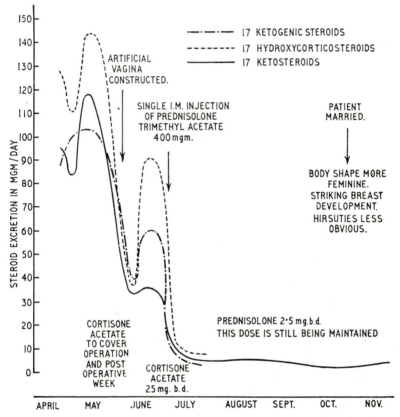

Fig. 96. Ketosteroid excretion of patient illustrated in Figs. 94 and 95, showing excellent response to corticosteroids. (This patient is now happily married following the construction of an artificial vagina by McIndoe's method.)

The vulval abnormality is simply corrected by a small plastic operation and as a rule it is wise to amputate the hypertrophied clitoris between 5 and 10 years of age.

Certain cases of virilisation of the foetus in utero have been reported following the use of progesterone in the pregnant mother. The synthetic progestogens ethisterone and nor-ethisterone are comparatively more potently androgenic. In fact all progestogens if given in sufficient dosage are suspect with the exception of 17α hydroxyprogesterone caproate, so that if progestogen is to be used at all on the pregnant woman this is the drug of choice at the present time of writing.

The effect on the foetus depends largely on the duration of pregnancy at the time of administration and on the dosage employed. If progestogens are given before the 12th–14th week of gestation the neonatal picture may be similar to that of the intra-uterine adreno-genital syndrome, i.e. enlarged phallus and imperforate perineal membrane.

(*b*) **Post-natal adreno-genital syndrome.** This can be due to an excessive output of ACTH from a basophil adenoma of the anterior pituitary (Cushing's syndrome) which gives rise to adrenal cortical hyperplasia. An adrenal tumour which can be benign or malignant has the same effect. An adrenal tumour is not dependent on pituitary influence.

(2) *Certain Virilising Tumours and Conditions of the Ovary* such as arrhenoblastoma, hilus cell tumour, Stein Leventhal syndrome and hyperthecosis. These ovarian causes of virilism produce a clinical picture somewhat similar to the post-natal adreno-genital syndrome.

In the post-natal variety of virilism, the genital tract is normal but the clitoris enlarges, the uterus atrophies with resulting amenorrhoea, the voice deepens, hirsutism is marked and the breasts atrophy. 17-ketosteroid excretion is raised only if the adrenal is hyperplastic or neoplastic, whereas with a virilising ovarian tumour it is unaltered.

Treatment of Female Pseudohermaphroditism

(1) If the fault is an enzyme block at the level of 17-hydroxyprogesterone, the exhibition of cortisone or synthetic corticosteroid will effectively control the excess production of ACTH. The external genitalia can be restored to a feminine pattern by plastic surgery, e.g. the formation of an artificial vagina by McIndoe's operation if the patient is engaged or married. Cortisone therapy, if successful, may restore menstruation in a patient with amenorrhoea. It is important in such patients to correct any anatomical defect of the lower genital tract in order to obviate the complication of retained menstrual products such as haematocolpos or haematometra.

(2) If the virilism is due to adrenal hyperplasia or tumour, surgical removal is the method of choice. This also applies to ovarian androgenic tumours or conditions.

(3) A regular maintenance dose of oestrogen is usually effective in restoring some of the secondary sex characteristics, e.g. breast development.

(4) The most effective treatment of facial hirsutism is shaving and cosmetics.

Summary of the Management of the Intersexual Patient

In the determination of a patient's sex, some of the following investigations will be used:

FIG. 97. A study of this admirable illustration—the Spectrum of Sex—reveals the various possibilities of sexual aberration in diagrammatic and tabular form. (By kind permission of Dr. C. N. Armstrong and the Hon. Editors of the *Proc. Roy. Soc. Med.*)

Comparative table of sexual characteristics across normal and intersex conditions. (Gonad and external-anatomy cells in the original are anatomical drawings rather than text.)

Condition	Nuclear Sex Chromatin	Oestrogens	Androgens	Phallus: Penis	Phallus: Clitoris	Micturition	Menstruation	Fertility	Psychological Sex	Aetiology
Normal female	+	normal F	normal F		normal size	normal	normal	+	F.	genetic
Simple constitutional masculinism	+ but lesser % in polymorphs		increased for female		normal size		irregular or amenorrhoea	+ or –	F.	genetic/or hormone
Adreno-genital masculinism	+		increased for female++		enlarged		absent	–	F.	genetic/or hormone
Female homosexual	+ occasionally – in polymorphs	normal F	normal F		normal to enlarged		normal or irregular	+	M. or F.	genetic or psychological
Female transvestism	+	normal F	normal F		normal to enlarged		normal or irregular	+	Neutral or M.	genetic
Female intersex I without adrenal disorder	+	normal F	normal F		enlarged++		normal	–	F or M	genetic
True hermaphroditism	+ or –		normal or low	normal penis...or enlarged clitoris			usually absent	–	F or M	genetic
Turner's syndrome	rarely +	low			normal size		absent	–	F.	genetic
Swyer's syndrome	?	high	normal		normal to enlarged		amenorrhoea	–	F.	genetic
Male intersex II "testicular feminisation syndrome"	–	normal M	normal M		normal size		absent	–	F.	genetic
Klinefelter's syndrome	rarely –	not increased	< normal	small to moderate size				–	Neutral or M.	genetic
Male transvestism	rarely +	n to >n for male	deficient for male	small				– or +	Neutral or F.	genetic
Male homosexual	–	normal M	normal M.	normal size				+	M, F, or both	genetic or psychological
Adreno-genital feminism	–	probably >n for male	increased++	normal size				–	M.	hormone
Simple constitutional feminism	–	diminished for male	diminished for male	small				+	M. or rarely F.	genetic/or hormone
Male with hypospadias	–	normal M	normal M	small (often mistaken for enlarged clitoris)				–	M.	genetic
Normal male	–	normal M	normal M	normal size				+	M.	genetic

(1) Genetic, chromosomal or nuclear sexing is simple and reliable from a study of buccal smears, skin biopsy or neutrophil examination.

(2) The external genitalia should be examined, preferably under an anaesthetic, when, for example, a vagina may be discovered concealed by fusion of the labia majora. Contrast radiography is sometimes helpful. By instilling a radio opaque fluid into the urethral opening in the perineal membrane a vagina may be demonstrated by the colpogram in a case of intra-uterine adreno-genital syndrome. At this examination, the pelvic contents can be investigated, e.g. the presence of uterus and appendages.

(3) Gonadal biopsy of the testis in an apparent male or

(4) Laparotomy and gonadal biopsy in the apparent female provide an opportunity for direct examination of the internal genitalia. The presence of rudimentary or under-developed Müllerian structures strongly suggest a female sex.

Culdoscopy and·or peritoneoscopy is an alternative to laparotomy but rarely as informative.

(5) Estimation of oestrogen and 17-keto steroids in the urine.

(6) Estimation of serum electrolytes.

(7) Intravenous pyelogram and pneumography of the adrenal.

(8) X-ray of the pituitary fossa and the skeleton.

(9) Psychological assessment of patient's sex.

The gynaecologist will naturally consult his endocrinological and psychiatric colleagues before finally deciding on diagnosis and treatment which is usually best deferred until after puberty when the pragmatic sex of the individual declares itself, that is the sex to which the individual shows greatest inclination and attitude. At this consultation the parents should be available as their co-operation and intelligent supervision is vital to the ultimate interests of the inter-sexual individual (see Fig. 97).

7 The Vulva

The vulva is a region in which three specialities are interested, namely, gynaecology, dermatology and venereology, and this unfortunate division of sovereignty has led in the past to multiplication of disease nomenclature with resulting confusion to the student. It is therefore proper to state that as part of the external genitalia the vulva primarily belongs to the province of the gynaecologist and that most lesions of this region will come to him in the first instance for diagnosis and treatment. Before referring them to his colleagues he must be capable of making an accurate diagnosis in his own right.

Anatomy

The boundaries of the vulva when viewed in the lithotomy position consist of the lower part of the mons veneris superiorly, the perineum inferiorly, and the labia majora laterally. The inner limit of the vulva is the introitus of the vagina bounded by the hymen, beyond which the vagina proper begins. The clitoris, urethral orifice and Bartholin's gland being contained in these boundaries are conveniently considered as part of the vulva. The labia minora are naturally contained in this area and form an important part of the vulva.

Congenital Abnormalities. Maldevelopment of the vulva is seen in the condition known as hypoplasia, when the pubic hair is scanty and the labia minora are small. It is not to be confused with the atrophic condition of kraurosis which is seen in postmenopausal women or in those who have undergone surgical or radiation castration, and to which it bears a superficial resemblance, apart from belonging to quite a different age group.

The condition of superficial vulval atresia is best regarded as an acquired lesion, the result of adhesive inflammation, which can occur at any age though it may be present at birth. In this condition the labia majora are adherent and the urine escapes from a small orifice situated anteriorly. The adhesions consist of granulation and fibrous tissue and can be quite readily separated by blunt or sharp dissection.

Hypertrophy of the labia minora and clitoris may be seen as a rare occurrence. Congenital hypertrophy of the clitoris is to be differentiated from that caused by the adreno-genital syndrome and virilising tumours of the adrenal gland and the ovary. Acquired hypertrophy of the labia minora is said to be the result of sexual malpraxis, though the evidence for this is slender. Hypospadias may involve the urethra, and the intersexual condition of pseudohermaphroditism has already been mentioned, in which the vaginal introitus is concealed by a persistent perineal membrane. Very rarely the vagina and anal canal may open into a common cloaca.

Abnormalities of the Hymen have already been described on p. 151. It may be of importance medico-legally to be able to state whether defloration has occurred. In most cases there is no difficulty, for the unruptured hymen has a small opening, shows no scars, and is not distensible sufficiently to admit a finger without causing pain. On the other hand, the opening may be congenitally wider than the normal and the hymen may be sufficiently elastic to allow coitus without undergoing laceration. It is very rare indeed for the hymen of a virgin to admit two fingers. A ring of hymeneal tissue can always be palpated in a virgin and inspection will show no evidence of laceration. Rigidity of the hymen may prevent sexual intercourse and an imperforate hymen leads to the development of a haematocolpos.

Injuries of the Vulva. Minor injuries to the hymen nearly always occur at defloration. Multiple small lacerations occur resulting in a small or moderate haemorrhage which ceases in a few minutes and requires no treatment other than reassurance. Healing is complete in 3–4 days and intercourse should be avoided during this time.

Severe injuries to the hymen resulting from intercourse occurs when a single laceration extends to beyond the hymeneal ring to involve a branch of the vaginal artery. Moderate haemorrhage occurs and continues for several hours so that the patient may become exanguinated. The treatment is to examine the patient under general anaesthesia and undersew the bleeding vessel with 00 plain catgut. No antibiotics are required.

Direct violence, childbirth injuries and ruptured varicose veins may lead to the development of a haematoma which may reach considerable proportions. A vulval haematoma may develop after a repair operation done for prolapse where inadequate haemostasis in the depths of the wound is combined with too tight a suture of the skin. Not only is a large superficial haematoma produced but the upward extent of the contained blood and clot may reach the retroperitoneal tissues of the pelvis.

One of the most remarkable examples of vulval haematoma follows enucleation of a Bartholin's cyst where the incision has been tightly closed by primary suture. There is a large unilateral swelling extending superiorly to the mons, laterally to the thigh and inferiorly to the buttock. It is a mistake to close such an incision, which should be packed or drained. The treatment of a haematoma resulting from suture is to remove the sutures, turn out the clot and pack the wound. Since the adoption of the Marsupialisation operation for Bartholin's cyst and abscess this complication is now rare.

Perineal Lacerations almost always result from rupture of the perineum during childbirth. If the laceration is complete the posterior vaginal wall communicates with the anterior wall either of the anal canal or rectum. The torn external sphincter retracts backwards and the severed edges lie beneath depressions on each side of the anal orifice. Incomplete tears of the perineum are represented by bands of scar tissue which involve the skin of the perineal body (see Fig. 98).

Oedema of the Vulva. This may occur in pre-eclamptic toxaemia and occasionally in nephritis and morbus cordis. Severe oedema is particularly characteristic of a primary syphilitic sore. Some degree of oedema can be recognised in all forms of inflammation of the vulva, and is sometimes a feature of moniliasis. Angioneurotic oedema may involve the vulva in a form which is sometimes referred to as menstrual oedema.

Varicose Veins of the Vulva. Varicosities of the external genitalia are fairly common, and are particularly well marked during pregnancy. The varicose veins involve the labia majora.

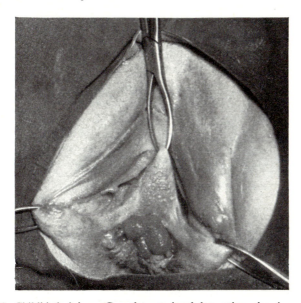

FIG. 98. Childbirth injury. Complete perineal laceration showing mucosa of anterior anal canal in direct continuity with posterior vaginal wall, no perineum intervening.

Inflammations of the Vulva

In vulvitis the vulva is swollen, reddened, tender, and covered with slight or profuse exudation. In severe cases the inflammation involves the skin of the adjacent areas of the thighs although the majority of diseases is limited to the vulva by the skin crease just lateral to the labia majora. The patient complains of burning, itching and tenderness. As the result of scratching and laceration of the skin, extensive excoriations develop.

Classification. It is very difficult to devise an accurate and serviceable classification of the inflammatory lesions of the vulva, and the author is conscious of the inadequacy of the following attempt since it includes lesions which are not strictly inflammatory, e.g. leukoplakia.

ACUTE AND CHRONIC INFLAMMATORY LESIONS:

(1) Inflammatory Lesions principally affecting the Vulva itself:
Pyogenic infection of the hair follicles of the mons and labia majora:

Folliculitis, furunculosis and intertrigo. The latter is due to irritation and infection of retained secretions in the skin folds, usually of the obese patient, and the friction of unhygienic underclothes or sanitary towels. These lesions exactly resemble those seen elsewhere in the body and the treatment is by general and local hygiene, local antiseptics such as Hibitane or pHisoHex cream together with local or systemic antibiotics.

Infected Sebaceous Cysts.

Infections resulting from Trauma—accidental, coital, obstetric and operative. An infected episiotomy or colpo-perineorrhaphy wound provides a good example. In these the best treatment is to cut out the superficial sutures and give frequent warm hypertonic saline baths, local radiant heat and systemic antibiotics if the patient has a pyrexia or systemic symptoms.

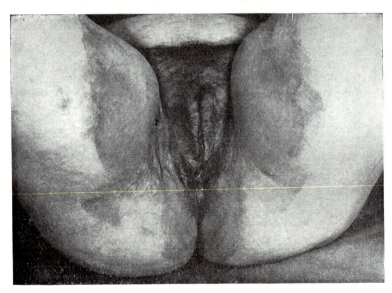

Fig. 99. Diabetic vulvitis. The illustration shows the distribution of the affected skin.

The most important traumatic cause of vulval infections is scratching with the nails, and this frequently converts a primary vulval condition into a secondary infective condition.

Venereal Infections of the Vulva. See Chapter 9.

Erysipelas of the Vulva, which is now a very rare disease and readily amenable to antibiotic therapy.

Vulvo-vaginitis in children—frequently gonococcal, see p. 227 and 243.

Senile Vulvo-vaginitis. These last two conditions are primarily vaginal and are discussed under vaginitis (see p. 228).

(2) Inflammatory Lesions primarily infecting Structures in the Vulva

Infections of Bartholin's Gland. In acute gonorrhoea, Bartholin's glands are tender and swollen, pus can be seen emerging from the duct, and in severe cases the gland suppurates to produce a Bartholin's abscess. Unless the abscess is incised it bursts on the inner surface of the labium minus and leads to the development of a temporary blind fistula. Subsequently, abscesses recur and the hard, indurated gland can always be felt in the presence of a fistula of this type. Bartholinitis is by no means invariably gonococcal and often results from the infection of a Bartholin's cyst with pyogenic organisms and *B. coli*.

Infections of the Para- and Sub-Urethral Glands, usually the result of chronic urethritis, often of gonococcal origin.

(3) **Secondary Inflammatory Lesions of the Vulva** (the primary site being elsewhere)

Trichomonas infection of the vagina. In this condition the vulva is frequently involved, being inflamed, oedematous and red. The profuse purulent vaginal discharge is characteristic and contains minute gas bubbles. The condition is fully discussed on pp. 223 and 253.

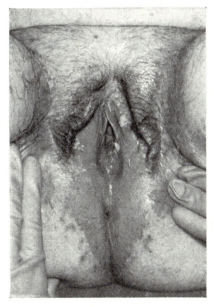

Fig. 100. Moniliasis of vulva. Note the glazed appearance of the vulva and the white cheese-like plaques.

Moniliasis. This fungal infection caused by candida albicans particularly affects the obese, hyperhidrotic, pregnant, diabetic patient and is a common sequel of systemic antibiotic treatment, after which the candida can be isolated from the anal canal, which may secondarily infect the perineum and vulva. While it is usually obvious in the vagina, the vulva may be the apparent primary situation. Well-marked erythema and oedema of the vulva with intense pruritus are suggestive. The diagnosis may be made by culture on Nickerson's medium which inhibits growth of bacteria, permitting Candida to grow in the form of dark brown or black colonies. The condition is always associated with vaginal candida infection so the treatment is the same as for vaginal moniliasis. Local antifungal cream (such as Mycostatin) will relieve the intense irritation very rapidly (Fig. 100).

Diabetic Vulvitis is often complicated by moniliasis. The vulva and adjacent skin are reddened and beefy in appearance, the skin is thickened and often brownish in colour. Pruritus leads to scratching and small abrasions are produced which exude discharge. Small infected hair follicles and furunculosis may present. The candida albicans and pyogenic organisms can be detected in the discharge.

The appearance of the vulva in diabetic vulvitis is characteristic. The inflammation is widespread and involves the surrounding skin. The skin of the labia majora has a peculiar grey colour with brownish patches, while small ill-defined ulcers involve the labia minora. Lastly, over the whole of the infected area are scales of coagulated discharge (see Fig. 99).

Vulvitis secondary to a chronic infected lesion of the cervix such as erosion or endocervicitis which cause profuse muco-purulent discharge.

Vulvitis Secondary to a Urinary or Bowel Fistula. Very severe degrees of secondary vulvitis result from urinary fistula. The skin becomes macerated and inflamed. The vulvitis often spreads and involves the skin around the anus and down the thighs.

(4) *Rare Inflammatory Lesions of the Vulva*

Vincent's Angina. This condition of the vulva clinically resembles that seen in the mouth with which it may be associated. The diagnosis is made bacteriologically by isolating the spirilla which is sensitive to large doses of penicillin.

Tuberculosis of the vulva is discussed on p. 265 and in Chapter 10.

Actinomycosis is extremely rare and presents the usual characteristic brawny lesion with typical sulphur granules in the discharge. Multiple sinuses may be present with fistula formation.

Skin Conditions Affecting the Vulva:

Tinea Cruris. Ringworm of the groin, thigh and vulva is extremely rare in the female. Ringworm was frequently seen in the groin, thigh and scrotum of the male but does not usually affect the female and when it does so is due to the organism tricophyton rubrum and usually similar lesions are present in the feet between the toes, the so-called athlete's foot. This fungus infection is encouraged by moisture from sweating and inadequate hygiene, and tends to be chronic and to relapse after treatment. The characteristic bright red circumscribed areas are found in the skin flexures of the thigh and outer aspect of the labia. A fine papular rash is usual and its area is sharply demarcated from the adjacent healthy skin. The intense itching provokes scratching as a result of which a secondary infection results and is superimposed on the primary lesion.

Treatment consists in meticulous hygiene, elimination of fungus infection elsewhere, frequently changed light underclothing, and dusting with a fungicidal powder or painting with half-strength Whitfield's ointment (benzoin and salicylic acid), or one of the new fungicidal agents such as Griseofulvin by mouth.

Pediculosis Pubis. This is especially an infection of the coarse hair of the body by the crab louse which can be seen with its eggs attached to the hair. The pubic hair is most frequently affected, but also the hair of the axillae or any other area of coarse hair on the body may be affected (except the head). It is encouraged by inadequate hygiene and transmitted by sexual contact or infected clothes. (It is not without reason that the disease in France is known as "Papillon D'Amour"—butterfly of love). It causes intense pruritus and secondary infection from scratching. Treatment used to consist of shaving the hair, frequent baths and disinfection of clothes by D.D.T., but now if the coarse hair is rubbed once weekly with one of the new compounds such as Lorexane Cream 1% (Gamma Benzene Hexachloride) the hair need not be shaved and the cure rate is very good.

Threadworms. Oxyuris vermicularis secondarily infects the vulva from the ano-rectal canal, especially in children. The parasite is easily detected in the stools, and the treatment is to eliminate it at its source by anti-helminthic drugs such as piperazine or gentian violet.

Herpes. Three types of herpetiform eruptions occur in the region of the vulva. Firstly *herpes zoster*, which follows the distribution of a nerve and is a unilateral, painful lesion similar to herpes zoster elsewhere and which resolves spontaneously in three weeks. This is treated by a sedative drug and a mild antiseptic powder or antibiotic cream to prevent infection of the vesicles.

Herpes simplex may occur in the *primary* form where the virus gains entry into the body, usually in the eye, mouth or vulva. The primary lesion is a red area of skin in which umbilicated vesicles are situated. Following the primary lesion antibodies develop and subsequently recurrent *secondary* herpes may develop. This annoying, rather painful, irritating recurrent lesion lasts for seven to ten days and is self limiting. No specific treatment is known for either primary or secondary herpes simplex infections. See also p. 185.

Contact Dermatitis. This is an acute local eczematous dermatitis resulting from contact with drugs (douches) applied locally, pessaries, creams, ointments, soaps, powders, even clothes washed in certain detergents, and condoms. The vulva is intensely inflamed and swollen with a vesicular or pustular eruption. Pruritus is a notable symptom. Treatment consists in the elimination of the cause and the application of local steroid ointment (Hydrocortisone ointment 0.5%).

Dermatitis Medicamentosa. This is a similar condition in which the reaction is more constitutional and generalised with nausea, fever, gastro-intestinal upset and generalised eruption in which the vulva is involved. It occurs in patients who are sensitive to antibiotics or to arsenic or heavy metals used in vaginal pessaries.

Neurodermatitis. Chronic lichen simplex is the result of prolonged chronic irritation from scratching due to pruritis. The ano-genital skin is thickened, sodden and excoriated, and other friction areas on the body may be affected, e.g. knees and elbows. Biopsy shows hyperkeratosis and has a characteristic appearance. Treatment is by sedatives and local hydrocortisone ointment, $\frac{1}{2}$ to 1%, or superficial X-rays.

Seborrhoeic Dermatitis may affect the vulva which is red and swollen with lichenification and a greasy, scaly eruption.

Lichen Planus. This condition, which may occur in the mouth, is very rarely seen on the vulva. It may affect the labia minora. A whitish or grey patch with a smooth, shining surface showing a fine, scaly eruption is seen.

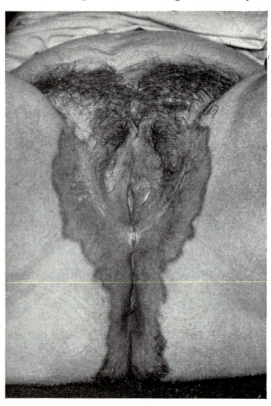

FIG. 101. Psoriasis of vulva. Note that the lesion extends laterally on to the inner surface of the thigh and posteriorly to involve the perianal skin and anal cleft.

It is liable to be misdiagnosed as leukoplakia and biopsy may be needed for diagnosis from this condition. It can cause pruritus. Treatment is designed to allay the pruritus, if present.

Intertrigo. This skin condition is seen in the obese where areas of skin are in contact and where sweating moistens the skin surfaces. It is often seen under the pendulous breast of a fat patient. The affected skin surfaces are reddened but not oedematous and give rise to a burning, itching sensation which promotes scratching and secondary infection. The area involved is well demarcated and has a bright red, glazed appearance with eventual pigmentation and lichenification. The sodden skin renders secondary infection likely apart from scratching.

Treatment is by weight reduction, scrupulous hygiene, light well-ventilated clothing and dusting with a starch and zinc oxide powder. Elimination of any vaginal discharge which moistens the vulva is important.

Psoriasis. This lesion, seen characteristically on elbows and knees, may affect the mons and labia majora. The scaly patches, sharply defined, are almost self-diagnostic. The plaques are covered with a silvery scale which can be readily scraped off to reveal a red papular underlying surface. The aetiology is unknown and the treatment (see Fig. 101) is by local steroids which are quite effective.

Vitiligo. Once seen, this area of pigmentary deficiency is unmistakable. The condition is asymptomatic and without any inflammatory basis, the skin texture being completely normal. Only the veriest tyro will mistake it for leukoplakia owing to its intense whiteness. No treatment is indicated or required.

Chronic Epithelial Dystrophy of the Vulva in which the inflammatory element is not predominant:

(*a*) Simple atrophic vulvitis (Kraurosis).

(*b*) Lichen sclerosus.

(*c*) Leukoplakia.

These conditions are considered in detail later.

VIRUS INFECTIONS PRODUCING CONDYLOMATA

Condylomata of the vulva are of several types. **Syphilitic condylomata** are flattened and are usually associated with small ulcerations, but it must be emphasised that not all flat condylomata are syphilitic.

Condylomata acuminata are small papillary warty growths spread diffusely over the whole of the vulval area (see Figs. 102 and 103). **A third form of condyloma** must be recognised. This takes the form of isolated pedunculated cauliflower-like excrescences which involve not only the labia but the area of skin around the anus. Almost always the development of such condylomata is preceded by profuse vaginal discharge. Many cases are found in pregnant women and a few patients suffer from chronic gonorrhoea. These warts are caused by a virus and are similar to warts occurring on the hands and other parts of the body.

An effective treatment for most varieties of warts is to paint them with 25% podophyllin in alcohol or liquid paraffin but if this is ineffective cauterisation of the individual warts with diathermy under general anaesthesia will usually result in a cure. If not achieved at one sitting the treatment can be repeated. Any source of vaginal discharge must be eliminated, e.g. a cervical erosion or chronic endocervicitis should be treated by cauterisation or diathermy conisation.

Summary of Diagnosis of Vulvitis

Most of the lesions described as vulvitis are sufficiently characteristic as to be diagnosed by inspection in a good light. It is always necessary to make a

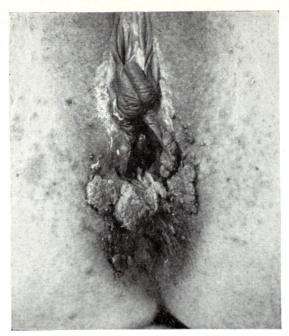

FIG. 102. Condylomata acuminata of the vulva.

vaginal examination, a bimanual pelvic examination and to inspect the vagina and cervix with a speculum. Any discharge must be examined bacteriologically. In all suppurative conditions and in the presence of moniliasis, the urine should be tested for the presence of sugar to exclude diabetes. The lower urinary tract should be examined and rectal examination and protoscopy performed. Skin biopsy of the vulva is helpful in obscure conditions, e.g. leukoplakia.

Treatment

The cause of the vulvitis should be diagnosed and treated. Apart from the specific treatment of the cause of the disease, general treatment should be employed. The pubic hair and the hair covering the labia majora should be clipped short. Bartholin's abscess should be treated by marsupialisation. In the vulvitis caused by intertrigo, the affected areas should be washed and dried and then powdered with a simple zinc powder. The vaginal discharge of gonorrhoea should be dealt with by appropriate treatment of the disease. The treatment of leucorrhoea and purulent vaginal discharge is discussed in Chapter 8.

If unresponsive to treatment by steroids or combined steroid-antibiotic cream, it may be necessary to admit the patient for stricter supervision and more regular and controlled treatment. After a day or two in bed improvement is to be expected, whereas if the patient is up and about the inflammation does not respond so well.

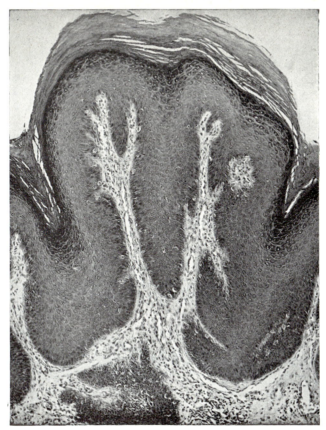

Fɪɢ. 103. Section of condyloma acuminatum showing marked hyperkeratosis of squamous epithelium and round cell infiltration of the corium. (×87).

Ulcerations of the Vulva

Traumatic Ulcerations. The best example of this type of ulceration is the **puerperal ulcer** resulting from infected tears of the perineum. Such ulcerations may persist for a long time. They are treated by irrigation with antiseptic solutions and by saline baths. Local application of antibiotic cream may be required and systemic antibiotics should be given if much induration is present. Other lacerations may lead to similar forms of ulceration if they become infected.

Herpes Genitalis. In herpes genitalis, small vesicles develop on the inner surfaces of the labia minora and in the region of the clitoris. The vesicles have an inflamed periphery, and are extremely tender. After rupture they give rise to small ulcerations which clear up with the application of antiseptic powders. Behçet's syndrome is a rare but well recognised condition in which cyclically recurrent ulceration of the vulva and mouth with uveitis is seen. Mono-articular joint lesions and the presence of skin nodules resembling erythema

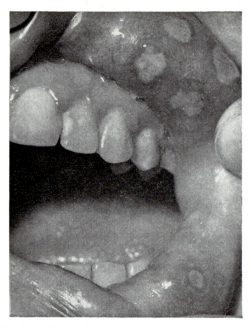

FIG. 104. Behçet's syndrome showing the oral ulceration. (Courtesy of D. L. Phillips and J. S. Scott.)

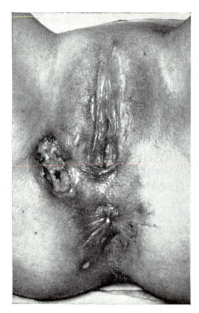

FIG. 105. Behçet's syndrome showing vulval ulceration.

nodosum have been described in Behçet's syndrome. The aetiology of this painful condition is unknown. It is certainly not infective; it may possibly be allergic and its cyclical recurrence suggests an endocrine basis. It has not been described in the pregnant, which adds weight to a possible endocrine explanation (Figs. 104 and 105).

Venereal Ulcerations (see section on Venereal Diseases, p. 9).

Tuberculosis of the Vulva. Two types are recognised, the ulcerative and the hypertrophic. Both forms are extremely rare. The ulcerative type is the more common of the two and gives rise to chronic ulceration with well-marked peripheral induration. In the hypertrophic form, indurated swellings develop in the vulval region. In both types the diagnosis is made by biopsy, although it should be remembered that tuberculosis of the vulva only develops in patients with advanced tuberculosis elsewhere in the body, especially in the upper genital tract. Treatment consists in wide excision using the diathermy (see Chapter 10), after eradicating the disease present in the upper genital tract.

Elephantiasis of the Vulva

Elephantiasis of the vulva is a rare disease in Great Britain. The disease most frequently involves the clitoris, but it may affect the labia minora, and in rare cases the labia majora. Very large tumours of this kind can be seen in most pathological museums. On section the tumour has a waxy appearance, while microscopically there is extreme hyperplasia of the papillae of the skin, together with thickening of the cutis. The disease is caused by lymphatic obstruction. The most frequent cause of the disease is tropical infection with filaria. The disease usually runs a chronic course and there is no difficulty in diagnosis.

CHRONIC EPITHELIAL DYSTROPHIES OF THE VULVA

There are three conditions affecting the vulva which are frequently seen in clinical practice. They are:

(i) Primary atrophy of the vulva or kraurosis.

(ii) Leukoplakia.

(iii) Lichen sclerosus vel atrophicus.

Much confusion has arisen in the past over the exact nomenclature of these conditions, largely because gynaecologists and dermatologists call the same condition by different names and give the same names to different conditions. For example, quite unjustifiably, any white-coloured lesion of the vulva has been called leukoplakia—for example, vitiligo. It should, therefore, be stressed at the outset that the only sure criterion of diagnosis is skin biopsy. In this account, the terminology of Wallace, whose work and experience in this subject is unique, has been followed.

(1) Primary Atrophy of the Vulva (Kraurosis)

This condition is one of *primary atrophy of the vulva*. It is a progressive sclerosing atrophy of the skin of the vulva, resulting in a gradual stenosis of the vaginal introitus. The labia minora, clitoris and frenulum, together with the vestibule and urinary meatus, are involved, but the condition does not spread to the genito-crural folds or onto the perineum. The affected areas are dry and shining, and the colour varies from a waxy white or yellow to red. Scattered over this area are prominent bright red vascular patches especially noticeable in the vestibule near the urethra. These bright red patches are often misdiagnosed as a caruncle and have been termed carunculoid. In the late stages of the disease there is well-marked atrophy of the inner part of the vulva, particularly of the vaginal orifice, so that coitus finally becomes impossible. The disease is most common in patients of menopausal or post-menopausal age though it can occur in quite young women often parous. It sometimes develops in patients who have received an artificial menopause by radio-therapy and it is seen in young patients when both ovaries have been removed by operation. It is because of its association with the natural or artificial menopause that an oestrogen deficiency has been suggested as causative and, for this reason, the condition has been treated by oestrogen substitution therapy. It is, however, sometimes seen in young patients who menstruate regularly and in whom there is no oestrogen deficiency.

The histological picture of primary atrophy of the vulva (kraurosis) shows, as the name suggests:

(a) A thinning of the epidermis, the deeper layers of which are flattened with almost complete absence of the rete pegs. Keratinisation is reduced.

(b) Immediately below the epidermis is a layer of chronic inflammatory cells.

(c) Elastic tissue in the dermis is reduced and the collagen ultimately becomes replaced by hyaline degeneration.

The progress of primary atrophy of the vulva has been carefully observed by Wallace over a ten-year period and he found that nearly half were either associated with leukoplakia or subsequently developed leukoplakia. The appearance of pruritus—not itself a symptom of primary vulval atrophy—was always a significant index of the presence of leukoplakia. It must now be stated that, contrary to most previous teaching, carcinoma of the vulva is just as likely eventually to arise in the atrophic as the hypertrophic lesions. In order further to confuse the issue it is worth mentioning that most European clinics regard kraurosis and leukoplakia as identical and some American authorities consider kraurosis to be the atrophic end result of leukoplakia. The student is advised to eschew these theories.

Symptoms. Local discomfort in the affected area, dyspareunia due to the stenosis of the introitus, and sometimes urinary symptoms are seen. Pruritus is not a symptom of simple vulval atrophy and, when it is, it suggests the development of leukoplakia or the more sinister import of malignant degeneration.

Treatment. This consists in making the exact diagnosis which is best done by a skin biopsy of the affected areas. Bland local applications such as zinc oxide ointment are harmless and often helpful. Oestrogen cream or oral oestrogen in small doses is worth a trial and may give remarkable if not permanent relief. Most important, however, is periodic observation at regular intervals and, should pruritus intervene, suggesting leukoplakia, then a simple vulvectomy should be performed to control the danger of cancerous change.

2. Leukoplakia Vulvae (also called leukoplakic vulvitis)

Leukoplakia vulvae is a pathological condition in which the skin is thickened and indurated and patches of white skin are scattered irregularly over the vulva. The affection usually involves the labia majora, and, to a lesser extent, the labia minora. It rarely extends beyond the perineum, unlike lichen sclerosus. The vestibule and the vaginal orifice are not involved.

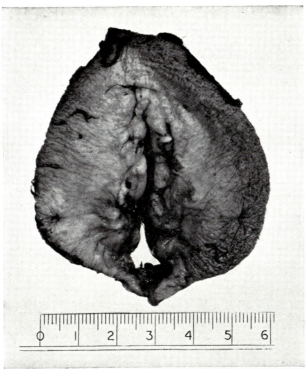

FIG. 106. Leukoplakia of the vulva treated by simple vulvectomy. Note the well-marked fissures in this essentially pre-cancerous condition.

The disease must be distinguished from vitiligo, a form of achromatosis of the vulva in which the same distribution is found but in which there is no thickening of the epidermis (Fig. 106).

The pathological characteristics of leukoplakia are as follows:

(1) The superficial layers of the epidermis show excessive keratinisation.

(2) There is considerable epithelial hyperplasia of the rete malpighii with irregular or branching hyperplastic rete pegs dipping deeply into the corium (Fig. 107).

(3) Chronic inflammatory cells infiltrate the upper layers of the corium

in which the elastic tissue is absent and the collagen replaced by hyaline degeneration.

(4) This hyperplasia of the epidermis may finally result in the development of a carcinoma, especially in a crack or fissure (see Fig. 107).

If these pathological criteria are accepted leukoplakia can then be regarded as a hypertrophic condition and its true incidence is rare. An atrophic variety of leukoplakia, histologically indistinguishable from primary atrophy and lichen sclerosus, has been described. This diagnosis is puzzling and causes confusion in a subject already sufficiently obscure. It is therefore best avoided.

Its relationship to the atrophies of the vulva is interesting. Wallace observed 100 patients with leukoplakia and found it:

Following or associated with primary atrophy of the vulva .	52
Following or associated with lichen sclerosus . . .	24
Following lichenification from scratching	11
Arising *de novo*	13
	100

Leukoplakia of the vulva usually arises in patients of post-menopausal age. In cases in which carcinoma of the vulva arises in pre-existing leukoplakia it is usually found that cracks and fissures have first formed in the

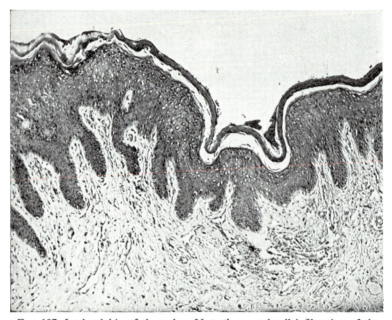

Fig. 107. Leukoplakia of the vulva. Note the round cell infiltration of the corium and excessive superficial keratinisation.

affected area; if such conditions are found an early carcinoma of the vulva should be suspected.

The symptoms of leukoplakia are local discomfort, pruritus and discharge. The prognosis depends upon the incidence of carcinoma. In some cases of leukoplakia vulvae the disease remains stationary.

Since leukoplakia is now recognised as a precancerous condition, if the diagnosis is certain both clinically and by biopsy, a simple vulvectomy should be performed with ½ in. of healthy skin round the affected area. Treatment by X-radiation is now recognised to be unjustifiable.

3. Lichen Sclerosus vel Atrophicus

This condition occurs in various parts of the body apart from the vulva and perineal area. It is an atrophic form of scleroderma.

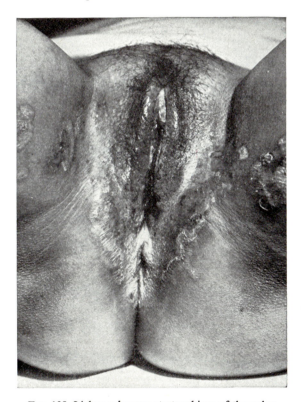

FIG. 108. Lichen sclerosus et atrophicus of the vulva.

The primary lesion starts as a small flat very white papule which, by fusion with other similar papules, forms a white confluent area involving the vulva and spreading over the perineal region and into the genito-crural folds into the thigh and buttock. The distribution of the lesion is thus wider than that of leukoplakia and this is one of the characteristics of lichen sclerosus. In a well-established example, a smooth shining atrophic surface which involves the vulva and adjacent skin results, and in which telangiectasis can quite often be seen; this latter feature is another characteristic of lichen sclerosus. As in primary atrophy of the vulva—kraurosis—the labia minora and clitoris, and sometimes the introitus, shrink so that dyspareunia and, ultimately impenetrability result (see Fig. 108).

Histologically, the skin biopsy of lichen sclerosus shows a thin atrophic epidermis with absence of rete pegs. In this, the condition resembles primary atrophy (kraurosis) but the cornified layer of the epidermis is thick and horny. The superficial layers of the epidermis show degeneration of the collagen which is hyaline and oedematous, and elastic tissue is absent. There is, in this region, a zone of chronic inflammatory cells.

The important point to realise about lichen sclerosus is that this essentially dermatological lesion has been misnamed in the past by gynaecologists as the atrophic phase of leukoplakia. The issue is still further confused by the fact that, in 25% of Wallace's patients who had leukoplakia, lichen sclerosus was the precursor. Lichen sclerosus causes as its symptoms discomfort, dyspareunia and dysuria, and pruritus. It responds very well to local application of steroids.

Summary of the Three Conditions—Primary vulval atrophy, leukoplakia and lichen sclerosus:

(1) These three obscure conditions present three different clinical pictures in distribution, gross appearance and histological characteristics.

(2) When observed over a period of several years, the atrophic conditions of primary vulval atrophy or lichen sclerosus may coexist with or develop into leukoplakia, respectively 50% and 25%. This interchangability suggests a common aetiology as yet unknown.

(3) Leukoplakia is a precancerous lesion in 50% of cases.

(4) The cardinal symptom of leukoplakia which is clinically diagnostic is pruritus.

(5) If, therefore, primary atrophy of the vulva or lichen sclerosus presents the symptom of pruritus, leukoplakia changes should be suspected and sought for by careful vulval skin biopsy.

(6) The treatment of leukoplakia, once diagnosed by biopsy, is indisputably local vulvectomy. Whilst the present authors still maintain this radical attitude, it is only fair to concede that there is a considerable dissentient voice which claims that only one tenth of all leukoplakias become malignant. Until one or other view is proven we prefer to be safe and remove the vulva.

(7) If, owing to the youth of the patient, vulvectomy is not performed, close and careful observation is essential at frequent intervals—certainly three-monthly.

(8) The lichen sclerosus of the dermatologist is almost certainly the atrophic phase of leukoplakia of the gynaecologist. This latter term should, therefore, be discarded and leukoplakia should be regarded as a hypertrophic, potentially malignant condition.

Pruritus Vulvae

The symptom of irritation or pruritus of the vulva is complained of by patients suffering from many different types of gynaecological disorder. It should be strictly defined and accurately localised as an irritive condition which provokes an intense desire to scratch and the area affected is the vulva—not the groin, anus or lower abdomen. Unfortunately the term is used rather loosely and inaccurately both by patient and clinician. The following is a list of the causes:

(1) *Vaginal discharge* due either to *trichomoniasis* or *moniliasis* accounts for 75% of all causes of pruritus. The causative organism may not be found at the first attempt, but culture will often reveal monilia where ordinary smears have failed to do so. Non-specific vaginitis and cervicitis, if associated with a profuse and persistent vaginal discharge, are less important than trichomonas or monilial infections.

(2) *Constitutional toxic states* which cause pruritus anywhere—jaundice, uraemia and Hodgkin's disease.

(3) *Deficiency diseases*—iron deficiency anaemia, pernicious anaemia, achlorhydria, hypovitaminosis A and B.

(4) *Diabetes*. A glucose tolerance test is essential in all cases where the diagnosis is not otherwise obvious. It is insufficient merely to test the urine for sugar which after a long fast in the out-patient waiting room may well give a false reading.

(5) *Skin Conditions Affecting the Vulva*. (*a*) Tinea. (*b*) Scabies. (*c*) Pediculosis. (*d*) Threadworms. (*e*) Herpes. (*f*) Contact dermatitis—local idiosyncrasy to soap, drugs, chemicals, pessaries or contraceptives. (*g*) Dermatitis medicamentosa. (*h*) Localised neurodermatitis—generalised drug reactions—penicillin. (*i*) Seborrhoeic dermatitis. (*j*) Lichen planus. (*k*) Psoriasis. (*l*) Intertrigo. (*m*) *Chronic epithelial dystrophy* is perhaps the most frequent and important local cause of pruritus vulvae. Primary atrophy, lichen sclerosus and leukoplakia are all responsible.

(6) *Carcinoma of the Vulva*. In a small but significant proportion of patients, pruritus is the presenting symptom or an associated symptom. (66 out of 314 patients in Stanley Way's series.) Bowen's disease and Paget's disease, which should both be considered premalignant, should be included under this heading.

(7) *Psychogenic*.

(8) *Cause Undiagnosed*.

It is found in clinical practice that when all possible causes for the pruritus have been excluded a group of cases can be distinguished of a nervous idiopathic essential pruritus which should be regarded as a manifestation of a psychoneurosis. In such patients scratching can be regarded as a kind of nervous tic and the habit once acquired is extremely difficult to break. Pruritus may be the manifestation of guilt, sexual frustration or insecurity centred on the vulva. It may be an effective defence against the attentions of an unwelcome or boring sexual union. It may be engendered by fear of cancer or venereal disease. These possibilities are particularly attractive to the baffled investigator and danger lies in their diagnosis before full investigation

7*

has been undertaken. It would be deplorable to treat a patient by psychotherapy when she in fact should have her blood sugar estimated or a biopsy of the vulva performed for a leukoplakia developing a cancerous change.

Pruritus becomes aggravated when the patient is under stress. It is always most marked when the patient is in bed, partly because of the warmth and partly because her attention is more concentrated on the pruritus than when she is up and about and is otherwise distracted. In severe cases the itching is constant both by day and night, and leads to scratching with subsequent damage to the skin of the vulva. The general health may suffer from the constant and intolerable annoyance of the irritation and the insomnia which results. There is hyperkeratosis of the skin of the labia which becomes greyish-white in colour and produces an appearance which is almost pathognomonic. In severe cases the hyperkeratosis may spread to involve the inner aspects of the thighs. In late cases the epithelium atrophies and hyaline changes can be demonstrated in the stroma. The labia become swollen, but it is exceptional to find signs of an active vulvitis with reddening and tenderness except in diabetes.

The diagnosis of idiopathic pruritus vulvae must be made with caution and primary local causes must be carefully excluded before the diagnosis is justified. When investigating an obscure case of pruritus, the following investgations should be performed:

(*a*) A blood count to exclude iron-deficiency anaemia.

(*b*) Gastric analysis to exclude achlorhydria.

(*c*) Glucose tolerance test to exclude hyperglycaemia and diabetes even if there is no glycosuria.

(*d*) Repeated and unremitting search for monilia and trichomonas.

(*e*) Skin biopsy of the vulva, especially in the presence of hyperkeratosis, since pruritus is often an early sign of incipient carcinoma.

Treatment. The treatment of pruritus vulvae is primarily a matter of accurate diagnosis, since 4 out of 5 patients will have trichomoniasis, moniliasis, diabetes or some local vulval lesion which when treated leads to a cure.

There is the residual 15–20% of patients in whom no satisfactory causative factor is found and in whom treatment is largely a matter of trial and error. Certain main principles, however, apply to all patients.

(*a*) Strict hygienic regimen, avoidance of all irritants, soaps, cosmetics, local chemicals, local and general allergens, not forgetting the synthetic fabrics of underclothing and the present cult of skintight underwear.

(*b*) It is essential to ensure that the patient obtains deep sleep at night, and, as in vulvitis, hypnotics must be freely used during treatment, as unless the patient sleeps deeply, there is a tendency for involuntary scratching, and the more the skin of the vulva is damaged the more marked is the symptom of itching.

(*c*) If an allergy is supected general and local antihistamines should be used.

(*d*) The most generally useful local application is $\frac{1}{2}$ to 1% hydrocortisone ointment which acts by a local anti-inflammatory effect. This is usually sufficient to overcome the habit of scratching and, once this has been achieved, the most vicious link in the cycle is broken. The effect of hydrocortisone is, however, unfortunately not permanent in every instance and further treatment by the drug may be disappointing. Simple powders of zinc and starch are often very helpful, not forgetting the time honoured calamine lotion.

(e) It is important to be quite certain that the pruritus does not spread forwards from the anal region. If the case is primarily one of pruritus of the anus there is no hope of cure until the anal condition has been cured by a proctologist. In idiopathic cases a great improvement can be expected from hospital admission, in-patient investigation and treatment.

(f) Removal of the patient from home worries, together with the atmosphere of hospital routine and careful supervision, is often followed by great improvement.

(g) Endocrine therapy has a very limited use and should be confined to the oestrogen deficient menopausal patient, in whom vulval biopsy showed an atrophic epithelial dystrophy.

(h) When secondary vulval changes have followed prolonged scratching, e.g. lichenification, or where an epithelial dystrophy is proved by biopsy, simple vulvectomy may be the final logical procedure. It must not be regarded as a certain cure since the dystrophy may recur in the skin peripheral to the excision or may transfer its activities to the perianal skin area. The patient is then commited to further operations more complicated, radical and of dubious permanent benefit.

Tumours of the vulva. Under this heading are included all swellings of the vulva whether of inflammatory or neoplastic origin.

Bowen's Disease of the Vulva

This is an intraepithelial carcinoma of the vulva in the pre-invasive state. It presents as a very slow-growing hard raised red patch on the vulva. It is at first well circumscribed with either a dry or eczematous surface. In some patients the local lesion is minimal and would pass unnoticed if the symptoms of pruritus did not draw attention to the vulva and lead to biopsy, when atypical prickle cells will be seen to invade the epidermis. Giant cells and corps ronds are characteristic of the lesion. Treatment consists in simple vulvectomy.

Rodent Ulcer of the Vulva

Rodent ulcer of the vulva (basal cell carcinoma) is a rare form of locally invasive cancer. Its behaviour is similar to the lesion seen on the face. The patient notices a small lump on the vulva which tends to ulcerate with a watery discharge and which refuses to heal in spite of various local medicaments. A biopsy should be performed, when the diagnosis is obvious (see Fig. 109). The treatment consists of a local excision and it is unnecessary to perform a radical vulvectomy. Wherever the situation of the tumour, it is important to have a good wide margin of skin and a reasonable depth of excision to obviate recurrences. The diathermy can usefully be employed in this operation. Radium treatment is effective in this condition but is rarely used because surgery is easier and more effective.

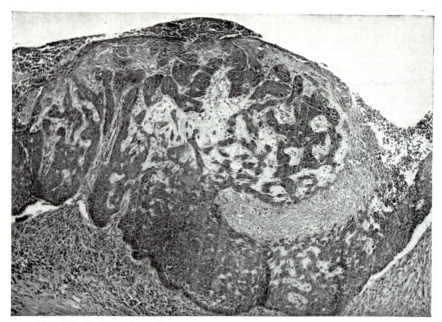

Fig. 109. Rodent ulcer of vulva (low power). This is a basal cell carcinoma which characteristically shows only local infiltration. A rare and relatively benign form of local cancer.

Paget's Disease

Paget's disease of the vulva is extremely rare and the diagnosis is unlikely to be made except by biopsy. In a recent patient of the author's, the presenting symptom was pruritus and a white, indurated, slightly elevated patch was found in the region of the clitoris; the distribution of this plaque was asymmetrical. Biopsy revealed the characteristic histological appearance illustrated in Fig. 110 on p. 197. It is, perhaps best to regard Paget's disease as an external manifestation of an underlying carcinoma, as in the nipple, and to treat the patient by a thorough local vulvectomy. Lymphadenectomy is not necessary.

Cysts of the Vulva

Bartholin's cyst is caused by occlusion of the duct of the gland by fibrous tissue as the result of Bartholinitis. The duct of the gland may be damaged or severed by a medio-lateral episiotomy incision. For this reason this particular incision should be avoided in favour of the posterior midline J-shaped incision. The cyst should be regarded as a retention cyst of the duct of Bartholin's gland. It lies in the substance of the labium majus and the labium minus passes over the convexity of the swelling. Bartholin's cysts are oval in shape and may become as large as $2\frac{1}{2}$ inches in length. They are usually adherent to the skin of the inner surface of the labium minus and are fixed posteriorly in the situation of Bartholin's gland, while anteriorly they are more movable beneath the skin. The cysts are treated by Marsupialisation under general anaesthesia which has replaced excision as the treatment of choice (see Figs. 111 and 112).

The operation of Marsupialisation is growing in popularity. It has the advantage of being very easy to perform, takes only a few minutes, is relatively bloodless and the patient need only stay in hospital for one night. The object of the operation is to provide a permanent fistulous track for the gland which thereby continues its function as a vaginal lubricant. This is a valid claim because patients who have had both Bartholin's glands excised

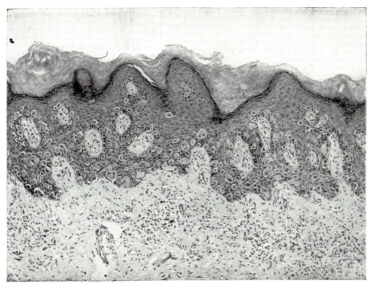

Fig. 110. Paget's disease of the vulva. Note the characteristic large clear Paget cells generously dispersed throughout the deeper layers of the epidermis.

do complain of lack of secretion and dryness of the vagina, leading to dyspareunia. (Fig. 113).

Apart from Bartholin's cysts, cysts of the vulva are seen infrequently. Nevertheless a large number of different types of vulval cysts have been described.

Rare cystic swellings of the labium majus are cystadenomata, arising from sweat glands, cystadenomata of Bartholin's glands, and cystic swellings containing blood comparable to chocolate cysts of the ovary which represent forms of heterotopic endometrial proliferations. Cysts of the labium majus have been described which are lined by ciliated epithelium. The cysts may be simple in type when they are regarded as arising from embryological rests of the urogenital sinus. A few cases of papilliferous cysts have been described which are microscopically identical with the papillary serous cystadenoma of the ovary.

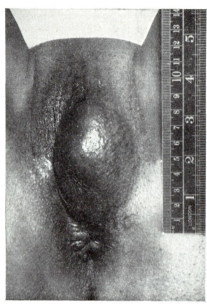

Fig. 111. A typical Bartholin's cyst grossly distorting the left labium majus and minus under which it lies.

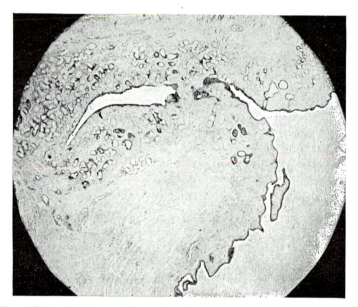

Fig. 112. Bartholin's cyst. The cavity of the cyst lies to the right and is lined by transitional epithelium. Above and to the left lies Bartholin's gland.

Sebaceous cysts and lymphatic cysts of the labium minus are seen occasionally. Small implantation dermoids are found fairly frequently in the scars of
old perineal tears and of old perineorrhaphy operations.

Small cysts of the hymen have been described. They are most common
in the new-born and are considered to arise from relics of Gartner's duct.

Cysts of the paraurethral region form rare swellings and arise from the

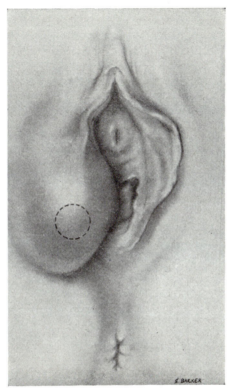

Fig. 113. Bartholin's cyst. Notice that the labium minus passes over the convexity of the cyst. The black circle indicates the extent of skin removed in
marsupialisation.

paraurethral glands. They are often termed sub-urethral cysts and, if infected,
can cause a sub-urethral abscess.

Cysts of the vulva must be distinguished from cysts of the canal of Nück,
from labial herniae and from fibroadenomata and adenomyomata of the
round ligaments. The diagnosis should be made without difficulty, for such
swellings are found in the substance of the labium majus, lateral to the cysts
of the vulva which have just been described.

Endometrioma. Endometriomata of the vulva are rare tumours, and only
a small number of cases has been recorded. They have been found on the

mons veneris, on the perineum, and on the labia majora. The tumours enlarge and become painful during menstruation. They are composed of tissue resembling the endometrium of the uterus and cyclical changes have been demonstrated in them during the menstrual cycle. The tumours are plum coloured, and the characteristic menstrual tenderness enables the diagnosis to be established. They are treated by excision.

Endometriomata of the vulva are difficult to explain on the theory of implantation since they are subepithelial (see Chapter 27, p. 682). Endo-metriomata have been found in the pelvis in association with the tumours of the vulva, and the theory of lymphatic permeation has been used to explain the development of endometriomata of the vulva. They are, however, much

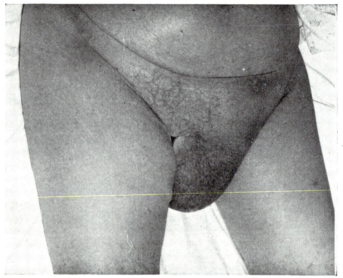

Fig. 114. Left labial tumour which was a left indirect inguinal hernia pro-truding into the left labium majus.

more conveniently explained by supposing that they represent a reaction of remnants of the Müllerian system to the stimulus which is responsible for pelvic endometriosis.

Endometrioma of the vulva must be distinguished from the more common tumours of the round ligament and of the inguinal canal. Endometriomata of hernial sacs are occasionally seen, but endomentrioma of the vulva is rare. The possibility of an inguinal hernia in this situation must never be forgotten (see Fig. 114.)

Papillomata of the Vulva. Two forms of papillomata of the vulva are recognised: condylomata acuminata and simple papillomata.

Condylomata acuminata have already been discussed on p. 183.

Simple Papilloma. Simple papillomata of the vulva are infrequent tumours, which usually arise on the mons veneris or the labium majus. The tumours are pedunculated and have a characteristic cauliflower-like appearance. They are covered by squamous epithelium, but the core consists of connective tissues and there is no induration at the base. Transition into malignant tumours is a very rare complication. Treatment consists in excision or diathermy coagulation.

NEOPLASMS OF THE VULVA

Connective Tissue Tumours of the Vulva

Fibroma. Fibromata of the vulva are infrequent tumours which arise during the child-bearing period of life, and because of the vascularity of the vulval

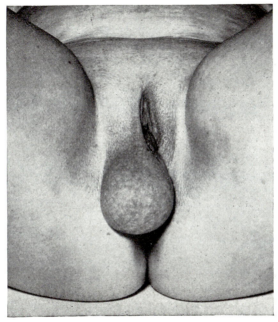

FIG. 115. Soft fibroma of the vulva. (Courtesy of Mr. G. F. Gibberd.)

region they may attain a large size, 15 lb. having been recorded. The tumours are encapsulated and take the form of spherical or ovoid swellings. The consistence is hard unless cystic degeneration has occurred. The tumours usually arise from the labia majora and more rarely, from the labium minus, the clitoris, the fascia of the pelvic diaphragm and from the tissues of the vesico-vaginal and rectovaginal septa. The tumours cause no symptoms except the discomfort of a large swelling. Eventually the tumour develops a long pedicle of skin and subcutaneous tissue. The diagnosis is usually made without difficulty and treatment consists in excision. The tumour should be examined histologically to ensure that it is not a fibrosarcoma (see Fig. 115).

Fibromyoma. Fibromyoma of the vulva is a rare tumour which possesses characters similar to those of a fibroma. The tumours grow slowly and give rise to no symptoms. They must be distinguished from myomata of the round ligament in the inguinal canal. They are treated by excision.

Lipoma. Lipoma of the vulva is a rare tumour which usually arises in the tissues of the mons veneris or of the labium majus. It may become very large and even obstruct delivery. The tumours may spread deeply along the vesicovaginal septum and into the paravaginal tissues. The tumours are easily recognised by their characteristic consistence and are treated by excision (see Fig. 116).

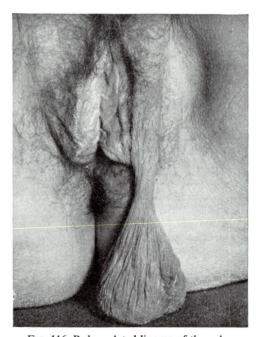

FIG. 116. Pedunculated lipoma of the vulva.

Neuromata, chondromata and haemangiomata of the vulva are rare tumours.

Sarcoma of the Vulva. Primary sarcoma of the vulva is a very rare tumour. The tumour usually arises in the labium majus or in the clitoris, and only rarely in the labium minus. A rare form of sarcoma of the urethral meatus has also been described.

Sarcoma of the vulva may give rise to either a diffuse swelling or a localised pedunculated tumour. Large tumours have been recorded which have broken down and ulcerated. The tumours infiltrate the surrounding structures and permeate into the inguinal glands. Generalised metastases subsequently develop. Most tumours are spindle-celled, and care must be taken in the differential diagnosis between fibroma and sarcoma of the vulva. The tumours may arise at any age; the average age of onset is 40, which is younger than in the case of malignant melanoma.

The tumour gives rise to no symptoms beyond swelling, irritation and pain. Treatment consists in radical vulvectomy with excision of the involved and potentially involved lymph nodes similar to that used in carcinoma of the vulva (see p. 212). Deep X-radiation may be employed as an adjunct to surgery. Local recurrence in the scar is frequent. The prognosis is bad because of blood borne metastases.

Grapelike Sarcoma. The grapelike sarcoma of the vagina which develops in young children may protrude at the vulva or may infiltrate the surrounding tissues to give rise to a tumour which appears to originate from the tissues around the vaginal orifice. These tumours will be described under the heading of grapelike sarcoma of the cervix. They are mixed mesodermal tumours comparable to the Wilms' tumour of the kidney and contain striated muscle fibres.

Malignant Melanoma. Malignant melanoma of the vulva is occasionally encountered when it arises from the clitoris, the labium majus or the labium minus. The tumour usually occurs between the ages of 50 and 60, and the average age of onset is 54, although a few cases have been recorded in patients under the age of 30. The tumour gives rise to a dark blue or dark brown swelling which is usually soft with a smooth shining surface. The tumour rapidly ulcerates when it causes irritation and discharge.

Pigment cells are represented in the normal skin of the vulva by the chromatoblasts of the basal layer of the epidermis and by the chromatophores of the papillary layer of the corium. The majority of malignant melanomata of the vulva arise from the chromatophore cells.

The tumour gives rise to few symptoms until ulceration causes a blood-stained purulent discharge. The prognosis of malignant melanoma of the vulva is bad and the average duration of life from the onset of symptoms is about eighteen months. The tumour spreads both by the blood stream, when it gives rise to generalised metastases, and also by lymphatic permeation, when it infiltrates the inguinal lymphatic glands and spreads upwards to the iliac and lumbar glands. Large swellings are sometimes produced in the inguinal glands. Treatment consists in wide excision of the primary growth together with the regional lymphatic glands, which can be followed by deep X-radiation therapy.

Epithelial Tumours of the Vulva

Hidradenoma Vulvae. These tumours are probably derived from cystadenomata arising from sweat glands. The tumours may be confused with adenocarcinoma of the vulva because of their peculiar histology. They arise from apocrine glands and can be shown to have a direct connection either with a sweat gland or with its excretory ducts. The tumours are innocent and complete excision is all that is required (see Fig. 117).

Carcinoma of the Vulva. Carcinoma of the vulva is a relatively rare form of carcinoma of the female genital tract. The incidence of carcinoma of the female genital tract is as follows:

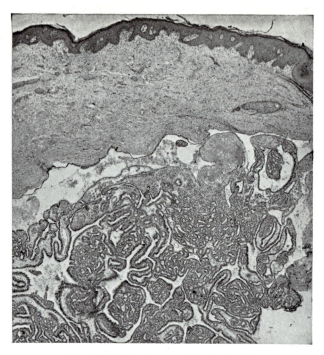

FIG. 117. Hidradenoma of vulva ($\times$33.)

Fallopian tube	.	.	.	.	0·2%
Vagina	.	.	.	.	2·0%
Vulva	.	.	.	.	4·8%
Ovaries	.	.	.	.	13·0%
Body of uterus	.	.	.	.	36·0%
Cervix of uterus	.	.	.	50·0%

The tumour usually arises in patients between the ages of 60 and 70 but it is sometimes seen in young women between the ages of 20 and 25. Parity is not concerned in the aetiology, although in Way's series of 264 cases only 12% were nulliparae. Three clinical types of tumour are recognised, the cauliflower growth, the flat induration, and the excavated ulcer. The tumour arises most frequently in the labia majora (in 43% of cases), and is seen less frequently in the labia minora (20%), the clitoris (20%), and rarely in the perineum. Carcinoma of the urethral meatus and adenocarcinoma of Bartholin's gland are rare tumours. It is interesting to note that the anterior half of the vulva is involved far more frequently than the posterior half in the ratio of $3\frac{1}{2}$ to 1 (Way) (see Figs. 118, 119, 122 and 123).

The symptoms of carcinoma of the vulva are few and fairly constant in that the patient notices a nodule, ulcer or sore place on the vulva. Pain is a relatively rare symptom though pruritus is a common complaint (see Fig. 120 and Table I).

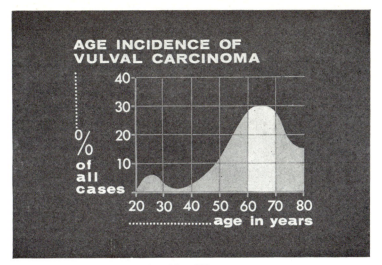

Fig. 118.

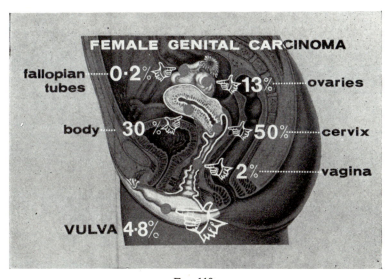

Fig. 119.

Diagnosis is straightforward and is made by inspection and palpation and in any case of the slightest doubt by biopsy of the growing edge of the tumour or ulcer. There are four conditions likely to stimulate carcinoma of the vulva; syphilis, tuberculosis, condylomata and rodent ulcer. Biopsy will always settle the question whereas a positive Wassermann reaction may be confusing, as cancer and syphilis may co-exist. Condylomata are histologically benign and tend to disappear spontaneously. (Fig. 102 and 121.)

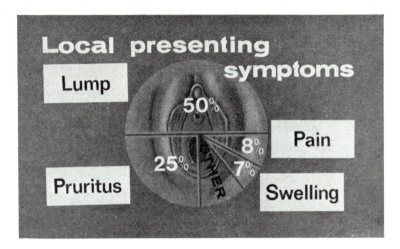

FIG. 120.

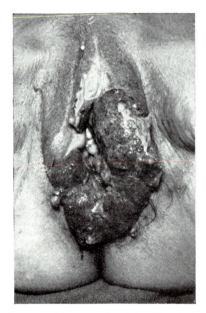

FIG. 121. A large hypertrophic cancer involving the whole of the left labium majus and minus, and extending onto the perineum and into the right labia.

TABLE I. *Symptomatology of Carcinoma of the Vulva*

Lump, sore or ulcer on vulva .	154	Vaginal discharge . . .	2
Pruritus vulvae . . .	29	Pain in the leg . . .	2
Pain in the vulva . .	22	Dyspareunia . . .	1
Generalised swelling of vulva	20	Injury to vulva . . .	1
Pruritus followed by a lump .	19	Incontinence of urine . .	1
Pruritus and a lump . .	18	Retention of urine . .	1
Dysuria	9	Prolapse	1
Lump in the groin . .	8	No information . . .	20
Post-menopausal haemorrhage	5		
			313

Histological Appearances. The commonest type is a well-differentiated squamous epithelioma with well-marked epithelial pearl (Fig. 124) formation. The anaplastic type is half as common and is said to grow more rapidly and produce metastases earlier. If Bartholin's gland is the site of the primary lesion, an adeno-carcinomatous pattern is seen. Intra-epithelial carcinoma in situ of the vulva (Bowen's disease), Paget's disease and rodent ulcer have all been considered already on pages 195–6.

The role of leukoplakia in the aetiology of vulval carcinoma is important. In 69% of the cases of cancer recorded by Taussig, 82% by Way, and all the cases of Berkeley and Bonney, leukoplakia was considered to be a precancerous lesion. The evidence of these authorities is convincing and it is now almost universally acknowledged that, once diagnosed, leukoplakia of the

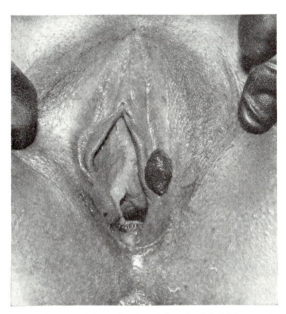

FIG. 122. Carcinoma of the vulva involving the left labium majus only.

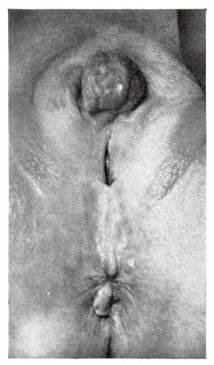

FIG. 123. Carcinoma of the vulva involving the clitoris.

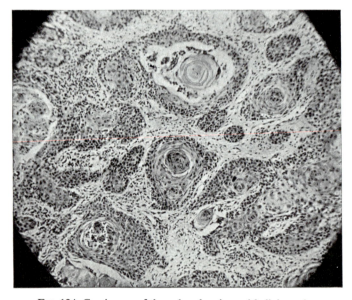

FIG. 124. Carcinoma of the vulva showing epithelial pearls.

vulva should be treated by a generous excision. If too conservative an excision is performed there is a danger of cancer developing at the edge of the excised area. In addition, leukoplakia is prone to recur after modest surgery and the new area of leukoplakia may give rise to a subsequent cancer. For this reason Way recommends a far wider excision of the vulva in leukoplakia than is commonly recommended and practised by most gynaecologists.

The importance of lymphatic spread in carcinoma of the vulva cannot be overstressed since lymph-node involvement is to be expected in 53.5% of all cases of this disease. Way's latest figures show a reduced incidence of node involvement—42% in 143 patients treated by radical vulvectomy. It is therefore essential in the understanding and treatment of this disease to have a thorough knowledge of the lymphatic pathways concerned in the drainage of the vulva (see Table II).

TABLE II.   *Incidence of Node Involvement*

Author	Total cases	Nodes involved	Nodes not involved	Percentage involved
Bassett	112	70	42	61
Rentschler .	71	39	32	54
Stoeckel	28	14	14	50
Sobre-Catas and Caranya . .	30	15	15	50
Ducuing	23	13	10	56
Cancer Institute, Louvain . .	40	20	20	50
Tumour Clinic, Brussels . .	23	14	9	60
Radium Institute, Brussels . .	25	11	14	44
Way	143	60	83	42
	495	256	239	53·5

The superficial inguinal group provides the main primary nodes for the vulva and is traditionally divided into longitudinal and vertical groups. The former is arranged along the line of the inguinal ligament, and the latter around the fossa ovalis of the saphenous opening and along the great saphenous vein. This group drains to the deep femoral nodes, the most important and constant of which is the gland of Cloquet or Rosenmüller, which lies at the upper end of the femoral canal under cover of the inguinal ligament, which must be divided for its adequate exposure. The gland of Cloquet is important for two reasons: first, it receives all the efferents from the superficial inguinal group and, secondly, it receives the direct efferents from the clitoris and upper half of the labia. Thus all vulval cancers must sooner or later permeate this node and its removal is the main object in the surgery of this condition. The next node group to be involved consists of the external iliac group, which ultimately drains into an important node or nodes at the bifurcation of the common iliac—known as the bifurcation node. Various inconstant nodes are to be found in the region of the round ligament and in the fat of the mons veneris. The lymphatic channels of the vulva are extremely rich and form a dense and intricate network with very free anastomoses across the midline in the anterior and posterior parts of the vulva. It is these

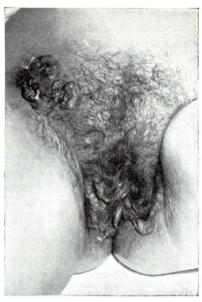

Fig. 125. Cancer of the vulva showing extensive involvement of the right inguinal nodes. Ulceration through the skin is already obvious.

anastomoses that explain the ease with which a cancer of the left labium may metastasise to the right inguinal group and vice versa, so that any operation for vulval cancer must always demand a bilateral gland dissection.

Node involvement in carcinoma of the vulva is extremely insidious.

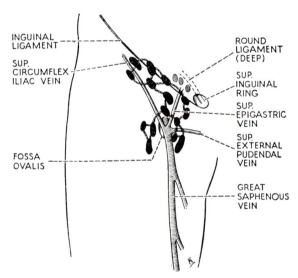

Fig. 126. The superficial inguinal and sub-inguinal lymph nodes. (Right side.)

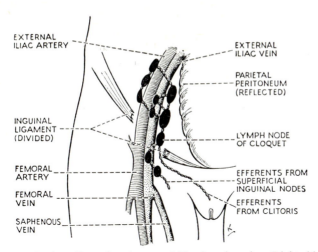

EXTERNAL
ILIAC ARTERY

EXTERNAL
ILIAC VEIN

PARIETAL
PERITONEUM
(REFLECTED)

INGUINAL
LIGAMENT
(DIVIDED)

LYMPH NODE
OF CLOQUET

FEMORAL
ARTERY

FEMORAL
VEIN

SAPHENOUS
VEIN

EFFERENTS FROM
SUPERFICIAL
INGUINAL NODES

EFFERENTS
FROM CLITORIS

FIG. 127. The deep femoral and external iliac lymph nodes. (Right side.)

Ordinary clinical examination is absolutely unreliable and the fact that no nodes are palpable must never be taken as a sign that none is involved. Nor is the size of the tumour any guide to node involvement, since a large tumour may be node free and vice versa. Even the length of the history is misleading, contrary to expectation, and cancer present for over twelve months shows a lesser node involvement than one present for under six months. An indication of node involvement may be the histology of the tumour—the anaplastic type of growth shows 58.5% of involvement compared with 24% for the differentiated (see Table III).

TABLE III.   *Length History of and Incidence of Node Involvement*

Number of patients with	*Duration of tumour*		
	Less than six months	*Six to twelve months*	*More than twelve months*
Nodes involved . . .	25 (55·5%)	21 (55·2%)	17 (40%)
Nodes not involved . . .	20	17	25

Life History of Cancer of the Vulva. In a typical case an area of leukoplakia may become fissured and linear ulcers appear. In one of these a small indurated plaque or ulcer develops, which at first is slow growing. In spite of its slow local growth inguinal node metastasis may be early and bilateral, but these metastases at first tend to remain localised to the inguinal group of nodes, and it is only in late cases that the higher groups of nodes, such as the external iliac, are involved. As the primary tumour grows it ulcerates and a foul evil-smelling pus bathes the vulva and adjacent skin. Pain and pruritus are a marked feature. If the urethra and anal canal are involved micturition and defaecation become difficult and painful and a severe cystitis develops. Later the inguinal nodes ulcerate and a general septic intoxication results (Fig. 125). Massive lymphoedema may result from blockage of the lymphatic channels of the leg so that walking becomes painful and then impossible. Sometimes severe and fatal secondary haemorrhages result from erosion of the femoral artery. Generalised extrapelvic metastasis is a rare event in this disease (see Fig. 128).

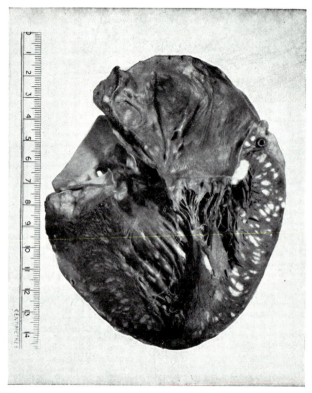

Fig. 128. Cancer of vulva in a patient who died with multiple widespread metastases. Photograph of left ventricular wall showing secondary cancer.

Treatment of Carcinoma of the Vulva. Owing to the poor results from radiation and as a result of the work of Bassett, Taussig and Way, the best method of treating this disease is undoubtedly an extensive surgical excision of the vulva and a careful dissection of all the affected and potentially affected nodes up to and including the bifurcation group of glands. A wide area of skin from the lower abdomen to include the whole of the mons veneris must be removed. All the inguinal nodes and the upper part of the saphenous vein are removed so that the external oblique fascia, inguinal ligament and fascia

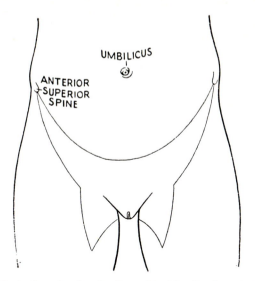

FIG. 129. Illustration showing the lines of incision for the extended radical vulvectomy.The area of skin bounded by the lines of incision is removed.

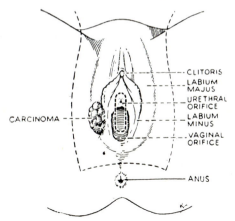

FIG. 130. Lines of incision for the removal of the vulva and primary tumour in the extended radical vulvectomy. In the case of larger tumours the lateral limits of the incision. may have to be widened.

of the thigh are left clean and bare. The abdomen is opened extraperitoneally by an incision 1 in. above the inguinal ligament and the peritoneum swept medially to expose the external iliac vessels. The inguinal ligament is divided over the femoral canal and all the nodes of the external iliac and deep femoral group removed. The extraperitoneal part of the round ligament is removed to eliminate the inconstant nodes in this vicinity. The abdomen is closed in layers and the skin wound in the groin sutured. The patient is now placed in

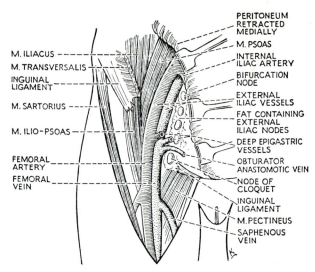

M. ILIACUS

M. TRANSVERSALIS

INGUINAL
LIGAMENT

M. SARTORIUS

M. ILIO-PSOAS

FEMORAL
ARTERY

FEMORAL
VEIN

PERITONEUM
RETRACTED
MEDIALLY

M. PSOAS

INTERNAL
ILIAC ARTERY

BIFURCATION
NODE

EXTERNAL
ILIAC VESSELS

FAT CONTAINING
EXTERNAL
ILIAC NODES

DEEP EPIGASTRIC
VESSELS

OBTURATOR
ANASTOMOTIC VEIN

NODE OF
CLOQUET

INGUINAL
LIGAMENT

M. PECTINEUS

SAPHENOUS
VEIN

FIG. 131. The exposure of the deep lymph nodes in the extended radical vulvectomy.

(Figs. 126, 127 and 129–131 are reproduced from Way: "Malignant Disease of the Female Genital Tract", 1951. Churchill.)

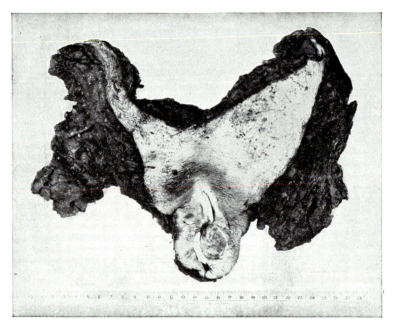

FIG. 132. Specimen removed by radical vulvectomy. Note the primary cancer in the left labium majus and minus and the generous area of skin and lymphatic watershed removed.

the lithotomy position and the vulva radically excised by diathermy. The mons is removed as far as the periosteum of the symphysis and the vulval wound packed with tulle gras. It is impossible to close the wound in the vulva by sutures and it must be allowed to heal by granulation, which may take up to three months (see Figs. 129–132).

Modifications of this radical operation may be used according to the indication. For example, if the growth does not extend onto the labio-crural fold or the perineum it is not necessary to excise the large area of skin lateral to the vulva, and this conservation of skin often permits a one stage closure of the vulval wound and certainly shortens convalescence by many weeks.

It is also sometimes justifiable in the frail, elderly or poor risk patient to abbreviate the gland dissection and confine it to the extraperitoneal inguinal groups provided Cloquet's gland is removed. When the dissection has reached this stage, if a frozen section report is favourable, the dissection of the external iliac glands is omitted.

Post-operative Progress and Complications. Convalescence can be expected to be stormy and highly skilled nursing is essential. Fluid and blood loss must be replaced and electrolyte balance maintained. Sepsis is inevitable and must be controlled by antibiotics. Early baths are the best method of cleaning a septic wound and the vulva is best treated by nursing the patient under a cradle naked from the abdomen downwards. A self-retaining catheter will be needed for the first week or more. Skin grafting of the raw area is not worth performing and it is surprising how well these mutilating wounds eventually heal by granulation and the ingrowth of skin from the periphery. Some patients can be expected to develop lymphatic oedema of the legs, but this should not last as a permanent disability and usually disappears after twelve to eighteenth months.

The operability rate should be in the region of 80% of all cases seen and the absolute five-year survival rate should be 86% if the nodes are free of growth and 48% if they are involved.

Secondary Growths of the Vulva

Secondary growths are sometimes seen at the vulva. In cases of chorion epithelioma, metastases are not unusual in the lower third of the vagina which spread to involve the vulval region. Similarly, in cases of carcinoma of the cervix, the growth sometimes spreads beneath the anterior vaginal wall to ulcerate in the region of the vestibule. Mention should be made of the suburethral metastasis seen in advanced carcinoma corporis uteri. This metastasis may be mistaken for a primary carcinoma of the urethra or vulva, and when such a growth is found a diagnostic curettage of the endometrium is always indicated. The suburethral metastasis occurs as a result of retrograde lymphatic permeation or embolic venous spread. Metastases in the lower third of the vagina and at the vulva are sometimes seen in carcinoma of the ovaries. The grape-like sarcoma of the vagina which arises in young children may also extend to the vulval region.

8 Diseases of the Vagina

BIOLOGY OF THE VAGINA

In healthy adult women in the child-bearing era of their lives, the vaginal contents consist of white coagulated material which, when examined is seen to consist of squamous cells, Döderlein's bacilli, and coagulated secretion. Döderlein's bacilli are large Gram-postive organisms which are sugar-fermenting. This ability to convert glycogen into lactic acid is partly responsible for the high acidity of the normal healthy adult vagina, pH4. The vaginal contents are mostly derived from the squamous cells of the vagina. In healthy women the cervical secretion is small in amount and there is little secretion from the endometrium of the body of the uterus even during the secretory phase of the menstrual cycle. In any case, the escape of endometrial secretions is largely blocked by the plug of mucus in the endocervix. When such pathological conditions as erosions and ectropion of the cervix are present, the mucous secretion is increased, so that patients may complain of a mucous discharge at the vaginal orifice.

The cornified cells produce glycogen under oestrogen stimulation and are continously desquamated. Subsequently, as a result of the breaking down of the cells, glycogen is liberated and is ultimately converted into lactic acid. In the new-born, before the appearance of Döderlein's bacilli, glycogen is broken down into lactic acid and there is some evidence that the process is brought about by enzyme action. After the appearance of Döderlein's bacilli the production of lactic acid is augmented by the action of the bacilli on simple sugars.

The amount of normal vaginal secretion varies with age, in health and in disease. Pregnancy increases it and it is maximal in the early days of the puerperium and, to a lesser extent, after abortion. It varies at different times in the menstrual cycle, increasing just before menstruation. In health it is dependent on the vascular state of the genitalia and this, itself, is largely oestrogen-dependent. Congestive conditions of the genitalia and the adjacent pelvic organs increase vaginal transudation apart from the increased secretion that such conditions themselves contribute to the vaginal contents. Simple examples are prolapse with a hypertrophied cervix and cervicitis, retroversion with a congested and myohyperplastic uterus and, apart from the genital tract, the pelvic congestion of chronic constipation.

It is not easy to decide when the vaginal secretion becomes excessive though it is usually simple to determine if it is pathologically infected because of the local symptoms and signs of such an infection, e.g. moniliasis.

(1) The normal moistness of the vagina is sufficient to lubricate the vagina

and labia minora but without staining or moistening the underclothes except at certain times when the secretions are increased. These times are at ovulation, the immediate pre-menstrual phase, during pregnancy and under the stimulus of sexual excitation. An uninstructed, apprehensive or highly fastidious woman may exaggerate this normal humidity into one of pathological significance and become obsessed with ideas of uncleanliness and actual disease.

(2) A moderate increase in vaginal secretion is one in which the underclothes are undeniably soiled and require changing and washing daily. Normal but excessive vaginal secretion tends, after drying on the underclothes, to become discoloured and this naturally supports the patient's fear of disease. She may say that she has a brown discharge or suggest that it is blood-stained.

(3) An excessive degree of vaginal secretion requires the wearing of some extra absorbent pad, diaper or internal tampon and is, at all times, to be classed as genuinely pathological. It is to be stressed, however, that this excessive discharge is not necessarily pathologically infected—though it may be.

The components of vaginal secretion are:

(1) The sweat and sebaceous glands of the vulva and the specialised racemose glands of Bartholin. The characteristic odour of vaginal secretion is provided by the apocrine glands of the vulva.

(2) The transudate of the vaginal epithelium and the desquamated cells of the cornified layer. This is strongly acid.

(3) The mucous secretion of the endocervical glands which is alkaline.

(4) The endometrial glandular secretions.

All play a varying part at different times of the menstrual cycle but the last two being most active just before menstruation.

Structure of Vaginal Epithelium. The squamous cells are divided for descriptive purposes into three layers: superficial, middle and deep. The deep layer consists of two types of cell, basal and parabasal. The basal cell is the less mature, smaller and more basophilic cell. It is a small round cell with a basophilic cytoplasm and a relatively large central nucleus which is uniform in shape and size. Vaginal smears where this cell predominates are typical of low oestrogen content, e.g. menopausal, lactating or postpartum smears (see Fig. 133).

The parabasal cell is similar to the basal but slightly more mature. This middle cell type is represented by a cell intermediate between the basal and the superficial or fully cornified cell. It is three times larger than the basal cell, and ellipsoid or quadrilateral in shape. The cytoplasm stains more faintly and the nucleus is smaller and less deep staining than in the basal cell. The presence of parabasal cells in a vaginal smear indicates a low but not absent oestrogenic influence as seen in the normal menopause or in the normal vagina after the menopause.

It is also characteristic of rapid desquamation of the vaginal epithelium which may result from vaginal infections or basal cell hyperplasia.

The superficial cells are of two types—precornified and cornified. The precornified cell is larger than the intermediate cell being a hexagonal or

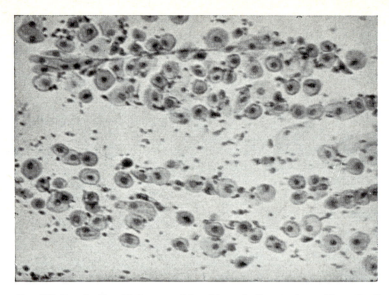

Fig. 133. Basal cells with large nuclei and basophylic cytoplasm. Normal cell picture of the postmenopausal woman. (Ayre. "Cancer Cytology of the Uterus." Grune and Stratton Inc.).

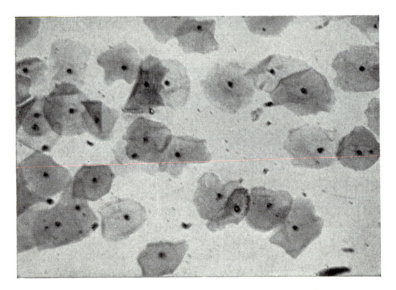

Fig. 134. Mature cornified squamous cells. These have acidophil cytoplasm with small dark pyknotic nuclei of uniform size. The cells are large, flat and wafer-shaped. (Ayre. "Cancer Cytology of the Uterus." Grune and Stratton Inc.)

octagonal flat wafer. Its main point of distinction from the fully cornified cell is that its cytoplasm is still faintly basophilic. Its nucleus is small and pyknotic.

The cornified or fully mature cell represents the final phase of complete oestrogenic maturity. It has a pink eosinophilic cytoplasm, the largest cytoplasm of any vaginal cell. The nucleus is remarkably uniform in size and staining throughout a large number of cells, and this nuclear uniformity is one of the most notable features of the fully cornified cell (see Fig. 134).

The maximum level of cornification is usually seen in the late proliferative phase of a normally menstruating woman whose oestrogen production is optimal.

Physiological Changes in the Vaginal Epithelium. It is possible to demonstrate cyclical variations in the vaginal epithelium during the menstrual cycle by cytological examination; this technique has now become so well authenticated that a competent cytologist can diagnose the date of the menstrual calendar from an examination of the vaginal smear with nearly the same accuracy as he can assess it from a study of the endometrium. The *cornification index* (the percentage of cornified cells) is one simple method of assessing oestrogen activity. Plotted on a graph over a complete cycle the daily cornification index gives a *cornification curve*. The appearances seen in vaginal cytology during the different phases of the menstrual cycle are as follows:

(1) *Menstruation*. Endometrial debris, red and white blood corpuscles and histiocytes are present. The vaginal squames are immature in that they have basophilic cytoplasm, are adherent or conglomerate, and their nuclei are larger than those of the mature cell.

(2) *Early Proliferative Phase*. Polymorphs are few and the squames tend to be discrete, more mature, their cytoplasm more acidophilic and their nuclei more pyknotic and smaller: cornification index rising.

(3) *Late Proliferative*. As the oestrogen activity reaches its maximum, the squames become uniform and mature, and the nuclei are all small and pyknotic. The cells are separate: cornification index is highest.

(4) *Early Secretory Phase*. The squames become clumped together in clusters. They are less mature, the cytoplasm is now largely basophilic, and the nuclei are bigger and less dark-staining. The cells are no longer flat but appear to be folded with a crinkled or crumpled appearance. Some are pointed and characteristically spear-shaped like an assegai. Cornification index falling.

(5) *Late Secretory Phase*. Intermediate precornified cells predominate. There is lack of cornification. Cytoplasm is basophilic—the cells are crumpled and folded. The nuclei are large, pale-staining and vesicular. Pyknosis and concentration of nuclear substance is absent. Polymorphs are on the increase.

The cyclical changes in the vaginal epithelium show that activity is at its maximum during the week before the onset of menstruation. The brown staining of the vagina, when the walls are painted with iodine, gives a rough indication of the oestrogenic titre of the patient's blood. The maximum glycogen content of the vaginal epithelium is found in the vaginal fornices, where it is present to the extent of 2·5–3 mg. per cent., and it is at its lowest in the lower third, where its value is 0·6–0·9 mg. per cent.

Cytology of the Vagina; Neonatal, Pubertal and Post-Menopausal

Cornification is well marked in the vagina of the new-born infant because of the high oestrogen level which has been transmitted from the mother. After about ten days the vaginal epithelium becomes thinner and remains in this state until the approach of puberty. At puberty the functional layer increases in thickness. In the first half of a normal pregnancy the cornification index is low and should not exceed 25%. A progesterone deficiency is shown by a rise in the cornification index and if the index rises over 50% the patient is liable to abort. In late pregnancy the cornification index falls even lower and at term may fall to 10%. After the menopause, although the ovaries have ceased to function, some degree of cornification is usually present, the oestrogens probably being derived from the adrenal cortex.

Vaginal Acidity. The vaginal acidity is due to lactic acid, which may be present to as much as 0·6%. The pH value is 5·7 in the new-born and reaches 6–8 in children, and falls to 4 at puberty. During pregnancy the pH value is usually 4. After the menopause the pH rises to 7. The normal pH for healthy women during the child-bearing period of life is about 4·5.

It is important to understand that Döderlein's bacillus is almost the only organism which will grow at a pH of 4–4·5. As the acidity of the vagina falls and the pH rises, normally non-resident pathogens are able to thrive.

Natural Defence Mechanism of the Vagina against Infection

The skin of the vagina is a tough stratified squamous epithelium devoid of glands. It presents a smooth unbroken surface to the attack of pathogenic organisms. There are no crypts where organisms can comfortably multiply as in the endocervix. The pH is low and the high acidity militates against bacterial culture. The thickness of the armour—the epithelium—and the hostile pH depends upon oestrogen and, therefore, it is only in extreme youth, before puberty and in senescence—after the menopause—that bacterial inroads are likely. During the era of sexual activity and maximum oestrogen production, there are certain times at which the pH is raised:

(a) During menstruation when the cervical and endometrial discharge which is alkaline, tends to neutralise the vaginal acidity.

(b) After abortion or labour when the alkaline lochia has a similar effect.

(c) When an excessive cervical discharge, such as occurs from an endocervicitis, has the same effect.

Apart from these exceptions, the vagina is naturally self-sterilising.

Flora of the Female Genital Tract

In healthy women the Fallopian tubes, the cavity of the uterus and the upper third of the cervical canal are free of micro-organisms. The lower third of the cervical canal always contains micro-organisms, as does the vagina. In healthy women Döderlein's bacillus is the only organism found in the upper two-thirds of the vagina, but in the neighbourhood of the vulva both saprophytic and parasitic organisms can usually be demonstrated. Döderlein's bacilli have been found in the vagina of the new-born within nine hours after delivery, although the usual time for them to appear is fifteen hours. The vagina of the new-born is probably inoculated during parturition.

During the puerperium the acidity of the vagina is reduced and foreign organisms such as coliform bacilli and other pathogens are present.

During the climacteric and after the menopause the number of Döderlein's bacilli is reduced and sometimes this organism cannot be demonstrated in the vagina.

The importance of Dĕderlein's bacillus is that its presence is associated with the production of lactic acid contained in the vagina and this acidity inhibits the growth of other organisms. In multiparous women when the vaginal orifice is patulous as the result of lacerations during childbirth, foreign organisms may be found in the lower part of the vagina, which by producing a low grade vaginitis may give rise to discharge.

Leucorrhoea

The term leucorrhoea should be restricted to those patients in whom the normal vaginal secretion is increased in amount. In such patients there will be no excess of leucocytes present when the discharge is examined under the microscope, and the discharge is macroscopically and microscopically non-purulent. Purulent discharges due to specific infections such as gonorrhoea, trichomoniasis and moniliasis, to ulcerated growths of the cervix and vagina and to discharges caused by urinary fistulae are of a different type and should be excluded from the term leucorrhoea. There is, however, much confusion in the use of the word leucorrhoea, and some clinicians use the term to describe any white or yellowish-white discharge from the vagina, strictly excluding the presence of blood.

An increase in the normal vaginal secretion develops physiologically at puberty, during pregnancy, at ovulation, and, in some women, during the premenstrual phase of the menstrual cycle. During pregnancy the normal discharge is increased in amount because of the vascularity of the female genital tract. During the latter part of the menstrual cycle the hypertrophied premenstrual glands of the endometrium secrete mucus which is discharged through the cervix into the vagina at the time of menstruation. The leucorrhoea of puberty is probably caused by the increased vascularity of the uterus, cervix and vagina at that time. It is of temporary duration and needs no treatment.

Non-pathogenic leucorrhoea, therefore, can be classified into (a) cervical and (b) vaginal.

Excessive Cervical Secretion. (Cervical Leucorrhoea.) Mucus discharge from the endocervical glands increases in such conditions as chronic cervicitis, cervical erosion, mucous polypi, and ectropion which is caused when the cervix has been badly lacerated during childbirth so that the cervix is partly everted to expose the cervical glands.

Cervical discharge is distinguished by being mucoid in type, causing the patients to complain of a mucous discharge at the vulva. When the mucous secretion of the cervix is produced in excess it undergoes little change in the vagina. The amount of mucus normally secreted by the cervix is small.

Probably the small quantity of cervical secretion which is normally discharged into the vagina is broken down so that the carbohydrate radical of the
glycoprotein mucin is split off and fermented into lactic acid. It seems,
however, that the number of Döderlein's bacilli found in the vagina is only
capable of dealing with the small amount of mucus normally secreted by the
cervix. If mucus is discharged from the cervix in excess, it causes a mucous
discharge at the vulva.

Excessive Vaginal Secretion. (Non-Pathogenic Vaginal Leucorrhoea.)
This form of leucorrhoea is seen when the discharge originates in the vagina
itself as a transudation through the vaginal walls. It is now established that
almost all the lactic acid of the healthy vagina is formed from the glycogen
contained in the keratinised cells of the vagina and the vaginal portion of the
cervix. The cells are constantly being desquamated, when their glycogen is
liberated to be fermented by Döderlein's bacilli, a process which results in the
production of lactic acid. This process is under the control of oestrogen, the
level of which determines the pH of the vagina, and it is likely that oestrogen
also influences the amount of vaginal transudation.

Local congestive states of the pelvic organs such as pregnancy, acquired
retroversion and prolapsed congested ovaries, chronic pelvic inflammatory
disease and even chronic constipation associated with a sedentary occupation
are all a reasonable cause of an increased vaginal secretion.

Leucorrhoea probably causes practitioners more trouble in diagnosis
than any other minor gynaecological ailment. Leucorrhoea must be distinguished from specific vaginitis by bacteriological examination and care must
be taken to differentiate between the cervical discharge of chronic cervicitis
and excessive vaginal secretion. It is useless to treat the cervix for chronic
cervicitis if the discharge is caused by an increased transduation from the
vaginal walls. A speculum examination of the vagina and cervix, if necessary
under anaesthesia, will usually decide the source of the leucorrhoea. If cervical
an excessive mucoid discharge will be obvious at the external os.

Specific Vaginal Infections

If the strict definition of leucorrhoea is accepted as an excessive vaginal
secretion in which the primary cause is not infective, any vaginal discharge
which is frankly purulent and contains pus cells and from which the causative
organisms can be isolated and cultured, should be considered as due to a
specific vaginal infection. The line of demarcation between a diagnosis of
leucorrhoea and that of vaginitis is often impossible since the two may co-
exist or the one develop into the other.

The following diagnostic points may be helpful:

(1) A full clinical history is taken. The amount and onset of the discharge
is noted: Its colour, odour and consistence recorded.

(2) A complete medical examination of the patient is made.

(3) A careful bimanual pelvic examination is then performed.

(4) During this the external genitalia are inspected and examined.

(5) Preferably in the lithotomy position, a speculum lubricated only with

warm water is passed and, as it navigates the vagina, the vaginal walls are inspected. The cervix is next inspected under a powerful light.

If this examination fails to reveal the presence of any pus, inflammation of the vaginal walls or cervical disease, a genuine leucorrhoea may be diagnosed provided the patient has not recently given herself a vaginal douche. Many sensitive women will refuse to present themselves for examination unless they have first thoroughly douched themselves so that they may be in a clean and fit state for examination by their practitioners. This misguided delicacy on the part of the patient is responsible for many negative findings and many negative cultures if an antiseptic douche has been employed.

If, however, pus is seen to be present in the vagina, swabs should be taken from the posterior fornix and from the cervix. If gonorrhoea is suspect, a urethral swab is also taken. In addition, a hanging drop preparation or a swab placed in moist saline is examined immediately for trichomonas or monilia.

From an inspection of the vaginal discharge, the state of the vagina and the direct smear, in conjunction with the bacteriological report, it should be possible to diagnose the cause of the vaginal discharge. The possibilities are as follows:

SPECIFIC VAGINITIS

Gonococcal and other Venereal Diseases. (See Chapter 9.)

Trichomoniasis. In clinical practice, this is the most important and one of the most common. Nearly half the patients who complain of pruritus vulvae harbour this organism. It is almost entirely a disease of the child-bearing era, though young girls and post-menopausal women are not at all immune. There is no doubt that this infection is sexually transmissible (see Chapter 9) but, in some instances, it can be acquired by inadequate hygiene or the use of an infected person's towels, bath or clothes. Its ingress to the vagina is favoured by a lowered state of general resistance and when the pH is raised as during a menstrual period.

The trichomonas is actively motile, slightly larger than a leucocyte and is anaerobic. Three types of trichomonad are known, namely, Tr. buccalis, which is found in the mouth; Tr. hominis, which is a normal inhabitant of the anal canal and rectum; and the Tr. vaginalis, which is found in the vagina. It has been shown by transplantation experiments that Tr. buccalis and Tr. hominis are unable to survive in the human vagina. Men harbour the trichomonas vaginalis in the urethra and prostate.

Symptoms. The vaginal discharge is profuse, thin, cream or slightly green in colour, irritating and frothy. The vaginal walls are tender, and the discharge causes pruritus and inflammation of the vulva. There are often multiple small punctate strawberry spots on the vaginal vault and portio vaginalis of the cervix and, sometimes, a superficial erosion of the cervix. The characteristic frothy discharge is almost self-diagnostic but the presence of a secondary infection may alter and mask this initial sign. The patient may also complain of urinary symptoms, such as dysuria and frequency, and a low-grade urethritis may be discovered on examination.

In all suspected cases it is necessary to examine a wet film preparation under the microscope. The preparation should be fresh and the temperature should be at least 35°C. The trichomonas is in constant motion, which distinguishes it from pus cells (see Fig. 135). The trichomonas is usually accompanied by a mixed group of secondary infecting organisms such as E. coli and pathogenic cocci. If the wet film is negative, the parasite can be cultured in a special medium to which antibiotics have been added to inhibit the growth of contaminants. Culture is claimed to be 98% reliable. Trichomonas may also be diagnosed on a smear stained for cytology.

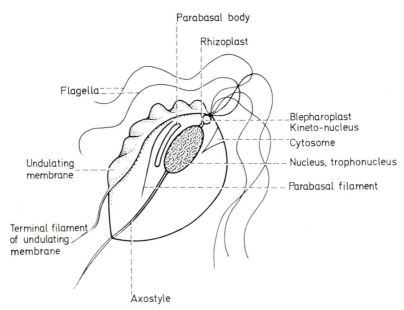

FIG. 135. Trichomonas vaginalis. The specimens are seen only in a wet film and are of varying shapes. They may be adherent to a squamous cell or they may be attached to pus cells. (Diagram after Glen Liston.)

Treatment of trichomoniasis (see page 253, Chapter 9). Metronidazole 200 mgms. by mouth three times daily for a week is effective in 85% of patients.

Moniliasis. This infection is due to a Gram positive fungus candida albicans which flourishes in an acid medium with an abundant supply of carbohydrate. It is, therefore, common in pregnancy and diabetes. Pregnancy favours infection because of the increased vaginal acidity and increased glycogen content. The progesterone-containing contraceptive pills also predispose to monilial vaginitis for the same reason. It is much commoner since the introduction of antibiotics and patients frequently will date their vaginitis from their treatment by one of these drugs for some other illness.

Symptoms. These are a profuse discharge and intense pruritus. There is often soreness and oedema of the vulva.

Signs. On vaginal examination, the following may be seen:

(1) Inflammation of the vulva, especially the labia minora and introitus, often with excoriation from scratching.

(2) White patches or plaques of cheesy material adherent to the vagina which when removed, leave multiple petechial-like haemorrhagic areas.

(3) A reddened vaginal wall with profuse watery discharge; it is muco-purulent but without cheese patches.

(4) Multiple ulcerated areas in the vagina without cheese patches and a profuse discharge causing intense pruritus.

Diagnosis. Direct smear done immediately and culture on Sabouraud's or Nickerson's media will confirm the diagnosis.

Treatment. Mycostatin, Nystatin or Sporostacin pessaries, one or two placed in the vagina nightly for at least fourteen days, including menstruation, and preferably for a further fourteen days if the clinical response is not satisfactory. Resistance of Candida Albicans to Mycostatin has not been recorded. Moniliasis is less resistant to treatment than trichomoniasis and, if it recurs, can usually be cured at the second attempt.

The vagina may not be the sole site of infection, the patient's finger nails being a possible source of reinfection from scratching due to the pruritus vulvae. Intestinal infection is another possibility and is suggested if the pruritus is perianal. If intestinal moniliasis is suspected, and this is particularly likely after antibiotic therapy, a swab taken from the anal canal and another from the perianal skin may be positive on selective culture media. Nystatin should then be given orally in tablet (500,000 unit) form. Finally, as in trichomoniasis the husband or other sex partner must not be forgotten. He may have a digital or genital source of reinfection. As with trichomoniasis it will then be necessary to treat both partners.

NON-SPECIFIC VAGINITIS

In this important group of disorders a variety of mixed pathogens is recoverable on smear and culture—staphylococci, streptococci both haemolytic and anaerobic, and E. coli.

Aetiology. Chemicals, drugs, douches, pessaries, tampons, trauma, foreign bodies such as rubber ring pessaries, and contraceptives, and even vaginal and cervical operations are all causative. Alteration in the pH towards alkalinity always favours non-specific infection—hence its common incidence in the puerperium. The association of coccal secondary infection with trichomoniasis is important, since the isolation of the secondary organism may mask the undetected presence of the trichomonas which is really responsible for the discharge. Hence it is important to use selective culture media in all cases where response to treatment is disappointing.

Symptoms and Signs. A red, swollen, tender vagina with irritation, burning and often dysuria and frequency. The vaginitis is mild or severe, acute or chronic, and the colour, consistency and amount of the discharge is variable.

Diagnosis is by smear and culture.

Treatment. This varies according to the responsible organisms and is general and local:

8*

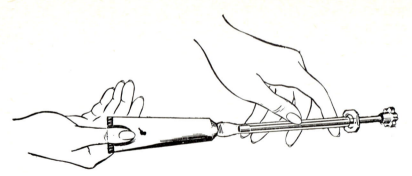

FIG. 136. Fill applicator by affixing it to the tube. Squeeze tube from its base forcing the gel or cream into the transparent cylinder until the plunger is pushed out to its fullest extremity.

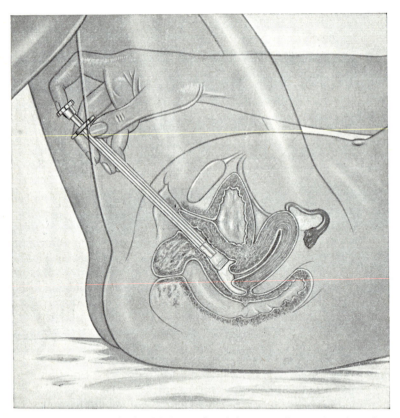

FIG. 137. Lying on back with knees flexed, insert applicator deep into the vagina. Depress plunger fully; thus depositing its entire contents high into the vagina, covering cervix. Keep plunger in closed position and remove applicator.

(*a*) General. All measures designed to improve the general health of the patient.

(*b*) Local. (i) The correction of the vaginal pH to 4·5 by a water dispersible buffered vaginal jelly which can be inserted in a graduated amount with a special disposable applicator. (See Fig. 136.)

(ii) A locally applied bacteriocidal cream such as triple sulpha (sulphathiazole 3·42%, N-acetyl sulphanilamide 2·86% and N-benzoyl sulphanilamide 3·70%; excipient to 100%). (See Fig. 137.) Or antibiotic pessaries when the organism and sensitivity is known.

(iii) The elimination of any reservoir of infection in the genital tract such as chronic endocervicitis by diathermy conisation. Failure to eradicate a chronic cervical sepsis condemns local vaginal therapy to failure and ensures recurrence.

OESTROGEN DEFICIENCY VAGINITIS

This is seen as vulvo-vaginitis in children and as senile vaginitis in the post-menopausal woman. In both these age groups, the vaginal epithelium is thin and ill-protected against infection, glycogen content is low, Döderlein's bacillus is thinly populated and the vaginal pH is higher than normal, approaching or exceeding 7·4.

Vulvo-Vaginitis in Children. The common age-group is in the first five years of life but any prepubertal girl can be affected. The infecting organism is the gonococcus, any pyogenic coccus or E. coli; trichomonas vaginalis and monilia may be present but are rare. Infection is transmitted from adults or another child by hands, toilet utensils or clothes. Thread-worms which encourage scratching are a fairly common causative factor. The possibility of a foreign body inserted in the vagina, the variety of which baffles enumeration, must not be forgotten. This primitive Freudian urge accounts for many otherwise inexplicable vaginal discharges in young children.

Symptoms and Signs. A reddened, oedematous vulva bathed in a profuse purulent discharge, with soreness and irritation. The child is fidgety and constantly handling or scratching the external genitalia.

Diagnosis. Examination under anaesthesia is probably the most effective method of excluding a foreign body, obtaining an adequate smear and inspecting the upper vagina.

Treatment. (1) Small doses of oestrogen by mouth, e.g. 0·25 mgm. of stilboestrol daily or every second day for two to three weeks. This increases the vaginal epithelial resistance and the vaginal acidity and, in itself, is often all that is needed to effect a cure.

(2) Specific chemotherapy to which the infecting organism is sensitive. This is best given systemically and not locally.

(3) No local treatment.

(4) Isolation from other children to prevent cross infection.

If not adequately treated and speedily eradicated, the infection can become chronic and resistant.

Senile Vaginitis. In many respects this is comparable to vulvo-vaginitis in children. As a result of oestrogen deficiency, the vaginal epithelium becomes thin and atrophic, the glycogen content and acidity of the vagina is lowered and the ever-present mixed pathogens obtain a footing.

Symptoms and Signs. A purulent and often slightly blood-tinged discharge is evident. The vagina is inflamed, sore and often slightly oedematous. The vulva readily becomes inflamed, tender and the skin is excoriated. Urinary symptoms of frequency and dysuria are common. On examination, the urethral meatus is pouting and shows a low-grade chronic urethritis often misdiagnosed as a urethral caruncle. There is a patchy granular vaginitis, the spots of which are red and bleed easily when swabbed. These raw, inflamed areas may become adherent and produce an obliteration of the canal in the region of the vault. The infection may spread upwards to involve the endometrium and produce a senile endometritis, and later a pyometra.

Diagnosis. The clinical features outlined above are easy of interpretation but certain reservations are of great importance.

(1) Senile vaginitis does produce a blood-stained discharge but this simple explanation may mask a cancer of the endometrium or even endocervix.

(2) Senile vaginitis and senile endometritis may co-exist.

It is, therefore, obligatory in patients who have postmenopausal bleeding to examine them under an anaesthetic and perform a diagnostic curettage to exclude a cancer of the endometrium or endocervix and, incidentally, a pyometra.

Treatment. (1) Oestrogen to improve the resistance of the vaginal epithelium, raise the glycogen content and lower the vaginal pH. Ethinyl oestradiol, 0·01 mgm. daily for three weeks should suffice.

(2) Local treatment by pessary containing oestrogen.

(3) As an alternative to pessaries which may be difficult for the patient to insert, a vaginal cream containing similar ingredients may be injected by the special applicator illustrated on p. 226.

This treatment should be effective and can be repeated if the symptoms are not cured.

SECONDARY VAGINITIS

In this section are included all varieties of vaginitis in which the primary cause is not essentially vaginal.

Foreign Body. The presence of a vaginal pessary to control prolapse or retroversion invariably causes a vaginitis. Contraceptives and vaginal tampons operate in a similar way, if neglected or forgotten.

Infective Conditions of the Cervix. Vaginitis is frequently secondary to a chronic infection of the cervix, usually an endocervicitis, the effective irradication of which is sufficient to clear up the vaginal infection. Childbirth injuries of the genital tract, such as complete perineal tears, provide another example.

Vesico-Vaginal and Uretero-Vaginal Urinary Fistulae and Recto-Vaginal

Fistulae are causes of vaginal infection though suprisingly the vagina is often resistant to such obvious portals of infection.

Malignant Disease of the Genital Tract is always infected and may involve the vagina.

Vaginitis Medicamentosa. Due to chemicals, douches, arsenic pessaries and, occasionally, contraceptives.

RARE FORMS OF VAGINITIS

Emphysematous Vaginitis. In this extremely rare condition, the vaginal walls are distended with gas-containing vesicles. The subepithelial tissues are indurated and oedematous, and the clinical picture suggests a malignant infiltration. There is, however, no ulceration. The main symptom, apart from a swollen vagina, is a profuse vaginal discharge. The aetiology is unknown except that the patients are usually pregnant and the treatment is expectant as the condition resolves spontaneously.

Less severe varieties of this emphysema have been described in which the gas-containing vesicles were found on a routine inspection of the vagina and caused minimal symptoms.

Treatment of Leucorrhoea and Vaginitis

In cases of vaginal discharge in which there is some local cause, such as a retained pessary, the cause must be removed. In vaginitis due to prolapse and secondary vaginitis caused by fistulae, it is useless to treat the vaginitis without first dealing with the primary cause. Specific infections of the vagina are treated by the appropriate antibiotic as soon as the causative organism has been identified.

There are various methods of treating vaginal discharge.

Vaginal Irrigations. One method of treatment of vaginitis consists in the use of vaginal irrigations. Patients and nurses should be given detailed instructions of the correct method of using the irrigations. An enamelled douche can, which can easily be cleaned and sterilised, should be used, and a long piece of rubber tube should pass from the douche can to the vaginal douche nozzle. The douche nozzle should be made of glass and should be sterilised by boiling before use. In domiciliary practice it is perhaps wise to dispense with the douche nozzle, which is liable to become chipped or cracked and could be a source of danger to the patient. It is perfectly satisfactory to insert the rubber tube direct into the vagina. Rubber containers for the irrigating solutions should be condemned, as they cannot be cleaned satisfactorily and can only be sterilised efficiently by boiling. This also applies to the rubber tube of the douche can but it is easily replaced.

The object of using the douche is twofold. First, it should irrigate away the vaginal discharge and secondly it should bring antiseptics into contact with the vaginal walls. The longer the antiseptic solution remains in contact with the vaginal walls the better. In hospital practice when a nurse administers the douche in the ward the patient should lie on her back, and during the irrigation the douche can should be raised to a level of about 1 ft. above the vagina. The most convenient form of douche nozzle is one which is two-way, with both inlet and outlet tubes, pyriform in shape, which can be inserted into the vagina and when pushed gently into position prevents the irrigating fluid running out of the vagina except through the exit tube. A long tube can be attached to the exit tube and passed to a receptacle under the bed. If the douche is self-administered in the home a simple and effective method is for the patient to lie in a bath with the douche can placed upon a bath tray, the exit fluid from the vagina passing into the bath. About twenty minutes should be spent over a vaginal irrigation and by compressing the rubber tube passing from the douche can to the nozzle the patient can ensure a slow flow of the irrigating solution. At least 2 pints of irrigating fluid should be used, the temperature of which should not be more than 100°F. Hot irrigations do more harm than good by damaging the vaginal walls. It will be found that most patients fail to understand the purpose of the vaginal irrigations, and believe that rapid vaginal douching is the correct method to employ. In cases of leucorrhoea and vaginitis, vaginal irrigations should be used at least twice every day at the beginning of treatment, and the frequency should gradually be reduced as the treatment continues.

Care must be taken in selecting the particular solution to be used for the vaginal irrigation. In cases of gross sepsis, such as is seen in the ulceration by retained pessaries, an alkaline solution containing 60 grains of sodium bicarbonate to the pint should first be used to remove purulent discharges. This alkaline solution is also useful when treating the mucous discharges of erosions and the mucopurulent discharges of chronic cervicitis. Ordinary salt (a teaspoonful to a pint of warm water) makes a simple, safe and non-irritant solution. The use of strong antiseptics such as lysol and chloroxylenol is not advised since such antiseptics tend to set up a secondary chemical vaginitis which is very difficult to eradicate. Patients tend to become over-enthusiastic in the dosage of antiseptic used and to use strong solutions in a mistaken belief that the stronger the solution the more quick and certain the cure. The authors have seen serious burns of the vagina and vulva from lysol and corrosive sublimate. Such burns may cause scarring and adhesive vaginitis during healing and present a serious problem in plastic surgery. It is important to avoid any douching under pressure, and for this reason any douche apparatus operated by a syringe of the Higginson or whirling-spray type is strongly to be condemned. In pregnancy the use of a douche under pressure carries a genuine risk of abortion, and the introduction of air bubbles in the douche fluid into a uterine vein may well cause a serious or fatal air embolism. Douching is not recommended during pregnancy.

In leucorrhoea the most satisfactory douche is plain water. Household vinegar one teaspoon to the pint is equally efficient.

The Introduction of Pessaries which contain:

(a) Oestrogen to promote keratinisation of the epithelium, increase glycogen content and vaginal acidity. Oestrone pessaries contain 0·1 mg. (1,000 international units) or 1 mg. (10,000 international units). Their efficacy is never comparable to oestrogen given by mouth.

(b) Antibiotic pessaries.

(c) Pessaries containing cortisone or bacteriostatic drugs.

(d) Specific fungicidal drugs, e.g. Penotrane (phenylmercurie di-naphthyl-methane disulphonate), Mycil (chlorphenesin) and Nystatin (100,000 units).

Bactericidal Creams, similarly applied, such as triple sulpha cream.

Hospital Admission. Rarely is it necessary to admit the patient for a few days, and examine her thoroughly under anaesthesia. Swabs should be taken for culture from the cervix, vagina and urethra and the appropriate antibiotic given systemically or locally as soon as the organisms and their sensitivities are known.

Ulcerations of the Vagina

Ulcerations of the vagina are rare. The type which is seen most frequently is that caused by a retained pessary, when the ulcer is usually situated high up in the posterior vaginal wall. The base of the ulcer is covered with granulations which discharge offensive pus. Such ulcerations are easily recognised,

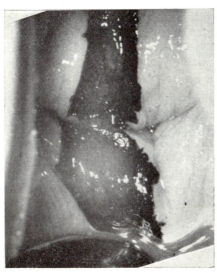

FIG. 138. Burns of the vaginal fornix photographed through a speculum. The result of potassium permanganate.

but it should be remembered that carcinoma of the vagina sometimes develops in ulcers of this kind, and if there is any suspicion of carcinoma, a biopsy should be performed.

Other forms of vaginal ulceration are as follows:

Venereal Ulcerations. These affections are dealt with in the chapter on Venereal Diseases (see Chapter 9).

Tuberculous ulceration of the vagina is extremely rare. The ulcerations are usually multiple, and are found in conjunction with tuberculosis either of the cervix or of the vulva.

Ulceration of the vagina is sometimes seen in association with prolapse, although it is usually restricted to the prolapsed cervix. The ulceration in cases of this kind is very characteristic: the surface epithelium is lost, the base is red, but discharges very little pus, and there is little if any induration at the periphery of the ulcer.

Ulceration after Radiotherapy. Ulceration of the vagina may develop after radium or X-ray treatment of carcinoma of the cervix. There is no difficulty in distinguishing between this form of ulceration and direct spread of the carcinoma to the vaginal walls. Ulcers of this kind give rise to a purulent bloodstained vaginal discharge, and during the process of healing the deposition of scar tissue often distorts the vagina. Adhesions between the vaginal walls is a common sequel, and the upper part of the vagina is sometimes completely obliterated.

Chemical Ulceration. During recent years there has been a growing practice amongst women desiring abortion of inserting tablets of potassium permanganate into the vagina. While inefficient as an abortifacient, the compound does produce deep circular apposition ulcers in the vaginal walls which may be mistaken for primary chancres. Occasionally a large blood vessel is eroded and profuse bleeding results. Healing of the ulcers may produce extensive scarring, especially if the cervix is involved (Fig. 138).

Scars, Stenoses and Atresia of the Vagina

Extensive scarring of the vaginal and paravaginal tissues is not uncommon. Possible causes are injuries during childbirth, operations for the cure of prolapse in which an excess of vaginal wall has been inadvertently or purposefully (as in colpocleisis) removed, scarring resulting from chemical burns, the radiotherapeutic treatment of malignant disease of the cervix and the development of adhesions following operation, or infection as after severe vulvovaginitis in children.

The application of forceps during labour prior to the full dilatation of the cervix often leads to splitting of the cervix, and the tear may extend along the vaginal walls ; as a result fibrous tissue is deposited which gives rise to firm bands deep to the vaginal walls. Lateral tears of the cervix may spread laterally to involve the vaginal walls, and it is not uncommon to see extensive scarring in this situation. Spiral tears of the vagina, which are usually produced at childbirth by deliberate rotation of the head with forceps, are also followed by deposition of scar tissue. The vulvovaginitis of children sometimes leads to extensive scarring so that stenosis of the vagina and even complete vaginal atresia may develop. Vaginal atresia gives rise to haematocolpos when menstruation begins. Stenosis of the vagina resulting from scar tissue may cause difficulty during coitus and during childbirth. Stenosis of this kind should be treated by surgery, in preference to the simpler methods of gradual dilatation which are unsatisfactory.

Cysts of the Vagina

Cysts of the vagina are uncommon. They may be found in any part of the vagina, but are most frequent in the anterior vaginal wall between the urethra

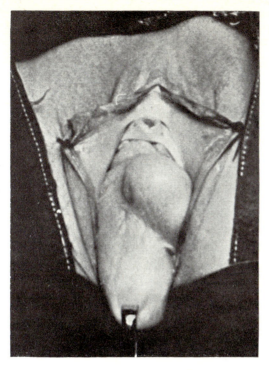

Fig. 139. A cyst of the anterior vaginal wall. The cyst lies between the vaginal wall and the bladder. After removal it was found to be an implantation dermoid.

and the vagina. The cysts are generally small, but they may be as much as 3 in. in diameter (Fig. 139).

The vagina contains no glands. The majority of vaginal cysts arise as simple retention cysts in relics of Gärtner's duct. Their epithelium is either cubical or flattened with plain muscle tissue in the cyst wall and they contain clear serous fluid (see Fig. 140).

Gärtner's duct can be traced from the lateral side of the uterus downwards and forwards over the lateral vaginal fornix, until it finally lies deep to the anterior vaginal wall just lateral to the urethra. Such a cyst may protrude at the vulva when the patient strains and must be distinguished from a cystocele. Gärtner's duct cysts are only rarely found in the upper part of the lateral walls of the vagina.

Small implantation cysts in the lower third of the posterior vaginal wall are not uncommon and result from perineal tears during parturition or episiotomy incisions. Such implantation cysts have a thin translucent wall and the contained fluid resembles that seen in sebaceous cysts, being thick, greasy and yellow. Theoretically an implantation dermoid cyst can occur anywhere in the scar of a repair operation or as a result of childbirth injury.

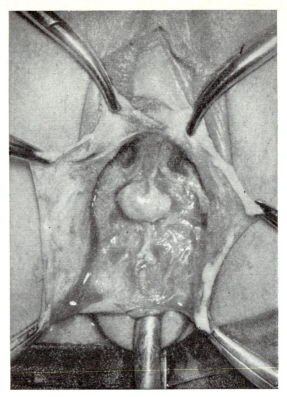

Fig. 140. Anterior colporrhaphy. The cervix is drawn out and the anterior vaginal wall has been opened up. The small cyst in the midline is thought to be derived from remains of Gärtner's duct.

Dermoid cysts of the rectovaginal septum are rare tumours. They give rise to discomfort in the perineal region and to protrusion of the posterior vaginal wall.

Vaginal cysts give rise to no symptoms unless they protrude at the vaginal orifice or cause difficulty during coitus. The cyst can usually be removed without difficulty.

Endometriosis

Endometriosis of the Rectovaginal Septum. Endometriosis is certainly not a neoplasm and its appearance in the posterior fornix is rare. It may produce multiple blue domed cysts in this situation and these sometimes ulcerate. It is therefore included here under vaginal cysts.

It is probable that endometriosis cysts in the posterior fornix are an extension of pelvic endometriosis involving the recto-vaginal septum and uterosacral ligaments and therefore an extra-abdominal extension of a pelvic endometriosis. The recto-sigmoid will almost certainly be involved and some stricture result. The tumours give rise to severe dyspareunia, as they are extremely tender; to pain on defaecation and in some cases to dysmenorrhoea. The condition is diagnosed by the presence of tender plum-coloured swellings beneath the posterior vaginal wall and of induration immediately behind the cervix uteri. Histologically the swelling consists of plain muscle and fibrous tissue, together with glandular elements similar to those of the endometrium of the uterus which undergo premenstrual hypertrophy and menstrual necrosis. The swellings usually contain small collections of altered tarry blood, derived from these glands. If ulceration has occurred the condition resembles a carcinoma and is only differentiated by biopsy.

If circumscribed the swellings can be removed by local excision. If the vaginal endometriosis is part of an extensive pelvic endometriosis involving recto-sigmoid, uterus, appendages and other adjacent organs surgical removal is a formidable undertaking, since it involves a very difficult total hysterectomy and bilateral salpingo-oophorectomy. A liberal cuff of vagina containing the endometriotic cysts must be mobilised and removed. If the recto-sigmoid is partially obstructed by endometriosis it may require local resection, though usually the condition improves once the ovaries have been removed. As an alternative to surgery oral progestogen is well worth a trial and preferable to a radiation menopause.

Tumours of the Vagina

Connective Tissue Tumours. Fibroma, myoma and lipoma are the only innocent connective tissue tumours of the vagina which have been described, and they are extremely rare. The tumours usually arise in the anterior vaginal wall and are covered by the vaginal squamous epithelium. They are sometimes polypoidal, and may grow to be as large as 3 in. in diameter. They probably arise from the plain muscle and connective tissues of the vaginal wall. Myomata may also extend from the uterus into the vesicovaginal septum, and myomata arising from the uterosacral ligaments may spread downwards into the rectovaginal septum. In most cases the diagnosis of these innocent vaginal tumours is made without difficulty and treatment consists in excision of the tumour (Fig. 141).

Sarcoma of the Vagina. *Primary sarcoma* of the vagina of the round-celled, spindle-celled or mixed-celled type arises as a very rare tumour in children. It rapidly ulcerates and causes a bloodstained discharge, and later infiltrates the cervix, the bladder and the rectum. Multiple metastases are infrequent, although the regional lymphatic glands are soon infiltrated. Treatment should consist in the application of radium or supervoltage radiation.

Grapelike Sarcoma. Grapelike sarcoma of the vagina develops in young children as a polypoidal tumour which fills the vagina and projects at the vulva. It rapidly infiltrates the surrounding structures. The tumour, like the grapelike sarcoma of the cervix, consists of undifferentiated mesodermal cells together with striated muscle fibres and is best termed a mixed mesodermal tumour. Cartilage, bone and fat have not been demonstrated in the grapelike sarcomata of the vagina of children, although these tissues are found in the comparable tumours which arise in the cervix of adults. The diagnosis of

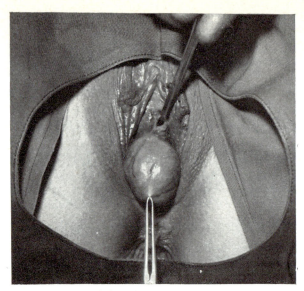

FIG. 141. Suburethral lipoma of the vagina.

grapelike sarcoma of the vagina in children is made without difficulty. The prognosis is extremely bad. Radiotherapy is the usual treatment.

Carcinoma of the Vagina. Primary carcinoma of the vagina is a rare tumour, and its incidence is only 1·9% of all genital carcinomata in the female. The tumour usually arises between the ages of 55 and 60, but it sometimes develops in young women between the ages of 20 and 30. The tumour is most often seen in the upper third of the posterior vaginal wall and produces either a cauliflower-like growth or an indurated ulcer (Fig. 142). In young patients, vaginal carcinoma usually develops in the lower third of the vagina. The tumour gives rise to well-marked induration, and the growth spreads, deep to the vaginal wall, either along the rectovaginal septum or in the vesicovaginal septum. Later, the growth infiltrates either the rectum or bladder and gives rise to fistula formation. Permeation of the carcinoma into the regional lymphatic glands is rapid, so that very soon the sacral, the hypogastric and the parametric glands are infiltrated with growth. Histologically the tumour is usually a squamous-celled carcinoma. It is known that carcinoma of the vagina may develop in the ulceration caused by retained pessaries (Fig. 143).

Secondary carcinoma of the vagina is common. It is the invariable sequence of a cervical carcinoma when it reaches stage II, it is the common site of a recurrence of carcinoma of the body (endometrial) following a panhysterectomy, and the suburethral region is one site of metastasis from the same endometrial growth. Chorion epithelioma quite frequently, and carcinoma of the ovary rarely, develop metastases in the vagina. By direct permeation a carcinoma of the bladder or rectum will ultimately involve the vagina.

Symptoms. Carcinoma of the vagina gives rise to pain and bleeding

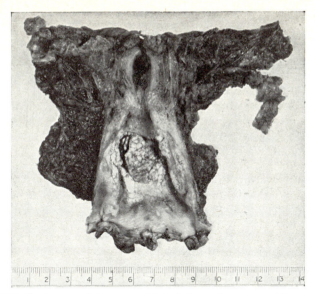

Fig. 142. Carcinoma of the upper third of the vagina removed by extended hystero-colpectomy.

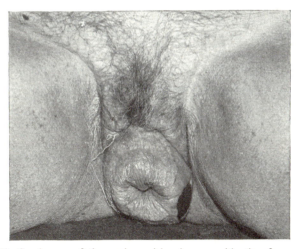

Fig. 143. Carcinoma of the vagina arising in a procidentia of many years duration. The carcinomatous ulcer lies to the left of the patient's cervix. Malignant change in a procidentia is rare.

following coitus, and later to a bloodstained offensive vaginal discharge. As the result of the spread of the growth, vesicovaginal and rectovaginal fistulae may be formed. Pain in the lower abdomen and in the back develops as the result of involvement of the sacral nerves or the lumbo-sacral plexus. The prognosis in cases of carcinoma of the vagina is much worse than in cases of carcinoma of the cervix because of the proximity of such structures as the bladder and rectum and because of the plentiful supply of lymphatics in the vagina, so that lymphatic permeation of the growth is rapid.

Treatment of carcinoma of the vagina is difficult because of the proximity of the rectum and the bladder. Early cases can be treated by performing an extensive Wertheim's operation and removing the whole of the vagina. The uterus and parametrium are dissected clear by the abdominal route, then the raw area in the pelvis is covered with peritoneum and the abdomen is closed. The vagina is now dissected away from the rectum and urethra from below, and finally the whole of the vagina, the uterus and its appendages and the parametrium pulled down through the vaginal orifice. A better method is the synchronous combined abdomino-vaginal approach advocated by Howkins, in which one abdominal and another vaginal team operate together (see under Carcinoma of the Cervix). In more advanced cases where the bladder and rectum are involved the only hope is some form of exenteration if surgery is to be used. Supervoltage radiation gives better results in the advanced case than surgery, but whatever the treatment the 5-year salvage is poor and unlikely to exceed 15%.

9 Sexually Transmitted Diseases in the Female

By C. S. NICOL, M.D., F.R.C.P.

Physician-in-Charge, Department of Venereal Diseases,
St. Bartholomew's and St. Thomas' Hospitals

This chapter will describe various diseases which may be transmitted by sex contact. These are the legally recognised venereal diseases, gonorrhoea, syphilis and chancroid, together with other undoubtedly venereal conditions such as lymphogranuloma venereum and granuloma inguinale. Non-gonococcal genital tract infection, including Trichomoniasis, is usually sexually transmitted. There are also a number of minor conditions such as pediculosis pubis, genital scabies, genital herpes simplex and genital warts which are usually sexually transmitted. Genital candidal infection in the female can be transmitted to her male consort.

GONORRHOEA

Aetiology. The causative organism is a member of the Neisserian group, the gonococcus (*N. gonorrhoeae*). In the female gonorrhoea may occur at any age, but is most commonly seen between the menarche and the menopause. It is usually transmitted by sexual intercourse, but in children may be transmitted accidentally (see p. 243). Gonorrhoea was diagnosed in 12,287 female cases attending treatment centres in England and Wales during 1968. This figure compares with 32,568 male cases diagnosed over the same period, i.e. a ratio of almost 1:2·7.

Incubation Period. This may vary between two to ten days, but is often difficult to assess as many women have no symptoms of the disease.

Pathology. (*a*) *Adult Female.* In the genito-urinary tract the gonococcus penetrates the columnar epithelium, producing a marked polymorphonuclear response in the tissues. Both transitional and stratified epithelium are much more resistant to the organism. Thus the glands of Skene and Bartholin, part of the urethra and the urethral glands, the cervix, Fallopian tubes and rectum are commonly involved, while the vulva, vagina, bladder and upper renal tract are much less often affected. In the untreated case resolution of the infection depends on two factors: the building up of local tissue immunity and, more important, adequate drainage. This drainage may be impaired in glandular tissue by inflammatory oedema of the gland ducts. Skene or Bartholin abscesses may form, and without treatment these may rupture or become chronic. In the cervix there is an endocervicitis with involvement of the cervical glands. The spread of infection from the cervix to the Fallopian tubes may be transmitted by the organism in regurgitated menstrual blood rather than by direct spread across the endometrium. Once infection has spread into one or both Fallopian tubes there is invasion of the lining epithelium with intense reactive leucocytosis and oedema of the stroma. The swollen plicae become adherent and there is exudation of pus into the tubal lumen. Intense hyperaemia of the tube and mesosalpinx is present; and localised or generalised peritonitis results. The persistence of chronic untreated infection produces disorganisation of the plicae and, usually, permanent tubal blockage. Occasionally the acute infection results in adhesions at the fimbrial end of the tube only, and a pyosalpinx forms, later developing into its chronic stage of hydrosalpinx. If the acute inflammatory process also involves the ovary a tubo-ovarian abscess may develop. Pus may become localised in the pouch of Douglas to form a pelvic abscess.

(b) *The Female Child.* In the child the vulva, vagina and rectum, and possibly the urethra, are infected. The glandular structures are not involved, nor does the organism spread to the Fallopian tubes.

Diagnosis. The laboratory diagnosis of gonorrhoea is of paramount importance. It depends on the examination of smears and cultures and may be aided occasionally by the performance of the Gonococcal Complement Fixation Test (G.C.F.T.). Fluorescent techniques show promise of future value.

There are four main members of the group Neisseria. Two, the *N. gonorrhoeae* and the *N. meningitidis*, are pathogenic, while two, the *N. catarrhalis* and the *N. pharyngis sicca*, are pharyngeal nonpathogens. The various members of the group can only be differentiated by sugar fermentation reactions. All other tests are common to all members of the group.

(a) *Examination by Smear.* Material from the site concerned is spread carefully on to a glass slide with a platinum loop; it is fixed by gentle heating and is then stained with Gram's stain, using 1% Safranin as the counterstain. The diagnosis is made by finding Gram-negative diplococci of typical reniform shape in an intracellular position in polymorphonuclear leucocytes. Many other Gram-negative organisms are seen in slides taken from the female genital tract, and short coliform bacilli, often in pairs and sometimes intracellular, may cause particular difficulty in diagnosis.

(b) *Examination by Culture.* This is most satisfactorily done in two stages, using (1) a carrying medium and (2) a growing medium.

(1) CARRYING MEDIUM. Stuart's medium is prepared in small screw-capped bottles which can be stored for long periods at room temperature. Material to be tested is obtained with a Stuart's swab, which is put into the medium and cut short so that the cap may be replaced. The medium is now stored in a refrigerator until the bacteriologist is ready to inoculate it on to freshly prepared growing medium.

(2) GROWING MEDIUM. McLeod's chocolate agar is preferred, but blood or hydrocoele agar may be used. The pH of the medium must be carefully adjusted to 7·5. Plates or slopes are inoculated from the carrying medium and are incubated in a moist atmosphere containing 5% CO_2. Incubation should be at 36°C. for forty-eight hours. Plates are then removed from the incubator, inspected with a plate magnifying glass and are flooded with

freshly prepared "oxidase reagent" (dimethyl *p*-amino phenylenediamine hydrochloride); Neisserian colonies turn purple and later become black. Colonies which do not change colour with the dye are not Neisserian, but some bacterial and candidal colonies may also change colour; therefore the organism must be identified by making a spread of the colony on a slide and staining with Gram stain. If subculture of the Neisseria is intended only part of the plate must be tested with oxidase reagent, which kills the organisms. When rectal cultures are examined various antibiotics are added to the culture medium to inhibit the growth of common intestinal bacteria such as E. coli and B. proteus. This selective medium may contain polymyxin, vancomycin or nystatin.

(3) FERMENTATION REACTIONS. A pure subculture of the Neisserian organisms must first be prepared. This is inoculated on to three hydrocoele agar slopes containing glucose, maltose and sucrose respectively. When the slopes are incubated an indicator (phenol red) contained in the medium demonstrates fermentation (acid formation) by changing from red to yellow. Table IV shows the fermentation reactions of the Neisseria:

TABLE IV

	Glucose	Maltose	Sucrose
N. gonorrhoeae . . .	+	—	—
N. meningitidae . . .	+	+	—
N. catarrhalis . . .	—	—	—
N. pharyngis sicca . .	+	+	+

When examining women with genito-urinary infection only a presumptive diagnosis of gonorrhoea can be made without performing these fermentation tests. Most laboratories, however, do not perform fermentation tests, and even if they are done at least seven days will elapse before a report is available. Thus in the majority of clinics gonorrhoea is diagnosed on the presumptive findings with the chance of a 2-3% error. It is essential to insist on fermentation reactions being done in cases when any legal action, e.g. rape or divorce proceedings, may result.

Gonococcal Complement Fixation Test. This complement fixation test employs a standard gonococcal antigen and tests for the presence of antibody. It may be performed as a quantitative test. It is usually only positive when the disease has been present for some weeks or when pelvic complications have ensued. The test may remain positive after treatment which has otherwise appeared effective. A positive fixation test alone is not sufficient to warrant a diagnosis of gonorrhoea, but in the absence of a past history of gonococcal infection, especially when the male contact is known to have gonorrhoea, a positive fixation test indicates that smears and cultures should be repeated.

Fluorescent Tests. These new diagnostic tests may become of great value in diagnosis. The immediate slide test is specific for the gonococcus, as is also the delayed test from an 18 hour culture. These tests are still being developed on a research basis.

ACUTE GONORRHOEA

Signs and Symptoms in the Adult Female

The signs and symptoms of acute gonorrhoea may be considered under the headings (i) Local, (ii) Pelvic and (iii) Metastatic.

Local. It should be emphasised that symptoms are absent in at least 50% of patients and that signs may be minimal. Many women only attend hospital on the advice of their male contacts who have developed gonorrhoea.

(*a*) URETHRITIS. The main symptom is dysuria, described by the patient as a scalding or burning pain when passing water. Women, unlike men, do not usually notice urethral discharge. On examination, after removing any vaginal discharge from the vulva, a yellow purulent discharge may be massaged from the urethral orifice by bringing the gloved finger down the anterior vaginal wall. Occasionally a peri-urethral abscess may form and is felt as a tender fluctuant mass through the anterior vaginal wall. On the other hand urethritis is often not obvious.

(*b*) SKENITIS. The two small paraurethral glands of Skene lie on each side of the terminal 2 cms. of the urethra, and the ducts open at the urinary meatus. When the glands are infected a small bead of pus may be expressed from the duct by massage as described for urethritis. Sometimes the gland tissue breaks down and an abscess is formed. This may be felt through the anterior vaginal wall as a small indurated mass to one or other side of the terminal urethra.

(*c*) BARTHOLINITIS. The glands of Bartholin lie in the posterior third of each labium majus, and the ducts open on the inner surface of each labium minus at the junction of the posterior and middle thirds. The patient usually complains of marked tenderness and swelling or of an abscess. On inspection there may be marked oedema of the labium minus and an inflammatory mass may be seen in the posterior part of the labium majus. This can be confirmed by palpation between one finger on the vulval skin and one finger in the vaginal introitus; pressure may express a small bead of pus from the duct opening, but this is often not possible as the duct may be blocked by the inflammatory reaction. If the gland substance has broken down and an abscess has formed, fluctuation of the mass will be felt. The abscess may have ruptured through the external or vaginal skin. It should be remembered that gonorrhoea is *not* the only cause of a Bartholin's abscess.

(*d*) VULVITIS. Acute vulvitis is relatively rare, but when it does occur the patient will complain of discomfort and swelling. On inspection the labia are oedematous with pus oozing from between the labia minora.

(*e*) CYSTITIS. A mild trigonitis is not uncommon and the patient will complain of increased frequency. On the other hand, a severe cystitis with strangury and haematuria is rarely seen. Cystoscopy should not be performed in this acute stage. Infection of the upper renal tract is very unusual.

(*f*) PROCTITIS. This condition, which occurs in over 40% of females with gonorrhoea, usually gives rise to no symptoms, but the patient may complain occasionally of rectal discharge with discomfort on defaecation or of rectal bleeding. Proctitis is usually caused by a spread of infection from the genital tract. There is no doubt, however, that the gonococcus is sometimes introduced directly as a result of anal coitus, and the patient should always be questioned on this point when gonococcal proctitis has been diagnosed. When a proctoscope has been passed frank pus or muco-pus will be seen on the rectal wall or may be adherent to hard faeces; there may be oedema and reddening of the rectal mucosa, but ulceration does not occur. If ulceration is seen the possibility of concomitant lymphogranuloma venereum should be considered (see p. 250).

(*g*) VAGINITIS. Patients with acute gonorrhoea often complain of vaginal discharge which may be due to a trichomonas infection, which occurs in over half the cases seen. There is evidence, however, that patients with acute gonorrhoea who do not have trichomonas infection may have a vaginitis which mainly affects the vaginal fornices, and a purulent vaginal discharge may be seen on passing a speculum.

(*h*) CERVICITIS. This condition is often symptomless, but patients may complain of low backache or of a vague feeling of lower abdominal discomfort. Increased mucopurulent cervical secretions may cause the patient to complain of vaginal discharge. On speculum examination, mucopurulent or purulent cervical secretion is seen flowing from the external os; it is not uncommon, however, for the secretion to be mucoid. There may be reddening around the external os and an erosion may or may not be present. There is no evidence that the cervical erosion is directly related to gonococcal infection.

Pelvic Infection. When the gonococcus has involved the Fallopian tubes and has produced various other pelvic complications the first step in diagnosis is to establish that there is local gonococcal infection by laboratory tests and then, by an assessment of signs and symptoms, to confirm the presence of pelvic inflammation. The G.C.F.T. is often but not invariably positive. Lastly, it is necessary as far as possible to establish the exact type of pelvic lesion present.

Metastatic. Metastatic complications such as arthritis, tenosynovitis and iritis, while relatively common in the male, are not due to the gonococcus but to a concomitant non-specific infection (see p. 253). A few cases of true gonococcal arthritis may occur in the female; an upper limb joint may be involved. Proof of the diagnosis is the finding of the gonococcus in the joint fluid. Cases of gonococcal septicaemia with acute bacterial endocarditis have been reported. Metastatic infection may result from operative trauma of the genital tract in women with undiagnosed gonorrhoea.

Signs and Symptoms in the Female Child

ACUTE VULVO-VAGINITIS. The child may complain of soreness or dysuria, but often she comes to the clinic because the mother notices a discharge on the child's underclothes. The mother may give some history of the child having had sex contact with an adult male or with a boy. Although there is evidence that infection may be transmitted from one child to another by rectal thermometers in a hospital or children's home, a commoner cause is due to the infected mother handling or washing the child, or to infected parents sharing the same bed with the child.

On examination the child is found to have an acute purulent vaginitis with some inflammation of the vulva; it is usually very difficult to assess whether urethritis is also present; proctitis is not uncommon. Skenitis, Bartholinitis, cervicitis and pelvic infection do not occur.

Gonorrhoea in Pregnancy

It may be very easy to miss the diagnosis of gonorrhoea in a symptomless pregnant woman, as routine tests to exclude gonorrhoea are not usually performed in antenatal clinics. The first evidence of infection may be the development of gonococcal ophthalmia in the new-born child. If this occurs, tests should be performed immediately on the mother.

Chronic Gonorrhoea

This condition is always difficult to diagnose as after a time the gonococcus tends to disappear from the inflammatory secretions in untreated patients, and if the organism cannot be isolated in smear and culture the signs and symptoms cannot be distinguished from those of non-gonococcal infection of the genital tract. Some presumptive evidence may be obtained either from a definite past history of gonorrhoea in the patient or in her male contact, or from a positive G.C.F.T. Proof of the diagnosis may occasionally be obtained by direct evidence of her ability to infect her present male sex partner.

Local. Patients complain of few symptoms except perhaps chronic backache. The only common residual signs are a cystic swelling of Bartholin's gland and chronic infection of the cervix with infected retention cysts of the cervical glands presenting on the vaginal portion of the cervix. Mild chronic urethritis, Skenitis or proctitis may also be present. A trichomonas vaginitis is often associated. Urethral stricture formation in the female is very rare.

Pelvis. Untreated gonococcal pelvic infection results in chronic ill-health. Such patients tend to have recurrent attacks of salpingitis with lower abdominal pain and low-grade pyrexia, and dyspareunia is a frequent symptom. Women who have had bilateral salpingitis are usually sterile as a result of tubal occlusion, and often suffer from menorrhagia with a resultant chronic microcytic anaemia. On examination there may be lower abdominal tenderness and bimanual examination often reveals that the cervix is pulled to one side by fibrous adhesions, and the uterus may be bound down in a retroverted position. The cystic mass of a chronic hydrosalpinx or of a chronic tubo-ovarian cyst may be felt in the lateral fornix.

Treatment

Antiobiotics have revolutionised the treatment of gonorrhoea. Many strains of gonococci have developed a partial resistance to penicillin, but a cure rate of over 90% can still be obtained if 2–5 mega units of a fortified penicillin is given. Oral penicillin therapy should not be used alone, though some advocate combined treatment (using ampicillin). Streptomycin is no longer of use as most strains have become resistant, but Kanamycin 2·0 G. in a single dose is highly effective, and has the advantage of not suppressing incubating syphilis. In addition the serological tests for syphilis are repeated up to three months after treatment.

The tetracycline antibiotics given by mouth in an adequate dosage are capable of curing gonorrhoea; recently Vibramycin 300 mgms. in a single oral dose has given good results. An interesting new development is the re-introduction of the sulphonamides as effective therapy. When a sulphonamide gantanol is combined with trimethoprim it is potentiated and is stated to become bacteriocidal. This new preparation (Septrin, Bactrim) given as two tablets twice daily for five days appears very effective in early trials, but it should not at present be given to pregnant women.

Antibiotic or chemotherapy alone is usually effective in curing the local manifestations of gonorrhoea in the female, but additional effective drainage of periurethral, Skene's and Bartholin abscesses, if present, must be obtained. A periurethral abscess is best opened through the anterior vaginal wall, when it quickly resolves and a fistula is very unlikely to form. An abscess of Skene's glands is best drained by electro-cautery. Bartholin's abscess should be marsupialised under general anaesthesia. No local treatment is needed for proctitis.

Pelvic Infection. A single injection of penicillin is never effective when pelvic inflammation has developed. The patient should be given benzyl penicillin intramuscularly 1·0 mega units six-hourly for three days to be followed by procaine penicillin 600,000 units daily for seven days. This is also a dosage sufficient to cure incubating syphilis. It has been reported that if small doses of oral steroid (prednisone) are given with the beginning of the penicillin course, this reduces the chances of tubal block. This is, however, doubtful. It is most important that the patient should be in bed, preferably in hospital.

Children. A single injection of procaine penicillin graded according to age and weight is usually effective in curing vulvo-vaginitis. Additional oestrogen therapy is sometimes indicated. This also applies to Septrin and Bactrim (see above).

Chronic Gonorrhoea. There is little evidence that antibiotics are effective unless the gonococcus can be isolated by smear or culture. The finding of a positive G.C.F.T. does not indicate the need for penicillin. A Bartholin's cyst or recurrent Bartholin's abscess requires surgical excision of the gland or marsupialisation; chronic Skenitis may be eliminated by destroying the gland with the electro-cautery. If chronic urethritis, cervicitis or proctitis are considered to be non-gonococcal they should be treated accordingly (see Non-gonococcal Genital Infections).

Pelvic. Although symptomatic relief may be obtained with pelvic diathermy, patients with recurrent or chronic pelvic inflammation are best treated surgically. Laparotomy and removal of the chronically inflamed pelvic organs should be successful in relieving symptoms.

Tests of Cure. Patients who have been treated for acute gonorrhoea should be tested twice weekly for the first month and then once monthly, after the period, for two months. Tests include urethral and cervical smears and cultures and a vaginal slide for the trichomonas vaginalis on each occasion. Rectal smears and cultures are taken after treatment when proctitis is present, and routinely at the end of the third month. Serological tests for syphilis (Wassermann and R.P.C.F. tests) are performed at the end of three months. If pelvic inflammation has been present, a bimanual examination should be made at each test of cure.

SYPHILIS

In this section only the lesions of syphilis which involve the genital tract will be considered. Syphilis is caused by the *Treponema pallidum* and has an incubation period ranging from ten to ninety days.

Early Syphilis (Primary, Secondary and Latent Stages)

In the clinics of England and Wales in 1968, 382 female patients were diagnosed as having early syphilis in the first year of the disease.

In recent years new blood tests for syphilis have been adopted. These demonstrate true syphilitic antibody in the serum in contrast to the Wassermann reaction which tests for "reagin," a non-specific lipoid substance which may occur in other diseases, after certain injections and also in some pregnant women. The new tests are the Treponemal Immobilisation test (T.P.I.) and the Reiter Protein Complement Fixation (R.P.C.F.) test and the Fluorescent Treponemal Antibody (F.T.A.) test.

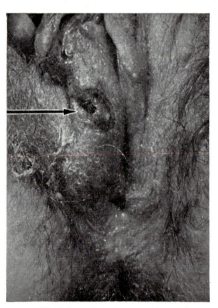

Fig. 144. Primary syphilis. Note the ulcer on the oedematous right labium minus.

PRIMARY STAGE. The diagnosis of a primary chancre is of vital importance. The typical primary lesion is circular and indurated, with a eroded base, and there is often marked oedema of surrounding tissue. Lesions are usually single but are multiple in 10% of cases. The chancre may develop on the labia majora or minora, at the fourchette, near the external urinary meatus, on the clitoris or on the cervix. Vaginal chancres are very rare, but an anal chancre

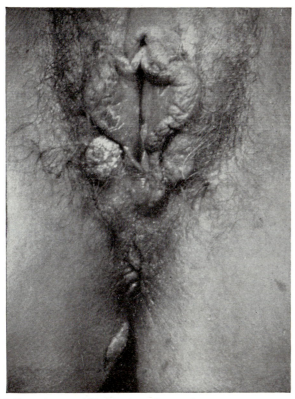

Fig. 145. Secondary syphilis. Note the flat condylomata on the right labium majus and the right buttock behind the anus. (Compare with Fig. 102.)

may sometimes be seen following anal coitus. In all types except cervical chancres the superficial inguinal glands are involved in the great majority of cases. There is unilateral or bilateral painless enlargement of the glands, which are discrete and rubbery in consistence (see Fig. 144).

Diagnosis. This is made by examination of serum from a sore by the method of dark-ground illumination. When the patient gives a history of applying an antiseptic or penicillin cream to a sore, diagnosis may be made by dark-ground examination of serum obtained by puncture of one of the enlarged inguinal glands. If the typical Treponema pallidum can be indentified on the dark ground then the diagnosis is established. Blood tests (Wassermann and R.P.C.F. tests) should always be taken, but it is several weeks from the first appearance of the chancre before the serological tests become positive.

SECONDARY STAGE. Six to eight weeks after the appearance of the primary chancre secondary manifestations may appear. Skin, mucous membrane and muco-cutaneous junctions are commonly involved. Papular lesions occurring on the vulva may be covered with scales (papulo-squamous), but because of the moisture the tops of the papules are rubbed off, leaving small circular erosions (eroded papules). On the skin of the vulva sodden white areas may develop similar to those seen in the mouth (mucous patches). In the perianal

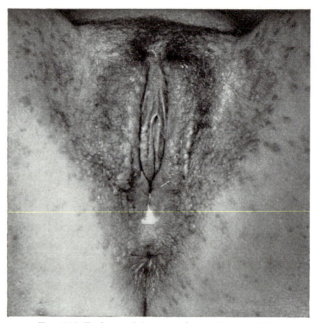

FIG. 146. Early condylomata of secondary syphilis.

region hypertrophic flat-topped condylomata lata may be seen; these condylomata may also occur on the vulva and spread out over the adjacent skin of the thighs; several lesions may fuse together to form large plaques. All these lesions are extremely contagious (Figs. 145 and 146).

Diagnosis. The treponema pallidum can often be identified in dark-ground examination of the serum of moist secondary lesions, especially condylomata lata. The serological tests (Wassermann and R.P.C.F. tests) are always positive. Condylomata lata must be distinguished from condylomata acuminata.

Late Syphilis (more than two years after infection)

Gummatous lesions of skin or mucous membranes may occur, but they are rarely seen on the genitalia. They appear as chronic punched-out ulcers with central healing; any scar formed is of tissue paper appearance. Dark-ground examination is always negative. There is no local adenitis. Gumma of the uterus has been described but is very rare. The Wassermann reaction may be negative, but the T.P.I. and R.P.C.F. tests are positive.

At this point the differential diagnosis of genital sores in the female will be considered. They may be listed as follows:

(1) Syphilis: (*a*) primary sore, (*b*) secondary lesions, (*c*) gumma (rare).
(2) Chancroid.
(3) Lymphogranuloma venereum: (*a*) primary lesion, (*b*) late ulceration.
(4) Granuloma venereum.
(5) Carcinoma (*a*) of the vulva, (*b*) of the cervix.
(6) Trauma: (*a*) physical, (*b*) chemical (potassium permanganate ulcers).
(7) Acute vulval ulcer (as part of Behçet's syndrome).
(8) Scabies.
(9) Herpes simplex.
(10) Herpes zoster of the genitalia and cervix (involving S.3 posterior nerve-root ganglion).
(11) Tuberculosis.

Treatment of Syphilis

Penicillin is the drug of choice, but other antibiotics may have to be given in penicillin hypersensitive patients.

Early Syphilis (Primary and Secondary Stages). Procaine penicillin 600,000 units intramuscularly is given daily for twelve to fifteen days. The serological tests for syphilis are done once monthly for the first three months, three-monthly for the next nine months, and finally at the end of the second year. The spinal fluid is examined at the end of the first year. The serological tests, if positive, should become negative in nine to sixteen weeks after beginning treatment. Treatment is successful in over 90% of cases. If clinical or serological relapse occurs the patient should be re-treated with a double length course of penicillin. A course of penicillin should be given during any subsequent pregnancy. Tetracycline 2·0 g. daily for fifteen days can be given if the patient is penicillin hypersensitive.

Late Syphilis. Prednisone 5 mg. is given before the first two injections of penicillin to prevent a Herxheimer reaction. The penicillin is given for fifteen to twenty days. Examination of the spinal fluid and X-ray screening of the aorta to exclude an aneurysm are performed before any treatment is given. The course of penicillin does not reverse the serological tests from positive to negative in the majority of cases. This does *not* indicate a poor prognosis or reason for further treatment. Tetracycline can be given in the hypersensitive patient (see above).

Chancroid (Soft Sore)

This disease is caused by Ducrey's bacillus, a member of the haemophilus group. It is not commonly seen in this country and only two women with chancroid attended treatment centres in England and Wales in 1968.

The disease is very much more common in males, who often acquire it abroad. The incubation period is from three to five days.

Multiple ulcers with irregular edges and yellow sloughing bases develop on the vulva. They are extremely painful but not very indurated on palpation; on handling they bleed easily. Occasionally there may be considerable tissue destruction (giant chancroid) or the lesions may be raised (ulcus molle elevatum). In a number of cases the inguinal glands are also involved in the inflammatory process and a bubo is formed, several glands matting together and later breaking down in the centre. The overlying skin becomes red and finally the contents of the bubo are discharged, leaving a large cavity which only heals slowly by granulation. The bubo, which is tender on palpation and later fluctuant, may occur in one or both groins.

Diagnosis. Identification of the causative organism from a genital sore or from the pus of a bubo is not easy. Occasionally the Ducrey bacillus may be seen as a fine Gram-negative rod on a Gram-stained slide; the bacilli may be arranged like a school of fish in a streak of mucus. The organism is sometimes cultured on defibrinated rabbit's blood and may be seen growing in chains. The most satisfactory test, however, is the Ito test, performed with B. Ducrey vaccine. The vaccine (0·3 ml.) is injected intradermally, and an area of erythema 8 mm. across at twenty-four to forty-eight hours is considered positive if a saline control is negative. The intradermal test will not be positive until the ulcers have been present for ten days, after which it remains positive for many years in spite of treatment.

Treatment. The sulphonamides and streptomycin are effective and the end results of treatment are generally satisfactory.

Genital Ulcers. Sulphadimidine 5·0 g. daily for ten days. If the ulcers do not resolve after five days, streptomycin 1 g. daily may also be given for the second five days.

Bubo. Sulphadimidine is used as above together with streptomycin 1 g. daily for ten days. In addition the bubo may have to be aspirated through normal skin with a wide-bore needle. Buboes should never be incised.

Lymphogranuloma Venereum

This disease is caused by an infective agent which belongs to the lympho-granuloma-psittacosis group. It is more common in the negro and is not often seen in this country. Only 55 male and female cases with this condition were reported during 1968. The disease is transmitted by sexual intercourse.

The incubation period is one to three weeks. The primary lesion is a very small, transient herpetic type of ulcer occurring on the genitalia. It is rarely found in women. Within a few weeks the inguinal glands become tender and indurated. Glands of both superficial and deep inguinal groups are involved and the external iliac glands may also be palpable. The inguinal glands become matted together, the overlying skin is involved, assuming a bluish-purple colour; later the glands break down and discharge through multiple sinuses. At later stages in the disease the lymphatics become blocked, and this may result in oedema and ulceration of the vulva (esthiomene). Involvement of the perirectal lymphatics produces proctitis and rectal ulceration, which is followed by stricture formation. Rectal stricture may cause intestinal obstruction many years after the initial infection.

Diagnosis. The infective agent may be identified in epithelial cells in Giemsa stained slides of pus discharged from the inguinal sinuses or from biopsy material. The most useful diagnostic test, however, is the Frei test, using "lygranum" antigen; 0·1 ml. of antigen and a similar amount of control

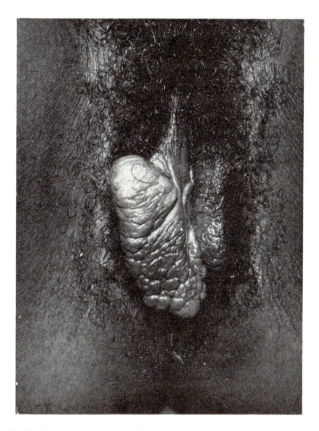

FIG. 147. Esthiomene. Oedema of the vulva secondary to lymphogranuloma venereum.

serum are injected intradermally. A papule at least 6 mm. across at forty-eight to seventy-two hours is regarded as positive. There is also a complement-fixation test using psittacosis antigen. The presence of antibody must be demonstrated at a titre of at least 1 in 32 to be diagnostic.

Treatment. The tetracycline antibiotics are effective. Tetracycline or oxytetracycline may be given in 1·0 g. daily dosages for twenty days. Vitamin B complex tablets may also be given. Rectal bougies will have to be used to dilate the stricture, or surgery may be necessary.

Granuloma Inguinale

This disease is caused by the Klebsiella granulomatosis, which is probably a bacterium. It invariably occurs in negroes and is usually transmitted by sexual intercourse. It is not often seen in this country; eleven cases were reported in 1968. It must be remembered, however, that the negro population in this country is rapidly increasing, and this fact may influence the prevalence of this disease and of lymphogranuloma venereum in the future.

The condition usually develops slowly as a massive granulomatous ulcer

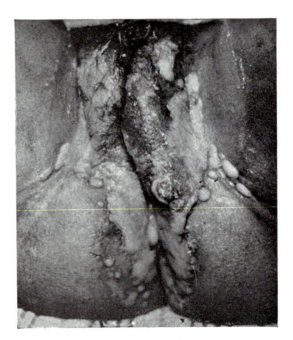

Fig. 148. Granuloma inguinale.

in the groin, but similar granulomata on the vulva or in the perianal region are not uncommon (see Fig. 148). After some years carcinomatous changes may supervene.

Diagnosis. A scraping from the edge of one of the granulomatous lesions is spread on a slide. After fixing it is stained with Wright's stain. Typical Donovan bodies (not to be confused with the Leishman-Donovan bodies of kala-azar) are seen in the cytoplasm of mononuclear cells.

Treatment. The tetracycline antibiotics are also effective in this condition. Tetracycline or oxytetracycline, 1 g. daily is given for two weeks together with vitamin B complex.

NON-GONOCOCCAL GENITAL INFECTION

It is now generally agreed that non-gonococcal (non-specific) genital infection is often a sexually transmitted condition. One cause of this type of infection is the *T. vaginalis*, but the majority of cases still remain of unknown aetiology.

Trichomoniasis

It has been demonstrated experimentally that inoculation of a pure culture of *T. vaginalis* into the healthy male urethra can produce urethritis. The organism is in fact found in up to 15% of male patients suffering from non-gonococcal urethritis, it may also occur in males with balanitis. In the female *T. vaginalis* is frequently found in the vagina, and may also be present in the urethra and the glands of Bartholin and Skene. Trichomoniasis occurs mainly during the years of sexual activity. It occasionally persists after the menopause and in rare cases may occur in female infants during the first week of life, when they are under the influence of the mother's oestrogens. Careful investigation will usually show that the mother or nurse handling the infant has trichomoniasis (Fig. 135).

In the past trichomoniasis has been reported in "virgins"; it is true that the *T. vaginalis* is sometimes found in a girl with an intact hymen, but careful questioning will reveal that she has had genital contact with a male sex partner. In certain cases the *T. vaginalis* may persist in the vagina for months or even years without producing any symptoms, and only be found on routine examination. In these patients a history of *recent* intercourse is not obtained, and the original sex contact may be forgotten. *T. vaginalis* infection in the female is very commonly associated with gonorrhoea. There is no evidence to support the idea that trichomonas vaginitis is caused by a transferred infection from the rectum. The *trichomonas hominis* which occurs in the bowel is morphologically different from the *trichomonas vaginalis* and does not survive when inoculated into the vagina.

Treatment. In the past local vaginal therapy resulted in a high relapse rate; acetarsol (S.V.C.) was the most popular drug, used in the form of a vaginal pessary. The main reason for this high relapse rate was the presence of *T. vaginalis* in other parts of the genito-urinary tract. Metronidazole (Flagyl) acts systemically and is excreted in the urine. It is highly effective when given in a dosage of 200 mg. t.d.s. for seven days, or 400 mgms. b.d. for five days. No local genital therapy is needed; no serious toxic effects have been noted. Reinfection has to be excluded in treatment failures, and similar treatment with Flagyl should be given to the male sex contact with trichomonas urethritis. The need for treating male patients who cause reinfection of their female partners must always be considered even if *T. vaginalis* is not found.

Non-gonococcal Genital Infection other than Trichomoniasis

While the aetiology of this group of infections remains obscure the following have been suggested as possible causes.

(*a*) A bacterium such as *E. coli* or *Haemophilus vaginalis*.

(*b*) A member of the Chlamydia (Bedsona) group (such as the TRIC agent).

(c) A member of the Mycoplasma group (such as the "T" strain).

Signs and Symptoms. All the signs and symptoms are similar to those occurring in gonococcal infection. In general they are less acute in their onset, longer in their course, with a greater tendency to chronicity.

Treatment. In a condition in which the aetiology is unknown, treatment must be empirical. The justification of treatment is twofold; first to control the patient's infection and secondly to prevent reinfection of the male. It seems logical to give the female the empirical treatment which is most successful in treating the non-gonococcal infection in the male. This is tetracycline or oxytetracycline 2·0 g. daily for up to ten days. Penicillin is not effective in the treatment of non-gonococcal infection.

Venereophobia

While there are a number of perfectly normal women who attend a treatment centre following a sex contact in order to be reassured that they have not acquired any infection, there is another group of women who may never have had any sex contact, or may have had a sex contact many years previously. They have a morbid fear of venereal infection and reassurance that their tests and blood tests are negative may not remove this fear. They will go from one hospital to another seeking examination. These patients, who are not necessarily just psychoneurotics, should be referred for a psychiatric opinion following two negative sets of tests. They are often found to be prepsychotic or actually psychotic with schizophrenia and may be in urgent need of psychiatric treatment.

Routine for all New Patients

History. Special attention must be paid to the recent history of sexual contacts and a note taken of the exact dates and the men concerned, *including the husband if the patient is a married woman.* The town in which intercourse took place in this country or abroad should be noted, and also details as to contraceptives employed by either sex partner. Any known details of disease in the male contact should be enquired for, and if he is attending another hospital a confidential letter should be sent to the doctor requesting a medical report. The duration and types of symptoms should be noted, with special emphasis on those referable to the genito-urinary system.

Any past history of venereal or allied diseases should be asked for together with details of treatment given. Past history of any other disease with dates of operations should also be noted. The usual menstrual history and the number and dates of live births, stillbirths and miscarriages should be recorded.

Examination. This should be performed with the patient in the lithotomy position. She should not have passed urine recently. It is convenient to examine the abdomen first, noticing any scars and palpating the lower abdomen for signs of tenderness. Genital examination is then made in a good light. First the pubic, vulval and perianal regions should be inspected for lice, any skin disease or areas of oedema or ulceration; serum for dark-ground examination should be taken from any suspicious ulcer. The inguinal regions are then palpated and any abnormality of the inguinal glands noted. The vulva is now inspected and the glands of Bartholin examined. Smears and cultures are taken from the duct openings only if the glands are tender and swollen. A speculum, lubricated only with water, is passed, provided the hymen is not intact, and the vaginal portion of the cervix is manipulated into view; the type of vaginal discharge and the appearance of the vaginal wall is noted. A wet film and culture (Oxo Trichomonas No. 2 medium is suitable) are made from the vagina and examined for trichomonas vaginalis, and a vaginal smear and culture (Sabouraud medium) examined for candida. A swab in a holder is used to remove the secretion from the external os and the appearance of the cervix is noted. Smear and culture are taken from the cervical canal to exclude gonorrhoea. The speculum is now withdrawn and the urethra massaged downwards along the anterior vaginal wall with the finger; any discharge from the urethra or from the paraurethral glands of Skene is noted. Smear and culture are taken to exclude gonorrhoea, with similar tests from the glands of Skene when indicated. A moist slide and culture may be taken to exclude trichomonas infection. A proctoscope lubricated with liquid paraffin is now passed and the appearance of the rectal mucosa and the presence of pus is noted; smear and culture are taken to exclude gonorrhoea and the proctoscope removed. A bimanual examination of the uterus and tubes is performed and any abnormality noted. Blood (7 ml.) is withdrawn for routine Wassermann and R.P.C.F. tests (G.C.F.T. if indicated).

When any venereal or allied disease is proved to be present the male partner should be encouraged to present himself for examination.

Examination of children is similar to that described above except that a vaginal speculum is not passed. The rectal tests are taken with a platinum loop or swab passed through the anal orifice.

10 Tuberculosis of the Genital Tract

In recent years clinicians have become increasingly aware of the incidence of this disease, largely due to the use of endometrial biopsy in the investigation of infertility. The fact that most of the patients were otherwise healthy and in their sexual prime has rendered the discovery all the more startling. The incidence amongst women attending the infertility clinics, and not of course the total female population, is assessed by most authorities (Halbrecht, Sutherland, Sharman and Stallworthy) to vary between 2%—5·5%, being high in an environment where pulmonary tuberculosis is high, e.g. Glasgow. The incidence may well be higher as this disease, apart from the infertility, is largely symptomless and the diagnosis involves a fairly elaborate laboratory technique. Furthermore, one isolated negative report does not mean freedom from genital infection, and at least three negative reports at monthly intervals are necessary before pronouncing a case of endometrial tuberculosis cured, and even then clinical supervision will be needed for a year or longer at regular intervals.

Primary Source of Infection. The method of infection of the genital tract is not entirely clear. In a few cases there is an active or recently active pulmonary lesion, and roughly 10% of all women dying of active chest disease will show genital tract involvement at autopsy.

In Sutherland's 325 patients with proved genital tuberculosis, 177 gave a previous history of extragenital tuberculosis as follows:

Pulmonary tuberculosis..	29
Pleurisy (presumed tuberculosis)	79
	——
Total pulmonary lesions	108
Abdominal tuberculosis	91
Bone and joint tuberculosis	11
Renal tuberculosis	1
Tuberculous abscess in groin	1
Erythema nodosum	1
Tuberculous cervical adenitis	1
	——
Total lesions in 177 patients	214*
	——

* This discrepancy is due to some patients having more than one tuberculous lesion.

The conclusion from Sutherland's figures is that by far the most important primary focus is either pulmonary or abdominal tuberculosis. When these 325 patients were examined clinically and their chest and abdomen X-rayed, a further 77 patients, in whom no history whatever suggesting tuberculosis infection was obtained, were found to have evidence of extragenital disease. So, 254 or 84·3% of the total number with pelvic tuberculosis were found to have a primary extra-genital lesion. It should be noted that the primary focus is often quiescent or healed by the time that the genital lesion becomes obvious and that long latent periods of many years may intervene.

Method of Spread. (1) The blood stream is by far the commonest method of spread—in fact, it may be the universal route, as suggested by Magnus Haines. One important piece of evidence to support this statement is that genital tuberculosis is almost invariably due to the human organism and, in 93 patients, Sutherland recovered the human mycobacterium in 90, the bovine in three. In childhood, tuberculous peritonitis is frequently due to the bovine organism so that, since the genital tract infection is nearly always human, it is illogical to suggest that it is secondary to the original bovine peritonitis.

(2) From the peritoneum by direct spread, or by lymphatics from infected mesenteric nodes. This theory is difficult to support or refute but the evidence given in the preceding paragraph is against direct peritoneal spread. In Jedberg's series of genital tuberculosis, 7% of bovine organisms were found and this possibly represents the average percentage in which the infection was directly derived from some type of abdominal primary focus, i.e. tuberculous peritonitis, infected mesenteric nodes or a bowel lesion.

Age Incidence. The maximum age incidence at diagnosis is 28 years with extremes of 16 and 53 (Sutherland).

Obstetric History. Only about 12% of patients with genital tuberculosis have had children. One important fact should be noted. Not infrequently genital tuberculosis is first diagnosed after abortion or delivery.

Pathology. As the Fallopian tube is the most frequently involved part of the genital tract and provides over 90% of all genital tuberculous lesions, it will be considered first. It has been estimated that of all inflammatory lesions of the tube tuberculosis is responsible for 5% (Novak) to 10% (Clifford White).

Various types of tuberculous salpingitis are recognised:

(1) *Tuberculous Endosalpingitis.* This is sometimes called the exudative type. The tube is thickened, enlarged and tortuous; the fimbriated extremity, unlike that of other inflammatory lesions of the tube, is not necessarily closed but may remain open, pouting and everted; the isthmic portion may suffer the brunt of the disease, and here the tube is nodular and distorted. Some of these tubes in the earlier stages are patent and the employment of diagnostic salpingography may result in a serious flare-up of peritoneal tuberculosis. This was a particular risk when lipiodol was employed as the radio-opaque fluid for diagnosis, and many cases are on record in the literature of pelvic tuberculous peritonitis resulting from its use. The risk, though present, is less from water soluble contrast media and carbon dioxide gas. Giant cell systems are seen in the tubal plicae which at a later stage undergo necrosis and become adherent to each other with destruction of the surface epithelium. Collections of caseous material may become walled off by fibrosis to form

9*

pseudo-dermoids in the tube. In more advanced cases the tube becomes filled with caseous material with thickened walls (Figs. 149, 150); dense adhesions often develop around such a tuberculous pyosalpinx and the adjacent large and small gut, omentum, parietal peritoneum, ovary and uterus are involved. Some tuberculous pyosalpinges, however, are remarkably free from adhesions and their clinical mobility leads to a diagnosis of ovarian cyst. A few tubercles may be seen on the peritoneal surface, but these are not always noticeable. Quite large swellings are thus produced, and in such cases the ovary may be secondarily involved and a tuberculous tubo-ovarian abscess result. During the process of healing in less advanced cases, areas of heterotopic tubal

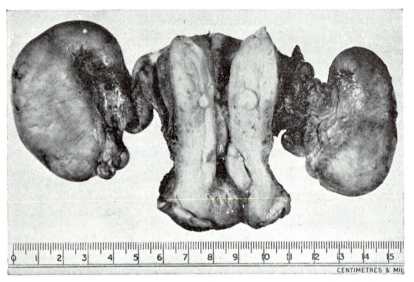

Fig. 149. Bilateral tuberculous pyosalpinx. Note the retort-shaped tubes and comparative absence of tubercles on the peritoneal surface.

epithelium are found in the tubal musculature, especially in the region of the isthmus—a form of false tubal adenomyosis known as salpingitis isthmica nodosa. This histological picture is not the prerogative of tuberculous endosalpingitis and may be seen in other forms of chronic tubal inflammatory disease (see Chapter 19, p. 422).

Although the contents of a tuberculous pyosalpinx are by nature sterile, such a lesion is particularly liable to recurrent attacks of secondary infection by the usual pyogenic organisms. Such an attack will be accompanied by severe lower abdominal pain, constitutional upset, fever and leucocytosis. A fair-sized palpable mass, usually more marked on one side of the pelvis, will be recognisable by bimanual examination. Such abscesses are liable to point to the surface or into the bowel and a chronic persistent fistula which is extremely debilitating may result. Sometimes surgeons not appreciating the

condition may drain these abscesses and the tract of the drainage tube
becomes a tuberculous fistula that refuses to close. Intestinal obstruction is
a not uncommon complication in this type of case.

(2) *Tuberculous exosalpingitis* or *perisalpingitis*, which is also called the
adhesive type, is a more obviously tuberculous condition in that multiple
tubercles are found studded all over the peritoneal surface of the tube, ovary,
uterus, pouch of Douglas and the adjacent bowel. Such cases are really

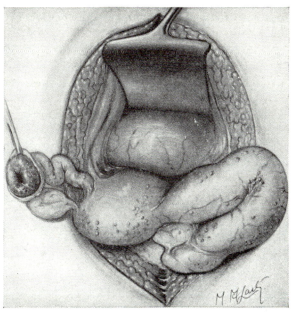

FIG. 150. Tuberculous uterus and adnexae. (Stallworthy, 1952. *J. Obstet.
Gynaec. Brit. Emp.*)

instances of tuberculous pelvic peritonitis and it is therefore not surprising
that the ampullary part of the tube is the most affected. Three types are
recognised:

(*a*) In the *miliary form* the tubercles are the diagnostic feature. There is
    some free fluid with a few fine filmy adhesions and fibrinous flakes in
    the fluid and the peritoneal surfaces have lost their glistening lustre.

(*b*) In the *caseating form* masses and abscesses appear in the pelvis with
    dense, hard fibrous adhesions involving all the adjacent viscera.
    This is the type of lesion liable to develop intestinal or bladder
    fistulae and ultimately intestinal obstruction. Secondary infection
    from the bowel results in periodic exacerbation with severe con-
    stitutional signs.

(*c*) The plastic or adhesive type of peritonitis results in a dense inextricable
    mass of intestinal adhesions to such a degree that the surgeon is
    almost unable to enter the peritoneal cavity at operation. Ascites is

not marked and, if present, is usually encysted in the pelvis. Obviously these dense adhesions are very liable to produce intestinal obstruction. Tubercles are not obvious in this type of peritonitis.

(3) There is a third type of interstitial tuberculous salpingitis in which tubercles are found in the wall of a thickened and nodular tube. In this type of salpingitis the lesion is more circumscribed and there is minimal constitutional reaction. In fact the diagnosis is only definitely established on the histological report.

Before leaving the pathology of tuberculous salpingitis it should be emphasised that there is no clear-cut division between the various types of lesion found. What starts as a tuberculous endosalpingitis may end up as a tuberculous peritonitis. The pathological compartments are therefore largely artificial.

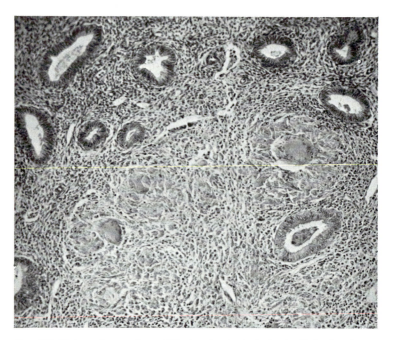

Fig. 151. Tuberculous endometritis showing typical giant cells in the stroma (×115).

Tuberculous Endometritis. From a study of biopsy material from the infertile patient the incidence of this variety of genital tract tuberculosis is probably 5%. Apart from infertility, there may be no abnormal physical findings. Although the tube is almost invariably involved, there may be no clinical evidence of this, but it is believed that a tuberculous endometritis is nearly always secondary to a tubal lesion. It is fair to state that tuberculous endometritis is almost invariably associated with tuberculous salpingitis and vice versa. The endometrial lesion may not be obvious and may evade diagnosis by biopsy in the first instance but persistence will eventually disclose its presence. In other words, tuberculosis of endometrium and tubes are one and the same disease entity. The early cases of endometrial disease may show only a few scattered tubercles with an almost normal and intact glandular pattern, while in the more advanced cases caseation, ulceration and destruction of the mucosa may end in a tuberculous pyometra (see Fig. 151). The disease spreads from the endometrium outwards through the myometrium and it may rarely traverse the uterine wall to reach the serosa. If this occurs, dense adhesions of bowel and omentum form round the uterus. Occasionally, extensive endometrial and myometrial involvement resembles macroscopically a carcinoma of the endometrium.

Diagnosis. If genital tract tuberculosis is suspected, the patient should be examined under an anaesthetic and the appendages and uterus carefully palpated. Enlargement, thickening or fixity of the appendages may be noted. Curettage should be performed just before menstruation when the tubercles have had an opportunity to mature in the superficial layers of the endometrium and the curettings divided into two specimens: (1) for histological investigation for the presence of the characteristic giant cell systems, (2) for inoculation of suitable culture media, or for guinea-pig inoculation. These investigations should be repeated in all cases where there is any doubt or when employed as a criterion of cure. Probably three negatives at one- to two-monthly intervals are necessary before pronouncing a favourable verdict. Suspect lesions of the vulva, cervix and tube should be similarly treated and culture and biopsy of sinuses that may be tuberculous should be made.

Symptoms of Pelvic Tuberculosis

Sutherland's analysis of 325 patients with genital tuberculosis is instructive:

Infertility	143
Abdominal pain	76
Menorrhagia or irregular bleeding	48
Amenorrhoea, usually secondary	26
Vaginal discharge (probably unrelated to the tuberculosis)	19
No symptoms	14
Total number of patients	325

Infertility. This has already been mentioned and is an extremely important symptom—in fact, it is often the only symptom. Pelvic examination is negative and the patient is a clinically fit woman, usually in her early twenties. In some cases there may be a past history of pleurisy or pleural effusion, and if this history is elicited the clinician should be doubly cautious before embarking on tubal patency tests until he has had negative results from endometrial biopsy and culture. The incidence of infertility is the main and often sole complaint in between 35% and 60%.

Menstrual Disorders. In less than half the cases there is some alteration of menstruation varying from mild menorrhagia in 40 % to amenorrhoea 10 %, this latter being a sign of extensive endometrial disease. If a young woman in her twenties complains of amenorrhoea and pelvic examination reveals an adnexal swelling, the likelihood of tuberculosis of the genital tract must be considered.

Pain. In all cases of genital tuberculosis pain is only present in 25 %. Unless there is an associated tuberculous peritonitis or tubo-ovarian abscess, pain is not a feature and is conspicuously absent in tuberculous endometritis. A cold abscess of the tube causes little discomfort apart from a vague lower

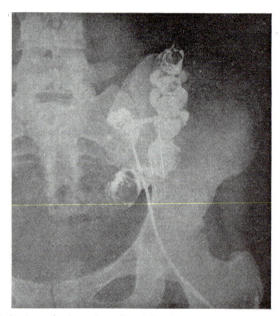

Fig. 152. Injection of tuberculous faecal fistula with barium enema. (Stall-worthy, 1952. *J. Obstet. Gynaec. Brit. Emp.*)

abdominal ache or mild congestive dysmenorrhoea, but a secondary infection of such a cold abscess will be characterised by all the symptoms and signs of a pyosalpinx—considerable pain, acute local tenderness, a tender fixed mass which is usually more marked on one side, fever, leucocytosis and constitutional upset with anorexia, nausea, vomiting and a furred tongue and constipation. Such cases are readily misdiagnosed as an appendix abscess or simple tubo-ovarian abscess and may be opened and drained with disastrous results. It is in these that tuberculous fistulae may develop. Stallworthy rightly stresses the point that a woman with an adnexal mass, unilateral or bilateral, acute or chronic, with no history of infection, should be suspected of tuberculous salpingitis. This especially applies to the virgin and the nullipara.

Signs of Peritoneal Involvement. The patient is obviously ill with fever, night sweats, loss of weight and gastrointestinal upset. The onset of the peritonitis may be acute and resemble an ordinary peritonitis associated with other forms of spreading pelvic inflammatory disease. Lower abdominal pain, distension of the gut and free fluid may be obvious on examination. In the chronic cases symptoms are insidious and a slow distension of the lower abdomen with associated pain is all that is found. Some of these patients exhibit signs of encysted fluid and a diagnosis of ovarian cyst is made. Such a cyst is, however, suspiciously immobile and the uterus and appendages are similarly fixed. The presence of free fluid and tubercles on the peritoneum will immediately betray the true state of affairs at laparotomy.

Fistula Formation. Any conservative operation on a tuberculous salpingitis or pyosalpinx is particularly liable to be followed by a fistula. The reason for this is that tuberculous tissue has been cut through when the tube is resected from the uterine cornu. The use of unabsorbable ligatures and sutures for ventrosuspension is a dangerous practice and the employment of any drainage is strongly to be deprecated. Drainage of a pelvic tuberculous abscess by posterior colpotomy is liable to be followed by a particularly chronic type of fistula with persistent and intractable vaginal discharge (Fig. 152).

No Symptoms. A few patients suffer from genital tract tuberculosis with no symptoms whatever and all experts on this disease will agree with this statement. The absence of symptoms does not mean that the disease may not become serious in the near future and the unexpected diagnosis is always an indication for prompt and thorough treatment.

Clinical Signs

In Sutherland's 325 patients with genital tuberculosis, the clinical findings were as follows:

Adnexal swelling, usually bilateral	156
Erosion of cervix (6 tuberculous)	44
Retroversion	36
Cystic enlargement of one ovary	7
Fibroids	4
Pyometra	1
No palpable pelvic swelling	111

(Multiple lesions in single patients account for a total greater than 325.)

Adnexal masses are usually small but fixed, though they can be sizeable and mobile, suggesting the diagnosis of an ovarian cyst. A virgin or nulligravida, with no history of infection, who presents with a pelvic mass that is fixed and often unilateral, strongly suggests a diagnosis of tuberculosis. If a patient complaining of infertility, when examined bimanually is found to have an adnexal swelling, tubal patency tests should be postponed until endometrial biopsy or curettage has excluded tuberculous endometritis. If, however, a hystero-salpingogram has been performed, it may show certain characteristic signs which strongly suggest tuberculous salpingitis (Moore-White):

(1) Fimbrial occlusion with small or large dilatations.
(2) A rigid non-peristaltic pipe-like tube.
(3) A jagged fluffiness of tubal outline.
(4) Beading and variation in filling density (Fig. 153).
(5) Coiling of the tube.
(6) Calcification of the tube.
(7) Cornual block.

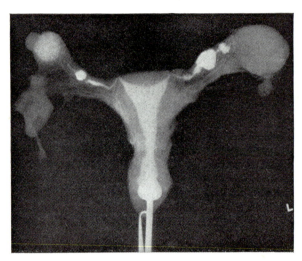

FIG. 153. Tuberculous uterus and tubes injected immediately after removal. (Stallworthy, 1952, *J. Obstet. Gynaec. Brit. Emp.*)

Treatment

Chemotherapy. Streptomycin, 1 gm. daily, combined with P.A.S., 12 gm. daily, for twelve weeks was the original course recommended. It is now agreed to be inadequate since the recurrence rate after two years observation was 24% (Sutherland). Some gynaecologists recommend streptomycin, P.A.S. and isoniazid for one year, followed by P.A.S. and I.N.A.H. for a further year. Thereafter an annual curettage should be used as a control of treatment. 14% of the patients will have serious drug reactions, vestibular disturbances being the most common and serious complication of streptomycin. Skin reactions and gastro-intestinal upsets can occur. This conservative treatment should be given a fair and patient trial in the hope that it may save the patient, who is a young woman, a dangerous and probably castrating operation. The great drawback is the prolonged course of intramuscular injections which is likely to test the endurance of the most patient and is bound to result in some defaulters. The advantage of sanatorium admission is therefore obvious in assessing continuity of observation and treatment.

Biopsy and curettage are not without the danger of a pelvic flare-up.

Results of Treatment

Streptomycin and P.A.S.:

Negative after two years' treatment	..	..	..	..		..	67%
Recurred	..	..	..	..	..	..	21%
Not followed	..	..	..	..	..	..	12%

Streptomycin and Isoniazid:

Negative	..	..	..	..	..	..	85%
Recurred	..	..	..	..	..	..	9%
Not followed	..	..	..	..	..	..	6%

Surgery. The indications for surgery are:

(*a*) Failure of chemotherapy to control a proved tuberculous genital tract lesion. The evidence of failure is enlargement of adnexal swelling during treatment or its recurrence after adequate treatment.

(*b*) Persistence of tuberculous fistulae or sinuses in spite of chemotherapy.

(*c*) Older women in the late thirties or early forties.

(*d*) Patients in whom secondary infection has resulted in recurrent attacks of pelvic inflammatory disease with gross disorganisation of the pelvic viscera.

If any surgical operation is to be performed on these patients it must consist of total hysterectomy and bilateral salpingo-oöphorectomy. Conservative operations such as simple salpingo-oöphorectomy will lead in most cases to spread of the disease and fistula formation.

The surgical treatment of tuberculous fistulae originating from the genital tract is one of the biggest problems in pelvic surgery. A full radiological investigation of the chest, urinary tract and bowel will be necessary. The exact extent of the fistula can be investigated by injecting it with radio-opaque fluid and X-ray photography in several planes. Cystoscopy may be informative and is essential. Pre-operative treatment and transfusion should not be stinted. The bowel should be sterilised by phthalyl-sulphathiazole or oral Neomycin. When the patient has been brought to a state of optimum fitness, the skin adjacent to the track is excised and the fistula dissected out intact to its origin. This may involve resection of one or more segments of bowel with end-to-end anastomosis. The pelvis must then be cleared by total hysterectomy and bilateral salpingo-oöphorectomy. Postoperative streptomycin and P.A.S. is advisable until the temperature chart and the E.S.R. warrant their discontinuation.

Pregnancy after treatment of proved Genital Tuberculosis. This is a rare event but there are 55 authentic full term pregnancies recorded in the world literature. Mostly, the result has been abortion or extra-uterine gestation.

Tuberculosis of the Vulva

While tuberculosis of the endometrium and tubes are relatively common lesions, that of the vulva is extremely rare. Children are not immune from this disease and two types are recognised—the ulcerative and the hypertrophic. In the ulcerative form the chronic characteristic tuberculous lesion is seen with raised epithelial margins and adjacent oedema. The end result of the ulcer is considerable destruction of the labia. In the hypertrophic type a condition like elephantiasis results. The diagnosis must be made from syphilis and carcinoma and rests on the result of the biopsy. If this is doubtful,

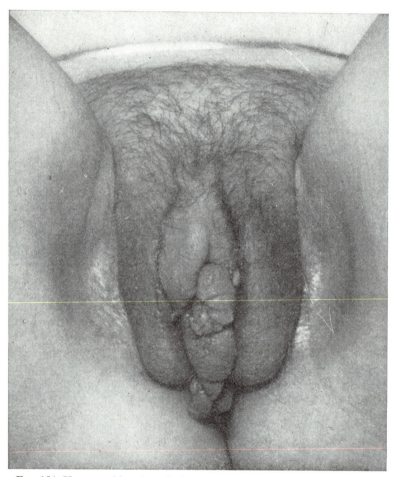

FIG. 154. Hypertrophic tuberculosis of vulva. Note considerable oedema of labia majora and elephantiasis-like appearance of labia minora (from McLeod and Read, *Gynaecology*, 1955. Churchill.)

animal inoculation may be necessary. The treatment is initially by chemotherapy. If unresponsive, a diathermy excision of the vulva should be considered provided that there is no active tuberculous focus elsewhere (Fig. 154).

Tuberculosis of the Vagina

This should always be considered to be secondary to advanced tuberculosis of the uterus and tubes. Treatment is by chemotherapy and exactly similar to that used in upper genital tract tuberculosis. It is worth noting that surgical removal of the primary genital lesion in the tubes or endometrium results in a progressive improvement of the vaginal focus and this was observed before chemotherapy became the mainstay of treatment.

Tuberculosis of the Cervix

While this is usually a late manifestation of the uterine and tubal infection, it may be seen as an apparently isolated primary lesion. It produces an ulcerative or hypertrophic lesion which may clinically be undiagnosable from carcinoma, except by biopsy. Occasionally it can cause pyometra. Its resemblance to carcinoma is further increased by the presence of a bloodstained discharge and absence of pain. The treatment consists in a full course of chemotherapy and total hysterectomy with bilateral salpingo-oöphorectomy if the uterus and tubes are involved.

Summary of Treatment

As most of the patients are young women, the initial treatment is a full course of chemotherapy. Relapse or recurrence may necessitate surgery, and if this is employed it must be radical. This involves complete pelvic clearance, since both tubes and the uterus are likely to be microscopically involved however innocent to the naked-eye appearance. Such a surgical castration is a serious step in young women and is only to be undertaken as a last resort. In fact some surgeons have refused to sacrifice both ovaries and have saved the most normal and healthy one, subsequently protecting it by a full course of antituberculous chemotherapy.

11 Injuries of the Female Genital Tract

OBSTETRIC INJURIES

Most injuries of the female genital tract occur during childbirth. In normal delivery the circular fibres which surround the external cervical os are torn laterally on each side so that an anterior and a posterior lip of the cervix become differentiated. As a result of stretching, the vagina becomes more patulous, and, through laceration, the hymen is subsequently represented by irregular tags of skin termed the carunculae myrtiformes. A superficial

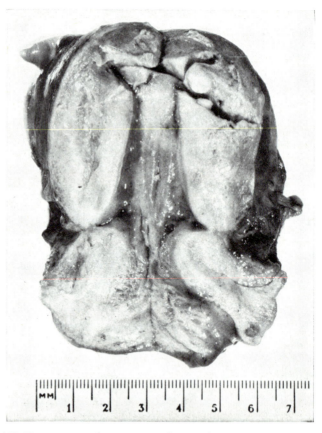

FIG. 155. Uterus removed many years after previous Caesarean section. The specimen clearly shows the transverse scar of a lower segment Caesarean section. Note the considerable thinning of the myometrium at the level of the scar.

laceration of the perineal skin of the first degree is common, even in uncomplicated deliveries.

In abnormal labour and when obstetrical manipulations have been carried out, or as the result of inexpert technique, injuries of the birth canal are frequent. Severe lacerations of the perineum are perhaps the commonest form of birth injury. Tears of the vagina may be caused by rotation of the head with forceps or may take the form of extensions of tears either of the perineum or cervix. Severe lacerations of the cervix are usually caused by violent uterine contractions at the end of the first stage of labour, others result from the delivery of a posterior position of the occiput and some from cervical dystocia. A vesicovaginal fistula may result from a difficult forceps delivery in cases of disproportion, while a rectovaginal fistula is the result of a complete tear of the perineum or a suture which perforates the rectal wall.

The majority of obstetrical injuries are theoretically preventable. Cases of disproportion should be recognised antenatally and if considerable treated by Caesarean section (see Fig. 155). Lacerations of the cervix and extensive tears of the perineum, although usually avoidable, should be treated by immediate suture.

Injuries due to Coitus

A slight amount of haemorrhage from the torn edges of the ruptured hymen is normal after defloration, but the haemorrhage is sometimes very severe, particularly when the tear has spread forwards to the region of the vestibule. Cases have been recorded in which alarming haemorrhage of this kind has occurred. The haemorrhage can usually be controlled by the application of gauze pressure, but suturing under anaesthesia is often required and blood transfusion may be necessary.

Bruising of the vaginal walls is not uncommon in the early days of married life, and a urethritis may result from bruising of the urethra. Such cases are seen frequently, and it is not uncommon for an ascending pyelo-nephritis to result.

Lacerations of the vagina caused by coitus are occasionally seen. Violent coitus or rape in young girls, postmenopausal atrophy and such malformations as an imperforate vaginal septum are all possible causes. The laceration usually takes the form of a longitudinal tear of the anterior vaginal wall. Cases have been recorded where the posterior vaginal wall has been torn through and the peritoneal cavity opened up and both bladder and rectum may be involved in serious coital injuries. Similar injuries may occur in patients upon whom vaginal operations have been previously performed, especially if coitus takes place too soon after operation. All patients who have had a vaginal operation should be warned to avoid coitus for two months. The same injury can occur after the operation of total hysterectomy where the recently sewn vaginal vault may be disrupted by coitus. Large or small bowel and omentum can prolapse into the vagina with resulting shock and later peritonitis. Severe haemorrhage follows injuries of this kind, and Neugebauer collected together 157 recorded cases with twenty-two deaths either from haemorrhage or from peritonitis caused by tearing through the posterior vaginal wall. When the injuries are small, treatment consists in plugging the vagina, provided thorough inspection has excluded the possibility of extensive or internal injury. In more severe cases it is necessary to suture the lacerations under anaesthesia. If the bowel has prolapsed, it is imperative to open the abdomen so that a complete inspection of the gastro-intestinal tract from jejunum to rectum can be made. Damage to bowel or mesentery can then be assessed and the correct treatment performed under direct vision. It is interesting to note that quite apart from coitus or direct injury, a spontaneous rupture of the vagina can occur in the upper posterior one-third. The patients are always elderly and the vagina is atrophic. The cause is usually a violent bout of coughing or some severe strain associated with a sudden rise in intra-abdominal pressure. The treatment is the same as for coital injuries.

Direct Trauma

Injuries to the vulva as the result of direct trauma are not uncommon. Such accidents as falling astride gates and chairs are frequent, and usually produce bruising of the labia majora. In more severe cases, such as result from automobile accidents where the pelvis may be fractured and its visceral contents very possibly injured, large haematomata develop in the labia majora, and the effused blood spreads widely in the lax connective tissues. Comparable haematomata of the vulva are sometimes caused by rupture of varicose veins of the labia majora during pregnancy, and the large swelling may obstruct delivery. An important complication of haematoma of the vulva is infection.

Injuries to the vulva due to direct violence usually cause only small haematomata which respond well to the customary treatment of rest in bed combined with the application of such lotions as lotio plumbi. With large haematomata it is sometimes necessary to incise the swelling under strict aseptic precautions, and to turn out the clot. Lacerations of the vulval region due to direct violence may be followed by severe haemorrhage if the laceration involves either the region of the clitoris or the erectile tissue around the vaginal orifice. More serious injuries are those caused when a woman falls on to a sharp protuberance, the point of which may penetrate through the vaginal walls into the bladder, rectum, or even the peritoneal cavity. Such injuries must be treated by immediate operation, the edges of the lacerations being excised and the injuries repaired. If there is the least suspicion of visceral injury or if the pouch of Douglas has been opened, laparotomy must be performed, and any perforation of the large or small gut sutured. If the rectum has been injured it may be necessary to perform a temporary colostomy though chemotherapy to sterilise the bowel is usually sufficient provided the suture line is efficient.

Injuries due to Foreign Bodies and Instruments

Vaginal. (1) An extraordinary variety of bizarre foreign bodies have been recovered from the vagina including safety pins, hair grips (see X-ray, p. 143,) pencils, small jam jars and Sir John Bland-Sutton's famous case of a small bust of Napoleon Bonaparte, presumably introduced as a supreme act of hero-worship. The patient is often mentally defective or a young child and in both these a persistent and malodorous discharge should always suggest the presence of a foreign body.

(2) Neglected or forgotten objects employed therapeutically. The most frequently found is the ring pessary used for prolapse, some of which have remained in the vagina for many years and have become encrusted with phosphatic deposits. These neglected pessaries can cause severe ulceration of the posterior fornix and a few cases have been recorded where a vaginal carcinoma has finally developed. Less traumatic are forgotten swabs and tampons which cause a most evil-smelling and purulent discharge with superficial vaginal ulceration. Menstrual tampons fall into this category.

(3) Contraceptive devices such as cervical caps and diaphragms, even a mislaid condom when retained, cause discharge and ulceration as above.

(4) Rubber, vulcanite and glass douche nozzles may become broken or detached and, apart from the direct initial trauma, may be retained. One of the authors has removed the rubber tip of a douche nozzle after twelve years residence in the vagina—which was ulcerated. The sole symptom was a blood-stained discharge.

(5) Instrumental damage caused by attempted criminal abortion. Sounds, gum elastic bougies, hatpins, knitting needles and the like have all caused perforation of the vagina into the bladder, rectum, pouch of Douglas and the parametrium.

(6) The authors have personal experience of two urethro-vaginal fistulae caused by inexpert catheterisation.

(7) Broken needle: During the actual confinement of a patient, one of the present authors tore his glove and cut his finger during the performance of a vaginal examination. The offending object was the pointed half of a large perineal needle used to sew a tear caused by the first confinement seven years before. There had been no intervening symptoms and no dyspareunia. The needle was easily withdrawn without the patient's knowledge.

Uterus. (1) Foreign bodies in the uterus are almost always contraceptive appliances (see X-rays, p. 143) such as the wish-bone, collar-stud or Gräfenberg ring and at the present time the popular loop or coil. These are inserted in the first place by a qualified practitioner but may be neglected or forgotten. They cause ulceration of the endometrium in the region of the isthmus but can give rise to a serious ascending infection with inflammatory appendage masses (Fig. 156). A foreign body is one cause of menorrhagia. One of the authors has recently treated a patient for intractable bleeding where not one, but two intra-uterine contraceptive devices had been introduced. The removal of one failed to cure the patient and at hysterectomy the second was unexpectedly demonstrated.

(2) The other foreign body met with in the uterus has usually been introduced in order to procure abortion. Serious intra-uterine infections often result in pelvic abscess from acute salpino-oöphoritis.

(3) Surgical perforation of the uterus will be considered under dilatation and curettage (see p. 447).

Treatment of vaginal foreign bodies is to remove them, if necessary under anaesthesia. Simple local antiseptic douches suffice for after-treatment. If, however, the vagina has been perforated, chemotherapy is indicated and, if there are signs of peritoneal infection or bowel damage, as with criminal abortion, laparotomy may be needed.

Uterine foreign bodies should be removed usually under anaesthesia and, if infection is present, a swab taken and the correct chemotherapy given Adnexal involvement if resistant to chemotherapy, e.g. large persistent masses with recurrent fever and constitutional upset, call for laparotomy and removal. In young women, it is sometimes possible to conserve the uterus and some of one ovary though the patient is likely to be permanently sterile, even if one

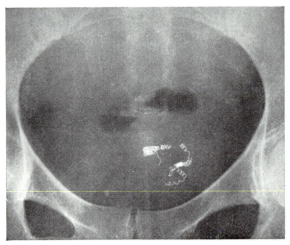

Fig. 156. A Gräfenberg ring in process of disintegration after many years in the uterus. Contrast with Fig. 74a.

tube can be saved, owing to salpingitis. When the pelvic organs are grossly disorganised by pelvic inflammatory disease, total hysterectomy and bilateral salpingo-oöphorectomy is the only logical answer. Fortunately, these severe infections from uterine foreign bodies are rare.

Chemical and Other Burns of the Vagina

(1) The commonest cause of these is the use of strong chemicals such as Lysol, permanganate or corrosive sublimate. The misguided but innocent enthusiasm of the patient is often to blame but some of these chemical burns are the result of self-administered abortifacients, e.g. permanganate. The dangerous complication of this type of burn is that, during healing, extensive vaginal adhesions and fibrosis will obliterate the canal and prevent coitus, and even cause retention of menstrual discharge with haematometra and pyometra. Plastic reconstruction is the only answer to this problem.

(2) Douches administered at too high a temperature. This is a culpable error on the part of the operator.

(3) During the operation of cauterisation of the cervix, by the actual cautery or diathermy it is quite easy to burn the vagina directly or by conduction. For this reason the authors always employ special non-conduction vulcanite-covered specula.

(4) It must be remembered that radium inserted into the vagina for carcinoma of the cervix always causes a radiation burn. During the process of healing, the vaginal vault frequently becomes obliterated by an adhesive vaginitis and subsequent fibrosis.

Treatment. Most vaginal burns, unless severe, heal with expectant treatment. Those resulting in extensive scarring and atresia will require plastic surgery.

Injuries of the Perineum

A minor degree of laceration of the perineal body often occurs during childbirth irrespective of the skill with which the delivery is performed. Some degree of perineal laceration occurs in nearly all normal deliveries while the incidence is greater if obstetrical operations have been performed. Lacerations are between five and six times more frequent with primiparae than with multiparae.

It is customary to grade lacerations of the perineum into three degrees. In the first degree the laceration is restricted to the skin of the fourchette. In the second degree the muscles of the perineal body are torn through, while in the third degree the tear extends backwards through the external spincter of the anus into the rectum and anal canal. A rare type of tear is the central tear of the perineum when the head penetrates first through the posterior vaginal wall, then through the perineal body and appears through the skin of the perineum. A central tear of the perineum is a rare complication of childbirth and usually occurs in patients with a contracted outlet.

Structure of the Perineal Body. It is important to appreciate the structure of the perineal body. The perineal body is roughly pyramidal in shape, the broad base being represented by the skin of the perineum and the apex by a point about a third of the distance up the posterior vaginal wall, where the bowel turns downwards and backwards to form the anal canal. The posterior vaginal wall limits the perineal body in front while posteriorly the perineal body is defined by the anterior wall of the rectum and anal canal. If the perineal body is dissected from without inwards, the following muscle layers can be identified. First is a superficial group of muscles which includes the superficial transverse muscle of the perineum, the bulbospongiosus and the external sphincter of the anus. These muscles are attached to the central point of the perineum. Secondly, deep to this layer of muscles lies the superficial layer of the triangular ligament, which is not well developed in the female, while more deeply lies the deep transverse muscle of the perineum. Thirdly, deep to the deep transverse muscle of the perineum lie the levator ani muscles, and fibres from the two puborectalis groups decussate between the vagina and the rectum. These decussating fibres lie high up, in part above the level of the apex of the perineal body.

Perineal Lacerations

First-degree lacerations, restricted to the skin of the fourchette, have no influence upon the integrity of the pelvic floor, but if the lacerations are not sutured after delivery, the vaginal orifice becomes more patulous. In practice, small lacerations of the fourchette are not always sutured unless they extend to the skin of the perineum, where they are more likely to become infected and to cause pain.

Second-degree lacerations should always be sutured carefully immediately after delivery, as the pelvic floor is weakened unless the injury to the muscles of the perineal body is efficiently repaired. If the decussating fibres of the levator ani muscles have been torn through, the hiatus urogenitalis becomes patulous because the two levator muscles separate from each other. As a result, prolapse of the vagina and uterus is more likely to develop than when the lacerations have been properly repaired immediately after delivery.

With extensive second-degree tears, the patient should be given a local, regional pudendal block or general anaesthetic, placed in the lithotomy position, and the torn muscles of the perineum identified and sutured together with catgut. The torn edges of the vagina and the skin of the perineum should then be sutured together with catgut. With smaller lacerations all that is necessary is to insert, with a large perineal needle, a few deep sutures which include the cut edges of the torn muscles. The essential part of the after-treatment of perineal lacerations consists in keeping the perineum clean. Frequent swabbing is therefore imperative during the puerperium. The wound should be irrigated after micturition and defaecation with an antiseptic solution, such as hydrogen peroxide, and then swabbed with a weak solution of spirit and finally powdered with zinc oxide and starch or sprayed with some chemotherapeutic agent such as polybactrin.

Third-degree tears are much more important, because unless they are efficiently repaired immediately after delivery, the patient becomes incontinent of faeces and flatus. Amongst the predisposing causes of complete tear of the perineum are forceps delivery in persistent occipito-posterior presentations, and extraction of the after-coming head in breech presentations in primiparae. Large heads and precipitate labour are also factors, but unfortunately the commonest cause is vigorous pulling in the wrong direction during forceps delivery, so that no opportunity is given for the head to be born by the natural mechanism of extension. A properly performed episiotomy will very largely eliminate the risk of a third-degree tear.

In complete tear of the perineum, repair should be performed as soon as possible after delivery. A practitioner should not undertake the repair of a complete tear of the perineum single-handed. The operation should be undertaken under anaesthesia with the patient lying in the lithotomy position in a good light and an assistant is necessary. The operation should be regarded as a surgical emergency and there is no excuse for delay. As the facilities available in the patient's home are inadequate she should be transferred to a hospital.

The immediate repair of a complete tear of the perineum is a relatively simple procedure, since the muscles of the perineal body, though torn, can be distinguished without much difficulty. The surrounding skin is first cleaned and the operation area isolated with sterile towels. A sterile pack is placed in the vagina and the limits of the laceration defined with tissue forceps. The rectum and the anal canal are first repaired with fine interrupted catgut sutures inserted with an atraumatic needle, the knots being turned towards the anal canal. A few Lembert's sutures are then introduced to invaginate the tear in the bowel wall. The muscles of the perineal body are now sutured together, and every effort should be made to obtain exact anatomical reposition. Particular attention must be paid to the sphincter ani muscle, and at least two catgut sutures should be used to draw the cut edges together. The tears in the vaginal wall and in the skin of the perineum are now repaired with interrupted catgut sutures. Care should be taken to avoid tying the sutures too tightly, as a moderate oedema of the perineum usually develops, and undue tension may afterwards lead to severe pain, and may cause the stitches to cut through. If a complete tear of the perineum is treated by immediate suture, the end results are good if correct anatomical reposition has been attained, although it is not uncommon for the superficial part of the wound to break down, particularly if the labour has been prolonged or if sepsis develops, in which case a swab is taken and the correct antibiotic administered. If primary union of the vagina and perineal skin is not obtained the practitioner need not despair. The wound should be kept clean and encouraged to granulate by frequent baths, and the instillation of 1 oz. of glycerine into the vagina after bathing will be found most helpful. The end results are often functionally good in spite of the initial breakdown of the suture line. The bowels should be confined for at least five days and intestinal antiseptics given.

Old-standing complete tears of the perineum usually result from careless attempts at immediate suture. Various degrees of complete perineal tears may be found. The rectal wall may be torn through as high as 2 in. or more along the posterior vaginal wall, but in most cases only the anal canal is involved. The appearance of the perineum in cases of complete tear is characteristic. The red glistening mucous membrane of the anal canal and rectum protrudes and fuses directly with the vaginal wall without any of the perineal tissues intervening. Laterally, on each side, on a level with the anus, is a depression in the skin which corresponds to the position of the severed edge of the torn external sphincter (Fig. 157). Behind the anus are radial folds in the skin which is corrugated by the underlying contracted subcutaneous sphincter.

One of the most interesting features of complete tear of the perineum is that it is very rarely, if ever, associated with prolapse, although the decussating fibres of the levator ani muscles have been torn through. The reason is that the patient continuously draws together the two levator ani muscles in an effort to close the bowel, so that by constant use the tone of the muscles becomes exceptionally good. This firmness and good development of the levator muscles is found on clinical examination when the levatores are palpated.

Treatment. The treatment of complete tear of the perineum is operative. The technical difficulties are much greater in old cases than in those operated upon immediately after delivery. The optimum time for operation in the case of old tears is three to six months after delivery. If operation is attempted earlier than this, healing by first intention is exceptional, while if operation is further delayed, dense scar tissue may be deposited which adds to the operative difficulties. Pre-operative preparation is of importance, and the patient

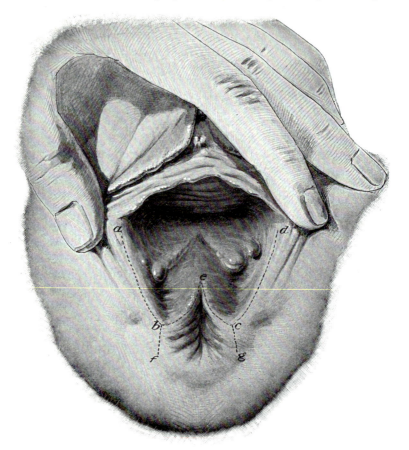

FIG. 157. Complete tear of the perineum. The dotted line illustrates the position of the incisions made in the operation of repair. The dimples adjacent to (*b*) and (*c*) mark the situation of the cut edges of the external sphincter. (Jellett and Tottenham.)

should be kept in hospital for several days before the operation, during which time the bowels should be emptied by aperients and enemata and the vagina disinfected by douching and by the insertion of gauze packs soaked in flavine 1 in 1,000. The bacterial flora of the bowel should be controlled by phthalyl-sulphathiazole or neomycin, given in large doses for three days before the operation. Various techniques have been described in the operative treatment of complete tears of the perineum, but the underlying principles are the same

in all. The rectum must be separated from the vagina by incising the intervening scar tissue, and by dissecting upwards in the rectovaginal septum.
Perhaps the most important step of all in the operation is to dissect the
rectum clear of scar tissue, and to mobilise it so that it can be brought down,
without tension, to the anal region. The tear in the rectum and anal canal
is now repaired by excising scar tissue, freshening the cut edges and suturing

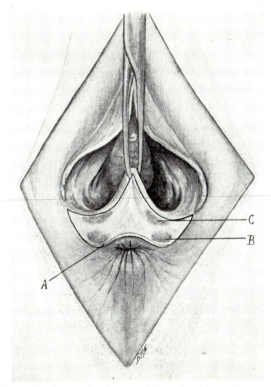

FIG. 158. Operation for repair of a complete perineal tear. An area of scarred
skin is excised and the mucous membrane of the anal canal freshened at the
edge. The rectum is then mobilised and pulled down. Three structures must be
defined, freed of scar tissue and mobilised—namely A, the mucous membrane
of the anal canal, B, the external sphincter, and C, the levator ani muscles. First
the edges of the anal canal mucosa must be sutured together, then the cut edges
of the sphincter and lastly the levator muscles. Afterwards the cut edges of
the posterior vaginal wall and the skin of the perineum are sutured.

them together with fine interrupted catgut sutures mounted on an atraumatic
needle and tied within the bowel. The needles, forceps and scissors used
during this step are now discarded. The wound in the bowel is now invaginated
with a layer of interrupted Lembert's sutures. Next, the deep muscles of the
perineal body and the levator ani are identified and sutured together with
No. 1 catgut. It is important to ensure that the muscles are dissected clear of
scar tissue, and are mobilised, as if any layer is sutured under tension because

of adhesions to scar tissue the operation is likely to be unsuccessful. The next important step in the operation is to suture together the torn edges of the external sphincter. These must be carefully defined, dissected clear of scar tissue and sutured together with three or four separate sutures. The remains of the superficial muscles of the perineum are now sutured together with catgut and then the cut edges of the vagina and perineum are repaired, interrupted catgut sutures being used. These principles are uniformly followed in the various methods described for the treatment of complete tear of the perineum. Modifications depend solely upon the position of the incisions made in the vaginal walls and in the skin of the perineum, and these, in their turn, depend not upon any particular technique, but upon the type of complete tear which is to be repaired (see Fig. 158).

After-treatment. The patient is nursed exactly the same as after the operation of colpoperineorrhaphy (*vide infra*). Prophylactic chemotherapy to control infection of the wound from the bowel is a reasonable precaution. An indwelling catheter, though not necessary, greatly facilitates nursing and adds to the comfort of the patient. The most important part of the after-treatment is to keep the wound dry. The perineum should be irrigated and swabbed after micturition and defaecation with flavine in spirit 1:5,000, and subsequently powdered. The bowels should be confined until at least the fifth day after the operation and a low residue diet given. On the fourth day the patient is given liquid paraffin by mouth and an olive oil enema. If the wound heals by first intention, the patient can leave hospital on the fourteenth day. If the wound becomes infected, the patient should be given the requisite antibiotics. If the wound breaks down and suppurates, the patient should be given hot baths and intra-vaginal glycerine. In spite of this complication, the end result is usually good, although it is not uncommon for a small vaginoperineal fistula to develop. A subsequent rectovaginal fistula is usually the result of faulty technique. As in all operations on the perineum, retention of urine is a common complication, so that it may be necessary to catheterise the patient for residual urine after the indwelling catheter has been removed.

Incomplete Tears of the Perineum. Old incomplete tears of the perineum are not usually treated surgically except when associated with prolapse of the vaginal walls.

Rectovaginal Fistula

The majority of rectovaginal fistulae result from obstetrical injuries, usually a complete tear of the perineum which has been imperfectly sutured immediately after delivery. It has already been pointed out that the repair of a complete tear of the perineum should be undertaken carefully, with the patient in the lithotomy position under anaesthesia. If, for instance, a few sutures are placed through the lower part of the anal canal and the upper part of the tear in the rectum is not accurately sutured, a fistulous opening may form between the rectum and vagina. Rectovaginal fistulae may occur after operations for old complete tears of the perineum if the wound breaks down or if the rectum is not properly mobilised before the repair of the wound in the rectal wall. Such fistulae occur after the operation of perineorrhaphy in thin, elderly patients when the anterior wall of the rectum is accidentally opened.

Other rarer causes of rectovaginal fistula are tuberculosis, carcinoma of the vagina and carcinoma of the rectum. In advanced carcinoma of the cervix when the growth has spread down the posterior vaginal wall a rectovaginal fistula eventually results. Occasionally such fistulae are seen after the radiation treatment of carcinoma of the cervix or vagina, or following extended Wertheim operations for the same condition. A malignant fistula is impossible to close and can only be treated by some form of posterior pelvic exenteration or a palliative colostomy. In cases of pelvic abscess when there is a collection

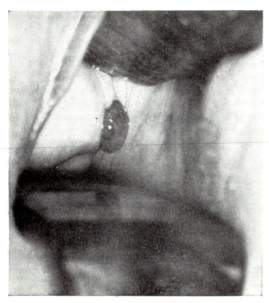

FIG. 159. Recto-sigmoid fistula opening into the vaginal vault, photographed with speculum in the posterior fornix. In this patient the fistula was caused by a diverticulous abscess and was successfully treated by left colectomy.

of pus in the pouch of Douglas, the abscess sometimes bursts into the rectum and a rectovaginal fistula may develop, particularly if the abscess is opened up through the posterior fornix of the vagina. Congenital rectovaginal fistula is rarely seen and is the result of maldevelopment of the lower part of the rectum and anal canal. In such cases it is customary to perform a preliminary colostomy before plastic operations (Fig. 159).

There is a form of rectovaginal fistula which follows infection in an anal crypt with resultant abscess formation, after which the abscess bursts into the vagina. These cases are difficult to treat surgically and good results cannot be expected until the whole fistulous tract into the anal canal has been excised. This necessitates division of the external sphincter, and follows the principles laid down in the treatment of fistula-in-ano.

Treatment

The traumatic form of rectovaginal fistula is treated by operation. Pre-operative treatment is important and the bowel should be emptied with purges and enemata, and the vagina disinfected with douches and gauze packs soaked in antiseptic solutions such as flavine and paraffin emulsion. Phthalylsulphathiazole should be given orally for a few days before operation or neomycin can be used to sterilise the bowel contents.

With a small recto-vaginal fistula above an intact perineal body—an unusual event—it is tempting and sometimes feasible to excise the fistulous track and close the defect by a local operation, and sometimes this is quite successful. It will, however, be more commonly found that the perineal body below the fistula is inadequate and that the levatores are not approximated. In fact, in many recto-vaginal fistulae, there is merely a thin skin bridge below the fistula and often the anal sphincter itself is incompetent. When, in addition to these perineal defects, the recto-vaginal fistula is itself large, the best treatment is to cut the skin bridge in the midline and convert the fistula into a complete perineal tear. This is then repaired exactly as described above and the results should be most satisfactory. In the unfortunate event of local sepsis causing a breakdown of the repair, some of the operation remains intact and a subsequent repair can be confidently undertaken with every prospect of success.

Vaginal Lacerations

Vaginal lacerations have already been mentioned. The most extensive lacerations are caused by forcible rotation of the head with forceps when spiral tears may be produced by the blades. In most cases the laceration is restricted to the vaginal walls and good union is obtained if the tear is immediately sutured with catgut. Suppuration in the wound may lead to the development of a cellulitis of the paravaginal connective tissues. Another form of vaginal laceration is really an extension from a cervical or perineal tear. When the cervix is deeply torn and the tear extends into the vaginal vault, there is danger that a large uterine vessel may be torn. If this possibility is not appreciated and the offending vessel underpinned and efficiently ligated with a suture ligature, and if the vaginal skin is merely approximated, a severe haematoma may develop and extend into the parametrium. This haematoma can reach a considerable size and is associated with shock. It is a serious complication and requires immediate evacuation by opening the vaginal wound and searching for the offending vessel which, if found, should be ligated. Usually it is impossible to identify the source of the haemorrhage and the cavity and vagina should be firmly packed with flavine gauze rolls.

It is not uncommon for laceration of the lower third of the posterior vaginal wall to be produced during childbirth, although the skin of the perineum remains intact. In such cases a small amount of haemorrhage before the birth of the head is usual. Such lacerations are often overlooked, because they cannot be seen unless the labia are separated and the posterior vaginal wall inspected. The muscles of the perineal body may be torn quite considerably although the skin of the perineum remains intact. Prolapse of the posterior wall often results from tears of this kind. The repair of this type of laceration is more difficult than that of the commoner form which involves the skin of the perineum. It should be undertaken immediately after delivery, with the patient in the lithotomy position. A good light and an assistant are essential for success.

Lacerations of the Cervix

A minor degree of laceration of the cervix during a first delivery is to be regarded as normal. The thin layer of circular fibres which surround the external os is torn through before the cervix becomes fully dilated so that an anterior and a posterior lip of the cervix subsequently become differentiated. Severe lacerations of the cervix are uncommon except as a result of obstetrical interference. Scars of the cervix, caused by such operations as trachelorrhaphy, may break down and lead to extensive tearing during childbirth. The most usual cause of severe laceration of the cervix is forceful dilatation of the thin cervix by violent contractions at the end of the first stage of labour, but the condition may result from rapid extraction of the breech and the after-coming head through the undilated cervix. If the laceration is restricted to the vaginal portion of the cervix a moderate amount of haemorrhage ensues which is usually spontaneously controlled either by clotting or by retraction of the muscle tissue of the cervix. If, however, the laceration extends to the vagina, the cervico-vaginal branch of the uterine artery may be injured and cause severe haemorrhage. In such cases, the diagnosis is usually made without difficulty, as the severe vaginal bleeding continues although the uterus is hard and retracted. Such haemorrhage cannot be controlled unless the patient is placed in the lithotomy position, the vaginal walls retracted and the lacerations repaired with sutures. As a temporary measure a pair of sponge forceps should be applied to each lip of the cervix, alongside the laceration, the haemorrhage thus being controlled until the patient can be anaesthetised and preparations made for suture of the laceration. The suturing of such lacerations must be carried out with respect for the proximity of the ureter.

The cervix may also be split either anteriorly or posteriorly if forceps are used before the full dilatation of the os. In lacerations of the anterior lip of the cervix, the tear is usually restricted to the cervix, but with tears of the posterior lip, the lacerations frequently extend backwards to the posterior vaginal wall. Such lacerations heal well if sutured immediately after delivery. The cervix is not always inspected after an instrumental delivery of this kind and the lacerations are left to heal by granulation, with the result that the cervix is eventually scarred, fibrotic, and chronically inflamed (see Fig. 160).

A rare complication of delivery arises when almost the whole of the vaginal portion of the cervix is detached during delivery. This annular detachment results in the undilated or only partially dilated portio vaginalis of the cervix being avulsed by the pressure of the presenting part behind it. Apart from this *vis a tergo*, the circumferential pressure of the cervix causes a weakening at the line of rupture with possibly some pressure necrosis.

This type of severe cervical tear is to be expected where some degree of obstructed labour is associated with very strong uterine contractions.

In addition to obstetric injuries the cervix may be torn during the operation of dilatation and curettage. Too rapid and forcible use of the larger sizes of dilator may lead to a sudden split in the circular fibres of the cervix. The danger of this tear lies in the possibility of tearing a branch of the uterine artery in the base of the broad ligament from which a large intraligamentary retroperitoneal haematoma soon forms. This presents as a swelling above Poupart's ligament which may extend to the kidney and down to the utero-sacral region. It is associated with shock and demands transfusion and instant laparotomy, and may even necessitate hysterectomy before the torn vessel can be controlled.

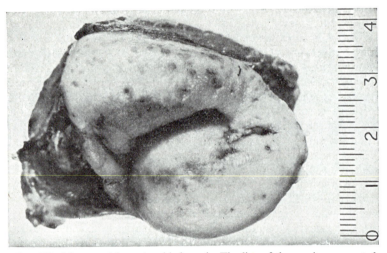

Fig. 160. A lacerated hypertrophied cervix. The lips of the cervix are everted to produce the condition called ectropion. In addition, the vaginal portion of the cervix is covered with a multitude of small Nabothian follicles.

End Results of Cervical Lacerations. Unless cervical lacerations are repaired by immediate suture, they become infected, and lead to chronic inflammation of the cervix. In other cases the inflammation spreads deeply into the parametrium and the paravaginal tissues to give rise to parametritis which, at a later date, owing to the deposition of scar tissue, is responsible for chronic backache and pelvic discomfort. Chronic cervicitis causes hypertrophy and fibrosis of the cervix, and inflammation of the glands produces a discharge of mucus and pus from the cervical canal. In the process of healing of cervical lacerations the columnar epithelium of the cervical canal grows over the raw areas of the vaginal portion of the cervix and produces an erosion of the cervix. Sometimes the cervix is extensively lacerated on each side so that both lips become everted, with columnar epithelium covering a large part of each lip of the cervix. This condition, termed **ectropion**, is extremely common. The treatment consists in repair of the cervix by the operation of trachelorrhaphy (p. 493). The treatment of chronic cervicitis and of lacerations of the cervix will be dealt with in Chapter 20.

Rupture of the Uterus. This is almost entirely a complication of pregnancy or labour and its discussion is not germane to this volume. Very rarely a pyometra or haematometra may rupture spontaneously as a result of distension and thinning of the atrophic myometrium.

Perforation of the Uterus in the non-pregnant state is discussed under the section dealing with dilatation and curettage. Perforation of the pregnant uterus is discussed under abortion.

Other Genital Tract Injuries. The injuries to the genital tract as a result of criminal abortion will be considered in some detail in the chapter on abortion. The vagina, cervix, uterine body, posterior fornix, rectum, bladder and even the remote contents of the abdominal cavity have all been bruised, damaged or perforated by a variety of instruments varying from slippery elm bark to needles of all sizes. Though severe haemorrhage may result from such injuries, the chief menace of the abortionist's instrument is sepsis.

Urinary tract injuries and fistulae will be considered in the subsequent chapter.

12 Diseases of the Urinary System

Urinary symptoms are frequently complained of by gynaecological patients. Sometimes the symptoms can be attributed to lesions of the genital tract; at other times they depend upon abnormalities of the urinary organs. In addition, they are occasionally unconnected with any genito-urinary disorder and are caused by some medical disorder, e.g. neurological. It is important, therefore, to indicate clearly which urinary symptoms are caused by gynaecological disorders and how such cases can be distingushed from diseases of the urinary and other systems.

Retention of Urine

(1) The commonest cause of retention is some operation on the vagina, usually for prolapse, and this is especially so if the operation includes an anterior repair for stress incontinence. Here the causative factor is largely obstructive due to post-operative oedema in the neighbourhood of the stitch-line. But any vaginal operation is liable to cause a reflex spasm of the bladder sphincters and this also follows operations on the anal canal. Abdominal hysterectomy should rarely be complicated by retention but extended Wertheim operations for cancer of the cervix are invariably followed by retention which may last for several weeks. The cause of this is denervation of the nerve supply of the bladder which travels in the parametrium from S.2, 3 and 4. In fact, a properly performed Wertheim leaves a patient with an insensitive bladder in which large quantities of residual urine accumulate. This denervated bladder is comparable to the neurological bladder of tabes or spinal cord injury. Overflow incontinence is, therefore, a common symptom after this operation. It may take many weeks for the bladder to recover its function after a Wertheim's operation. One interesting cause of post-operative retention occurs when the vagina has been firmly packed to arrest or control haemorrhage. In fact if the vagina has been efficiently packed a self-retaining catheter is essential if the pack is to remain in position for more than twelve hours. The vaginal pack operates in the same way as any other space-occupying lesion in the pelvis.

The treatment of post-operative retention is continuous or intermittent catheterisation, urinary antiseptics and catheterisation for residual urine until this is less than 100 ml. Posture and comfort when passing urine are most helpful and the bed pan should be abandoned for the portable wheel-chair ward commode. Sensitive patients are allergic to passing urine in public and their troubles soon resolve when they can enjoy the privacy of the ordinary lavatory. Continuous encouragement from the ward staff and surgeons is important for their morale as some post-operative patients seriously wonder if they will ever pass urine again.

(2) Puerperal retention is comparable to the post-operative variety and the bruised, tender vagina or episiotomy wound plays a similar part in causation.

(3) Obstructive conditions intrinsic to the urethra are extremely rare causes of retention. Strictly intrinsic are cicatricial stenosis following operations for the repair of a urethro-vaginal fistula or stenosis following operations for caruncle. Inflammatory stricture after gonorrhoea is very rare in women. Extrinsic stenosis is caused by the urethro-vesical angulation of a prolapsed cystocele which always responds to digital manipulation. After sling operations for stress incontinence, retention is not uncommon and may be so severe as to necessitate cutting the sling. Cancer of the urethra, bladder neck, vulva or vagina sometimes causes retention.

(4) Space-occupying lesions of the pelvis which obstruct or embarrass the urethra (these are conveniently, though only approximately, grouped according to the age of the patient):

(a) Haematocolpos in young girls (15 years old).
(b) Retroverted gravid uterus at fourteen weeks, and the pelvic haematocele of extra-uterine gestation in young women (25 years old).
(c) Cervical or juxta-cervical myoma or a myoma of the posterior wall impacted in the pelvis (35 years old).
(d) Ovarian tumours—often malignant in older women (45 years old).
(e) Obstetric—during labour—due to the pressure of the descending presenting part.

(5) Neurological causes: Spinal cord lesions, disseminated sclerosis and tabes dorsalis; after Wertheim's operation.

The treatment of retention in the presence of an organic lesion is the removal of the primary cause.

Retention due to a retroverted gravid uterus is encountered relatively frequently. It develops between the 12th and 14th weeks of pregnancy, when the enlarged retroverted uterus lies in the pelvic cavity. The anterior vaginal wall and the attached urethra are stretched as the body of the retroverted pregnant uterus sinks low into the pelvic cavity. Sometimes the urethral meatus itself may be drawn upwards into the vagina. The retention is probably not produced by direct pressure on the urethra, because a soft catheter can be passed into the bladder without difficulty. Stretching of the urethra and of the neck of the bladder are responsible for the retention; whether by occlusion of the lumen of the urethra or by disturbance of the reflex mechanism of evacuation of the bladder is uncertain, though the latter is the more likely explanation. After the 15th week of pregnancy the uterus is too large to be contained in the pelvis and has risen out of it, so that there is no longer danger of retention. The diagnosis of retention of urine, due to a retroverted gravid uterus, depends upon the identification of the abdominal tumour as the distended bladder and the pelvic tumour as the pregnant uterus. In pelvic haematocele due to ectopic gestation, a similar picture may be produced, for retention of urine may develop through the presence of a large swelling in the pouch of Douglas, and the haematocele may be mistaken for the retroverted gravid uterus. The uterine haemorrhage of ectopic gestation may be mistaken for the moderate amount of haemorrhage which not uncommonly appears in cases of retroverted gravid uterus. A history of severe abdominal pain is invariable in cases of ectopic gestation, and the characters of the swelling in the pouch of Douglas in the case of pelvic haematocele are palpably different from those of the retroverted gravid uterus. The diagnosis can be established once the bladder has been emptied with a catheter, when, in cases of pelvic haematocele, the uterus can be palpated separate from the swelling in the pouch of Douglas.

The treatment of retention of urine due to a retroverted gravid uterus is **slow** evacuation of the bladder. The patient should be put to bed, a self-retaining catheter inserted into the bladder, and connected by sterile tubing to a drainage bag. The rate at which the bladder is emptied is controlled by means of a screw clip attached to the tubing. The evacuation should be controlled so that at least twenty-four hours is spent in the process. The patient should be instructed to lie on her face so that posture and gravity can assist the anteversion of the gravid uterus. It will then almost always be found that the uterus has righted itself spontaneously to its normal position of anteversion and anteflexion. If the bladder is emptied rapidly, there is a possible danger of haemorrhage from the urinary tract, though this has been much exaggerated in the older textbooks, but the uterus will remain retroverted with the possible development of further retention, unless the uterus is replaced. The replacement of a retroverted gravid uterus large enough to have caused retention of urine is extremely difficult. The method usually adopted is to push up the uterus with two fingers in the posterior fornix, with the patient placed in the genupectoral position. Another method is the application of traction on the anterior lip of the cervix with volsellum forceps, the body of the uterus being pushed upwards by two fingers placed in the posterior fornix. A third method is to insert a large ring pessary in the vagina in order to effect continuous pressure in the posterior fornix. All these methods are open to the criticism that the trauma to the uterus may cause abortion and this is especially so if an anaesthetic is employed. These procedures are usually unnecessary, as the uterus will right itself spontaneously in the large majority if the bladder is emptied slowly.

Difficult Micturition

Difficulty in emptying the bladder is a symptom present in those conditions already mentioned which eventually produce retention of urine. It also arises in cases of new growths of the bladder and urinary calculi. One of the commonest of the gynaecological causes of difficulty of micturition is a severe degree of prolapse of the anterior vaginal wall and procidentia. When such patients strain to micturate, the anterior vaginal wall prolapses and the bladder descends so that a large sacculation of the bladder comes to lie below the level of the external urinary meatus. The more the patient strains, the less likely is she to empty her bladder, as the bladder urine is forced down into the cystocele instead of through the urethra. The only way the act of micturition can be started by the patient is by her own digital manipulation pushing back the prolapsed anterior vaginal wall and uterus. Treatment consists in anterior colporrhaphy combined with a pelvic floor repair and vaginal hysterectomy if indicated.

Painful Micturition

Pain may be present either during or immediately following the act of micturition. Pain during micturition is usually of vesical origin due to infection but may be of urethral origin and referred to the urethra itself, whereas an intrinsic lesion of the bladder gives rise to bladder spasm felt in the mid-hypogastrium so that, as soon as the patient has voided urine, she must try to pass urine again though the bladder is empty. Gonococcal urethritis causes scalding pain as the urine passes over the inflamed mucous membrane. Other causes of painful micturition are tender caruncles at the meatus, prolapse of the urethral mucous membrane, diseases of the vulva such as kraurosis and carcinoma, and carcinoma of the urethral meatus. The recently consummated marriage somewhat traumatises the urethra and leads to pain and frequency of micturition. This has been called honeymoon cystitis or less accurately pyelitis. All operations performed upon or near the urethra and instrumentation of the canal, even with a soft catheter, cause some degree of dysuria. Painful micturition is a prominent symptom in cystitis; the pain is experienced at the end of micturition when the inflamed surfaces of the bladder come into opposition. Other conditions which cause painful micturition are papilloma, carcinoma, tuberculosis and stone. One important cause of dysuria and pain is radiation cystitis which in severe degrees can cause a small capacity, irritable bladder. This is seen after a radium menopause as well as radium treatment for carcinoma of the cervix, and can be very distressing. The urine should be examined in all cases where the symptom is present, and the presence of infection excluded or confirmed by culture. Cysto-urethroscopy must always be performed to exclude the presence of the more serious causes of dysuria. The post-radiation bladder often shows telangectasis of the vessels in the region of the trigone.

Increased Frequency of Micturition

Frequency of micturition is one of the commonest symptoms complained of by gynaecological patients, and although many causes of frequency lie in the urinary tract, a large number are gynaecological. The possibility of disease not arising in the genito-urinary tract must be remembered, where there is an increased urinary output due to, for example, diabetes mellitus or insipidus, or characterising one phase of incipient renal failure. In some an even simpler explanation, purely physiological, is suggested by the habit of ingesting large quantities of tea as a nightcap before retiring to bed. Frequency of micturition is present when the patient passes small amounts of urine at short intervals and it is often associated with other symptoms of bladder irritability such as urgency of micturition and urgency incontinence. The symptoms always develop with cystitis, whatever the cause of the cystitis may be, whether a E. coli infection, tuberculous infection, stone or growth.

Frequency of micturition is a normal symptom of early pregnancy and develops again during the last few weeks when the presenting part has entered the pelvis. Pressure upon the bladder by pelvic tumours such as myomata of the uterus and ovarian cysts also causes frequency. The symptom is often complained of by patients with cystocele, mainly because a chronic cystitis is usually coincident. Inflammatory swellings around the bladder such as parametritis and inflamed appendages also lead to frequency. Infiltration of the bladder by carcinoma of the cervix or of the vagina will cause frequency of micturition. Apart from urological causes, the symptom also develops in retention overflow when the bladder is over-distended. One very important cause of frequency is bladder neurosis. A bladder makes a good servant but a bad master and bad habits are easily acquired. Everyone knows that one symptom of a minor nervous crisis is a desire to pass urine and neurotic, introspective patients soon self-diagnose the cause as a weak bladder. This weak bladder is probably a non-existent entity from an organic point of view but it is certainly weak as far as the patient is concerned. In the fully established bladder neurosis, the patient's life is ultimately dominated by her bladder—though this at first only happens in the day-time. She may even undergo several operations for prolapse repair, urethra-buttressing, sphincter plication and even sling operations. The condition is readily misdiagnosed as stress incontinence. The urine is sterile, cystoscopy normal and no local cause discoverable. Treatment is by simple applied psychotherapy, bladder discipline and sedatives. Increased frequency due to an organic lesion, usually cystitis, occurs equally at night as during the day and the nocturia score gives a rough indication of the severity of the condition. Light sleepers or poor sleepers naturally appreciate the slightest bladder distention and pass urine as a habit but, when the bladder wakes an otherwise good sleeper, it is significant.

The investigation of frequency of micturition requires in addition to the usual gynaecological examination, a complete examination of the urine, cystoscopy and intravenous pyelography.

Incontinence of Urine

In true incontinence of urine, due to a vesicovaginal or uretero-vaginal fistula, the urine is discharged involuntarily and continuously so that the patient is constantly wet, and the bladder is always empty, without residual urine, in the case of a vesico-vaginal fistula and only contains half the expected normal in the case of a uretero-vaginal fistula. True or complete incontinence of urine is present in cases of urinary fistulae, in malformations such as ectopia vesicae, ectopic ureter opening into the vagina and in some diseases of the spinal cord.

False or partial incontinence is much more common. It is exemplified by the nocturnal enuresis of young girls when the urine is voided during sleep and when such local reflex causes as threadworms may be found. One of the commonest types of partial incontinence is the stress incontinence of patients with prolapse of the anterior vaginal wall, when the patient voids very small quantities of urine involuntarily while sneezing, coughing or laughing. The condition often develops during pregnancy or immediately after delivery during the first weeks of the puerperium, although the majority of cases are seen at a later date. The cause of stress incontinence is incompetence of the sphincter at the base of the bladder produced by prolapse of the anterior vaginal wall, and loss of the posterior urethro-vesical angle. Stress incontinence will be described in detail below.

An important condition that is readily confused with stress incontinence is **urge incontinence.** In this condition the patient must pass urine at a moment's notice and, unless she is quick about it, she is unable to control her bladder which empties itself of some of its contents before the patient can reach the lavatory. As a point of differential diagnosis from stress incontinence the amount of urine lost in urgency incontinence is always considerable and sometimes the bladder is completely emptied involuntarily. This catastrophe is preceded by an extreme desire to pass urine. Whereas in stress incontinence the amount of urine lost is minimal and measurable in a few millilitres, nor is there a previous desire to pass urine. As a matter of interest urgency incontinence is much commoner than true stress incontinence with which it is unfortunately and all too commonly confused, to the detriment of the patient who undergoes an operation for stress incontinence with the expected disappointing results. The condition is essentially due to a bladder spasm which overcomes the sphincter which is normal. Cystoscopy is normal apart from a decreased bladder capacity. The condition is largely functional but there may be an organic basis. For example, urge incontinence is often present with true cystitis or urinary infection.

Partial incontinence is seen very rarely in patients without local abnormality, when it may be due to a congenital weakness of the vesical sphincter. Various types of plastic operations have been performed to tighten up the sphincter muscle, and good results have been reported after faradism and remedial exercises to the pubococcygeus muscle have been used to stimulate and increase its tone. Bladder discipline and re-education is important, the patient being taught to hold her urine for longer and longer periods. Simple psychotherapy is often useful.

Stress Incontinence of Urine

Symptoms. Stress incontinence is an extremely common symptom, particularly in patients who have borne children and in whom careful questioning will reveal its presence in over half. A very small quantity of urine, not more than a few millilitres, is lost when the patient raises her intra-abdominal pressure during laughing, coughing, sneezing, lifting a weight or even running and walking. The amount of urine lost at one time is very small but the repetition of the leakage soon wets and stains the underclothes. Stress incontinence can also occur in the nulliparous at any age, though in this group it is less incapacitating. The psychological importance of stress incontinence should never be under-estimated. It undermines a woman's self esteem, curtails or even prevents all her social activities because, ever conscious of her insecurity and the odour of urine, she is forced to retire into a shell, seldom leaves the house and becomes a self-dictated outcast.

10*

Jeffcoate has rightly pointed out that she overeats to comfort herself—one form of psychogenic obesity—and this obesity increases her intra-abdominal pressure and so aggravates the condition.

Aetiology. In some patients stress incontinence is a purely functional disorder and is in fact a form of enuresis which started with bad habits developed in childhood. The basis of this condition is psychological and, as such, is unlikely to benefit from a surgical attempt at correction. In a few other patients there is a genuine neurological lesion such as disseminated sclerosis which is equally unrewarding to a surgical approach. Careful questioning will show that these patients with a neurological bladder suffer from urgency incontinence or retention with overflow and not stress incontinence at all. It is, therefore, essential to conduct a full general examination in all patients suffering from imperfect control of micturition before considering operative correction, and failure to obey this rule will result in a percentage of surgical disappointments.

No patient should be operated upon for correction of stress incontinence unless certain conditions are fulfilled:

(1) *A patient, careful and accurate history* will confirm that the loss of urine at any one time is minute and occurs without a desire to pass urine. The history alone should segregate stress from the commoner urgency incontinence.

(2) *The demonstration of the ejection of a small quantity of urine* when the patient coughs and the ability of the patient to repeat this demonstration. It is here important to state that the patient should have a full bladder at the time of examination, since most gynaecological out-patients are instructed to empty their bladders as part of the drill of examination. This is the reverse of what the patient with stress incontinence should do. It may be necessary to have a second consultation with a full bladder before this vital test can be made.

This demonstration of stress incontinence is usually made in the dorsal or left lateral position and may fail to be positive. An intelligent patient will volunteer that she is never wet when lying down but only when standing erect or rising from the sitting position. The explanation is that it is only the maximal rise of intra-abdominal pressure which overcomes the incompetent sphincter mechanism and if this particular patient is requested to stand up and cough the stress incontinence previously absent is now all too obvious. Failure to make this test has resulted in many stress incontinences being labelled in the past as neuroses.

(3) *The exhibition of Bonney's test.* After the above test has proved to be positive the examiner then places two fingers, one on each side of the urethra, and exerts upward pressure against the subpubic angle; the patient is again requested to cough, and if no urine can escape while pressure is maintained digitally, operative correction can be confidently assumed to be practical. This simple test should be applied in all patients complaining of stress incontinence and, if positive, is a strong indication for operation.

(4) The gynaecologist should not neglect the possibility of a small congenital or acquired **urinary** fistula and *a full urological investigation* is an

important part of the pre-operative treatment of stress incontinece. This includes cystoscopy and intravenous pyelography. Such rarities as an ectopic ureter opening in the vagina will thereby be disclosed.

(5) *Lateral urethro-cystograms* are extremely valuable provided that expert facilities are available. The presence or absence of the posterior urethro-vesical angle, the demonstration of incompetence of the bladder sphincter or a patulous bladder neck are most helpful in providing additional diagnostic accuracy to the obscure or recurrent case of stress incontinence. Radiography is often helpful and revealing after operative failures. But to be useful cystography requires the interpretation of a gynaecologist who is something of a radiologist or vice versa. Few possess this rare dual qualification and thereby much valuable information is lost.

(6) *Cystometry*. Measurement of pressures within the bladder and the urethra during artificial filling of the bladder also help to differentiate true stress incontinence, urgency and other types of incontinence. The relationship between the bladder and urethral pressures can be most helpful in planning the correct treatment for a patient who presents a difficult problem.

Anatomy. When studying the anatomy of stress incontinence certain conclusions may tentatively be accepted.

(1) Probably the most important structure, on the integrity of which continence depends, is the lisso-sphincter which consists of two loops of smooth muscle which embrace the bladder neck, one drawing it anteriorly and the other posteriorly; when these two loops are contracted the urethro-vesical angle becomes more acute and the internal urethral orifice is constricted.

(2) The specialised fascia of the endopelvic system is particularly well developed around the bladder neck and has been designated as the pubo-urethro-vesical fascia. It is the anterior part of the structure called Mackenrodt's ligament, and when intact it supports the bladder neck and the urethra between the cervix and the pubic bone—the so-called pubo-cervical fascia or ligament. It is particularly prone to childbirth injuries, and when these are well established the urethrovesical angle becomes obliterated and cysto-urethrocele is clinically demonstrable (see Figs. 161 and 162).

(3) The anterior fibres of the puborectalis are similarly important in the control of the urogenital hiatus, and divarication of them due to childbirth injuries is in part responsible for anterior vaginal prolapse in the same way as a similar divarication between the rectum and vagina is responsible for rectocele and posterior vaginal wall prolapse.

(4) The wall of the urethra is composed of smooth muscle arranged spirally, the function of which is to close the urethra. Relaxation of the coiled spirals allows the urethra to dilate. This muscle is antagonistic to and synergistic with the bladder detrusor, i.e. when one is contracting the other is relaxed and vice versa.

(5) The rhabdosphincter is a voluntary muscle and part of the musculature which lies between the two layers of the urogenital diaphragm, and of which the deep transverse perineal muscle is the other member. The exact function of this voluntary muscle has been exaggerated in the past and its importance

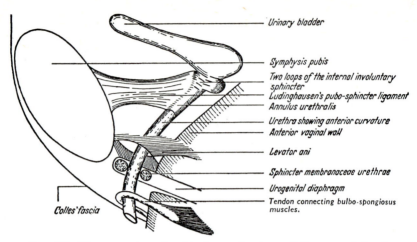

Urinary bladder

Symphysis pubis

Two loops of the internal involuntary sphincter
Ludinghausen's pubo-sphincter ligament
Annulus urethralis
Urethra showing anterior curvature
Anterior vaginal wall

Levator ani

Sphincter membranaceae urethrae

Urogenital diaphragm

Tendon connecting bulbo-spongiosus muscles.

Colles' fascia

FIG. 161. The supports and sphincter mechanisms of the normal female urethra (diagrammatic).

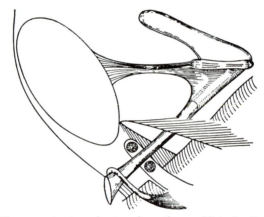

FIG. 162. The same structures in stress incontinence. Note the divarication of the levator ani, the attenuated Ludinghausen's ligament, the stretched internal sphincter, and the loss of anterior curvature of the urethra. (J. J. O'Sullivan in "Surgical Progress 1951." Butterworths.)

in urinary incontinence is small. It can, for instance, be excised in operations for carcinoma of the vulva without causing incontinence.

(6) The superficial perineal muscles, bulbospongiosus and ischiocavernosus, also voluntary, form an accessory external sphincter to the urethra and, like the rhabdosphincter, play an unimportant part in the control of micturition.

The important structures in order of merit are the lissosphincter, the smooth muscle of the urethra, the pubocervical fascia and the puborectalis muscle. Traumatic or functional inefficiency of these structures may result in stress incontinence, and the surgical correction of this condition should therefore be primarily aimed at the repair of any demonstrable damage to them. The radiographic end result of a successful stress incontinence repair will be the restoration of the posterior urethro-vesical angle where previously none existed. The details of this repair will be discussed later.

Radiographic Investigations of Stress Incontinence

Jeffcoate and Roberts (1952) published an important paper in which they assessed the significance of cysto-urethrography as previously described by

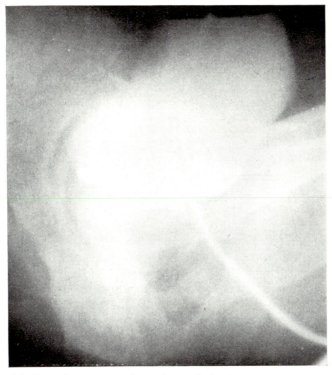

FIG. 163. Lateral cystogram of a patient suffering from stress incontinence, taken at rest with two contrast media in the bladder: (1) 200 ml. of 9% Hypaque solution to outline the bladder and (2) 20 ml. of Neo-Hydriol to define the bladder neck. This heavier medium is seen in the lower part of the bladder with a catheter in position in the urethra.

Roberts (1952). Lateral X-rays were taken in which the bladder, filled with contrast medium, was outlined at rest, straining and during micturition. In twenty-four normal controls without stress incontinence a well-marked posterior urethrovesical angle was seen, normally measuring about 100 degrees. In sixty-seven patients who had stress incontinence significant changes were seen in sixty-five, and fifty-four showed loss of the posterior urethrovesical angle. Twenty-three patients were next studied in whom there was considerable prolapse but no stress incontinence. In spite of descent of the urethra and bladder, the posterior urethrovesical angle was maintained in all but one of these patients. Jeffcoate and Roberts therefore concluded that continence does not depend on the position of either urethra or bladder

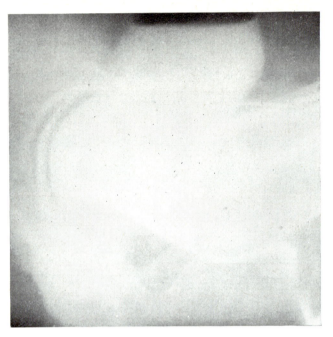

FIG. 164. The same patient straining. Note the funnelling of the bladder neck and loss of posterior urethro-vesical angle.

but on their relationship one to the other and that the anatomical correction of a urethrocele or cystocele was insufficient to cure stress incontinence unless it also restored the posterior urethrovesical angle. This proposition explains the success of the Aldridge sling and the Marchetti operation (Roberts, 1952). The work of Jeffcoate and Roberts was later confirmed by Bailey (1956) who has designed a modified colporrhaphy for stress incontinence which incorporates their radiological principles (Figs. 163 and 164).

The conclusion to be drawn from all this work is that lateral cystourethrography is an essential part of the diagnosis and treatment of stress incontinence and is particularly indicated in the obscure and complicated case and in those in which the standard anterior colporrhaphy has failed to effect a cure. The failure rate after anterior colporrhaphy is difficult to assess largely because insufficient time is allowed to elapse before initial success degenerates into ultimate failure. Bailey suggests that only 50 per cent. of patients with severe stress incontinence will be cured by the Manchester operation and reaches this figure after a stringent follow-up over six years. It is at least reasonable to expect an ultimate failure rate of 20 per cent. in all patients who have stress incontinence and in whom a vaginal operation alone is performed, and that the optimistic reports of most writers will be modified by the passage of time.

The present position may perhaps be summarised as follows:—

(1) Careful investigation must establish the accuracy of the diagnosis.

Stress incontinence is stress incontinence and not urgency incontinence. The tests outlined above (p. 290) must be stringently applied. Inaccurate diagnosis spells certain operative failure.

(2) The primary treatment of stress incontinence is a carefully performed anterior colporrhaphy and this operation should cure 80 per cent. of patients though a prolonged follow-up may well reduce the permanent cure rate.

(3) Lateral cysto-urethrography is a most helpful method of investigation and should be more frequently used.

(4) In severe degrees of stress incontinence and in those in which a purely vaginal operation has failed, some other method must be used to restore the posterior urethrovesical angle if it is demonstrated to be deficient or absent on lateral cysto-urethrography.

In many cases of stress incontinence the patient suffers from prolapse of the anterior vaginal wall, bladder and urethra. The surgical repair of the cysto-urethrocele with special reference to plication of the bladder neck sphincter should restore the posterior urethro-vesical angle and cure most patients; in the first instance this is the operation of choice. If the operation is performed by a competent surgeon whose anatomical dissection is accurate and if the musculo-fascial sutures are correctly placed, the cure rate should be in the region of 85%. The secret of success is to provide a stout sub-urethral support, and most vaginal operations are a modification of this cardinal principle.

For those patients who have undergone some such anterior colporrhaphy and whose symptom has recurred a number of operations have been devised, the number and complexity of which is testimony to their inadequacy. Most of these operations use the principle of the fascial sling, whereby a transverse strip of fascia is dissected from the external oblique. This strip is fashioned as long as possible and about 1 cm. wide: it is detached laterally but not at its medial end where it remains fixed to the anterior rectus sheath. The fascial incision is closed by interrupted catgut sutures. The transverse Pfannenstiel incision in the skin is left temporarily unclosed while the surgeon proceeds in the lithotomy position to display the urethra and bladder neck by the usual anterior colporrhaphy technique. A tunnel is now excavated from the vaginal approach lateral to the urethro-vesical junction via the cave of Retzius and through this is passed a pair of curved forceps, the point of which emerges through the anterior abdominal wall lateral to the inferior boundary of the rectus muscle. The forceps grasps the fascial sling at its lateral end and draws this down to lie under the urethro-vesical junction. This manoeuvre is repeated on the other side and the two ends of the sling are now sutured together under the urethra with sufficient tension to grip a number 4 cervical dilator but no more and no less. Too much tension can cause retention of urine and even pressure necrosis of the urethra. The vaginal and abdominal incisions are then closed. These operations are associated with the names of Aldridge, Millin and Shaw. After enjoying a great vogue when first introduced their popularity is now undoubtedly on the decline, partly because the operative procedure is a fairly major one and partly owing to a number of unfortunate complications such as haemorrhage, sepsis, urethral stricture and damage, and even in rare instances urethro-vaginal fistula. In the hands of the expert the results are adequate, but these operations are not for the occasional and less experienced operator.

A much simpler, safer and more satisfactory procedure is the operation of retropubic vesico-urethropexy. In this the cave of Retzius is opened by a small transverse lower abdominal incision and the bladder neck secured by a number of sutures to the periosteum of the symphysis. This anchors and elevates the bladder neck and restores the posterior urethrovesical angle if absent. The results from this operation are satisfactory. It is associated with the names of Marshall, Marchetti and Krantz in the U.S.A. and with Everard Williams in this country. It cannot be too strongly emphasised that it should not be employed as a primary procedure until and unless any anterior vaginal wall prolapse has been corrected by an anterior colporrhaphy, and that if this has been properly and carefully performed retropubic vesico-urethropexy will be required only in the 10%—15% of failures from the vaginal operation, or in those patients in whom the musculofascial tissues are too feeble and inadequate to offer a proper suburethral support.

Results

(Marchetti, Marshall and Shultis, 1957)

Patients operated upon 132
Previous vaginal operations, i.e., failures 65
Subsequent pregnancy and delivery without recurrence . . . 4
Success rate over nine-month to nine-year period of follow-up (84%.) 111
Infection—periostitis, cellulitis. (All responded at once to antibiotics) 2
Haematomas 4
Wound dehiscence 1
Temporary fistula (healed in three weeks spontaneously) . . . 1
Incisional hernia 1
Death (pulmonary embolism, aged 75) 1

Results of Marchetti Operation compared with other Authors

	Number of Cases	Failures	Per cent.
Marshall, Marchetti and Krantz (1949) .	132	21	16·0
Chalmers (1952)	30	1	3·3
Gallaher (1952)	11	1	9·1
Gillam, Hunter and Darner (1952) . .	20	1	5·0
Jeffcoate and Roberts (1954) . . .	19	2	10·5
Ullery (1953)	24	2	8·3
TOTAL . . .	236	28	11·8

Summary of Surgical Treatment of Stress Incontinence. The Marchetti operation at the time of writing is the most frequently used of all secondary procedures in the treatment of stress incontinence and gives as good results as the Aldridge operation with far less trouble to patient and surgeon. The Aldridge sling operation has, however, a small but useful place in the treatment of that small percentage of failures following anterior colporrhaphy and retropubic vesico-urethropexy. Properly performed by a surgeon conversant with the technique the Aldridge sling should cure 85% of patients.

Surgical perseverance will therefore be ultimately rewarded. A careful anterior colporrhaphy with suburethral buttressing and sphincter plication should control 80—85%. Of the 15—20% of failures retropubic urethro-vesicopexy should cure four out of five. Of the remaining unhappy four or five patients an Aldridge sling should cure all but one or two.

Palliative Treatment of Stress Incontinence. Before using surgical correction in young recently delivered mothers, in patients in whom for various valid reasons operation is inconvenient, in patients whose operation has not proved entirely satisfactory or in patients with poor pelvic muscular and fascial tone it is often worth while to try the effect of physiotherapy. This includes instruction in pelvic floor exercises, faradism to the bladder neck and more recently the experimental use of buried or intravaginal electronic devices.

The results of palliative treatment are not spectacular but sufficient benefit may be attained to postpone operation and to render the patient's life tolerable.

Cystitis

The female urethra always contains micro-organisms, and coliform bacilli, streptococci, staphylococci and Döderlein's bacilli should be regarded as its normal inhabitants. These micro-organisms, however, do not cause urethritis unless the urethral tissues are damaged, nor do they spread upwards to the bla dder unless they are transported by catheterisation. The catheter is undoubtedly the commonest cause of a lower urinary tract infection. However gentle and meticulously aseptic the technique, no matter of what material the catheter is constructed, once it has been passed there is a danger of infection. As the catheter is almost an integral part of all deliveries and of all gynaecological operations the incidence of cystitis must be accepted at a figure in the region of 80%, naturally highest in those patients requiring frequent catheterisation or an indwelling catheter. The logical answer is to abolish the use of catheters as a routine pre-operative measure in minor pelvic surgery and only to use them when strictly indicated, in which case a urinary antiseptic is a prudent prophylactic precaution.

Another method of infection of the bladder is by a descending infection from the kidney, such as may occur with renal tuberculosis and chronic pyelonephritis. Organisms may also spread to the bladder from adjacent structures, such as an inflamed cervix and parametric infections. The bladder may perhaps be infected by way of the blood stream, and in other cases by lymphatic spread from the genitalia or bowel. The organisms found in the urine in cystitis are the E. coli, streptococci, staphylococci, the B. proteus, the tubercle bacillus and occasionally other organisms, such as Ps. pyocyaneus. Gonococcal cystitis is relatively rare, and almost invariably follows instrumentation. The organism which is found most frequently is the Escherichia coli. This organism is now supposed to attack the bladder secondarily to an original infection by other organisms and subsequently to overgrow and replace the primary infection. On the other hand, it is well established that cystitis due to a primary E. coli infection is occasionally encountered. As the result of antiobitic treatment the Ps. pyocyaneus sometimes becomes the dominant infecting organism because of its resistance to antibiotics relative to the other infecting organisms.

The symptoms and signs of cystitis are painful and frequent micturition, pain over the bladder, strangury and the passage of pus in the urine. As the bladder fills up with urine its sensitive inflamed mucous membrane causes pain and a desire to micturate. Pain is also experienced at the end of the act of micturition when the adjacent inflamed surfaces of the bladder come into contact. In urethritis pain is experienced during the act of micturition, whereas in cystitis pain is felt after the urine has been voided. Frequency of micturition may be extreme, the patient having to pass urine every fifteen minutes. The symptoms of acute cystitis are severe, and patients are deprived of sleep and soon become exhausted. The temperature is raised, but it soon falls if proper treatment is employed. A persistent high temperature is usually due to the infection ascending to the kidney, causing pyelo-nephritis when constitutional symptoms are more marked and rigors may occur. With pyelo-nephritis the kidney is always tender to palpation in the costo-vertebral angle, and the patient will often localise pain to the loin which radiates down the ureter into the lower quadrant of the abdomen.

In chronic cystitis, pain and strangury are less prominent symptoms, but frequency of micturition and pyuria are always present. Chronic cystitis may persist for months or even years without causing symptoms and signs other than frequency of micturition and pyuria.

The diagnosis of acute cystitis is made from the characteristic symptoms and by an examination of the urine. Difficulty may be experienced in distinguishing between acute urethritis and acute cystitis. In acute urethritis, pain is experienced during the act of micturition. There is no abdominal pain or tenderness, and frequency is not extreme. In both conditions the urine contains pus and organisms. In acute urethritis harm may be done by catheterisation or cystoscopy, since the instrumentation may carry infection to the bladder. Similarly the inflamed mucous membrane is readily damaged and bleeds easily. Urethritis can be diagnosed by massaging the urethra against the back of the symphysis pubis, when pus will be expressed from the external meatus. Another simple method of distinguishing between acute urethritis and cystitis is the three-glass test, when in urethritis the third specimen will be clear of pus, but more contaminated with pus in cystitis. Instrumentation should be avoided as far as possible in acute urinary infections because of the risk of an upward spread of the infection to the kidneys.

Treatment. Cystitis must be treated by the administration of large quantities of fluids by mouth, at least 5 pints being taken every twenty-four hours. Plain water, alkaline drinks, milk and weak tea should be given. Alcohol in any form is contraindicated, as it aggravates the symptoms. In the acute phase the patient must stay in bed and some relief may be obtained by the application of a hot water bottle over the bladder region. The pain is best treated with codeine and belladonna. Opium and morphia should be used sparingly, although they need not be withheld if pain is severe. Large quantities of citrates should be given by mouth, as much as 3 grams of potassium citrate being given two-hourly by day.

The organisms, which have been cultured, are as a routine tested for sensitivity against the various antibiotics, and the bacteriological report, as soon as available, will indicate which drug should be used for a given patient. If the organism is sulphonamide sensitive this drug should be used in the first instance rather than the appropriate antibiotic, which should be kept in reserve for resistant or recurrent infections. If sulphonamides are used it should be remembered that certain sulphonamides are relatively insoluble, and there may be a risk of crystalluria if the dose is large and the urinary output small. For this reason it is safer to use one of the combined preparations of different sulphonamides, as the total effect is related to the sum of the agents and the solubility only to the proportion of each.

Since most lower urinary tract infections are due to E. Coli, which is nearly always sensitive to nitrofurantoin this drug is particularly useful as a prophylactic and as specific therapy for the established infection. The authors use it as a routine post-operatively in any patient who requires intermittent or continuous catheterisation.

Chronic cystitis caused by descending infections from the kidney is a urological problem and such patients should be handed over to the urologist.

Special forms of Cystitis encountered in Gynaecology

Some degree of injury to the bladder can often be detected on cystoscopic examination during the early days of the puerperium. Small submucous haemorrhages are not uncommon and Stoeckel has described oedema of the sphincter vesicae. This may be one cause of the so-called puerperal stress incontinence, which is largely a symptom of increased bladder irritability and hypertonus of the detrusor muscle.

Similar injuries are common after such operations as anterior colporrhaphy and total hysterectomy. In fact any operation which involves the dissection of the vesico-cervical space must cause some small haematoma formation in the adjacent bladder muscle. Sutures placed in the pubo-cervical ligament have the same effect and the presence of the sutures provokes a moderate local inflammatory reaction. After all prolapse operations, but especially those involving sphincter plication at the bladder neck, there is some retention of urine or some residual urine left in the bladder after micturition. This incomplete emptying of the bladder with persistence of residual urine is the most significant factor in encouraging urinary infection and, when combined with intermittent or continuous catheter drainage, the likelihood of a post-operative urinary infection is as much as 80%. For this reason many gynaecologists routinely employ chemotherapy as a prophylaxis after all prolapse operations.

Acute parametritis, usually puerperal or following a septic abortion, is rarely permitted to reach the stage of suppuration since chemotherapy should control it in the earlier stages. The neglected or untreated patient will very occasionally be seen where a pelvic abscess may point towards or even burst into the bladder.

The same applies to acute salpingitis resulting in the formation of a pyosalpinx, a tubo-ovarian abscess or pelvic peritonitis. In the pre-antibiotic era the abscess did occasionally discharge into the bladder, but this extreme complication should never occur now. The exception is a tuberculous pyosalpinx which remains a rare cause of a complicated internal fistula involving the bladder. Ovarian dermoids sometimes adhere to the bladder and a fistulous communication may develop and sebaceous material, and even hair, may be voided with the urine. Cases have been described in which ectopic gestations have become fixed to the bladder, so that foetal parts have subsequently been passed in the urine. Malignant ovarian tumours often infiltrate the peritoneal surface of the bladder, although it is rare for the growth to ulcerate through the bladder wall.

In carcinoma of the cervix infiltration of the bladder is common, and can be detected by cystoscopic examination. In the early stage a bullous oedema develops above the trigone owing to infiltration of the bladder lymphatics with the growth. Later an irregular depression can be detected, while in advanced cases the growth ulcerates into the bladder cavity and may result in severe attacks of haematuria.

In cystocele, the part of the bladder which prolapses is that which lies above the level of the inter-ureteric ligament and a well-marked pouch can be detected on cystoscopic examination. Residual urine is retained in this pouch and readily encourages urinary infection. The frequent association of urinary infection with prolapse is well recognised and it is a cardinal rule that no patient should be submitted to operation until a mid-stream specimen of urine has been centrifuged and examined for pus cells. If pus cells are present, a catheter specimen of urine should be obtained and cultured and the appropriate chemotherapy used to sterilise the urine before operation.

Pyelonephritis (Pyelitis)

Pyelonephritis is a complication of the urinary infections which are encountered in gynaecological practice. The urinary infections of post-operative and of puerperal cystitis often spread to the kidney to cause pyelonephritis. Pyelonephritis of pregnancy is not uncommon and the infecting organism is usually the E. coli. Ascending pyelonephritis is a common complication of late carcinoma of the cervix and vagina, either as the result of the growth ulcerating into the bladder or through involvement of the ureter in the growth, and a large number of patients, at least 60%, with carcinoma of the cervix die from uraemia induced by pyelonephritis. Recurrent attacks of pyelonephritis also occur in patients who have had a ureterocolic transplantation, either for the relief of incurable fistula or because the bladder has been removed in some exenteration operation for advanced pelvic cancer. The signs and symptoms of pyelonephritis are pain and tenderness in the loin, with high temperature and frequent rigors, headache, vomiting and furring of the tongue. Frequency of micturition is present due to the associated cystitis. In acute pyelonephritis the affected kidney region is exquisitely tender, while, in chronic pyelonephritis, pain is elicited by pressure in the costovertebral angle, and, if the kidney can be palpated, it is found to be tender. In acute pyelonephritis tenderness and rigidity along the course of the ureter can often be detected on abdominal examination. The urine is turbid and contains pus cells and organisms. In pyelonephritis, toxaemia is well marked, the blood urea is raised and casts are found in the urine.

Treatment consists in keeping the patient in bed lying on the unaffected side to prevent pressure upon the tender renal angle. The bowels must be opened freely with saline purges and copious fluids must be administered. The same drugs are given as in cystitis.

Pyelonephritis which does not respond to the usual methods of treatment or which recurs after initially successful treatment becomes a urological problem and the patient should be transferred to the care of a urologist.

DISEASES OF THE FEMALE URETHRA

Maldevelopments, such as epispadias and hypospadias, have been briefly described in Chapter 5. Treatment consists in plastic operations if the defects are small. In severe cases implantation of the ureters into the sigmoid colon may be justified to prevent incontinence of urine. Other malformations of the urethra are rare. It is sometimes duplicated, or it may be stenosed or abnormally patulous. In suitable cases plastic operations may be performed to remedy the defects.

Stricture

The lumen of the urethra may be congenitally small, but fibrous stricture is always acquired. A minor degree of stricture is not uncommon, but extreme degrees are very rare. Minor degrees of bladder neck obstruction are more common than previously considered, giving rise to frequency, residual urine and recurrent urinary infections. Inflammatory strictures such as occur after gonococcal urethritis in the male, are extremely rare in the female. Malignant growths such as carcinoma of the vagina, carcinoma of the urethral meatus, and carcinoma of the vulva may infiltrate the wall of the urethra and lead to stricture. Some degree of stenosis of the urethra may follow gynaecological operations on the anterior vaginal wall. One cause of urethral stricture is caused by excessive tension from a fascial or other sling which has been used in the operative cure of stress incontinence. Excision of a caruncle, especially by diathermy, may lead to stricture formation, and simple excision of the vulva for leukoplakia is sometimes followed by this complication. The symptoms of urethral stricture are difficulty in micturition combined with frequency. The diagnosis is easily made because of difficulty in catheterisation. Treatment consists in bougie dilatation when the underlying cause is simple.

Urethral Diverticula and Periurethral Abscess

In addition to Skene's tubules, a series of simple tubular glands and crypts are found along the course of the urethra which are regarded as being homologous with the prostate. In urethritis, small collections of pus may accumulate in these crypts and lead to periurethral abscess, which usually bursts into the urethra itself. Similarly, small cysts of Gärtner's duct deep to the anterior vaginal wall may become infected and burst into the urethra. If the epithelium of the mucous membrane of the urethra grows into these communications a diverticulum of the urethra results. Some urethral diverticula are regarded as congenital and cases have been described in which an accessory ureter has terminated in such a diverticulum. According to some authorities, the majority of urethral diverticula result from injuries to the urethra during childbirth.

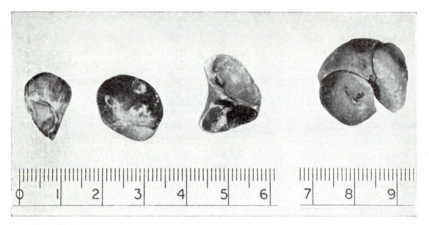

FIG. 165. Three faceted stones from a urethral diverticulum. On the right of the illustration they are shown in apposition.

The diagnosis of urethral diverticulum is made because the swelling can be emptied into the urethra. In addition, a small catheter or probe may be passed through the urethra into the diverticulum, and urethroscopy allows the opening into the urethra to be seen. Treatment consists in excision of the diverticulum through an incision in the anterior vaginal wall, but extreme care must be taken to repair the urethra, otherwise a urethrovaginal fistula may develop. Infection in a diverticulum may result in the formation of a calculus (see Fig. 165).

Prolapse of the Urethral Mucous Membrane

Prolapse of the urethral mucous membrane at the external meatus may be total, when a circular ring of mucous membrane prolapses, or partial, when the prolapse is restricted to the posterior part. The prolapsed mucous membrane is plum-coloured and vascular and bleeds easily. Circular prolapse of the urethral mucous membrane is usually seen in children or in women after the menopause. Sixty per cent. arise in children, 25% in women after the age of the menopause, and only 15% in women of the child-bearing period of life.

Little is known of the aetiology. Almost invariably a history is obtained that the prolapse suddenly develops after straining or a severe bout of coughing.

The symptoms complained of are burning pain on micturition, urgency and in some cases frequency. As the result of the vascularity of the mucous membrane a minor degree of haemorrhage is sometimes complained of. The circular form of prolapse of the urethral mucous membrane is diagnosed because the swelling is arranged symmetrically around the meatus, whereas with caruncle and polypi the tumour is restricted to the posterior part. In partial prolapse of the urethral mucous membrane there is often difficulty in distinguishing the condition from caruncle, for in both abnormalities the swelling is restricted to the posterior part of the meatus. A typical caruncle is pedunculated and forms a projecting swelling. Caruncles are far more tender than simple prolapse of the urethral mucous membrane. It is fair to state that a large proportion of caruncles diagnosed as such are in fact partial prolapse of the urethra. Carcinoma of the urethral meatus can be distinguished by its induration, and later by fungation and ulceration. Treatment of prolapse of the urethral mucous membrane consists in excision of the redundant mucosa, care being taken to insert sutures in such a way as to prevent subsequent stenosis of the meatus. With children, such conditions as worms and constipation must be treated, otherwise the prolapse is apt to recur. Recurrences are nevertheless not infrequent after operation upon children, and for such more elaborate operations have been devised. These patients come within the province of the urologist.

Urethral Caruncle

The true urethral caruncle is a swelling varying in size from a matchhead to a cherry stone, brilliant scarlet in colour with a smooth, glistening surface. Caruncles are always attached to the posterior part of the mucous membrane of the urethral meatus and like a polypus should be stalked. The swellings are exquisitely tender and bleed easily; they cause local tenderness and dyspareunia, and are responsible for extreme pain on micturition.

Practitioners tend to diagnose urethral caruncles with more readiness than strict accuracy; in fact, any lesion near the urethra which is red in colour is usually labelled a caruncle. Complicated pathological subdivisions have been readily manufactured so that descriptions are found of granulomatous, adenomatous, angiomatous, papillomatous and even malignant caruncles. These terms are largely artificial and should not be retained. The confusion is partly explained by the varied histology of the granulomatous caruncle which is extremely vascular and, therefore, looks angiomatous. Small polypoid papillomata do occur in the urethra in association with chronic urethritis, as is well recognised by urologists.

Clinically, urethral caruncles have not been clearly distinguished from localised prolapse of the urethral mucous membrane or from the bright red patches seen in the vestibule near the urethral orifice in the atrophic condition of the vulva, commonly called kraurosis. In localised prolapse of the urethral mucous membrane the tenderness is not of the exquisite degree that is present with urethral caruncle nor is a pedunculated swelling produced. In women of postmenopausal age the red area which develops around the meatus is usually restricted to the posterior part and forms a reddened prominence which is covered by a thin layer of epithelium. Such granulations are extremely common and cause no symptoms except those due to the chronic urethritis which is the real cause of the condition.

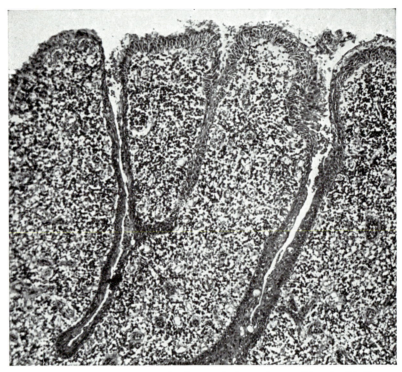

FIG. 166. A granulomatous urethral caruncle. Note the transitional epithelium and intense round cell infiltration ($\times$ 85).

True urethral caruncles are covered by transitional epithelium with invaginations of the epithelium into the subjacent stroma. A common error is to mistake the histological appearances for those of a squamous-celled carcinoma, for the transitional epithelium superficially resembles actively malignant squamous epithelium and the invaginations may be regarded as malignant infiltration of the stroma. Beneath the epithelium, the connective tissue core of the caruncle consists of connective tissue with a large number of dilated capillaries. In addition, there is always a well-marked infiltration with plasma cells, together with an accumulation of lymphocytes. Pathologically a caruncle should be regarded as the representation of a chronic inflammatory process. The majority of urethral caruncles are seen in patients past the age of 50, but occasionally they develop in young women. Sometimes a history of past urethritis can be elicited, while other cases are associated with persistent vaginitis, often senile and frequently associated with a chronic trichomoniasis (see Fig. 166).

The treatment of urethal caruncle is diathermy with the diathermy needle. Caruncles show an obstinate tendency to recur and patients are not uncommonly seen who have had as many as half a dozen operations. The

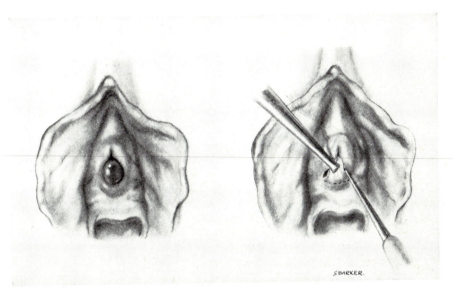

FIG. 167. A urethral caruncle.

FIG. 168. Operation for removal of a urethral caruncle by diathermy excision.

liability to recurrence can be largely obviated if the diseased area of the posterior urethra from which the caruncle arises is adequately diathermised together with the base of the caruncle. If care is taken to diathermy only the caruncle and the posterior aspect of the external urethal meatus subsequent stenosis will *not* occur. (Figs. 167 and 168.)

Urinary Fistulae

In women, most urinary fistulae result either from injury to the urinary tract during gynaecological operations or from obstetric damage. In Moir's series of 350 vesico-vaginal fistulae, the proportion of gynaecological to obstetric fistula was 268 to 82. As Moir's most recent report was in 1966 this ratio can be accepted as representative, though improvements in the obstetric services should reduce the obstetric contribution. The commonest form of fistula is vesicovaginal, in which there is a communication between the bladder and the upper third of the anterior vaginal wall. Next in order of frequency is ureterovaginal fistula which is usually caused by injury to the ureter during gynaecological operations. Urinary fistula can be classified as follows:

Vesical Fistulae

Vesicovaginal.
Vesicocervical.
Vesicoabdominal.
Vesicointestinal.

Ureteric Fistulae

Ureterovaginal.
Ureterocervical.
Ureteroabdominal.

Vesico-vaginal Fistula

A vesicovaginal fistula in this country is most commonly the result of some gynaecological operation (see Table below).

Gynaecological Causes of Fistula

Hysterectomy—abdominal or vaginal . .	111
Wertheim's operation	24
Colporrhaphy, including Manchester operation .	63
Radium	14
Congenital abnormality	5
Millin or Aldridge sling	10
Bladder neck resection (6 in young girls) . .	7
Urethral diverticulum or cyst	7
Abdomino perineal resection of rectum . .	4
Neglected pessary	4
Artificial vagina	3
Miscellaneous gynaecological	16
Total . .	268

Obstetric causes

Prolonged labour or forceps delivery . . .	70
Caesarean section	6
Rupture of uterus	5
Symphysiotomy	1
Total .	82
Grand Total .	350

Mahfouz, the greatest fistula expert in the world with a personal experience of more than 1,000 urinary fistulae, states that the majority of urinary fistulae in Egypt are the result of pressure necrosis following a long and difficult labour. The head is delayed in its descent through the pelvis and compresses the anterior vaginal wall or the undilated cervix against the back of the symphysis pubis. As the result of prolonged pressure the tissues undergo necrosis and slough about the fifth day of the puerperium, which leads to a fistulous communication between the bladder and vagina. Similarly, in cases of disproportion, if the membranes have ruptured prematurely the cervix may become compressed against the back of the symphysis pubis so that its anterior lip undergoes necrosis and a vesicocervical urinary fistula results. It is rare for ureterovaginal or urethrovaginal fistulae to be caused by direct compression during childbirth, as the ureter is usually displaced upwards above the brim of the pelvis and the urethra lies below the site of pressure at the level of the brim of the pelvis. These obstetric fistulae will be rarely seen in modern obstetric practice because of a readier resort to Caesarean section in all cases of difficult labour. Vesicovaginal fistulae may also be caused during obstetrical operations such as forceps delivery, the use of perforators and cranioclasts, and by spicules of the foetal skull from direct trauma. In such cases the fistula develops immediately after delivery. These traumatic obstetric fistulae fortunately become rarer every year.

Vesicovaginal fistula may follow gynaecological operations such as anterior colporrhaphy, total hysterectomy or Wertheim's operation, if the bladder has been injured and imperfectly sutured. Similarly, urinary fistulae may develop after operations of this kind if a ligature has included part of either the bladder or ureter. Moir states, and the authors agree, that inexpert catheterisation is one cause of a urethro-vaginal fistula. Congenital urinary fistulae between the bladder and vagina are sometimes seen, and impalement injuries in which pointed objects penetrate into the bladder from the vagina may also lead to a vesicovaginal fistula. This type of fistula is sometimes seen as a result of unskilled criminal abortion. Vesicovaginal fistulae develop in late carcinoma of the cervix and carcinoma of the vagina and very rarely as a complication of carcinoma of the bladder. In advanced cervical cancer, where the bladder is already involved, the application of radium is more likely to result in a vesicovaginal fistula than treatment with supervoltage radiation.

Ureterovaginal Fistula

A brief résumé of applied ureteric anatomy will illustrate some of the common surgical hazards.

(a) The ureter enters the pelvis at the brim, close to the bifurcation of the common iliac vessels and runs retroperitoneally along the lateral pelvic wall in close relationship to the internal iliac vessels and their branches. It is crossed by the ovarian vessels contained in the ovariopelvic fold of peritoneum and, while there is a healthy distance from these in the normal, in the case of pelvic inflammatory disease, endometriosis or adnexal tumours this is not so and the ureter may be cut or clamped at its very entry into the pelvis. This is danger point No. 1.

(b) It is an axiom of pelvic surgery that the ureter always clings to the peritoneum and inflammatory or malignant lesions which infiltrate the pelvic wall in the region of the ureter may cause a tear when dislodged, though it is more likely that ill-advised attempts to staunch bleeding by blind clamping will result in injury. This is danger point No. 2.

(c) After reaching the region of the ischial spine, the ureter passes downwards, forwards and medially towards the bladder in the base of the broad ligament, to reach the ureteric tunnel in Mackenrodt's ligament where it passes beneath the uterine vessels, 1·5—2 cm. from the cervix. Here it is at greatest peril in all hysterectomies and here it is strangled by parametric malignant infiltration. This is danger point No. 3.

(d) After tunnelling through the lateral part of Mackenrodt's ligament, the ureter traverses the anterior part of the same structure, the so-called pubo-cervical ligament and here it is in especial danger in all radical operations for cancer of the cervix since it has to be dissected quite free from the involved parametrium in this region. This is a common but little publicised site of injury—danger point No. 4.

(e) A further menace to the ureter almost anywhere in the pelvis is the needle and suture of enthusiastic reperitonisation and, even if not pierced or occluded, the tension of a continuous suture to ensure a neat and watertight peritoneal scar may kink, compress or embarrass the ureter and, more important, its tenuous blood supply. Interrupted tacks placed without tension are far better than the continuous stitch when closing the pelvic peritoneum.

(f) It is important here to consider the blood supply of the ureter since many surgeons who spare the organ the actual insult of knife, clamp and ligature, mortally injure the blood supply and a fistula results from ischaemic necrosis in seven to ten days after operation. This is particularly the case in the radical operation for cancer of the cervix where the the ureter must be extensively dissected from the parametrium. The ureter derives its blood supply from the renal, lumbar, iliac, uterine (an important and constant branch) and vesical arteries. These vessels anastomose longitudinally up and down the ureter and the ligation of too many of the parent trunks will lead to ischaemia. Equally important, however, is the trauma which results in haematomata of the ureter with thrombosis in the long collaterals. Hence the importance of gentle dissection and retraction—and the danger of the ureteric tape which angulates the ureter under tension. The ureter also derives many fine twigs from the peritoneum and should not be dissected from this structure further than is absolutely necessary. Ureteric fistulae will always be a risk of pelvic exenteration since the ligation of the internal iliac artery at its root is an essential step in the operation and deprives the ureter at one fell swoop of the bulk of its pelvic blood supply.

Ureterovaginal fistula is usually caused by injury to the ureter during gynaecological operations, when the ureter may be either divided, wounded, or included in a ligature. If the lumen of the ureter is opened a urinary fistula develops immediately, the urine leaking either through the vagina or through the abdominal wall if the peritoneal cavity has been drained. If the ureter is completely occluded by the ligature the kidney atrophies provided the urine is sterile. More frequently, however, after inclusion of part of the ureter in a ligature the patient develops a high temperature immediately after the operation, with pain in the loin on the affected side and a urinary fistula develops seven to ten days after the operation as the result of sloughing of that part of the ureter included in the ligature.

The **symptoms** of urinary fistula are caused by the continuous flow of urine from the vagina. The incontinence of urine is a true incontinence and must be distinguished from the imperfect control of micturition due to a relaxed sphincter, from the frequent micturition of cystitis and from retention overflow. There is often difficulty during the puerperium in determining whether incontinence of urine is caused by a fistula or whether it is due to imperfect control. Imperfect control of micturition, caused by laxity of the sphincter at the base of the bladder and by a relaxed anterior vaginal wall, is not uncommon during the puerperium, and the urine dribbles away when the intra-abdominal pressure is raised during coughing or straining. If such patients are questioned, it will be found that they are able to retain urine for short periods of time and to pass urine voluntarily, although the amount passed may be small. Similarly, there may be difficulty in diagnosis in cases of stress incontinence of urine at a later date, but again it will be found that such patients are able to retain urine in the bladder and to void it voluntarily although the amount retained may be small.

The constant trickle of urine down the vagina produces vaginitis and vulvitis with attendant soreness. Incrustations of phosphates may form in the vagina, and in old-standing cases there may be extensive excoriation of the skin of the vulva, groins and thighs.

The **diagnosis** of urinary fistula requires thorough investigation. Care must be taken to distinguish between imperfect control due to a relaxed sphincter and the true incontinence of a fistula. With a urinary fistula the urine continuously dribbles away and the patient has no control of any kind. A vaginal examination may enable a vesicovaginal fistula to be palpated or seen. With puerperal patients a large fistula may be present which is easily palpable through the anterior vaginal wall, and in severe cases most of the anterior vaginal wall may have sloughed. In most puerperal patients the fistula measures about $\frac{1}{4}$ in. across. The fistula may be seen during speculum examination and a vesicovaginal fistula can be diagnosed if a sound is passed through the urethral meatus into the bladder and by way of the fistula into the vagina. If the fistula is small and surrounded by scar tissue, further investigations must be made. The vagina should be swabbed dry and a solution of methylene blue run into the bladder by means of a catheter. If the blue solution can be seen to trickle into the vagina the diagnosis of vesicovaginal fistula is established. If, on the other hand, urine still trickles into the vagina but is not stained blue, the fistula must be ureterovaginal. A simple method of investigation is to insert two gauze swabs into the vagina, then to empty the bladder with a catheter and to introduce a methylene blue solution into the bladder by means of a catheter and to wait a few minutes. The first swab is usually contaminated with the blue solution when the bladder is being filled. This swab should be removed and the second swab examined.

If the second swab is stained blue the fistula must lie between the bladder and the vagina or cervix. If, on the other hand, the second swab is soaked with clear urine, the fistula must be ureteral. Cystoscopic examination will enable the diagnosis of ureterovaginal fistula to be established, for in such cases there will be either no efflux from the affected side or the efflux will be scanty and irregular. Small vesical fistulae can be recognised by cystoscopic examination, but the method of investigation is useless with large bladder fistulae because of the impossibility of distending the bladder.

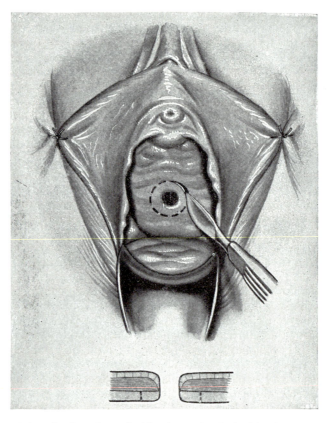

FIG. 169. Repair of a vesicovaginal fistulae. A circular incision is made through the vagina around the fistula.

In ureteric fistula an intravenous pyelogram will almost invariably show some hydronephrosis on the affected side. Retrograde catheterisation of the affected ureter is impossible and the catheter can only be made to pass up the damaged ureter as far as the site of injury.

Treatment. Small urinary fistulae sometimes heal spontaneously during the first few weeks of their existence. For this reason operations for repair should be delayed for at least six weeks after the fistula has developed. Ureteric fistulae following Wertheim's operation should be left for at least three and preferably six months before being treated by surgery. While awaiting operation the patient is best treated in hospital, where she can be kept comfortable and dry by inserting a large Foley catheter into the vagina, where it is lightly packed in position with "Vaseline" gauze. The catheter is connected to a low-pressure suction pump which removes the urine from the vagina. If necessary, a second catheter can be inserted into the bladder. Chemotherapy is used to keep the urine sterile.

Surgical Repair of Vesicovaginal Fistulae

Vesicovaginal fistulae which do not heal must be treated surgically. Before operation is undertaken local sepsis must be cleared up by vaginal irrigations and by chemotherapy. If the operation is performed carefully with correct technique the results are good. If, on the other hand, the operation is performed too soon, if the wound becomes infected, or if the wrong operative technique is employed, the fistula may recur. Later attempts at closure are always difficult, and the more unsuccessful operations previously performed to heal the fistula, the worse the prognosis. Several of Chassar Moit's patients had undergone many previous unsuccessful operations, quite a few reaching double figures. If dense scar tissue of cartilaginous hardness surrounds the fistula as the result of previous attempts at closure, the prognosis must be guarded, however skilful the operator and however ingenious his technique.

It is essential to obtain a good exposure of the fistula. An exaggerated lithotomy position with the pelvis raised above the level of the head provides good access. Vaginal retractors are required, and, if the vagina is small, it must be enlarged by means of a Schuchardt's incision through the lateral part of the perineum. Another method of exposure is to employ the Kraske position, with the patient lying on her abdomen with the buttocks raised. A Sims' speculum is used to retract the perineum upwards. The most difficult bladder fistulae are those following total hysterectomy when the fistula lies amongst the scar tissue at the top of the vagina.

The best method to adopt is to make a circular incision around the fistula and to separate the vagina from the bladder. The next step, the most important of all, is to mobilise the bladder through this incision so that the wound in the bladder can subsequently be invaginated without tension. After the bladder has been adequately mobilised the edges of the fistula are freshened. The simplest technique is to insert two guiding sutures through the bladder wall at two ends of the fistula and then to excise the scar tissue at the rim of the fistula with a sharp tenotomy knife. The bladder is now closed by a layer of interrupted sutures of fine catgut which do not include the mucous membrane but which pass through the muscle wall of the bladder along the freshened edges. A second reinforcing series of interrupted Lembert sutures should now be inserted. The vagina is then closed with interrupted catgut sutures (see Figs. 169—171). Suture material throughout the operation should consist of catgut, though Moir uses nylon and removes it after three weeks.

In some cases of vesicovaginal fistula it may be necessary to open the abdomen before the bladder can be adequately mobilised. When the bladder has been mobilised it is opened either retroperitoneally or transperitoneally. The fistula is then closed from inside the bladder under direct vision and the bladder drained by a suprapubic cystotomy for ten days in addition to drainage by an indwelling urethral catheter.

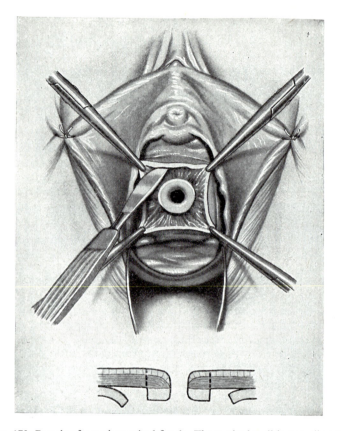

Fig. 170. Repair of a vesicovaginal fistula. The vaginal wall is now dissected away from the bladder with the utmost care to obtain a maximum degree of mobilisation of the bladder.

Surgeons such as Chassar Moir who have had a large experience of vesico-vaginal fistula claim that almost all can be closed successfully by the vaginal route.

Operations employing large and elaborate skin and muscle grafts should rarely be needed except for big bladder defects—usually the result of radiation treatment for carcinoma of the cervix. The effect of the radiation is to impoverish the local blood supply. It is in this class of case that the operation of colpocleisis or ureterocolic implantation has been occasionally used.

The after-treatment of operations for vesicovaginal fistula is important. A self-retaining catheter should be used for at least fourteen days and its patency checked at frequent intervals by observing a satisfactory flow of urine into the receptacle. If there is any suspicion of blockage the catheter must be renewed at once. During this time the patient should be given

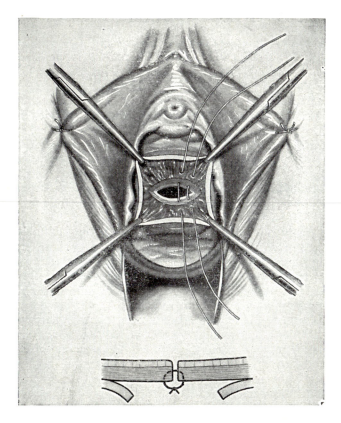

Fig. 171. Repair of a vesicovaginal fistula. The opening in the bladder is now closed. Interrupted sutures are passed through the muscle wall of the bladder. (*From Shaw's* "Operative Gynaecology," *Edinburgh, E. & S. Livingstone.*)

urinary antiseptics and large quantities of fluid. Care must also be taken to prevent infection of the vaginal wound, which must be safeguarded by the appropriate chemotherapy.

Ureteric Fistula

In the anatomical considerations, the various situations in which the ureter is likely to be damaged have been considered. The knife, scissors, clamp (partially or completely applied), needle, ligature and avascular necrosis can all operate to the detriment of the ureter. Finally, the surgeon may deliberately resect a part of the ureter in order to overcome the risk of leaving a small area of malignant infiltration, or he may deliberately cut the ureter in order to implant it into the bowel. All these accidents and procedures may result in a subsequent fistula. The most likely cases in which the ureter may be damaged are those of carcinoma of the cervix, body and ovary, endometriosis, pelvic inflammatory disease (not forgetting tuberculosis) and tumours which have burrowed into the broad ligament under the ureter and lifted it over the dome of the tumour or displaced it laterally. Sometimes ovarian cysts burrow retroperitoneally and may actually surround the ureter which lies in a tunnel in the cyst. Such cases obviously cause ureteric obstruction, but the chief danger lies in the distortion of the normal ureteric anatomy. The cardinal rule which should never be broken in these operations is to cut nothing and clamp nothing until the ureter has been identified and isolated in its entire extent. An excellent safety measure, when in doubt, is to identify the ureter high up at the brim of the pelvis, where it is readily found, and to follow it down to the bladder. During the operation, it frequently happens that large friable veins are torn in the uterine and vaginal plexus. Rapid and alarming haemorrhage wells up in the wound and the surgeon may call for a clamp and blindly plunge it into the morass of haemorrhage to staunch the bleeding vessel.

A competent pelvic surgeon will almost always recognise that he has cut the ureter the moment he has done so and, if the position in which it has been cut is in the region of the uterine vessels, ureterocystotomy should be immediately performed and as a rule the end results will be satisfactory although such an anastomosis demands periodic assessment to obviate the danger of stricture formation. If the ureter is cut too high to be implanted in the bladder, the surgeon has a choice of performing uretero-ureteric anastomosis over a ureteric catheter or of implanting the ureter in a convenient adjacent piece of bowel according to his own convictions and the indication of a given case. Drainage to the site of the anastomosis in these cases is usually unnecessary, but it is wise to provide drainage to bladder or bowel by an indwelling catheter for ten to fourteen days, until the junction becomes secure. It is important to remember that there must be no tension on the anastomosis whether it be bladder or bowel and it is better to put a ureter in the bowel without tension than to place it in the bladder on the stretch.

The problem of the immediately recognised injury from cutting or clamping is therefore not a great one and the end results are, on the whole, satisfactory. Damage from clamp or ligature, however, whether partial or complete, may may not be recognised at the time and subsequently may result in fistula formation. If the ureter has been clamped for a short period and this is immediately recognised, removal of the clamp and inspection of the area of damage may be all that is required, but it is wise to provide separate stab drainage to the site of the injury. Such a ureter is liable to stricture formation and may need subsequent implantation. If the surgeon is in any doubt as to the viability of the clamped area, he had better cut it proximally and implant it immediately. If a ligature has been passed round the ureter, in a few fortunate cases the affected kidney, if sterile, will undergo a quiet aseptic necrosis and apart from some pain in one loin little untoward will be noticed. If, however, the disaster is bilateral, the patient will, of course, have complete surgical anuria and exploration will be performed within twenty-four hours. Attempts to deligate the ureter may be unsuccessful; the operative area is oedematous and the anatomy is obscured by the recent trauma; the removal of the offending ligature may result in severe haemorrhage. In such a case, a quick bilateral nephrostomy may be the safest procedure and this can be followed by a subsequent ureteric transplantation when the local reaction has subsided and the anatomy has again become more normal. The wise surgeon will allow at least three, and preferably six months to elapse before undertaking such a procedure and will only consider it then if full urological investigation is favourable.

Ureteric Obstruction

Ureteric Compression and Obstruction from Extraneous Sources

It is unfortunately not well recognised by gynaecologists that many conditions in the female pelvis are associated with moderate degrees of ureteric obstruction:—

(a) *Uterine Prolapse.* In complete procidentia of the uterus, the main supporting structure of that organ, namely Mackenrodt's ligament, is greatly elongated and in its descent with the uterus a loop of the ureter is drawn down and lies outside the vaginal orifice. This process causes an acute angulation of the ureter and it is not surprising that it gives rise to hydroureter and hydronephrosis. The uterine arteries may also compress the ureter as they become elongated by the descent of the uterus. Many of these patients have a chronic urinary infection and this, associated with ureteric obstruction, may seriously impair their renal function and render them bad operative risks.

(b) *Pelvic Tumours.* These may cause compression and obstruction of the ureter, and this is especially true of a tight-fitting myoma which lies firmly embedded in the pelvis. Ovarian cysts, benign and malignant, and even pelvic inflammatory disease produce the same picture. Such patients should have a thorough urological investigation before operation since roughly half of them would show some ureteric obstruction, and this may well account for post-operative urinary infection in such patients. Removal of these tumours will restore the urinary tract to normal in 70% of cases. The worst offenders are those in which the obstruction is due to pelvic inflammatory disease, where permanent stricture formation has occurred in a segment of the ureter.

(c) *Carcinoma of the Cervix and other Malignant Infiltrations of the Broad Ligament.* Although the ureter is guarded by a tough sheath in the ureteric canal against actual malignant infiltration, its situation in this tunnel is a grave danger since it is particularly subject to compression. It is an absolute dictum of the authors that no case of cancer of the cervix should ever be treated by surgery or radiation until a preliminary urographic study has been made. Those patients who show ureteric obstruction have a definitely poorer prognosis and it must be remembered that 60% of cases of carcinoma of the cervix die, not of their primary disease, but of bilateral renal obstruction. In these patients, the surgeon's knife has been regarded in the past as the great menace to the ureter, but effective radiation of an infiltrated parametrium is an equal if not greater menace since the resulting fibrosis eventually strangles the ureter. This process is not immediate or spectacular and may develop over months or even years and the patient may well be cured of the local disease to succumb, at a later date, to the urinary obstruction.

(*d*) *Obstruction at the Site of a Fistula.* Many ureteric fistulae heal spontaneously and, while this is a gratifying process to surgeon and patient, the net results of such a cicatrix may be disastrous to the affected kidney. By the same token, uretero-ureteric anastomosis of a ureter sectioned too high to be implanted into the bladder is, unfortunately, too often followed by stricture formation at the site of the junction. Such a patient should be carefully followed up by a competent urologist and frequent pyelograms should control the conduct of the case. A periodic dilatation may well save the kidney but many of these patients end up with a nephrectomy. It is questionable whether uretero-ureteric anastomosis is a good operation, and it is possibly better to implant a ureter sectioned at a high level straight into the bowel as a primary procedure.

(*e*) *Pregnancy.* All gynaecologists are conversant with the fact that pregnancy has a profound effect on the ureter and kidney pelvis. This is due to the specific action of progesterone on all smooth muscle throughout the body. The gastrointestinal tract and gall bladder, the musculature of the veins and the ligaments of the spine and pelvis are all affected. The changes are most remarkable, however, in the urinary tract and appear by the fourth month to reach a maximum at term. After pregnancy this process of hydroureter slowly involutes and should have returned to normal at the end of the puerperium, certainly by the third month. If, however, a severe infection results in a pyelonephritis of pregnancy, the process of involution may never be completed and permanent damage may result in a chronic pyelonephritis. The cause of this ureteric dilatation is not compression from the growing uterus since it occurs before such obstruction can operate. It is more frequently noticed on the right than the left and is probably due to some distortion of the ureteric canal by the dextro-rotation and dextro-position of the pregnant uterus which is so frequent a finding at operations such as Caesarean section. This physiological hydro-ureter calls for no treatment and is only of real interest as being a probable cause of pyelonephritis of pregnancy.

13 The Pathology of Conception

Conception results from the fertilisation of the ovum by a spermatozoon. Much information has been obtained of the biological process whereby the spermatozoon enters the ovum, as fertilisation can easily be studied in lower animals. Specimens of young human fertilised ova obtained by Rock and Hertig have shown conclusively that fertilisation occurs in the Fallopian tube, and that the fertilised ovum remains four to five days in the Fallopian tube, during which time it develops into the blastocyst. At about the sixth day after fertilisation it reaches the cavity of the uterus and becomes embedded in the endometrium.

The mechanism whereby the spermatozoa pass along the uterus is not properly explained, as ciliary movement of the cervical and endometrial epithelia is downwards so that spermatozoa must migrate against the ciliary current. In addition to this adverse ciliary current, spermatozoa encounter the peristaltic waves in the Fallopian tube, the direction of which is against their upward progress. It can only be assumed that spermatozoa which live in an attractive medium of seminal fluid (pH 8), find the acid environment of vaginal secretion (pH 4·5) inclement and lethal in a matter of two to four hours. The cervix has the same pH (8) as seminal fluid and is undoubtedly and demonstrably attractive to the spermatozoa. Spermatozoa are powerful, fast swimmers whose behaviour resembles the determination of a spawning salmon. It has been experimentally estimated that from the time of ejaculation to the time of arrival in the ampulla of the tube, it takes about sixty minutes for the spermatozoa to cover the intervening 20 cms. This distance when compared to the size of a spermatozoon represents rapid and purposeful travel.

In order to understand the powers of fertilisation, it is essential to know the limiting period of viability which governs the useful life of a spermatozoon after ejaculation, during which it is capable of penetrating and fertilising the ovum. In the past estimates have erred on the generous side and spermatozoa have been credited with a wholly unjustifiable longevity. It is now generally accepted that, though a spermatozoon after ejaculation may remain motile for a longer period, its useful life span is limited to twenty-four hours and that, after this short interval, it is incapable of performing its biological duty. The period of survival of a mature ovum is probably even shorter than that of a spermatozoon and the time which elapses after its escape from a ripe Graafian follicle and its entry into the Fallopian tube during which it is potentially fertilisable, is estimated at twelve hours. The significance of this statement is that coitus, to be capable of fertilisation, must take place within twelve hours of ovulation. This theory, if correct, naturally shortens the chances of successful conception and it certainly explains why some married partners who are potentially fertile, fail to conceive for the simple reason that coitus does not coincide with ovulation. In other words, unless intercourse occurs frequently enough to cover the short time during which the ovum is viable, it may be months or years before a chance encounter achieves successful fertilisation.

This theory has been elaborated by Knaus who, from observation of the menstrual cycles of many hundred of patients, concluded that ovulation most commonly occurs fourteen days before the onset of the next period, no matter how short or how long the intermenstrual interval. Thus in a twenty-eight day cycle, ovulation occurs on the 14th to 15th day, in a twenty-one day cycle on the 7th and in a thirty-five day cycle on the 21st day. This calculation of ovulation time is the basis of the so-called safe period whereby unguarded intercourse which avoids the days near ovulation is considered to be safe from the risks of conception.

There are, however, two undoubted fallacies about the accurate prediction of ovulation time. The menstrual behaviour of a woman is not regulated by a chronometer and even the most exemplary and regular cycles are liable to unpredictable aberrations. This applies to healthy women, but derangement is even more likely in a woman suffering from minor ailments. The second fallacy is that evidence is accumulating that ovulation may be advanced or retarded by many extraneous factors which operate on the various agents responsible for menstrual function—cerebral cortex, hypothalamus, pituitary and ovary. This latter hypothesis will explain those authentic case histories in which women have conceived on any day in the menstrual cycle and the understandable limitations of the so-called safe period.

Little is known of the method of transport of the ovum from the ruptured follicle to the abdominal ostium. It is generally believed that ciliary movement induces currents which carry the ovum towards the abdominal ostium. Recent research has shown that the fimbriae of the Fallopian tube, by muscular contraction, become spread out over the ovary at the time of ovulation, a movement which simplifies the transport of the discharged ovum into the lumen of the Fallopian tube. Furthermore, the musculature of the Fallopian tube undergoes rhythmical contractions, especially at the time of ovulation, and these contractions can be recorded by kymographic tracings. It is most likely that a form of peristaltic contraction of the Fallopian tube determines the transport of the ovum towards the cavity of the uterus. It is not easy, however, to understand how the fertilised ovum passes through the interstitial portion of the tube to reach the cavity of the uterus.

It is a popular misconception to attribute infertility and difficulty during coitus to the female, but on general biological principles the blame should be shared between the two partners. It is not uncommon for patients to complain of difficulty during coitus when they have little knowledge of the correct method to be employed. During sexual intercourse the erectile tissues around the vaginal orifice become engorged and the vaginal orifice becomes more patulous. There is a discharge of mucus from the ducts of Bartholin's glands which acts as a lubricant. The female orgasm is induced by stimulation of the clitoris partly during the penetration of the penis and partly as the result of the clitoris being rhythmically pressed against the male after penetration. The importance of the extra-genital areas of sexual stimulation must not be forgotten. These erogenic areas vary with the individual and their susceptibility to stimulation is equally variable, but their aggregate response is cumulative and plays a vital part in the ultimate achievement of an orgasm. Little is known of the factors which constitute the female orgasm. It has been suggested hypothetically that both the uterus and the Fallopian tubes undergo rhythmical contraction, though a more likely explanation is a rhythmic spasm of the muscles of the pelvic floor. The uterine contribution to orgasm cannot be at all significant, since women who have undergone total hysterectomy continue to experience as full a satisfaction as before the removal of the uterus. There is some evidence that the mucous secretion contained in the cervical canal is extruded into the vagina during the orgasm. The seminal fluid is mainly deposited in the posterior fornix of the vagina, but it is possible that some of it is ejaculated directly into the cervical canal. It is also believed that the contractions of the uterus and the Fallopian tubes during the female orgasm cause seminal fluid to be aspirated into the cavity of the uterus, and it is possible that this aspiration effect is responsible, in part at least, for the migration of spermatozoa upwards into the Fallopian tubes. If this is so, it postulates the doctrine of reverse peristalsis since the normal wave of utero-tubal peristalsis is from above downwards. A more likely suggestion is that rhythmic contractions of the pelvic muscles direct the seminal ejaculate towards the cervix, whereafter the propulsive power of the spermatozoa provide the forward momentum. The female orgasm is not essential for conception, and it is not uncommon to see women who have conceived without full consummation of the marriage and in whom the hymen is intact. In such cases the spermatozoa, having been deposited around the hymen, migrate through their own motility along the whole length of the vagina and uterus.

It must, therefore, be conceded that the uterus need not be present in order to achieve an orgasm. Many women after hysterectomy actually confess to an improved orgasm and this is explicable on the grounds of disinhibition due to the removal of the fear of pregnancy. The explanation is therefore psychological and not physical. The value of the ovary is, however, far more important than the uterus. Removal of both ovaries in a young and sexually active woman may have unpredictable results. In some, ovarian deficiency leads to a premature menopause and possibly frigidity, while in a more favoured few the results are negligible and intercourse and orgasm continue to occur unaltered. Extragenital sources of oestrogen are undoubtedly compensatory to the loss of ovarian hormone, just as extra-genital erogenic zones are important in the achievement of orgasm. A great deal depends on the attitude of mind of the patient and not a little on the handling of the situation by her partner.

Vaginismus

Vaginismus can be regarded as a hyperaesthesia which leads to spasm of the sphincter vaginae and the levator ani muscles during attempted coitus or when an attempt is made to examine the patient vaginally. It should be sub-divided into primary vaginismus, in which there is no organic lesion present that can be considered causative, and secondary vaginismus in which some obvious painful lesion in the region of the genital tract can be found on examination. While this classification is helpful, it somewhat over-simplifies the problem since in most instances both factors are operative. In primary vaginismus, when the patient is being examined in the left lateral position and an attempt is being made to inspect the vulva by separating the labia, a muscle spasm is induced whereby the thighs are drawn together, the woman turns over on her back, and by spasm of the muscles of her back assumes a state of mild opisthotonos. The levator muscles become tonically contracted, and commonly the patient cries out and endeavours to push the medical attendant away from her. In secondary vaginismus, a minor degree of spasm may be brought about by painful local lesions such as small infected lacerations of the hymen, urethral caruncles, vulvitis and as a sequel of vaginal operations for the repair of prolapse. As a result of the operation the calibre of the introitus and the vagina is narrowed. The operation scar is naturally sensitive for some weeks after the repair and premature attempts at coitus are painful. It is thus easy for organic dyspareunia to lead to a protective spasm in order to avoid the pain of coitus. The spasm is not unlike that seen in primary vaginismus, although it is never of the same degree. Removal of the cause will cure this condition whereas in true vaginismus treatment is prolonged and the results not always satisfactory.

Typical vaginismus always has a psycho-neurotic basis. Frequently a history of mental trauma during adolescence can be traced, and in most women with vaginismus there is a subconscious dread of sexual intercourse. This distaste for coitus is often misinterpreted as frigidity whereas in actual fact the patient is normally orientated towards coitus and would gladly accept it if she could only overcome her anxiety neurosis. This anxiety neurosis is all too often the result of enthusiastic but clumsy technique on the part of her husband, dating from the time of the first consummation of her marriage. Sometimes it dates from a guilt complex engendered by an early, clandestine and extra-maritial association. Faulty parental advice or the active instruction from a frustrated and unsatisfied parent that all sex is slightly repugnant to decent intelligent people has been responsible for the gradual conditioning of the adolescent to regard coitus as shameful or even degrading. It would be expected that the parous woman would be immune to this complaint, yet this is not entirely true. A woman who has experienced a difficult labour or one ending in some obstetric tragedy fears the outcome of the next pregnancy. It is simple logic to avoid the issue by invoking a protective spasm and vaginismus results. Whatever the primary cause of the condition, subsequent attempts at coitus are associated with local pain and tenderness which result from bruising of the introitus. The final state of the patient is one of frustration and disgust that the ultimate physical pleasure of her marriage should become a travesty of pain and discomfort. She feels cheated of her physical rights as a woman and becomes convinced that she is unlikely to conceive. Her patience and that of her husband gradually become exhausted and she finally regards herself and her marriage as peculiar and unnatural. A grave strain is placed upon the husband who, convinced of his wife's physical incapacity, is strongly tempted to seek physical solace by extra-marital relationship. Unless the spiritual bond is stronger than the physical, such a marriage is in jeopardy of disruption. Equally culpable is the gentle over-indulgent husband who is too considerate to persevere in overcoming his wife's inhibition and rather than inflict the slightest trauma gradually desists altogether from any attempt at coitus.

If a patient suffering from vaginismus is examined under an anaesthetic, bimanual pelvic examination will most likely reveal no organic abnormality whatever. The capacity and calibre of the vagina is normal in that, if the anaesthesia is sufficient, it easily admits two fingers. Occasionally the hymen is incompletely ruptured and the introitus inadequately dilated but these findings are rare and their correction by plastic enlargement, though logical, does little to relieve the subsequent spasm since it is psychogenic rather than organic.

Treatment

(1) The first essential of treatment is to win the confidence and co-operation of both husband and wife, interviewed separately. This interview demands great tact and experience, and is time-consuming, but, if conducted correctly, is most rewarding. Once the confidence of the couple is won, the true cause of the trouble will usually be disclosed and simple instruction in its rectification may often be given.

(2) It may well be impossible to convince the patient that her difficulties are not due to some anatomical abnormality, e.g. she may be obsessed with the idea that her genital tract is mal-developed. In this case, she should be admitted for a night so that an examination under an anaesthetic can be performed. At this examination, the normality of her lower genital tract is confirmed and the vagina stretched to three fingers after which a large plastic dilator is inserted.

(3) When the patient recovers from the anaesthetic, this large dilator is removed and its visual presence demonstrates to her beyond argument that her vagina is of normal capacity. She is then instructed by demonstration to pass a slightly smaller dilator and is supplied with one to pass daily at home. This regular passage of a dilator will, or should, convince her that there is no obstruction to coitus which, after an interval of a week or two, she is encouraged to essay.

(4) If, when the patient is examined under an anaesthetic, a rigid hymen, often appreciated as a sickle-like band resistant to stretching in the region of the fourchette, is encountered, the operation of perineotomy (or Fenton's operation) should be performed. A longitudinal incision is made in the midline through the lower third of the posterior vaginal wall and skin of the perineum, when, after undercutting the tissues on each side and dividing the superficial muscles of the perineum, the wound is closed by interrupted sutures so that the scar lies transversely. The incision should be made of a length such that the vaginal orifice subsequently admits three fingers.

After this operation of plastic enlargement of the introitus, it is useful to pass a medium-sized plastic dilator daily and, when the patient is discharged to her home, she should be supplied with one and instructed in its use (as above). Coitus should not be attempted until the perineotomy wound has healed soundly, usually in three or four weeks.

(5) The patient should be kept under observation and encouraged to persevere with her treatment until normal coitus is established.

Dyspareunia

The term dyspareunia is loosely used for both difficult and painful coitus. The following classification of the causes of dyspareunia is suggested:

(1) Due to the male partner:
   (a) *Gross congenital abnormality* of the penis.
   (b) *Impotence*, usually partial, e.g. failure to maintain an erection long enough for penetration.
   (c) *Premature ejaculation.*
   (d) Complete and surprising *ignorance* in the technique of coitus.
(2) Due to the female partner:
   (a) *Painful lesions* in the region of the introitus, such as vulvitis (acute and chronic), urethral caruncle, Bartholin's cyst or abscess, tender scars from obstetric trauma or operation, and painful lesions of the anal canal, notably fissure.
   (b) *Obstructive conditions at the vaginal introitus:—*
      (i) Rigid or imperforate hymen and painful carunculae myrtiformes giving rise to spasm.
      (ii) Narrow introitus due to congenital hypoplasia, kraurosis or lichen sclerosus.
      (iii) Traumatic stenosis due to obstetric injury followed by scarring, but most commonly due to surgical interference, such as painful episiotomy scar or, most important, a too tightly sewn perineum after obstetric tears or perineorrhaphy operations.
      (iv) Cicatrisation due to chemical burns—usually permanganate tablets inserted to procure an abortion, and occasionally lysol.
      (v) The functional spasm of vaginismus (see above).
      (vi) A large tender Bartholin's cyst is occasionally obstructive to entry.
   (c) *Obstructive conditions above the vaginal introitus:*
      (i) Congenital stenosis and the various mal-developments—in the extreme case a partial non-canalisation of the vagina.
      (ii) Acquired stenosis—chemical burns are rare but the important causes here are the result of surgical operation. Vaginal hysterectomy and all prolapse repairs, Wertheim's operation, radium insertion and radiation therapy can all result in narrowing and shortening of the vagina. The great offender is the top stitch inserted in the levatores ani during a colporrhaphy operation. If too tight, an hourglass vagina results with a septum halfway up which resists all efforts at penetration and

is, in addition, painful. Sometimes the anterior and posterior suture lines of a colporrhaphy become densely adherent and fuse to form a stout septum which allows only partial penetration.

    (iii) Benign and occasionally malignant tumours of the vagina are rare causes of obstruction.

(d) *Uterine conditions* which are not obstructive but because they are painful, give rise to collision dyspareunia:

    (i) Cervicitis. Most chronic inflammatory lesions of the cervix are painless but, if associated with parametritis, they can cause pain.

    (ii) Chronic parametritis and parametrial scars.

    (iii) A bulky retroverted uterus, the body of which is demonstrably tender on bimanual examination. Retroversion causing dyspareunia is nearly always secondary and acquired. Primary congenital retroversion is usually symptomless.

    (iv) A fixed retroversion associated with chronic pelvic inflammatory disease.

(e) *Lesions of the uterine appendages:*

    (i) Prolapsed ovaries associated with retroversion.

    (ii) All types of acute and chronic salpingo-oophoritis.

    (iii) Endometriosis of the pouch of Douglas, recto-vaginal septum and utero-sacral liagments. Ovarian endometriosis of itself is not always associated with dyspareunia, since it is often a painless condition.

(f) *Extra-genital lesions* in the bowel, such as diverticulitis of the sigmoid colon, usually adherent to the left appendages and uterus.

Difficult Coitus. Difficult coitus may be caused by many of the same factors that are responsible for painful coitus. If the cause is insuperable, such as bony ankylosis of the hip in extreme adduction, consummation may be impossible and the correct term is not dyspareunia but apareunia. The latter naturally occurs with severe developmental defects of the vagina such as partial or complete failure of canalisation.

Clinical investigation of the problem of dyspareunia should be conducted along similar lines to that of vaginismus and here again the husband should not be neglected, especially if examination of the wife reveals no obvious organic cause. It must be always remembered that the utmost delicacy is needed to gain the frank confidence of both partners and more than one consultation may be required to gain full co-operation. Assuming that the husband is normal, the history elicited from the wife may be revealing if, for example, the dyspareunia follows a repair operation for prolapse. Clinically dyspareunia is divided into:

(1) **Superficial,** where the pain occurs immediately penetration is attempted and the causative lesion is therefore to be expected at or near the introitus (see previous list of causes).

(2) **Deep seated,** where the pain is not associated with penetration but is appreciated only after this has occurred and is usually localised by the patient as being in the depth of the vagina.

(3) There is a third and less well known entity—**post-coital dyspareunia,** sometimes associated with the deep seated variety. Here the patient complains of an aching soreness which lasts for several hours after the completion of the act.

Deep seated dyspareunia is usually organic and often associated with some ovarian pathology such as prolapsed and tender ovaries in association with retroversion, endometriosis or chronic pelvic inflammatory disease. These conditions can also cause post-coital dyspareunia, although the latter if not associated with deep dyspareunia at the time of intercourse may well be functional and a protective mechanism to avoid an act which has become unsatisfying, tedious or even repugnant with a partner who has forfeited his physical attractions. It has been cynically but somewhat truthfully remarked that dyspareunia only occurs with husbands and never with lovers. It might be added that with the latter it can only occur in the process of disenchantment.

When making a vaginal examination of a patient complaining of deep seated dyspareunia it is often found that the ovaries are fixed and tender on bimanual examination. In fact the patient may volunteer that this examination almost exactly reproduces the pain experienced at coitus. Hence the term—collision dyspareunia—is sometimes used to describe this variety. In the extreme instance the pain may be so genuine that coitus is eventually abandoned and infertility results.

Organic dyspareunia should be regarded as a symptom of the primary abnormality, and treatment consists in dealing with the cause. Local abnormalities at the vulva can usually be cured by appropriate treatment, but when dyspareunia is caused by such abnormalities in the pouch of Douglas as prolapsed tender ovaries, an abdominal operation is necessary. The ovaries may then be freed from adhesions, chocolate cysts can be excised, and the uterus fixed in a position of antiflexion by a ventro-suspension operation. This is one of the few occasions where this operation is justifiably indicated, especially if infertility is an additional complaint to the dyspareunia.

When all possible organic causes of the dyspareunia have been eliminated the psychogenic possibilities must be considered. Patient enquiry may then elicit the true cause, such as fear of pregnancy, frigidity, marital disharmony or some unhappy sexual experience in the past.

Infertility and Sterility

Although the terms infertility and sterility have literally the same sense, the inability to conceive, each has come to possess its own meaning in the lay mind. This has justified the distinction that infertility implies the failure to conceive, and sterility the inability to conceive. Infertility is, therefore, relative whereas sterility is absolute. Fertility in the human species is so related to the coincidence of ovulation and coitus that the term infertility escapes precise definition, and as no agreed convention exists there is no room for such terms as subfertility.

Sterility may exist when there is some fault either of the male or female which prevents fertilisation of the ovum. Such conditions as failure of the uterus or vagina to develop provide examples in the female, while in the male failure to produce spermatozoa as the result of castration, injury, operation, disease or imperfect development of the testes illustrate this condition. Infertility is termed primary if conception has never occurred, and secondary if the patient fails to conceive after having produced a child or had an undoubted miscarriage. One-child infertility is relatively common and is usually the result of an ascending infection of the Fallopian tubes during the puerperium so that tubal occlusion is produced. Similarly one-miscarriage infertility may be the result of post-abortional endosalpingitis.

Physiological sterility is present before puberty and after the menopause. It must be remembered, however, that a girl may conceive before menstruation develops, if the first ovum to be shed is fertilised, though this is very rare because the first cycles are usually anovular. At the menopause, it is possible that an ovum may be shed and fertilised within the first few months following the cessation of menstruation, which if it had not been fertilised would have given rise to a menstrual period. This occurrence is very rare.

A physiological sterility is present during pregnancy because ovulation is inhibited as soon as conception occurs.

The infertility of the lactation period should be regarded as relative. Only 60% of lactating European women have amenorrhoea. If a woman menstruates during lactation she is capable of conceiving and, even if she has lactation amenorrhoea, she cannot be considered absolutely infertile, although it is possible that the first few cycles are anovular. If the first ovum to be discharged from the ovary during lactation is fertilised, the woman will conceive without menstruating. The duration of amenorrhoea after childbirth is frequently overestimated, and the usual figure of six months is far too generous. Two months' amenorrhoea is the usual average, though in exceptional cases it may be less.

Pathology of Infertility

It has already been pointed out that conception depends upon the fertility of both the male and the female and that it is a popular misconception to attribute failure solely to the female. In one-third of all cases of infertility the male is directly responsible, in one-third both parties are at fault, and in the remaining third only can the cause of failure be attributed entirely to the female. These figures are perhaps extreme and it might be more accurate to distribute the fault evenly between the two partners.

Faults of the Male. Testicular function depends upon several factors. Androgens are produced in the interstitial cells of the testes as a result of stimulation by the gonadotropic hormone of the anterior pituitary. Spermatozoa are developed from the germinal epithelium lining the seminiferous tubules, largely under the influence of the anterior pituitary. The administration of male sex hormone to a patient will improve his erectile capacity and increase his libido but will not favourably increase his sperm count. For adequate spermatogenesis the testicle must lie in its correct position in the scrotum, where the temperature is slightly cooler than elsewhere in the body. Factors which raise scrotal temperature can adversely influence spermato-genesis, e.g. the occupation of men who work as stokers or in blast-furnaces and are subjected to excessive heat, the wearing of a tight scrotal support and the presence of a varicocele. The ectopic or undescended testicle provides the best example of the effect of temperature on spermatogenesis; testicular biopsy of such an abnormally situated testicle will very often show absence of function.

It is not enough, however, that spermatogenesis should be satisfactory, since it is a far cry from the seminiferous tubule to the Fallopian tube and many hazards beset the journey. The collecting apparatus of the epididymis may be damaged by trauma or inflammatory disease—notably gonorrhoea or tuberculosis. The vas deferens itself may be occluded, and this is especially to be suspected if there is a herniorrhaphy scar, and doubly so if the scar is bilateral. Chronic inflammatory disease of the prostate and seminal vesicle may be associated with male infertility, and congenital lesions of the penile urethra such as hypospadias provide an obvious mechanical explanation for imperfect insemination.

The importance of these facts will be apparent when the male partner is examined. A history of mumps, venereal disease or tuberculosis may suggest testicular atrophy or obstruction. Accidental or operative trauma, e.g. a blow on the testicle with haematoma formation and subsequent atrophy, or operation for hernia, varicocele or hydrocele may suggest a degenerative lesion of the testes or obstruction to the vas. To this list of organic causes of male infertility should be added a new hazard of modern life. Under the stress of overwork the husband undergoes a slow but progressive diminution of physical powers. The lithe athletic figure of the newly married has degenera-ted into the heavy smoking, heavy drinking business executive. Obesity and the motor car have undermined the physical powers and the once sexually active husband is too tired to fulfil his partnership role. Coitus becomes progressively less frequent and the chances of conception steadily decline. The treatment of this success symbol is drastic discipline in alcohol, cigarettes, business luncheons and dinners and a reversion to ambulation in preference to internal combustion engine propulsion. If the steel trap of success has closed around our victim there is little hope for improvement in his sexual capacity, unless he is prepared radically to modify his habits of living and business.

The general examination of the patient may show a pituitary failure, such as Fröhlich's syndrome, and the local examination may disclose some obvious defect such as hypospadias. Careful and tactful questioning may elicit a complete ignorance of the sexual act or some such functional disorder as ejaculatio praecox or frigidity. It cannot be too strongly emphasised that the husband should be interviewed alone and examined with tact and patience.

The most important part of the male examination is the semen analysis, and certain points regarding the methods and timing of the collection of the specimen are noteworthy. The best specimen is one obtained by masturbation in the vicinity of the laboratory, since this guarantees its freshness. If this method is uncongenial to the patient coitus interruptus into a wide-necked vessel such as a Petri dish may be employed. The production of a condom specimen is to be discouraged as condoms contain a spermicidal chemical and false readings will thereby be obtained. The best specimen will be produced after a short period of abstinence—not less than three days. It should be emphasised most strongly at this point that the sperm picture of a man should never be assessed on one specimen unless exceptionally good, and that the average of three readings is required to establish a definite defect. Quite often a poor initial showing is the result of anxiety or overwork, and a subsequent sperm count taken a month later may show a considerable improvement.

In ordinary clinical practice a typical specimen should show the following features when examined within two hours of production:

(1) Total volume, 3—5 ml. (average 3·5 ml.).
(2) Sperm count, 60,000,000—120,000,000 per ml. (average 100,000,000).
(3) Motility, 80%—90% (average 80%).
(4) Morphology, 80% or more normal (average 80%).

Viscosity and pH of the seminal fluid is more of academic than practical interest and need not concern us. The most important factor is the density of the sperm population, and counts below 40,000,000 are usually associated with infertility. Counts of 10,000,000 and lower are often encountered. Though such patients are infertile they should never be told that they cannot father a child. A repeat count in two or four months may show a startling

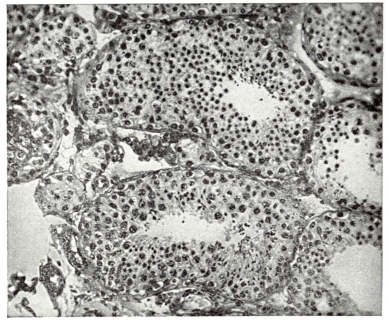

FIG. 172. Testicular biopsy. Normal seminiferous tubules. Note spermatozoa in lumen. (× 250.) (*From* "Gynaecology," 5th Ed., *MacLeod and Read*.)

improvement in their oligozoospermia. If therefore a patient shows oligozoospermia or azoospermia he should be told that his specimen is below average and instructed to produce another after an interval of a month. During this time he should be instructed in general hygiene, exercise and spacing of coitus, given a high protein, high vitamin diet and limited in the consumption of alcohol and tobacco. Unlike the ovary the male gonad is meant to function at a temperature slightly below that of the rest of the body. Modern living with tight underwear, hot baths, central heating, electric blankets and deep-sprung mattresses is designed to depress spermatogenesis. He should be

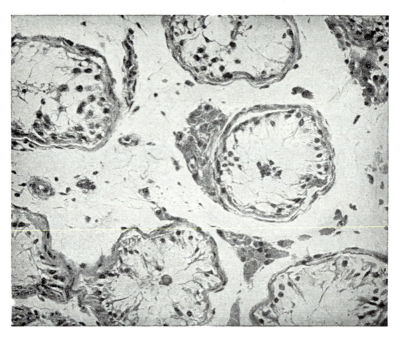

FIG. 173. Testicular biopsy. Tubular atrophy showing Sertoli cells only. (× 250.) (*From* "Gynaecology," 5th Ed., *MacLeod and Read.*)

advised to take a tepid or cold bath every morning and to avoid hot baths altogether, to discard tight underwear, electric blankets and excessive bedclothes. This type of thermoregulative treatment will cause remarkable improvement in many seminal counts. Only after three negative counts should he be pronounced to be azoospermic.

If azoospermia has been found on three occasions at two- to four-monthly intervals the next step is to establish if the seminiferous tubules are non-functional or if there is an obstructive lesion of the vas or epididymis. The simple out-patient operation of testicular biopsy will demonstrate which of these two factors is at fault (Fig. 172).

If testicular biopsy shows an obstructive lesion of the collecting mechanism the opinion of a urologist should be sought concerning the advisability of a short-circuiting operation on the vas and epididymis, provided of course that spermatogenesis is adequate. If testicular biopsy shows complete degeneration and atrophy of the testicles the patient may be pronounced sterile and, if desired, adoption of a child advised (see Fig. 173).

A word of caution is, however, necessary about the dangers of declaring a husband permanently and absolutely sterile. The clinician who thus commits himself may be called in evidence in a case of disputed paternity which but for his assertion might never have been brought.

Faults of the Female. Congenital defects of the female may prevent spermatozoa from ascending to the Fallopian tubes. Examples are afforded by maldevelopment of the vagina, such as non-canalisation, or occlusion by a septum. In extreme cases the vagina is not developed at all. If the uterus fails to develop, or if it is of the foetal type without canalisation, the woman must be sterile. Congenital defects of the Fallopian tube and stenosis also lead to sterility although this fault in the upper Müllerian system is extremely rare.

Sterility may be caused by less severe degrees of maldevelopment, such as rigid hymen, elongated conical cervix with a pinhole os, and acute ante-flexion and retroflexion of the uterus, but in these conditions the associated hypoplasia genitalis may also be a factor in producing infertility.

One of the commonest causes of infertility is salpingitis, when, as the result of acute inflammation, adhesions form around the abdominal ostium, while within the lumen of the tube the plicae become adherent and the passage-way between the uterus and the abdominal cavity is blocked. Gonorrhoea, salpingitis following septic abortion and salpingitis following puerperal infection are the three common causes of sterility of this type. Tuberculosis of the tubes also causes sterility for the same reasons.

Recent studies of endometrial biopsies have demonstrated that tuberculous endometritis is more common than has been previously believed, and that 5% of all patients attending an infertility clinic have this lesion though otherwise symptomless. Furthermore, tuberculous salpingo-oöphoritis is more frequently seen at the present day than before the last world war. Although chronic inflammations of the cervix might be expected to prevent the upward migration of spermatozoa, it is exceptional to see cases when the sterility can be attributed to this cause.

In recent years attention has been paid to chronic leucorrhoea as a cause of infertility. That this is largely hypothetical can be demonstrated by examining the cervices of multiparous patients, when every variety of inflammatory lesion of the cervix will be seen, including large erosions, infected lacerations and even polypi. Such highly fertile patients have a considerable muco-purulent discharge. It is, therefore, fair to state that a muco-purulent discharge may not hinder conception in the fertile though it should be eliminated in the patient who complains of infertility and in whom it is discovered in the course of the investigation. A high degree of acidity of the vaginal secretion also destroys the human spermatozoa. It is, however, exceptional to see cases in which the cause of the infertility can be attributed to abnormalities of the vaginal secretion. Inflammations of the vulva may indirectly lead to infertility because local tenderness may act as a bar to coitus.

It is well known clinically that if the uterus of an infertile woman contains a myoma and the myoma is removed, the woman may subsequently conceive. Such cases are difficult to explain unless it is assumed that the myoma distorts or elongates the cavity of the uterus. The discharges from tumours such as carcinoma of the cervix and infected myomatous polypi are inimical to spermatozoa, and yet patients with both these conditions do become pregnant. It has already been pointed out that dyspareunia is an important factor in the causation of infertility, and other factors on the part of the woman which lead to dyspareunia are retroversion with prolapsed tender ovaries or inflamed appendages, pelvic endometriosis, together with local abnormalities at the vulva such as urethral caruncle and vulvitis.

In recent years attention has been paid to disturbances of ovarian function as being the cause of infertility. Women with pathological amenorrhoea due to ovarian deficiency are usually infertile and with less severe degrees of ovarian dysfunction, for example, when the woman has menstruated irregularly with a prolonged menstrual cycle, infertility is not uncommon. A comparable state of affairs exists after the creation of an artificial menopause with X-rays or radium, and the production of a temporary artificial menopause has been employed in Germany as a method of birth control. Endocrine disorders, by inhibiting ovarian function, may lead to infertility, and a common clinical type is the woman aged about 30 with scanty and irregular periods, obese, with a masculine distribution of hair, who complains of infertility. Such endocrine causes will be considered later (see Chapter 18), and the clinical investigation of ovarian dysfunction in infertility is described in detail on pp. 337 and 425. Women with morbus cordis are exceptionally fertile, and it is a common belief that phthisical patients are apt to conceive easily, but with these exceptions chronic ill health and chronic disease reduce the fertility of the individual.

General Causes

The influence of hygienic factors on human fertility has been studied. They are in many ways comparable to the measures taken to ensure prolific breeding in cattle. It is now well established in those cases of infertility when both partners have been found to be normal in spite of the exhaustive investigations of modern gynaecology, that close attention to the habits and hygiene of both partners may result in conception. This is particularly so in the case of the male partner. Many men have insufficient sleep, work strenuously and anxiously for long hours and relax by the consumption of tobacco and alcohol. Often they overeat and exercise is taken in the form of violent physical exertion at spasmodic intervals. Adjustment of these factors is most important in this type of individual.

The timing of coitus is a simple but important factor in achieving conception. Many couples have totally erroneous ideas of the most fertile days in a given cycle and they expend their best endeavour on an infertile target. The most likely day of ovulation should be calculated, and intercourse should be reserved so that this period is adequately covered. This simple procedure often results in success, especially in those marriages where coitus is infrequent or random.

It is a common experience at infertility clinics that, in spite of exhaustive investigations, both partners prove to be perfectly normal, yet are infertile. There is a suggestion that these cases represent true incompatibility, so that both partners may be fertile with other consorts. On the other hand, normal people may be infertile for many years, and yet quite late in the child-bearing period of life the female conceives. Many years ago Matthews Duncan investigated the fertility of women of different ages and showed that the maximum fertility was reached between the ages of 19 and 25. The fertility of young girls was shown to be small and the chances of a woman conceiving for the first time after the age of 35 are far less than when she was between the ages of 20 and 25.

Clinical Investigation

We have seen that there is no definite standard by which the degrees of infertility can be judged. It is common practice to begin the investigation of a couple when a year has elapsed without conception in spite of normal coitus. Some authorities prefer to wait two years, as many marriages are fruitful during the second year, and thus many unnecessary and expensive investigations and false claims of success for these are avoided.

It is usually the woman who presents herself for investigation of infertility, because it is she who feels the stronger procreative impulse. Before starting any investigation certain aspects should be discussed and fully understood by the patient and her husband, if he will attend. First, only very exceptionally is it justifiable to investigate one partner if the other is unwilling to submit to any tests. Secondly, it must be clearly understood that the tests have no established therapeutic value and that they merely serve to discover any abnormality which may be present and which may or may not be remediable. Thirdly, both parties must have considered the possibility that investigation may show either to be sterile and be prepared to accept this situation, otherwise the clinician may find himself the unhappy cause of a broken marriage.

In the course of the investigations it is essential to discourage any sense of blame which may be attached to one partner who is found faulty by the other; in an issue so intensely personal as the ability to procreate it is almost impossible for the defective individual to preserve a philosophical view and escape a sense of guilt which may mar a previously happy marriage. If infertility is discovered in one partner and the fertility of the other has been found to be low, the couple will be helped to face the situation more easily if it is pointed out that both have a share in the failure of the union.

History. A careful menstrual history should be taken, for scanty menstruation occurring at long intervals is suggestive of pituitary or ovarian dysfunction. Previous labours and miscarriages should be enquired into; a history of puerperal fever, persistent lochial discharge or a history that the patient had to stay in bed for several weeks after parturition or abortion suggests the possibility of infection of the uterine adnexa. It may be possible to obtain a history of symptoms suggestive of gonorrhoea, such as acute vaginal discharge associated with scalding micturition, or of Bartholin's abscess. The Fallopian tubes may be bound down by adhesions as the result of past peritonitis caused, for example, by acute appendicitis or tuberculous peritonitis. Any history of chronic chest disease, persistent cough, pleurisy or pneumonia should always suggest the possibility of pulmonary tuberculosis as the primary focus of a genital tract tuberculosis.

Enquiries should then be made as to whether difficulty has been experienced during coitus, and it is customary to ask if this difficulty has been experienced during penetration or whether deep-seated abdominal pain accompanies sexual intercourse. Many women attribute their infertility to **fluor seminis,** when the seminal fluid runs out of the vagina immediately after coitus. Fluor seminis is extremely common, and is not of itself a cause of infertility.

General Examination of the Female. In view of the importance of genital tract tuberculosis in the aetiology of infertility in the female, a thorough chest examination, which should include an X-ray of the lungs, is an essential part of the general examination. This becomes all the more imperative if there is any significant history of pleurisy or lung disease. Endocrinopathies should be eliminated. Apart from diabetes and thyrotoxicosis which are both associated with lowered fertility, there may be evidence of pituitary or ovarian dysfunction from a history of menstrual irregularity, oligomenorrhoea and hypomenorrhoea. Gross disorders, such as Cushing's syndrome and adrenogenital syndrome, are not likely to be missed from the history and the clinical examination and these, and other endocrine conditions, will be considered in greater detail in the chapter dealing with menstrual abnormalities. Operation scars in the abdominal wall lead to questions being asked as to what operation was performed, if peritonitis had been present, whether it was of a severe degree and whether a pelvic abscess had been drained. The gynaecological examination will reveal such abnormalities as vaginismus, vulvitis, and abnormalities of the vulva, rigid hymen and maldevelopment of the vagina. A bimanual examination should then be made to determine whether the cervix is small and conical with a pinhole os and whether the uterus is ill developed or malformed. Examination of the appendages should detect such conditions as pyosalpinx and hydrosalpinx, chocolate cysts or prolapsed ovaries in the pouch of Douglas.

It will be found possible after a simple examination of this kind to state whether there is a clear cause for the infertility on the part of the female, or whether no obvious local cause can be found. In the first group are such conditions as vaginismus, maldevelopment of the vagina and bilateral salpingitis. Similarly, if there is good evidence of disease of the endocrine system, the infertility can often be attributed to ovarian dysfunction. In conditions such as gross maldevelopment of the vagina and foetal uterus, the prognosis can be regarded as hopeless, and there is no indication for further investigation or treatment. With vaginismus, rigid hymen and retroversion associated with prolapsed tender ovaries the infertility may very well be cured by operative treatment.

It should be taken as a principle in the investigation and treatment of infertility to exclude any fault of the male before undertaking any operative procedure or such investigation as insufflation of the Fallopian tubes on the female. It has already been strongly emphasised that the male partner is at fault in a large number of cases of infertility, and there is no justification for subjecting a woman to operation which, though not greatly inconveniencing her, will not be followed by conception if the male partner is primarily at fault.

After the clinical examination of the female partner the male should be examined and investigated as already stated on p. 325.

Detailed Investigation of the Female. After a general and pelvic examination of the infertile female partner, investigations are made to determine whether there is patency of the Fallopian tubes and whether ovulation is taking place.

Tests for Tubal Patency

Insufflation. The test is carried out in the interval between the end of menstruation and the fourteenth day of the cycle, assuming a normal twenty-eight-day cycle. If performed later in the cycle, insufflation might disturb a fertilised and implanted ovum. The gas used is carbon dioxide because of its high solubility should it enter the blood stream through the uterine veins. The

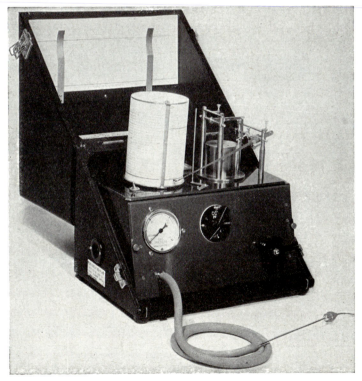

FIG. 174. Sharman's kymograph for tubal insufflation. (*Kelvin and Hughes Ltd., London.*)

use of air is absolutely condemned because of the danger of causing an air embolism. The apparatus consists of a cylinder of carbon dioxide which supplies a steady flow of gas through a reducing valve, a control valve by which the rate is determined and a safety valve which prevents the pressure exceeding 240 mm. of mercury. The pressure at the delivery end of the system is recorded by a tracing pen on a rotating drum; the mechanism is sufficiently sensitive to record alterations in intrauterine pressure due to peristalsis in the Fallopian tubes (see Fig. 174).

Insufflation may be done as an out-patient procedure without anaesthesia unless the patient is very apprehensive. First a vaginal examination is made to determine the position of the uterus at the time of the test. A speculum is then passed with the patient in the left lateral position and the vaginal portion of the cervix thoroughly cleaned. If there is any evidence of vaginitis or cervicitis the test should be deferred until this has been eliminated. Next, the anterior lip of the cervix is seized with a single-bite volsellum, which may cause momentary pain, and the cannula attached to the kymograph is introduced through the cervical canal into the uterine cavity. This cannula and the connecting rubber pressure tubing should first have been purged with CO_2. The cannula is equipped with a conical rubber collar, and when this is held firmly against the external cervical os with simultaneous traction on the volsellum a gas-tight closure is obtained. A recent refinement to ensure a gas-tight joint between the cannula and the cervix is the use of the Maelmström

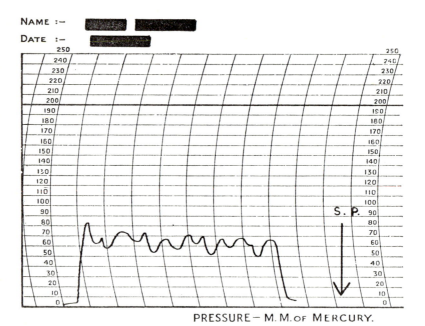

PRESSURE – M. M. OF MERCURY.

FIG. 175.   Normal tracings with patent tubes.   Note the peristalsis at low pressure.

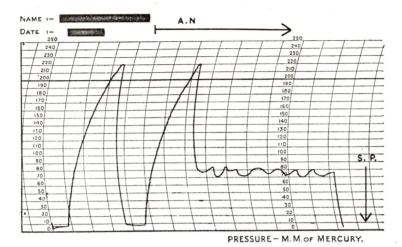

FIG. 176. Tubal spasm. Note the initial failure and normal tracing after administering amyl nitrite. A.N.=amyl nitrite. S.P.=shoulder pain.

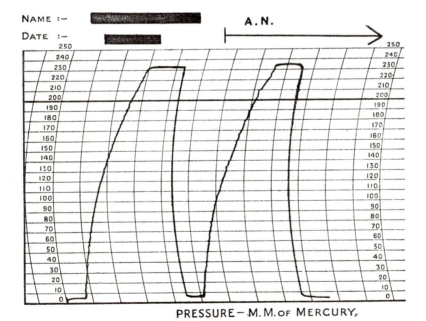

FIG. 177. Complete tubal occlusion. Note the failure with administration of amyl nitrite.

suction apparatus, employing a similar principle to that used in obstetrics for traction on the foetal scalp.

The kymograph is now started and is set to deliver gas at a rate of 60 ml. per minute. If one or both Fallopian tubes are patent and healthy there will be an initial rise of pressure to about 60 mm. of mercury followed by a wave pattern horizontal tracing indicating tubal peristalsis. If the tubes are closed by light adhesions and affected by previous salpingitis the initial pressure rise may be high (150—220 mm. Hg) and be followed by a smooth descending tracing indicating patency without tubal peristalsis. Not uncommonly, spasm of healthy tubes is encountered and the pressure will rise to the maximum allowed by the safety valve without any gas passing. If the patient is then given amyl nitrite vapour a sudden descent of the tracing occurs, followed by a peristaltic pattern at a normal level. Insuperable tubal blockage will be shown by failure to obtain passage of the gas in any circumstances. Additional evidence of success may be obtained by auscultation over the lower abdomen during the test, when bubbling or squeaking sounds may be heard. Finally, if a quantity of the gas has passed into the peritoneal cavity the patient may experience referred pain at either shoulder, usually the right, when she sits up after the test (see Figs. 175—177). A crescentic gas shadow under the diaphragm can be demonstrated by radiography as an additional refinement in cases of doubt.

When insufflation is unsuccessful it should be repeated at least once more, and if again unsuccessful the site of the tubal blockage should be investigated by radiographic methods. It should be emphasised that a failed tubal insufflation by gas is as likely to indicate spasm as organic obstruction.

Hysterosalpingography. Visualisation of the uterine cavity and the Fallopian tubes should be carried out by screening with the use of an image intensifier in an X-ray theatre with the co-operation of a radiologist. A general anaesthetic is desirable but not essential and the investigation is performed between the end of the menstrual period and ovulation (usually the 14th day of the cycle). After thoroughly cleaning the lower genital tract and with full aseptic precautions, a radio-opaque dye is injected through a cannula into the cervical canal under direct vision with the X-ray screen. The best fit with the cervix is obtained by means of a cannula held in position by the Maelström suction apparatus; 15 ml. of the medium is used—only as much being used as is necessary to outline the uterine cavity and tubes satisfactorily. If the tubes are patent the medium will be seen to spill out of the abdominal ostia and smear the adjacent bowel. A hydrosalpinx will show as a large confined mass of dye without peritoneal spill. If either tube is blocked the site will be shown. At any stage of the examination X-ray pictures may be taken for a permanent record of the result. A viscous water-soluble solution, 50% diodone with 6% polyvinyl alcohol in water, is the medium usually employed for hysterosalpingography. It is rapidly absorbed and the risk of tissue reaction and adhesion formation in the pelvis is minimal. Even when intravasated into the uterine venous system, it is harmless. It is, therefore, always to be preferred to iodised poppy-seed oils which, though giving a better radiographic detail, are not devoid of risk from adhesions and pelvic inflammatory reactions (Figs. 178

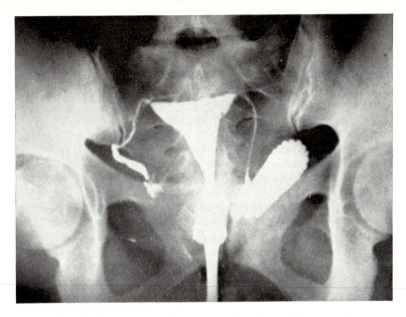

FIG. 178. Normal hysterosalpingogram. Note both Fallopian tubes are patent with spill into the peritoneal cavity.

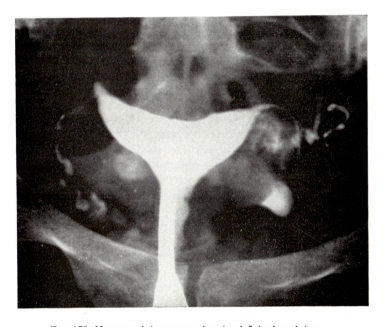

FIG. 179. Hysterosalpingogram showing left hydrosalpinx.

and 179). Maximum X-ray screening time must not exceed 30 seconds using an image intensifier, and only two X-ray plate exposures are permitted in order to minimise radiation to the female gonad.

Apart from tubal anatomy and function this examination should exclude congenital abnormalities of the uterus, such as uterus bicornis, arcuate, septate and subseptate uterus and the presence of endometrial polypi and submucous fibroids.

After completing these two tests, gas insufflation and X-ray hysterosalpingography the examiner should be able to say if the tube or tubes are blocked and, if so, where. On this it should be possible to give a reasonably accurate prognosis of the results of corrective surgery.

Tests for Ovulation

Basal Body Temperature. It is established that the basal body temperature falls at the time of ovulation by about $\frac{1}{2}$ degree Fahrenheit. Subsequently, during the progestational half of the cycle the temperature is slightly raised above the pre-ovulatory level, and the rise is of the order of $\frac{1}{2}$ to 1 degree. Moreover, if the patient conceives, the temperature remains at this level and does not fall as it would at the onset of menstruation. This phenomenon is due to the slight pyrogenic action of progesterone and is, therefore, presumptive evidence of the presence of a functioning corpus luteum and hence ovulation. Accurate recordings will therefore indicate whether the ovarian cycle is ovulatory or not and will denote the timing of ovulation. The patient must be capable of reading the thermometer to $\frac{1}{10}$th degree, and she must be able to make the recording scientifically without prejudice. Oral temperatures are accurate, provided the patient has not had either a hot or cold drink before taking the temperature, which should be done first thing after waking. The patient must be instructed how to record temperatures on a graph (Fig. 180).

Cytology. A scrape preparation obtained from the upper lateral vaginal wall and examined under the microscope after staining should show cytological evidence of corpus luteum activity if taken any time after ovulation has occurred and before the next period is due. The cells are predominantly of the basophilic intermediate type with vesicular nuclei. They show edge curling and folding, the so-called envelope effect, and are clustered together. Cytology can thus provide useful and readily obtainable evidence that ovulation has occurred and this technique is likely to be more widely used in the future.

Endometrial biopsy consists of curetting small pieces of endometrium from the uterus with a small endometrial biopsy curette one or two days before the onset of menstruation. The material removed should be fixed immediately in Bouin's fluid. Secretory changes prove that the cycle has been ovulatory. The technique has already been described on p. 62. The interpretation of the appearance of the endometrium requires the services of a trained gynaecological pathologist. Not only the superficial layer, but the middle layer of the functional endometrium must be identified. The incidence of anovulatory menstruation in the human female is disputed. The most reliable work is that of Rock and his co-workers who found in 392 infertile patients that approxi-

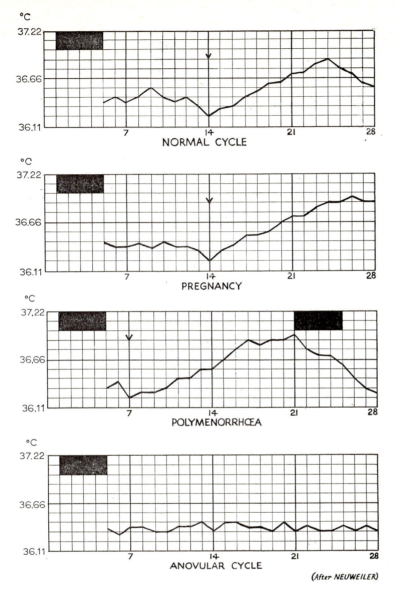

FIG. 180. Specimen charts of basal body temperatures. The arrow illustrates
the ovulation time. The dark zones indicate the time of menstrual bleeding.

mately 9% had occasional anovulatory menstruation and that 4% only were
habitually anovulatory.

The **corpus luteum function** can be determined by pregnandiol excretion
values. The estimation is not difficult but unfortunately the laboratory

facilities are somewhat limited, though increasing. If ovulation has occurred and the resulting corpus luteum is active, levels of 2—5 mgm. in the total 24-hour urinary output are presumptive evidence of ovulation. The specimen should be obtained seven days before the next expected menstruation.

Fern Test. If a specimen of cervical mucus is obtained by platinum loop or pipette and spread on an absolutely clean glass slide and allowed to dry, when viewed under the low power microscope it shows during the oestrogenic phase a characteristic pattern of fern formation. This ferning disappears after the 21st day of the cycle and if previously present its disappearance is presumptive evidence of corpus luteum activity.

The physical character of cervical mucus also alters with the dates of the cycle. At the time of ovulation cervical mucus is at its most profuse. So much so that patients may notice a clear discharge—the so-called normal ovulation cascade. This ovulation mucus has the property of great elasticity and will withstand stretching up to a distance of over 10 cm. This phenomenon is called spinnbarkeit or the thread test for oestrogen activity. During the secretory phase the cervical mucus becomes more tenacious and its viscosity increases so that it loses the property of spinnbarkeit and fractures when put under tension. The observation of this change in a menstrual cycle is one more piece of evidence that ovulation is occurring normally.

Sims' or Huhner's Test

Post-coital Examination of Cervical Mucus. (Sims' or Huhner's test). This test should be employed at the time the woman is ovulating, when the cervical mucus has a chemotactic influence on spermatozoa which enables them to penetrate through the cervical plug to reach the cavity of the uterus. The test is useless if the cervical secretion is infected and purulent. Obviously, if the patient is infertile and has an endocervicitis, the cervix must be treated with diathermy cauterisation.

The test should be performed within sixteen hours after coitus—preferably after two hours, and the patient must not have used contraceptive chemicals or douching. The patient is placed in the lithotomy position, the cervix exposed and a quantity of cervical mucus removed with small sponge-holding forceps and transmitted immediately to a warm glass slide. A cover slip is placed on the mucus and the material examined microscopically under a high-power lens. In normal cases between ten and fifty motile sperms should be found in each high power field.

Operations for Infertility

It is unjustifiable to subject a woman patient to any operation unless the husband has first been excluded as the cause of the infertility.

An obvious fault of the female may be present. For example, the hymen may be rigid and prevent penetration. Although conception is possible in such cases, the chances are small and the obvious procedure is to excise the hymen and to enlarge the introitus. If a myoma is present, and only if the clinician is convinced that its presence is contributory to the infertility, treatment consists in myomectomy by the abdominal route and care must be taken to ensure that the interstitial portion of the Fallopian tube is not damaged during the operation. With chocolate cysts and pelvic endometriosis abdominal operation is necessary, when the uterus should be ventro-suspended, adhesions around the Fallopian tube broken down, and the chocolate cyst resected from the healthy ovarian tissue. The prognosis in pelvic endometriosis is

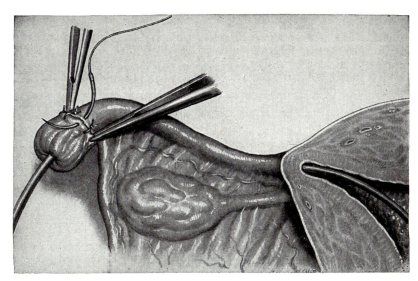

FIG. 181. Diagram to illustrate the operation of salpingostomy for tubal occlusion situated at the fimbrial extremity. A solid polythene rod has been passed through the tube into the cavity of the uterus and out through the cervix. A cuff of the fimbrial end of the tube is turned back and sutured as illustrated so that the fimbrial opening is permanently everted. A fine atraumatic needle is being used. (*From* Shaw's "Operative Gynaecology," 2nd Ed., E. and S. Livingstone.)

usually regarded as being poor, but recent figures have shown this attitude to be incorrect as the conception rate after conservative resection of ovarian endometriosis is stated by Te Linde to be 40% and by Whitehouse & Bates to be 45%. In salpingitis the prognosis as regards subsequent pregnancy is bad. If each Fallopian tube is replaced either by a pyosalpinx or a hydrosalpinx the prognosis is almost hopeless. If, on the other hand, the Fallopian tubes are bound down by adhesions and if the abdominal ostium is closed, it may be possible to fashion an artificial abdominal ostium by the operation of salpingostomy (Fig. 181).

Hysterosalpingography is first employed to determine the site of occlusion in the Fallopian tubes so that before operation the operator knows the exact position of the obstruction (see p. 336). In some cases, light adhesions surround the abdominal ostium. These can be easily broken down with the fingers, but it is important to ensure complete haemostasis before the abdomen is closed, otherwise fresh adhesions may re-form. If there is occlusion of the interstitial portion of the tube, determined by hysterosalpingography, and provided that the rest of the tube is healthy and patent, the isthmic end of the tube can be detached from the uterus after the occluded part has been excised. After incising the myometrium and exposing the cavity of the uterus the healthy remaining portion of tube is re-implanted. The technical difficulties of salpingostomy are great, but successes are obtained in a few cases. The operation is a delicate one and it is essential to ensure complete haemostasis, otherwise fresh adhesions will form and the artificial abdominal ostium become blocked. For this reason insufflation with CO_2 gas should be performed fourteen days after the abdominal operation. In order to discourage intratubal adhesions at the site of the new utero-tubal junction Green-Armytage recommended the use of an indwelling polythene catheter, which is passed from the abdominal ostium through the utero-tubal anastomosis and uterine cavity into the vagina and left in situ for some weeks.

Endocrine Treatment of Infertility

Endocrine treatment in the male is disappointing. Testosterone will improve virility but does little or nothing to increase a low count. In some circumstances Clomiphene citrate will raise the sperm density, but the reason for this is not known.

Genital hypoplasia in the female may be treated by oestrogens in small doses, but it is important to remember that normal genital development depends upon ovarian oestrogen. Genital hypoplasia may be the result of slow maturity, which does not require treatment, or of hypoplasia of the ovaries themselves when exogenous oestrogen may be indicated. Ovulation may be induced by giving Follicle Stimulating Hormone (F.S.H.) together with Human Chorionic Gonadotropin (H.C.G.) as described on p. 482 if there is evidence of pituitary dysfunction as shown by low F.S.H. levels. When F.S.H. levels are normal and the ovaries contain ova but ovulation does not occur as in Stein-Leventhal syndrome (hyperthecosis ovarii) then ovulation may be induced by Clomiphene citrate in a dose of 50—100 mgm. daily for seven days each month starting on the fifth day of the period. In true ovarian agenesis the residual ovaries do not contain any ova so that attempts to induce ovulation are pointless.

Artificial Insemination

There are two types of artificial insemination. In the first the semen of a donor is employed, and few British gynaecologists will countenance this method for legal, ethical and religious reasons. In the second, the semen of the husband is used, and in cases of hypospadias and ejaculatio praecox this has a certain small indication in selected cases. The technique is relatively simple. A fresh specimen of the husband's semen is obtained in a Petri dish by masturbation. This is aspirated into a 10 ml. syringe and injected into the posterior fornix. Intra-vaginal insemination is simple to perform and intra-uterine injection has no advantages over it.

Habitual Abortion

It is not uncommon to see patients who have no difficulty in conceiving yet who repeatedly abort in the early months of pregnancy. It is best to define habitual abortion as spontaneous abortion occurring at least three times in succession.

The Investigation of Habitual Abortion. The general history and examination of the patient may reveal some simple explanation, such as the presence of essential hypertension or chronic nephritis, thyrotoxicosis or diabetes. The obstetric history may, in itself, be significant as, for example, if the abortions occur in the middle months of pregnancy following a difficult first confinement with cervical laceration, or a dilatation and curettage—this type of history always should suggest cervical incompetence which is further confirmed when the patient, on closer questioning, describes the abortion as being preceded by a loss of watery discharge due to premature rupture of the membranes. A history of some gynaecological operation, usually for prolapse, which has involved a high amputation of the cervix, gives rise to one sort of cervical incompetence and a similar middle trimester abortion. Syphilis, the aetiological mainstay of our fathers when confronted with an habitual abortion problem, is hardly worth mentioning now except for historical interest in the changing pattern of causative disease.

Having performed a general examination which includes certain special investigations such as Rhesus blood group in husband and wife, Kahn reaction, urine-testing for albumin and sugar, a sugar tolerance test even when diabetes is not suspected, blood cholesterol or protein bound iodine if there is any suggestion of hyperthyroidism, local abnormalities in the genital tract must be excluded.

A careful bimanual pelvic examination will reveal the more obvious possible causes for the recurrent abortions such as retroversion of the uterus or the presence of fibroids. There are, however, certain less obvious but certainly important possibilities which cannot be diagnosed except by special investigation:—

(1) Cervical incompetence can usually be confirmed by the fact that the cervix allows the passage of quite high numbered dilators, e.g. Hegar of 8 or over, without gripping the instrument.

(2) Hysterosalpingography may reveal the presence of a small submucous myoma undetected by clinical examination.

(3) Hysterosalpingography may demonstrate a unicornuate, bicornuate, septate or arcuate uterus, all of which deformities are of considerable importance in causing abortion (Fig. 182 A and B).

(4) Whilst it is true that patients may habitually abort because of endocrine deficiency or imbalance during pregnancy there is no means whereby this can be estimated before the onset of pregnancy. Assuming in habitual abortion that a patient gets pregnant with relative ease her pre-pregnant hormone balance must be normal, or, if slightly abnormal, it obviously does not require correction. These pre-pregnant levels bear no relation whatever to the hormone levels that may develop during the ensuing pregnancy. Endocrine assay of the habitual aborter in her non-pregnant state has become a popular method of investigation, but we consider it unnecessary since the results bear no relation to any treatment that the patient may require during her subsequent pregnancy.

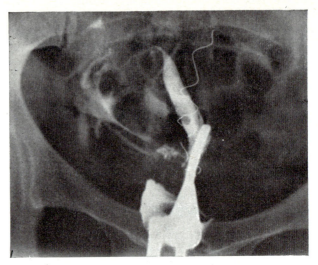

A

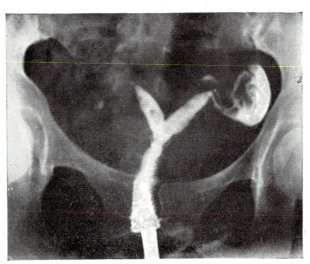

B

FIG. 182. (A) Hysterosalpingogram demonstrating a unicornuate uterus. The Fallopian tube is patent and dye is present in the peritoneal cavity. The wire which had been used to repair the rectus sheath at a previous operation is also visible. (B) Hysterosalpingogram demonstrating a bicornuate uterus. The dye which is present in the peritoneal cavity demonstrates patency of the left Fallopian tube.

Treatment

(1) The patient who habitually aborts soon develops with each abortion an anxiety state which, unless overcome, will continue to be one very significant factor in the recurrence of her abortions. Above all else, she needs a restoration of her confidence in herself and her doctors.

(2) The best drug is, therefore, Luminal 30 mgm. t.d.s. started as soon as she misses a period.

(3) Rest, avoidance of all psychological, social and physical stimuli, heavy

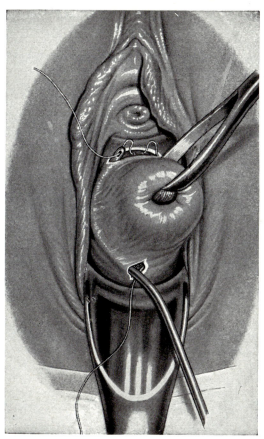

FIG. 183. Shirodkar's operation for cervical incompetence. The cervix is drawn downwards with a volsellum. A small incision has been made in the anterior fornix and a similar one in the posterior fornix. An aneurism needle has been passed from the posterior incision round the cervix so that its point presents in the anterior wound, where it is threaded with the ligature. When withdrawn through the posterior incision one half of the cervix is circumnavigated by the ligature and a similar manoeuvre on the other side will completely enclose the cervix in the ligature which is then tied with the requisite degree of tension, thus effectively closing the incompetent canal. (*From* Shaw's "Operative Gynaecology," Edinburgh: E. & S. Livingstone.)

work and long journeys. Coitus should be completely forbidden until all danger is past or, better still, until safe delivery is effected.

(4) The intramuscular implantation of 150—200 mgm. of progesterone in pellet form in the buttock or thigh, while largely empirical, is certainly valuable as a form of applied psychotherapy. Even if scientifically questionable, it gives the patient that confidence which helps to control her anxiety neurosis and, as such, is justifiable treatment. A more modern and refined therapy is the weekly intra-muscular injection of 17α-hydroxy-progesterone caproate in oil as a depot source of progesterone.

This particular drug is the one recommended as it is non-virilising to the foetus, unlike certain other synthetic progestogens.

As soon as pregnancy is confirmed vaginal smears are examined for evidence of progesterone influence. If progesterone deficiency is present the number of keratinised epithelial cells in the smear will be higher than normal. The number per 100 total cells is expressed as the Karyopyknotic Index (K.I.). A high K.I. (above 20) is an indication to commence administration of 17α-hydroxy-progesterone caproate by injection of 250 mgm. weekly. This dose should be increased by 250 mgm. weekly up to 1 g. weekly until a satisfactory smear pattern is obtained. Progesterone administration may be stopped at the twentieth week. Some workers doubt if progesterone exerts any beneficial effect on the pregnancy other than psychogenic, in which case the injections ought perhaps to be continued up to the twenty-eighth week by which time the patient has confidence in her pregnancy.

(5) Cervical incompetence can be treated by a plastic operation on the non-pregnant cervix by which the canal is reduced to normal calibre or, if pregnant, by Shirodkar's operation which, briefly, consists of passing a sub-cutaneous suture round the cervix at the level of the internal os and tying it tight enough to obstruct the extrusion of the foetal membranes. Stout nylon or nylon ribbon is used and the suture left long so that it can be cut when the patient starts labour (Fig. 183).

(6) Myomectomy is indicated if it is felt that any fibroid present is causative and very occasionally ventrosuspension is performed to correct a retro-version. If a suspension operation succeeds, it is again largely due to its functional rather than anatomic value.

Bicornuate or other septate deformities can be corrected by a plastic operation in which the uterus is split down the mid-line and a wedge containing the septum excised. The two halves are then resutured. This simple operation is well worth a trial if the hysterogram clearly demonstrates the deformity.

STERILISATION

In certain diseases affecting the female partner, such as severe heart disease, hypertension and chronic nephritis, it is often advisable in the mother's interest not only to terminate the pregnancy but also to sterilise her. This important decision should only be undertaken in those diseases in which the prognosis is adversely affected by any future pregnancy, and any disease, such as pulmonary tuberculosis, in which there is a reasonable chance of ultimate cure, does not provide an adequate indication for permanent sterilisation.

The operation of sterilisation is usually undertaken in conjunction with a termination of pregnancy, where the indication for the termination is the indication for the simultaneous operation of sterilisation.

Certain precautions, similar to those recommended for therapeutic abortion, should be taken.

(1) Sterilisation should be recommended by a consultant in the disease which provides the indication for the termination of pregnancy.

(2) Both partners of the marriage should understand the exact indication and nature of the operation and should signify their consent in writing and append their signatures.

(3) The general practitioner should be informed and should add his consent and approval also in writing..

(4) The patient and her husband must be informed that the operation is irreversible.

(5) The patient and her husband must be informed that there is a small risk of pregnancy if the tubes are simply divided but almost none if the tubes are excised.

Male sterilisation is increasing in popularity and over 6,000 have been done in this country in the last two years. Similar precautions should be followed as in female sterilisation with the husband and wife giving written consent, etc., except that the vas can be successfully rejoined if required in about 50—70% of instances. At least three months must elapse after the operation before performing seminal analysis for the first time. Spermatozoa are usually present for from three to five months after operation and a negative test must be obtained before allowing intercourse to resume.

Operative Procedure for Termination and Sterilisation

(1) *Vaginal Method.* The uterus may be emptied before the twelfth week of pregnancy by a dilatation and curettage. The pouch of Douglas can then be opened and the tubes drawn down and excised or tied in the region of the isthmus. This method is only really suitable for multiparous patients who have some degree of vaginal laxity.

Vaginal termination by suction curettage is gaining in popularity. Providing the usual precautions are observed it is a safe procedure. Aspiration of the uterine contents is performed at a negative pressure of up to 20 lb. per square inch and is generally used in pregnancies up to twelve weeks. The risks of sepsis, haemorrhage and retained products are less with aspiration than with ordinary curettage, but if the suction curette should perforate the uterus immense damage to extra-uterine structures can rapidly occur.

Injecting hypertonic saline or glucose into the amniotic cavity between the 16th—20th week of pregnancy will produce abortion in nearly every instance, but several deaths have occurred due to uterine infection so that the use of this method is steadily declining.

Recent work has suggested that prostaglandins may have a value in

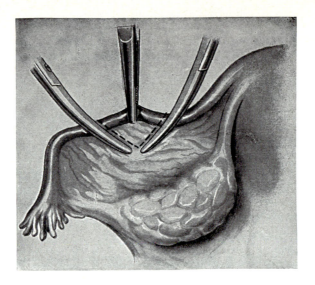

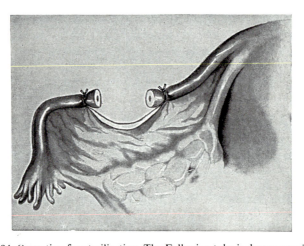

Fig. 184. Operation for sterilisation. The Fallopian tube is drawn up with dissecting forceps in a position where the broad ligament is relatively bloodless
and curved clamps are placed in position each side. The tissue enclosed by the
two clamps is then excised with a scalpel. Subsequently the tissues enclosed in
the clamps are ligatured. No effort is made to bury the cut ends of the Fallopian
tube. Although the operation is simple, it gives excellent results and subsequent
adhesions have been shown to cause no trouble. (*From* Shaw's "Operative
Gynaecology," 2nd Ed., E. & S. Livingstone.)

termination of pregnancy and may therefore lessen the need for surgical intervention.

(2) *Abdominal Method*. The uterus is emptied of its gestation sac by the operation of anterior hysterotomy—a miniature Caesarean section—and after the uterine incision has been closed by accurate suture, the Fallopian tubes are occluded by (*a*) simple ligature of their isthmic portion, (*b*) wedge excision of the isthmus, (*c*) bilateral total salpingectomy; (*b*) and (*c*) give a high degree of reliability, but (*a*) has been succeeded by many recorded instances of subsequent recanalisation and pregnancy. In fact, all methods of tubal ligation have been reported to fail in certain instances, though if the operation is carefully performed the failure rate is infinitely small (Fig. 184).

(3) Some surgeons perform a total hysterectomy of the pregnant uterus, and in certain instances this operation is the most satisfactory, e.g. if small fibroids are also present and provide in themselves an indication for the hysterectomy. Total hysterectomy of the uterus with the pregnancy in situ is the only absolutely certain way of sterilising a woman. The ovaries should always be conserved unless hopelessly diseased, e.g. malignant ovarian tumour associated with pregnancy.

14 Birth Control

The desire to exercise voluntary control over conception and the resulting demand for advice on methods of contraception is rapidly increasing. Higher standards and the increased cost of living, lack of accommodation and the great reduction of infant mortality are some of the factors that make spacing of pregnancies and limitation of family size a necessity for most married couples today.

On medical grounds, many women are advised against conception, although not always given the necessary instructions on how to carry out this advice. In certain medical conditions pregnancy may be a threat to health, or even life, and is contraindicated temporarily or permanently. Such conditions include active pulmonary tuberculosis, renal disease, severe cardiac disease, severe toxaemia in previous pregnancies and puerperal insanity. Limiting the number of pregnancies may be necessary in established Rhesus incompatibility. Temporary postponement may be advisable after an operation or debilitating illness. The spacing of pregnancies is indicated on medical grounds, for it has been shown that with birth intervals of less than two years there is a considerable increase in the incidence of prematurity and thus of neonatal deaths. But medical grounds cannot be limited by too narrow or too rigid an interpretation. Fear of the unwanted pregnancy may have serious effects on the health of a woman, may cause much marital discord with far-reaching effects on the health of the whole family and can be a contributory factor in the breakdown of a marriage. In extreme cases this fear may lead to attempts at abortion with all its attendant dangers.

The question of possible ill effects caused by the use of contraceptive methods frequently arises. However, it should be noted that the use of any contraceptive method may hide subfertility, and this danger should be made clear to the nulliparous woman. Increasing age, especially after the 30th year, decreases fecundity and makes prolonged postponement of the first pregnancy inadvisable.

Ideally, a child should be born because it is wanted, not because it cannot be prevented, and this can be made possible by the constructive use of methods to control conception.

The old idea that contraception implies the prevention of conception must be replaced by the newer concept of control of conception in order that a couple may produce the number of children which they desire at a spacing which they consider expedient according to their economic circumstances. The National Health Service in Great Britain has not yet accepted full responsibility for the control of conception, but it is slowly moving in that direction. Voluntary organisations, namely the Family Planning Association together with clinics established by the local authorities, do provide contraceptive advice for the majority of the population. An increasing number of hospitals are also providing advice in those instances where there is a medical indication for the control of conception. The medical profession, which has by tradition also failed to accept responsibility for this aspect of the requirements of its patients, is being slowly forced to change its ideas largely because the modern methods of conception control demand medical supervision.

The control of conception may be considered to be either personal or economic. The necessity of control of conception at a personal level is obvious and has already been referred to above. The necessity for the control of conception in the economic interests of a community are also obvious, when it is remembered that world population has doubled in the last fifty years and will be doubled again in the next thirty years. This particular aspect of conception control is particularly applicable to the underdeveloped or emerging nations of Asia and Africa, where population level has hitherto relied upon control by death. As modern medical science reaches these nations the control of their population by an early death rate no longer applies and therefore control of birth rate must be applied if the growth of their populations is not in future going to be limited by starvation.

It is a sad reflection upon modern methods of birth control that the majority of these is dependent upon the intellect of their users. The more intellectual members of the community realising the difficulty that faces them do, therefore, practise birth control and limit the size of their families, whereas the less intelligent members of the community produce large numbers of offspring, thus gradually diluting the intellectual capacity of the community. If this trend is allowed to persist unchecked it must inevitably lead to a general lowering in the standards of intelligence and ability.

Contraceptive Methods

By modern standards any method of birth control must be related to the fertility of the community at large, in order that some criterion may be established regarding the efficiency of the different methods which are available. When uninhibited intercourse is allowed in fertile women between the age of 20 and 40 a high pregnancy rate may be expected. This is expressed as the number of pregnancies per hundred woman years, or the number of pregnancies which would be expected to occur in a hundred women over a period of one year of sexual exposure. A normal figure, which varies from 75 to 90 may be anticipated. Any method or system which allows intercourse to occur and yet reduces the rate of conception may be considered to be a method of contraception.

METHODS
Abstinence
    1a. Total abstinence.
    1b. Abstinence during fertile phase.

Female 2a. Spermicidal substances in the vagina.
            2b. Douching.
            2c. Occlusive diaphragms.
            2d. Altering cervical mucus.
            2e. Intrauterine contraceptive devices.
            2f. Suppression of ovulation.
            2g. Surgical sterilisation.

Male   3a. Withdrawal (coitus interruptus).
            3b. Condom or sheath.
            3c. Drugs to suppress spermatogenesis.
            3d. Vasectomy.

ABSTINENCE.

1a. *Total Abstinence*

This is the only real certain way of preventing conception. It must be remembered, however, that spermatozoa deposited at the vulva may migrate up the vagina and result in eventual conception.

1b. *Abstinence during fertile phase*

This is the rhythm method or the use of the safe period, which depends upon the avoidance of sexual intercourse during the probable dates of ovulation. In a 28-day cycle ovulation occurs on the 14th day of the cycle. Seldom, however, is the menstrual cycle accurate to within an exact day and equally seldom is the time of ovulation accurately restricted to the 14th day. Even with a relatively regular 28-day menstrual cycle ovulation may occur anywhere between the 12th and 16th day. Spermatozoa deposited in the female genital tract may survive for up to three days, so that intercourse which occurs at any time from the 9th day to the 16th day could theoretically result in conception. The ovum itself may well live for 24 hours, so that intercourse between the 9th and 17th day results in a theoretical possibility of pregnancy. The safe period is, therefore, calculated from the first day of the menstrual period until the 8th day of the cycle and from the 18th to the 28th day. An alternative method is to calculate the danger period, which is from five days before ovulation to three days after ovulation. In a 35-day menstrual cycle, therefore, ovulation will occur on the 21st day (that is 14 days before the next period) so that the danger period is from day 16 to day 24; or alternatively the safe period may be calculated as from day 1 to day 15 and from day 25 to day 35.

The use of this method of contraception will result in approximately 25 pregnancies per 100 woman years. The failures result from irregular ovulation or from an irregular menstrual cycle, which in turn leads to ovulation occurring at an unexpected time. As most women do not have completely regular cycles, particularly during the early postnatal months and prior to the menopause, exact calculations of the date of ovulation are by no means easy and the method is, therefore, often unreliable. Some couples prefer to use this method on religious grounds or because they find mechanical methods unacceptable. As in every method of conception control, an explanation must be given to the patient of the failure rate and also the reasons for them.

FEMALE

2a. *Spermicidal substances in the vagina*

Chemical contraceptives containing spermicidal agents may be used in the form of soluble pessaries, creams, jellies or foaming tablets which are inserted into the vagina prior to intercourse. Used alone they are most unreliable, but used in conjunction with some mechanical barrier such as a sheath or an occlusive cap they give reliable contraception. A list of such chemical preparations which have been tested and found to be non-toxic and reach the required standard of efficiency is published by the Family Planning Association. This particular method relies upon a chemical substance being able to kill or immobilise spermatozoa before they can gain access to the cervical canal. Inevitably, of course, ejaculation direct in to the cervical canal will eventually occur and may result in a pregnancy, unless of course some mechanical barrier is used.

The use of sponges or tampons which are soaked in a spermicidal chemical and placed in the upper vagina prior to intercourse is designed to overcome the disadvantage of direct ejaculation into the cervical canal. Such devices, however, frequently get displaced and are, therefore, relatively inefficient. In order to be effective they must be bulky and therefore cause discomfort and must be discarded after use. There is nothing to recommend them. The pregnancy rate is approximately 30 per 100 woman years.

2b. *Douching*

Immediate post-coital douching of the vagina with a spermicidal solution for the purpose of washing away the sperms is a fairly common method. This method can only be effective if it is applied immediately after intercourse and before the spermatozoa have had an opportunity to gain access to the cervical canal, from which they cannot be dislodged by douching. As well as being highly inefficient, this method has obvious aesthetic disadvantages. The pregnancy rate is approximately 40 per 100 woman years.

2c. *Occlusive diaphragms*

These provide a barrier in the vagina against direct insemination, but they are not sufficient to prevent the sperm passing round the edges to reach the cervical canal. The diaphragm, therefore, is only effective when used in conjunction with a chemical spermicide in the form of a jelly or cream, and when sufficient time is allowed for complete destruction of the sperm before the diaphragm is removed. In practice, the diaphragm, liberally covered with spermicide, can be inserted at any convenient time and is left in position for a minimum of eight hours after coitus. It causes no discomfort and no douching is required when these precautions are taken.

Accurate fitting of the diaphragm is essential, and the size required is difficult to assess at the first vaginal examination of the patient, when there is so often some degree of vaginal spasm present due to nervousness. For this reason an approximate fitting is made and instructions in inserting and re-

12*

moving the diaphragm are given at the first visit of the patient. At a subsequent visit, after a few days, the patient returns with the diaphragm in position, when the vaginal muscles are usually found to be relaxed and the required size can be estimated with accuracy, and also the patient's ability to use the cap in the correct position can be checked. Alterations in the size and type of diaphragm required may occur as a result of changes in weight, debilitating illness and for other reasons, so that routine checking is advisable at suitable intervals, usually six months to one year. A refitting of the diaphragm is always required after childbirth and can usually be carried out about six to eight weeks after confinement.

Types of Occlusive Cap. There are three main types, and others which are modifications of these and have a more limited use.

The Dutch Cap or Diaphragm. This consists of a dome-shaped diaphragm of thin rubber, with a rubber-covered metal rim, which may be either a watch spring or spiral spring. These are made in a wide range of sizes and fit obliquely in the vagina, stretching from just behind the pubic ramus into the posterior fornix, thus covering the cervix. The diaphragm is held in position

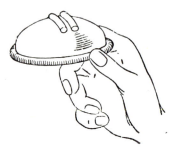

FIG. 185a. Two strips of contraceptive paste are placed over the dome of the cap.

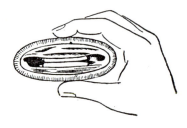

FIG. 185b. The rim is squeezed together so as to enclose the paste.

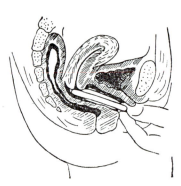

FIG. 185c. Insertion of Dutch cap—first stage.

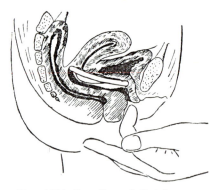

FIG. 185d. Insertion of Dutch cap—second stage. The anterior rim is pushed up well behind the symphysis pubis.

(By courtesy of **Dr. Helena Wright** from " Contraceptive Technique ".)

by the tension of the spring rim and cannot be retained where the vaginal tone is lax. It is contraindicated therefore in the presence of a cystocele or rectocele, sometimes during the early post-natal period, and occasionally after repair operations in those cases where the anterior wall of the vagina is flattened or lacking in elasticity because of scarring. It is the easiest type of cap for the patient to use, fits in the majority of cases, causes no discomfort to either partner when correctly chosen and fitted accurately, and therefore is the cap most frequently used (Fig. 185).

The failure rate of the Dutch cap is about four to six per 100 woman years and is nearly always associated with poor fitting due to a retroverted uterus when the diaphragm is placed in error in the anterior fornix.

The Dumas Cap. This is a cup-shaped rubber or plastic cap with a thickened rim, fitted to the vault of the vagina so that it encloses the cervix and is maintained in position partly by suction. It is available in five sizes. It can only be used in those cases where the patient can locate the cervix accurately, and fits most adequately where the uterus is retroverted and the cervix points forward in the vagina.

The Cervical Cap. This is a rubber cap shaped somewhat like a thimble, with a solid rolled rubber rim. It fits closely to the column of the cervix. It is indicated in similar conditions required for the Dumas cap and is suitable where the cervix is long and firm. Both these types of cap can sometimes be used where a diaphragm is contraindicated. Some patients prefer them despite the fact that they are often a little more difficult to manipulate, as they are smaller and cover less of the vaginal wall.

2d. *Altering Cervical Mucus*

It has been observed that the continuous administration of chlormadinone acetate acts as a contraceptive agent by causing a local alteration in the genital tract without suppressing ovulation.

Chlormadinone acetate is taken in a dose of 0·5 mg. daily continuously regardless of the menstrual cycle or the onset of bleeding. In approximately 60% of patients who are taking chlormadinone normal ovulation occurs and is accompanied by a mid-cycle surge of luteinising hormone associated with the other criteria of ovulation. In a normal menstrual cycle the cervical mucus undergoes characteristic changes at the mid-cycle which are associated with rapid sperm penetration of the cervical mucus and ready access to the upper genital tract. Under continuous chlormadinone administration these changes are suppressed and are associated with impaired sperm counts and sperm motility in the cervical mucus, as shown by examination of the mucus at post-coital tests. Chlormadinone results in biochemical changes in the cervical mucus at the time of ovulation, particularly in the protein concentration, so that the cervical mucus resembles that which is normally found in the luteal or late phase of the menstrual cycle There is also evidence that the endocervical pH becomes more acid under chlormadinone administration and therefore reduces sperm motility and penetration.

The disadvantage of the continuous administration of a low dose progestational agent such as chlormadinone is that there is lack of control of the menstrual cycle itself, so that menstrual irregularity and intermenstrual bleeding become relatively common. However, it appears to be a method devoid of most of the side-effects associated with oral-contraceptives.

2e. *Intrauterine Contraceptive Devices*

These have been used for many years in both animals and man. They were first popularised, however, in recent time by Grafenberg, who developed a silver coiled wire ring which could be inserted into the uterine cavity and left there undisturbed for approximately one year before it needed to be removed and changed. Prior to this, various types of intrauterine conceptive and intra-cervical contraceptive device had been used, the majority of which consisted oı some type of wishbone or stem pessary, a part of which protruded through the cervical canal in order that the device could be easily removed. The great disadvantage of the Grafenberg ring was that it required an anaesthetic for its insertion, since the cervix had to be dilated, and subsequently required an anaesthetic for its removal.

The Grafenberg ring earned for itself an undeservedly bad reputation, not only because it was said to be inefficient but also because it was supposed to cause pelvic infection and lead to carcinoma of the endometrium. In its day the Grafenberg ring was by far the most efficient form of contraception with a pregnancy rate of approximately two per 100 woman years. There is no evidence that the ring itself ever actually caused infection; indeed it is difficult to see how it could possibly do so. It is obvious, however, that if infection gains access to the uterus then the presence of a foreign body lying therein will make it more difficult for the uterus to eliminate that infection and if an infection has once become established then the presence of a foreign body will make that infection more extensive and more severe. There is no evidence that the Grafenberg ring was a predisposing factor in carcinoma of the endo-metrium, unless by causing nulliparity it automatically predisposed the uterus to endometrial carcinoma, which is traditionally more common in those who have not had children. The whole problem of contraception is bedevilled by bigotry and many generations of medical men have condemned the Grafen-berg ring because of its supposed complications.

The pressing need for population control after the Second World War resulted in a further and more critical examination of intrauterine contra-ceptive devices. The Japanese were the first to use plastic intrauterine contra-ceptive devices, mostly shaped as a circle, some having supporting struts rather like the steering wheel of a car. There followed a rapid development of intrauterine contraceptive devices using any material which was both flexible and cheap. These materials included wire, stainless steel, nylon and plastic of which eventually plastic became the most reliable and popular and is now most commonly used in the form of the Lippes Loop, Margulies Spiral and Birnberg Bow. These are manufactured from polyethylene which has been impregnated with barium sulphate in order to render it radio opaque. It is strange that the plastic device is now accepted as a reliable contraceptive agent in almost every community which had previously condemned the Grafenberg ring. The change from metal to plastic has been the excuse for acceptance.

Plastic intrauterine devices are flexible so that they can be straightened and fitted into introducers by which they are passed through the cervical canal and then released within the cavity of the uterus to take up their previous shape. The plastic must have sufficient elasticity to enable it to accommodate to a certain extent to the contours of the uterine cavity and yet resist the attempts of the uterus to expel it by uterine contractions. The Lippes Loop has two thin nylon threads attached to its lower end and these threads protrude down through the cervical canal into the vagina, where they may be palpated by the patient herself or the examining doctor in order to ascertain that the device is still within the uterus. The Margulies Spiral has a beaded nylon stem which protrudes through the cervix for a similar reason.

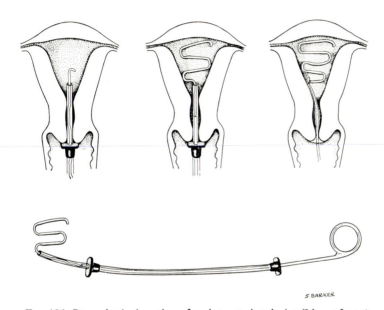

S BARKER

FIG. 186. Stages in the insertion of an intrauterine device (Lippes Loop).

The insertion of a plastic intrauterine contraceptive device is relatively simple and easy and requires very little training. It is essential, however, that any person who is going to insert a device into a uterus should be well acquainted with accurate methods of pelvic examination and should be well skilled not only in examining the patient but also in handling the patient, and must also be capable and dextrous in the use of surgical instruments. A gentle and skilful operator can insert these devices into the uterus of almost any multiparous patient without the need for an anaesthetic.

For the insertion of an intrauterine contraceptive device the patient may be placed either in the lithotomy position or in the left lateral position. A gentle but thorough pelvic examination is performed in order primarily to determine the position of the uterus and to ensure that the bladder has been previously emptied. Needless to say the presence of any uterine, tubal or ovarian pathology precludes the insertion of an intrauterine device. The vagina and cervix are then inspected by means of a speculum. Any vaginal discharge, vaginitis, cervicitis, cervical erosion or other cervical pathology must be treated and cured before a device is inserted. The cervix is then grasped with a tenaculum forceps in order that it may be steadied and a uterine sound is passed to assess the length of the uterine cavity. This, together with the size of the uterus as measured on bimanual pelvic examination, will determine the size of the intrauterine device to be inserted. The appropriate device, which has been previously sterilised in 1% Savlon or 1:1,000 chlorhexidine, is selected and is mounted by a no touch technique into the introducer (also previously sterilised). A number 3 Hegar dilator is now passed through the cervical canal in order to detect the position of the internal cervical os. The stop on the introducer is then adjusted to the length of the cervical canal. The introducer is then passed through the cervical canal and as the plunger is pressed home the device uncoils within the uterine cavity. (Fig. 186.) The

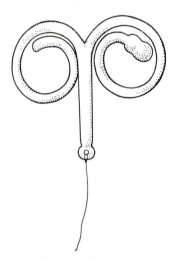

FIG. 187. Saf-T-coil.

introducer is then removed and the length of the threads or the stem of the Margulies Spiral are cut to the required length with scissors. The tenaculum forceps and the speculum are removed and a further vaginal examination performed to confirm that the nylon threads are easily palpable in the vagina. The patient is then instructed how to examine herself in order that the threads can be palpated.

The Saf-T-Coil is a more recently introduced intrauterine contraceptive device which can be obtained already mounted in its introducer and pre-sterilised by gamma radiation. (Fig. 187.)

Some patients experience some uterine cramp immediately after the insertion of an intrauterine device and this may be relieved by the administration of codeine or by a uterine antispasmodic. It is important that devices should be inserted either during menstruation or shortly after the cessation of a period in order to ensure that they are not inserted into the pregnant uterus. The patient is warned that she may experience some intermittent bleeding for the next few days and that her first few periods may be unduly heavy and prolonged.

Patients in whom a device has been inserted should be seen at intervals of one month, three months and then yearly. Providing a device is causing no symptoms there is no indication for its routine removal after one year, but most authorities would agree that a device should be changed after it has been *in situ* for three years.

The acceptance rate of intrauterine contraceptives varies widely. In the authors' series approximately 25% of devices had to be removed within three months because of pain, discomfort, continuous or heavy bleeding, or vaginal discharge. The pregnancy rate in those patients in whom the device has proved acceptable varies from two to six per 100 woman years. In the authors' series of over 500 patients in whom Lippes Loops have been inserted the pregnancy rate is 4·7 per 100 woman years.

Mechanism. The mechanism whereby an intrauterine contraceptive device works is not understood. The following reasons have been proposed:

1. In those instances where nylon protrudes through the cervix the pH of the cervical canal may be altered.

2. The presence of a device within the uterus renders the migration of spermatazoa more difficult.

3. A foreign body within the uterus provokes not only uterine contractility but also tubal contractility, so that the fertilised ovum is propelled down the Fallopian tube more rapidly than is normal and it reaches the uterine cavity before the development of the chorionic villi and is therefore unable to implant.

4. The normal preparation of the endometrium is prevented by the presence of the device.

5. The device may irritate the uterus to such an extent that it expels the newly implanted ovum.

Contraindications. Intrauterine contraceptive devices are contraindicated in the presence of pelvic pathology as indicated above. They are also contraindicated in the presence of prolonged or heavy periods. It is doubtful if intrauterine contraceptive devices should be used in the nulliparous patient and they are certainly contraindicated in those patients who suffer from primary spasmodic dysmenorrhoea, since the device will undoubtedly make this pain considerably worse.

Indications. For those multiparous patients who can tolerate an intrauterine contraceptive device it is undoubtedly a relatively efficient contraceptive. Few people, however, would advise the use of an intrauterine contraceptive device in a patient who can satisfactorily use a vaginal diaphragm or an oral contraceptive, but since many patients object to the use of a vaginal diaphragm and do not wish to use an oral contraceptive the intrauterine device has a large place in modern conception control. The ideal use of the intrauterine contraceptive device, however, is in the population control of communities rather than for the random protection of a particular individual.

Pregnancy. As stated above the pregnancy rate varies from two to six per 100 woman years in those patients in whom the device remains *in situ*. Pregnancies are more common shortly after insertion of the device and are relatively infrequent after a device has been *in situ* for one year. If pregnancy does occur there is a 30% chance that the pregnancy will end in abortion. Such an abortion is liable to be incomplete and to be associated with considerable haemorrhage. In those pregnancies which proceed to term the device will eventually be found after delivery to be embedded in the chorion, usually in the placenta. The presence of a device during pregnancy does not cause congenital abnormality of the foetus.

2f. *Suppression of Ovulation*

Undoubtedly oral contraception is the most effective of all contraceptive methods as yet available. It is estimated that approximately one million women in Britain are taking some type of oral contraceptive. Some oral contraceptives are more efficient than others in suppressing ovulation and pregnancy rates have been variously reported between 0·01 and 1·0 pregnancies per 100 woman years.

Two main forms of oral contraceptive agent are available. They are either the combined type of synthetic oestrogen/progestogen mixture, or the sequential type in which synthetic oestrogen is followed by synthetic progestogen.

1. The combined type of oral contraceptive agent usually consists of a mixture of ethinyl oestradiol or mestranol in a dose not greater than 50 micrograms, together with an orally active progestogen which is usually a 19-nor steroid or a 17-hydroxyprogesterone derivative. If the first day of the period is counted as the first day of the menstrual cycle then the tablets are taken for 21 days, starting on the fifth day of the cycle and finishing on the 26th day. Bleeding usually occurs on the 28th day, but a new course of tablets should be commenced seven days after the cessation of the previous course regardless of whether withdrawal bleeding has occurred or not.

2. The sequential type oral contraceptive agent which has been withdrawn from the British market because the daily dose is greater than 50 micrograms of oestrogen, consists of either ethinyl oestradiol or mestranol administered for 14 to 16 days, followed by an oestrogen/progesterone mixture for five to seven days. It was argued that the sequential type of tablet produces a more physiological withdrawal bleeding than does the combined type of oral contraceptive tablet. In the dose administered, however, the sequential type of oral contraceptive is not as efficient as the combined variety.

The exact mode of action of the oral contraceptive agents is still in doubt. Although their efficiency is accepted and is widely exploited in their favour, the exact reason for this efficiency is not precisely understood. The administration of a mixture of oestrogen and progesterone certainly exerts an influence on the hypothalamic-pituitary axis and evidence suggests that the amount of follicle stimulating hormone produced by the pituitary is not diminished during the first half of the menstrual cycle, but that the release of luteinising hormone is considerably reduced or even suppressed completely.

The administration of oestrogen alone, as in the sequential type of oral contraceptive, results in diminution in the production of follicle stimulating hormone by the pituitary.

Page 477 indicates how the body may convert progestational steroids into oestrogens and it may well be that part of the action of progestational steroids when administered as contraceptive agents is that they are converted in the body into oestrogens, which in turn suppress the production of follicle stimulating hormone. Meanwhile, the unconverted progesterone exerts an action upon the endometrium preventing satisfactory endometrial development and thereby preventing implantation of the ovum should fertilisation happen to occur. It is also suggested that even cyclic administration of a progestational steroid starting on the fifth day of a cycle will alter the pH and the chemical constituents of the cervical mucus to such an extent as to render it impenetrable by spermatazoa.

Choice of Oral Contraceptive Agent

It is difficult to lay down accurate rules and regulations regarding the choice of an oral contraceptive agent for a particular patient, but as a rough working rule the lowest possible dose should be administered. The dose of progestational steroid varies by as much as five times. The lower dose pills are equally efficient as contraceptives as the high dose tablets, but breakthrough bleeding does occur occasionally with those containing a lower dose so that a higher dose has to be administered in order to maintain a satisfactory menstrual cycle. Conversely, a high dose pill may cause complete suppression of menstrual bleeding and ought, therefore, to be replaced by a tablet containing a smaller quantity of hormone. The dose of oestrogen in a daily dose should not exceed 0·05 mg. (see below).

Menstrual Cycle. Most patients taking either the combined or sequential type of pill will have a regular 28-day menstrual cycle. The bleeding which occurs is not true menstruation but is withdrawal bleeding and will be less in amount and shorter in duration than a normal menstrual period. The actual blood itself will be darker in colour and patients should be warned of this fact lest it cause them some concern. As stated above, if a period does not commence after the cessation of one course of oral tablets the next course should commence seven days later.

Pregnancy Rate. The combined type of pill is more efficient than the sequential type. The pregnancy rate of the combined type is approximately 0·1 per 100 woman years, whereas with the sequential type the rate is approximately 1·0 per 100 woman years. If the patient forgets to take a tablet she should be instructed to take two tablets the following day. If the patient fails to take three tablets during a course then she must consider herself no longer protected and should take other contraceptive precautions until she has had a period, when she can commence her next full course of pills. The majority of failures undoubtedly occur as a result of the incorrect administration of the pill, rather than a fault in the pill itself.

Breakthrough Bleeding. The incidence of breakthrough bleeding or intermenstrual spotting varies considerably and this is considered to be one of the major complications of oral contraceptive therapy. People who suffer from break-through bleeding whilst taking the combined contraceptive pill usually commence spotting or bleeding on about the seventeenth day of the cycle. if spotting alone occurs the tablets should be continued and the spotting usually ceases after two or three days. If actual bleeding occurs then it is better to discontinue the course of treatment and start a further course after a gap of seven days. Patients taking the sequential type of tablet, however, should continue the course of treatment regardless of spotting or bleeding that may occur, since the progestational fraction of the administered hormone is in the last five to seven days of the cycle.

Side Effects. The modern contraceptive pill contains approximately 10% of the dose which was originally administered in oral contraceptive tablets fifteen years ago. The side effects of the modern low dose preparations are therefore very much less severe and fewer in number than those previously encountered. Some side effects related to hormone imbalance may occur during the first few days or even the first few cycles, but these gradually correct themselves without difficulty. The oestrogen element may give rise to nausea and actual vomiting, whilst both oestrogen and progesterone may cause fluid retention resulting in headache, migraine, oedema of the ankles and rapid weight increase, together with depression, irritability and a general sensation of lethargy. Some progestational steroids are undoubtedly anabolic agents, resulting in actual weight increase as well as fluid retention. The oestrogen/progesterone mixture usually causes some increase in breast size, an increase which may on occasion become sufficiently marked to be unwelcome. Intermenstrual spotting and bleeding has been mentioned above and the exact cause of this haemorrhage is unknown. Amenorrhoea, or lack of withdrawal bleeding, may also occur, especially where the dose of administered hormone is large.

The psychological effect of the pill upon patients is difficult or impossible to foretell. Whilst some have an increase of libido others undoubtedly have a suppression of sexual desire. These changes in sexual behaviour appear to be related to the constituents of the pill rather than to the pill itself, because changing from one particular brand to another may eliminate this symptom.

Dangers

The Genital Tract. The continuous administration of progestational steroids undoubtedly predisposes a number of women to monilial infections of the vagina. Recurrent attacks of vaginal moniliasis are relatively common in patients taking the combined pill. An individual attack can be cured by either nystatin or sporostacin and recurrent attacks can be prevented by inserting one of these pessaries one night each week for an indefinite period. The endocervical glands are influenced by oestrogen levels, so that an increase of mucoid discharge from the cervical canal is a fairly common complaint. Similarly, cervical erosions are also oestrogen-dependent and may occur especially in those patients who are taking the sequential type of oral tablet. There is no evidence that either the combined or sequential type of tablet has any permanent effect upon the endometrium, nor do they predispose the endometrium to the development of carcinoma. In fact there is some evidence to show that administration of progesterone decreases the incidence of endometrial carcinoma. There is no evidence that either the combined or sequential type of tablet has any carcinogenic effect on the cervix.

The Breasts. Breast enlargement is a fairly common complication of the pill. This enlargement may be accompanied by discomfort together with increased sensitivity or even pain. There is no evidence that oral contraceptives are a causative or even a predisposing factor in carcinoma of the breast. Nevertheless the use of oral contraceptives is contraindicated in any patient who has suffered from malignant disease and this is especially applicable to carcinoma of the breast.

Carbohydrate Metabolism. Carbohydrate tolerance may be impaired and the renal threshold for glucose decreased. There is no evidence that oral contraceptives alter the course or severity of diabetes as measured by present-day standards. The risk of hastening the onset of diabetes in the pre-diabetic patient is probably less than from pregnancy.

Liver. Oral contraceptives may alter liver metabolism but not to a degree which can be recognised as being clinically significant. Oral contraceptives, however, should not be given to a patient with advanced liver disease or to someone who has been recently jaundiced.

Heart Disease. Oral contraceptives are not contraindicated in heart disease, except where the fluid retention which may be caused by the oral contraceptive would exert an adverse effect upon the progress or the symptoms of the heart disease itself.

Varicose Veins. A number of patients who take an oral contraceptive complain that veins in their legs become more prominent or that actual varicose veins may develop. The presence of varicose veins is not a contraindication to the administration of the pill.

Thrombo-embolic Disease. Both oestrogen and progestogen cause changes in the clotting mechanism of the blood, but although the clinical importance of this has been difficult to assess there is increasing evidence that disturbances of clotting mechanism are associated with a relatively high oestrogen intake. It is possible that some of the progestogen is metabolised in the body into oestrogen and it is the resulting oestrogenic substances which exert an influence on the clotting mechanism. Some types of thrombo-embolic disorder are associated with the use of oral contraceptives. Women between the ages of 16 and 40 who are taking the pill are five times more likely to be admitted to hospital with deep venous thrombosis or pulmonary embolus than control patients not taking an oral contraceptive. Approximately one in every 2,000 women who are taking the pill is admitted to hospital each year for treatment of venous thrombo-embolism, whereas in the controls who are not on an oral contraceptive the figure is about one in every 20,000. There is also a strong relationship between the use of oral contraceptives and deaths from pulmonary embolus and cerebral thrombosis in otherwise healthy women, and this risk is about seven times greater in patients using oral contraceptives than in the controls. There is no evidence that oral contraceptives predispose patients to coronary thrombosis. The risk of thrombo-embolic disease to the patient on an oral contraceptive is difficult to assess, but it is certainly less than the risk of thrombo-embolic disease during pregnancy.

Sufficient evidence has been accumulated by the Committee on Safety of Drugs to demonstrate a broad relationship between the oestrogen content of oral contraceptive drugs and thrombo-embolic disorders. Pulmonary embolism is three times as frequent among women taking oral contraception containing 75 micrograms or more of oestrogen than among those taking products which contain 50 micrograms or less of oestrogen per day. All oral contraceptives containing more than 50 micrograms of oestrogen have been withdrawn from the British market. The reduction in oestrogen content does not diminish the efficacy of the combined pill.

Conclusions. There are risks in every form of medication and there are certainly risks in pregnancy. The risk inherent in taking the oral contraceptive pill must be weighed carefully for each individual patient and must be carefully considered against the relative unreliability or the unacceptability of alternative methods of contraception and also against the known hazards of pregnancy.

2g. *Surgical Sterilisation*

Surgical sterilisation may be performed by removing the ovaries, all or part of the Fallopian tubes or the uterus itself. It is obvious that the most frequently performed operation is the removal of part or all of the Fallopian tubes, or the interruption of their lumen by coagulation diathermy via the laparoscope. Sterilisation by interruption of the tubal lumen is an operation which must be considered to be irreversible. It should never be performed without full and frank discussion with the patient and her husband, both of whom must sign forms of consent before the operation.

MALE

3a. *Withdrawal*

Coitus interruptus is an extremely common practice to which patients usually refer when they say that pregnancy has been avoided by "being careful". Coitus takes place in a normal manner but the penis is withdrawn immediately before ejaculation. The unreliability of this method is obvious, but it has two great advantages. It costs nothing and it requires no equipment. Nevertheless it has a failure rate of approximately 25 per 100 woman years. The main cause of the failure is not that ejaculation occurs within the vagina but that the prostatic fluid secreted prior to ejaculation frequently contains active spermatozoa. This practice imposes a great strain upon the husband and is thought to be a causative factor in some anxiety states. It is also a common cause of failure in the wife to enjoy intercourse fully. As the failure rate is high, anxiety about the unwanted pregnancy produces an additional strain, and this is therefore not a method which can be recommended. Some couples seem to prefer this method, however, and make no complaints of suffering from strain or anxiety as a result.

3b. *Condom or Sheath*

In this method the penis is completely covered by a rubber sheath, which may be of very thin rubber (the condom), which is used only once, or a thicker rubber (washable sheath), which can be used repeatedly. A lubricant is advisable, and where the highest degree of security is desired a spermicidal jelly or a soluble pessary is used in addition, giving further protection if the sheath should slip or break.

This method is only partially reliable, having a failure rate of approximately 10 per 100 woman years, but it has the advantage of requiring no fitting or instruction. The use of the sheath, however, can cause psychological disturbances sufficient to interfere with potency in some men, and many couples object to this method because of the impairment of sensation or because of the inevitable interruption due to the adjustment of the sheath.

3c. *Drugs to Suppress Spermatogenesis*

Several drugs have been developed which either suppress spermatogenesis or reduce sperm motility. These have so far proved too toxic to use in man but undoubtedly some form of male pill will be developed in the near future.

3d. *Vasectomy*

The operation of vasectomy is discussed on page 346.

CHOICE OF METHOD

The contraceptive of choice depends on the particular requirements of the patient. It is strange how even the most enlightened patient or doctor will become extremely biased with regard to contraceptive methods.

The reliability of a method must always be discussed with a patient and it must be remembered that published figures are often prejudiced by vested interests or by personal enthusiasm. It is essential that the patient be given a contraceptive method which she finds acceptable, otherwise the results on either her sex life or the contraception are bound to be bad. The choice of a contraceptive can only be the result of enlightened and frank discussion between the patient and her adviser.

15 Pathology of Pregnancy

Abortion

Abortion refers to the termination of pregnancy whether it be spontaneous or induced before the twenty-eighth week, after which the child is considered to be viable. If pregnancy terminates between the twenty-eighth and the fortieth week, the term premature labour is employed. The word miscarriage is widely used, perhaps because the lay public is apt to regard abortion as suggesting a criminal procedure. The present tendency is to use words abortion and miscarriage synonymously.

The incidence of abortion is far higher than is generally believed: accurate statistics are impossible to obtain, but it is probable that at least more than 30% of pregnancies terminate spontaneously in abortion, and in fact some authorities state that it may be as high as 50%. These figures include criminal abortions, the incidence of which is even now impossible to calculate since all parties concerned are involved in a conspiracy of secrecy and silence. The number of police prosecutions is but a tiny fraction of the whole and the Registrar-General's returns in which maternal mortality includes deaths due to abortion are not completely reliable because a number of maternal deaths is certified as due to haemorrhage or sepsis with no mention of the primary cause which was really responsible. Recent legislation has made an attempt to tighten up certification.

AETIOLOGY

(1) Abnormalities of the Foetus

Maldevelopment. Approximately 50% of abortion material of the first two months of pregnancy show errors of development of the foetus. If abortion specimens are carefully examined, such abnormalities as hydatidiform degeneration of the placenta and maldevelopment of the embryo will be found in 50% of cases according to Hertig and Shebbon. If all abortion material available were histologically examined, the percentage of abnormalities from early abortions would be even greater than 50 and might reach 75. It is interesting to note that 25% of spontaneous abortions have chromosomal abnormalities. Looked at from another angle congenital malformations account for 20% of all infant deaths.

Intra-Uterine Death

Infections. If a pregnant woman contracts some infection such as pneumonia, malaria, typhoid, dysentery, smallpox, syphilis or, in fact, almost any except the mildest infectious fever, the foetus is liable to die *in utero*. With the exception of syphilis, rubella and smallpox, the infecting organism or virus does not pass the placental barrier and it is the pyrexia which kills the foetus and not the infection.

Poisons. The most dangerous and most effective abortifacient drug is lead, though quinine has great virtues in the eyes of the lay public. Before the ovum is adversely affected the mother is usually gravely ill, though cases of abortion have occurred after the use of quinine urethane for the injection of varicose veins. It is unlikely that cytotoxic drugs will be used on a patient who is pregnant unless the pregnancy is unrecognised at the time of treatment when the therapy will be lethal to the embryo.

Radiological Effects. It occasionally happens that a patient being treated for malignant disease by radiation is not known to be pregnant. If, in the first trimester, the abdomen receives sufficient dosage, abortion will result from intra-uterine death of the foetus. If the foetus does not receive sufficient radiation to kill it, there is a grave risk of foetal gonadal damage or developmental abnormality. For this reason diagnostic X-rays must always be limited in the pregnant (see Chapter 26).

(2) Abnormalities of the Placenta and Membranes

Acute hydramnios sometimes causes abortion, and hydatidiform degeneration has already been mentioned. A fairly common, and as yet not generally accepted, cause of abortion is placenta praevia. This is particularly to be suspected if the abortion is preceded by repeated haemorrhages. Such an abortion may be accompanied by severe and dangerous bleeding when it occurs later in the second trimester. Infarction of the placenta and accidental haemorrhage is the operative factor in hypertension and chronic nephritis affecting the mother.

(3) General Diseases of the Mother

Generalised Acute Infections. In measles, scarlet fever, cholera, typhoid, diphtheria, smallpox and malaria, there is a well-marked tendency for the pregnancy to end in abortion or premature labour. It is well established that severe degrees of pyrexia always tend to be followed by abortion, and it may be that the high temperature of specific fevers is the cause of the abortion rather than that the virus of the disease permeates into the foetal circulation.

Localised Acute Infections of the Mother. In pneumonia there is the same tendency to abortion, and with pneumonia it is not uncommon for pneumococcal peritonitis to develop subsequent to the evacuation of the uterus. Severe upper respiratory tract infections such as influenza are also important. Specific and effective chemotherapy has considerably modified the risks of abortion from all varieties of infection and if applied early should save the ovum.

Chronic Infections. *Syphilis.* Syphilis is fortunately of decreasing importance in the aetiology of abortion and never causes an abortion before mid-pregnancy. This enables almost all pregnant women, who have a routine serological test for syphilis at their first ante-natal visit, to receive adequate antibiotic protection for the foetus before it is infected.

Tuberculosis. Tuberculosis is not a common cause of abortion, which occurs only if infection is widespread and rapidly progressive.

Chronic Medical Diseases. It is a surprising fact that few medical diseases, however severe, cause abortion. Obstetricians know too well that a patient with completely decompensated morbus cordis may reach full-term pregnancy. There are very few medical diseases which actually cause abortion and the only really important diseases are hypertension and chronic nephritis which operate by interfering with placental circulation and foetal oxygen supply.

(4) Local Abnormalities of the Mother

Local Abnormalities of the Genitalia. In the past, the so-called condition of genital hypoplasia was stated to be a common cause of abortion. This largely hypothetical state of under-development of the uterus is very rare and is only seen in association with a gross ovarian deficiency. As such patients are sterile in any event, the question of abortion does not arise. Genital hypoplasia may, therefore, now be relegated to a very insignificant place in the aetiology of abortion.

There are, however, certain congenital abnormalities of the uterus which undoubtedly do cause abortion in certain patients and most of these comprise partial duplication of the upper part of the uterus—bicornuate uterus, septate, subseptate and arcuate uterus. They have already been mentioned in detail in a previous chapter. (See Chapter 5, p. 156.)

Displacements of the Uterus. Retroversion in the past has been grossly exaggerated as a cause of abortion and it is now considered by most enlightened gynaecologists to be only occasionally responsible, when the pregnancy usually terminates during the third month. The uterus rises out of the pelvis during the fourth month, so that abortion cannot be attributed to retroversion after that time. Misguided attempts to correct a retroverted gravid uterus, especially under an anaesthetic, are a potent cause of abortion.

Fibromyoma. The presence of a myoma is *per se* no bar to conception unless the tumour is submucous or polypoid. If conception should occur in such a uterus the liability of abortion is increased. Removal of the tumour by myomectomy is frequently followed by successful pregnancy.

Cervical Incompetence. Any injury which renders the cervix patulous, e.g. a cervical laceration resulting from a difficult forceps delivery or precipitate labour, a simple dilatation and curettage, or an amputation of the cervix is liable to leave the cervix incompetent. Congenital incompetence of the cervix, if it exists at all, is a very rare event. Abortion from this cause results in the middle trimester and is preceded by premature rupture of the membranes (see Chapter 13, p. 343).

Surgical Operations. Any operation, however trivial, or anaesthesia, however short, involves a risk of abortion. This risk increases the nearer the operation approaches the genital tract so that myomectomy in pregnancy carries the greatest risk of all. It is, perhaps, fair to say that it is not so much the nature of the actual operation which is the real factor but the susceptibility of the patient. A nervous woman liable to habitual abortion is likely to miscarry after having a tooth extracted while a more phlegmatic individual will tolerate bilateral partial oophorectomy and even removal of the corpus luteum without mishap to the pregnancy. The anaesthetised pregnant woman must never be allowed to become anoxic.

Drugs. Phosphorus, lead, quinine, ergot, pituitrin and mercury, when administered in large and poisonous quantities during pregnancy, may lead to abortion. Drastic purgation during the early weeks of pregnancy may also be followed by evacuation of the uterus. Many drugs are used illegally as abortifacients; amongst them are ergoapiol and pennyroyal. Very large doses of such drugs must be administered, however, before abortion takes place, and it is probable that none of the drugs mentioned has ever produced abortion in a healthy woman unless it has been administered in doses sufficient to produce a toxic effect on the mother or unless the patient is prone to abortion whether drugs are administered or not.

Injuries. Accidents and injuries to the lower abdominal region and the vulva may lead to abortion either because of the formation of haematomata in the region of the uterus, or because the placenta is directly dislodged during the injury. The local trauma of criminal abortion will be considered later. The disturbance of vaginal manipulations to correct a retroverted gravid uterus has been mentioned. The trauma of coitus has not, however, received its due attention, and there is no doubt that in the retroverted gravid uterus it is a possible cause of abortion. The fatigue and jolting of a long car journey and violent physical exercises such as riding, swimming and the modern pastime of water skiing and other sports are other less recognised causes. If a pregnant woman who is a susceptible abortion risk must travel, let her go by rail where she can rest and walk about in comfort. There is no reason to incriminate air travel except again in the susceptible subject.

Disturbances of the Endocrine System. It is established that the secretions of the corpus luteum are essential for the embedding of the fertilised ovum, so that pregnancy terminates in abortion unless a healthy corpus luteum is present in the first few weeks of pregnancy. After the first few weeks, probably the twelfth to the fourteenth, the functions of the corpus luteum are replaced by the placenta, and both ovaries may then be removed, and yet the patient go to term. It is possible, though not yet fully corroborated, that repeated abortions in early pregnancy may be caused by defects in the function of the corpus luteum. Similarly, in severe degrees of endocrine dysfunction, such as diabetes and thyrotoxicosis, there is usually a well-marked tendency to abortion, although the precise factors which lead to abortion are little understood.

Psychiatric Causes. It is well known that frights and acute mental disturbances may cause abortion. Little is known of the exact aetiology, and it is difficult to assess the frequency of this type of case. A woman, who, as a result of repeated abortion, develops an acute anxiety neurosis is a good example of this vicious circle.

(5) Faults of the Male

When, during the investigation of the problem of infertility or repeated abortion, the seminal analysis shows some abnormality, it is tempting to attribute the condition to this factor. For instance, a large number of abnormal forms in the sperm population suggests a ready explanation for the occurrence of foetal abnormality. So far this ingenious explanation has no scientific backing.

THE MECHANISM OF ABORTION

The general features of the evacuation of the uterus during the process of abortion correspond to what happens during normal labour at term, in that the body of the uterus contracts and retracts and the cervix dilates. Sometimes, however, the mechanism of separation and discharge of the ovum from the uterus is quite different, particularly in the early weeks of pregnancy.

(1) Expulsion of the whole ovum in one piece. In this method, which is only possible in the early weeks of pregnancy, the vera and basalis layers of the decidua separate from the uterus, so that the entire decidua and ovum are together expelled during the abortion. The method was familiar to Matthews Duncan. Specimens of abortion material of this kind show the relation of the decidua vera and the decidua reflexa to the ovum.

(2) Expulsion of the whole ovum by inversion of the decidua vera. The more common method of typical abortion consists in a primary detachment of the ovum by means of a retroplacental clot. The ovum is pushed into the cavity of the uterus and is extruded from the cervix: the inverted decidua vera, still attached to the ovum, being last to be born. In most cases the lower pole of the ovum first appears through the cervical canal, then follows the amniotic cavity and the placenta, and finally the inverted decidua vera. The method is similar to the Schultze's method of separation of the placenta. This mechanism of abortion is the one which usually occurs in the early months of pregnancy.

(3) Incomplete expulsion of the ovum, the placenta and membranes being retained. All varieties and combinations are possible but the one that is clinically important is where the foetus is expelled, either with or without the decidua capsularis, and where the decidua basalis and the placenta are retained. This type of abortion is often preceded by the initial premature rupture of the membranes and is the one to be expected with an incompetent cervix. This is the condition of incomplete abortion and always gives rise to subinvolution of the uterus and uterine haemorrhage. Sometimes the placenta is expelled but the decidua vera and amnion are retained. The symptoms are less severe than when the placenta is retained, but similar.

The above classification is not altogether satisfactory because it omits reference to the clinical condition, **missed abortion,** first described by Matthews Duncan in 1879. In missed abortion, the ovum is separated from its attachment to the uterus to a degree sufficient to kill the embryo, but the detached ovum, instead of being extruded from the uterus, is retained. Matthews Duncan pointed out that the ovum might be retained in the uterus until the end of the normal period of gestation of forty weeks, without increasing in size from that which it had attained when dislodged from the decidua.

In missed abortion the signs of pregnancy disappear. There is no further enlargement of the abdomen. The symptoms of early pregnancy disappear and foetal movements are not felt. The enlargement of the breasts regresses to the normal non-pregnant size. Often a brown discharge is lost from the uterus. Pregnancy tests, previously positive, become negative. Missed abortion will be considered in detail later when carneous mole is discussed. In due course the uterus contracts and expels the ovum and no satisfactory explanation has been suggested of the factors which determine the onset of uterine contractions.

PATHOLOGICAL ANATOMY OF ABORTION

Many types of degenerative processes can be recognised if abortion material is examined. If the foetus has been retained *in utero* for any length of time after death, it undergoes maceration. Between the third and sixth months the foetus may undergo mummification, while very occasionally, as the result of an extreme degree of maceration, the foetus may eventually be represented by a macerated skeleton. Lithopaedion formation, in which the foetus becomes calcified, is also described, although seen far less frequently than with ectopic gestation. In many cases of abortion the placenta is infiltrated with blood clot, the chorionic villi are matted together, and large white infarcts are commonly found. An endarteritis obliterans is invariably found in syphilis, but it is also seen apart from this disease.

Blighted Ovum. The term blighted ovum is used to describe those pregnancies in which the foetus itself does not develop. A pregnancy normally consists of foetus, umbilical cord, amniotic fluid, amnion and chorion and up to the twelfth or thirteenth week is dependent on progesterone from the corpus luteum for its continued survival. In a blighted ovum the foetus and umbilical cord do not develop but the amniotic fluid, amnion, chorion and chorionic villi are initially normal, so that an apparently normal pregnancy commences. The deficient conceptus does not enlarge normally after the eighth week and bleeding may occur any time thereafter, culminating finally in the abortion of the blighted ovum.

Placental Polypus. In some cases of abortion a small piece of placenta is retained in the uterus through adhesion to the uterine wall. Placental polypi vary between the size of a pea and that of a walnut, and project downwards towards the internal os. The polypi are plum coloured, soft and friable, and when the cut surface is examined, placenta-like tissue can be distinguished. The polypi contain degenerate chorionic villi, although in some cases the chorionic tissues appear to be healthy. Usually, however, the epithelial cells show pyknosis and karyorrhexis, and the majority of the villi are denuded of epithelium. Little is known of the aetiology of placental polypi, and there is great difficulty in explaining the attachment of the polypus to the uterine wall. It is reasonable to regard them as an immature example of the retained cotyledon of the adult placenta or even a succenturiate lobe. Their retention is perhaps due to some morbid adhesion as occasionally occurs in the full-term placenta. Placental polypi lead to severe uterine haemorrhage and discharge and rarely may cause pyrexia through infection.

Carneous Mole. In carneous mole the pregnancy is either a blighted ovum or one in which the foetus is destroyed by a subchorial haemorrhage, which is spread diffusely around the ovum, but which does not involve the amniotic cavity. In the early stages, when the blood is soft, the term blood mole is used. Later, when the blood clots fibrose, the term fleshy mole is employed, while the end result is sometimes a stony mole as the consequence of the deposition of calcium salts in the blood clot around the ovum.

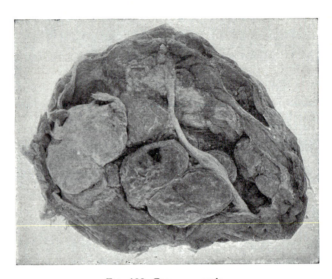

FIG. 188. Carneous mole.

Carneous mole was accurately described in 1892 by Breus. Breus emphasised three characteristics of the carneous mole:—

(1) The presence of circumscribed haematomata in the choriodecidual space, which give a lobulated or fibrous appearance to the inner surface of the amnion (see Fig. 188).

(2) A disproportion between the size of the embryo and the size of the amniotic cavity. In typical cases the embryo is far smaller than would be expected from the size of the mole, and in some cases the embryo disappears completely.

(3) A disproportion between the size of the embryo of the abortion and the pregnancy. In some cases the mole may be retained in the uterus as long as eleven months after the last menstrual period, yet when the specimen is examined the embryo is seldom more than 2 cm. in length.

Little is known of the aetiology of carneous mole. Breus's terminology of subchorial haematoma is no longer accepted, for it is now established that the clots are formed in the intervillous space. A carneous mole is **easily** recognised on microscopical examination by the presence of large deposits of calcium salts in the blood clot (see Fig. 189). It is quite clear that Matthews Duncan included cases of carneous mole in those he grouped together under the name "missed abortion." Carneous mole is a rare complication of pregnancy. There is one aspect of intra-uterine foetal death at any stage of pregnancy which should be remembered—namely, the occurrence of hypo- or afibrinogenaemia due to the release and absorption into the maternal circulation of placental degeneration end products and thromboplastin-like

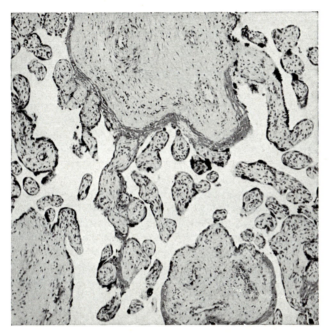

Fig. 189. A carneous mole. The mole consists of degenerate chorionic villi. These are sometimes called "ghost villi".

substances. Afibrinogenaemia is important clinically as the cause of un- controllable haemorrhage after emptying the uterus and only a timely trans- fusion of whole blood and plasma fibrinogen will restore the dangerous situation. Hypofibrinogenaemia is easily recognised by observing the behaviour of withdrawn blood in a test-tube when its clotting mechanism is seen to be deficient or absent. If the fibrinogen level is estimated it will be found to have fallen from a normal 400 mgm. per cent to 100 mgm. per cent or less.

Post-abortum Endometritis. Subinvolution of the Endometrium

One of the commonest complications of abortion is persistent uterine bleeding after the foetus and placenta have been discharged from the uterus.

The cases must be distinguished from those of septic abortion when there is well-marked pyrexia and purulent offensive bloodstained discharge. In many cases of persistent haemorrhage subsequent to abortion no obvious cause for the bleeding can be discovered. The uterus may be of normal size, anteflexed and freely movable, and the appendages may be normal. Sometimes the uterus is retroverted, but it does not follow that the retroversion of itself is responsible for the persistent bleeding.

Cases of this kind are very frequent and in the absence of localising signs it is customary to explain them by assuming a low grade inflammation of the endometrium. It is well known clinically that the haemorrhage usually clears up spontaneously after about six to eight weeks, and that the administration of ergometrine is a useful therapeutic measure. If the uterus is curetted, a placental polypus may be found, which is of itself sufficient to explain the symptoms, and the removal of which is followed by the cessation of bleeding. Placental polypi, however, are relatively rare, and the majority of cases of this clinical group have to be explained in some other way. Examination of the curettings often shows relics of chorionic villi and decidual cells with extensive infiltration of the stroma with leucocytes and plasma cells. The chorionic villi are mainly degenerate with loss of epithelial covering and fibrosis of the stroma. If a large amount of chorionic tissue has been retained it is not uncommon to find an extensive leucocytic infiltration together with an infection by saprophytic organisms. In such cases the symptoms are caused partly by the retained products of conception, and partly by a true infection of the endometrium. Heuck examined 47 cases of persistent bleeding following abortion, and found chorion and decidua in 15 cases, decidua alone in 22, and neither chorion nor decidua in 10. It seems, therefore, that two types of case can be distinguished, one when there are retained products of conception, the other when chorionic tissues cannot be demonstrated in the curettings. The aetiology of this second group is very obscure. There is usually no direct evidence of an infection of the mucous membrane of the uterus, although there may be a leucocytic and plasma cell infiltration, and the cases should be regarded as representing subinvolution of the endometrium. Possibly, there is endocrine disturbance affecting pituitary ovarian interrelation.

Severe haemorrhage after an abortion is almost always due either to retained products or to a placental polypus, and there should be no hesitation in curetting the uterus in such cases. Minor degrees of bleeding should be attributed to subinvolution of the endometrium, and in such cases curetting is not always a satisfactory method of treatment. Treatment should be conservative, and in due course the haemorrhage will clear up spontaneously.

In all cases of persistent uterine bleeding following abortion, the possibility of the development of chorion epithelioma should be borne in mind. The presence of small cysts in the ovaries and of a positive pregnancy test are very suggestive of this possibility. Chorion epithelioma will be described in detail in Chapter 16.

CLINICAL ASPECTS OF ABORTION

Classification of Abortion

Degree	Cause	Infection
(1) Threatened	(1) Spontaneous	(1) Septic
(2) Inevitable	(2) Habitual or	(2) Non-septic
(3) Incomplete	recurrent (already	
(4) Complete	discussed in a	
(5) Missed (carneous	previous chapter)	
mole)	(3) Criminal or	
	induced:—legal	
	illegal	

Every abortion has a degree, a cause and the possibility of infection. The above classification is meant to indicate that any degree of abortion may be spontaneous, habitual or induced and that each of these permutations may be septic or non-septic.

Threatened Abortion

In the majority of cases, the symptoms of threatened abortion develop during the early weeks of pregnancy. The main symptom is a moderate, painless vaginal haemorrhage accompanied by discomfort only. On examination, blood is seen to be discharged through the cervical canal, but the os is closed. The uterus has the normal characteristics of a pregnant uterus of that stage of gestation. In many cases of this kind the bleeding clears up under appropriate treatment, or no treatment at all, and the pregnancy continues to term. On the other hand, the syndrome of threatened abortion may represent the early stages of an abortion which will become inevitable, and there is no method of distinguishing between the two types of case except by expectant supervision. Severe bleeding, or painful uterine contractions, however, indicate that the abortion is becoming inevitable.

The diagnosis of threatened abortion may be difficult. First and foremost in the differential diagnosis comes ectopic gestation, for in both conditions a history will be obtained of early pregnancy followed by uterine bleeding. In ectopic gestation there is always a history of severe abdominal pain which often causes fainting and vomiting. Moreover, the vaginal bleeding in ectopic gestation is small in amount, and the discharged blood is dark and often coagulated. All patients with the symptoms of threatened abortion should therefore be subjected to a careful bimanual examination to exclude the presence of an adnexal swelling which has the sign of acute local tenderness. Apart from ectopic gestation, vaginal bleeding in early pregnancy may be produced by such local abnormalities of the cervix as mucous polypus, vascular erosion, and early carcinoma. The cervix should, therefore, be examined with a speculum in all cases of vaginal bleeding in early pregnancy. It has already been pointed out that some patients develop slight vaginal bleeding at times corresponding to the suppressed periods during the early months of pregnancy. It is impossible to distinguish such cases from those of threatened abortion.

Treatment of threatened abortion consists in absolute rest in bed, combined with the administration of such drugs as morphine, mgm. 15, initially, followed by phenobarbitone, mgm. 60 t.d.s. Drastic purges are contra-indicated as are enemata and hot baths. If the abortion becomes inevitable the bleeding persists, and in due course the uterus discharges the ovum. If, however, the abortion is only threatened the haemorrhage ceases. The patient should subsequently be examined carefully in case the ovum was killed at the time of the vaginal bleeding, to be retained in the uterus as a missed abortion. It has been customary with threatened abortion to insist upon the patient remaining in bed for seven days after all bleeding has ceased, that is, all bright active bleeding. This elective policy is rarely practical now and only acceptable where a woman is prepared to take no chance in order to ensure the continuation of her pregnancy. There is likely to be a sero-sanguinous brown-coloured discharge for some days after the bright loss has ceased and this is due to the slow expulsion and disintegration of blood clot retained in the uterus. It is not necessary to confine the patient to bed during this period of discharge.

It has been customary to treat cases of threatened abortion with pro-gesterone. The theoretical basis for treatment is the possibility that pro-gestin secretion is deficient. As a general rule, the treatment is empirical. Gynaecological opinion is divided on the advisability of using progesterone and it is probably best to reserve it for those cases in which a deficiency of progesterone can be demonstrated by an inadequate progesterone response in the vaginal smear (p. 133). If used at all probably as good a method as any is to give a weekly injection intramuscularly of 250 mgm. of hydroxy-progesterone caproate in oil. This is certainly convenient and time-saving for patient and doctor and better than more frequent smaller dosage. Some gynaecologists actively criticise the use of progesterone and allege that its employment is not only ineffective but increases the risk of inevitable abor-tion by stimulating uterine contraction. There is no doubt, however, that it has a most reassuring effect on the patient's psyche. She now feels that something active is being done and that her doctors are taking an intelligent interest in her problem and doing all they can to save the baby she may so desperately desire.

An equally debated method of treatment is the use of large doses of synthetic oestrogen on the assumption, quite hypothetical, that it stimulates placental development, and therewith progesterone production. As much as 100 mg. may be used daily during the time that abortion is most expected, and the dose is gradually tapered off in the later months of pregnancy.

When treating a patient with threatened abortion many gynaecologists forbid all vaginal examinations, but if any doubt remains whether the diag-nosis is an abortion or an extrauterine gestation a gentle vaginal examina-tion should always be made. When skilfully performed it cannot do harm but it must always be remembered that if the patient should subsequently abort she is very liable to blame the vaginal examination. At all events the patient must be examined vaginally before being discharged from hospital. No alarm need be occasioned by the presence of a brown discharge of old altered blood for some days after the original bleeding as already mentioned.

The prognosis in threatened abortion whatever the treatment is that one quarter of the conceptions will be lost, so that the outlook must always be guarded.

Inevitable Abortion

In inevitable abortion the vaginal bleeding is usually severe and the uterine contractions are painful. In typical cases the cervical canal is dilated so that a finger inserted into the cervical canal palpates the lower pole of the ovum. If convincing evidence can be obtained of the discharge of liquor amnii the abortion must be regarded as inevitable. In such cases bimanual examination detects that the globular feel of the uterus is less marked than in normal pregnancy, and the uterus feels flattened anteroposteriorly. If the umbilical cord prolapses, or if the foetus is discharged, the abortion obviously must be inevitable.

Two lines of treatment are available:

(1) *Conservative*. The patient is given 0·5 mg. intramuscular ergometrine and, thereafter, 0·5 mg. b.d., by mouth, until all bleeding is controlled after the completion of the abortion. Ergometrine should not be given for more than five days at a time for fear of peripheral vascular spasm. The patient must use only the ward commode or bedpan and everything passed must be carefully scrutinised and any products of conception sent to the laboratory for dissection. With good fortune, it is possible to pronounce the abortion as complete from this examination and, if all bleeding ceases and there is no fever or constitutional upset, the patient can go home in about five days. She is advised to report for examination at the out-patient department after her next period and to avoid conception for three months.

(2) *Surgical*. The conservative treatment of inevitable abortion is satisfactory provided that there is every indication that the abortion will be speedily completed without severe or dangerous blood loss. It is this factor of haemorrhage, so often insidious and progressive, which determines the correct treatment. It is foolish to persist in conservative treatment if the haemoglobin is falling to dangerous levels. If, therefore, in spite of ergometrine, a patient in the process of abortion continues to bleed, it is far better to give her an anaesthetic and explore the uterus by finger, ovum forceps or curette than to wait until she is in a state of haemorrhagic shock. In the severely shocked patient who has had a severe haemorrhage at home resuscitation and blood transfusion must be instituted and she must never be moved by ambulance until fit for the journey. Exactly what applies to post partum haemorrhage in domiciliary practice applies here with equal force. The risk of converting a clean abortion into a septic one by surgical interference has been greatly over-stressed and it can be reasonably stated that, in modern practice, the dangers of haemorrhage far exceed those of sepsis. Once a uterus is completely empty, it ceases to bleed and the only certain way of emptying a uterus is by surgical evacuation. It is certainly correct to state that

surgical evacuation of the pregnant uterus entails certain risks, such as perforation and the introduction of sepsis. The danger of perforation can be lessened by the skill and experience of the surgeon and, in expert hands, the large curette is probably less dangerous than the ovum forceps. The fingers of the surgeon who wields the curette acquire a certain indirect tactile sensitivity which the ovum forceps never transmit to the operator. As for the introduction of sepsis, this can be considerably controlled by aseptic technique and chemotherapy. One further argument favours the active evacuating of an inevitable abortion and that is that the retained necrotic placental tissue may become infected without any surgical interference, so that a post-abortional salpingitis results in infertility from tubal occlusion. The timely evacuation of the abortion by surgical means will obviate this additional danger.

Incomplete Abortion

It has already been pointed out that retention of the placenta is one of the common complications of abortion. In such cases the patient complains of vaginal haemorrhage, which takes the form of a continuous ooze of blood and which may lead to a severe degree of anaemia. The haemorrhage comes from the placental site, since the placenta has usually separated partially, so that the sinuses of the placental site bleed when the uterus relaxes. In many cases, the administration of ergometrine, by leading to contraction of the uterine muscle, causes expulsion of the placenta, and this method of treatment should first be tried unless the vaginal bleeding is very severe. If the vaginal haemorrhage is severe the uterus should be evacuated by operation and no time should be wasted in conservative treatment. A further haemorrhage, in addition to what has already been lost, may be not only dangerous but lethal, and the anaemia if severe should be corrected by prompt transfusion before, during and after the operation.

The signs of incomplete abortion are clinically most reliable and their elicitation on pelvic examination should be definitely diagnostic. On making a vaginal examination, the cervix is found to be dilated and obstinately patulous in spite of the fact that the abortion may have occurred some weeks before the examination. If, in conjunction with a patulous cervix, the uterus is found to be oedematous, softened and enlarged, it is strongly suggestive of retained products. Incidentally, such a subinvoluted uterus is frequently retroverted. In association with persistent, continuous bleeding, these two signs of cervical dilatation and subinvolution of the uterus seldom mislead the clinician.

Missed Abortion

The clinical history of missed abortion is very characteristic. At first, the patient suffers from the normal symptoms of early pregnancy, such as morning vomiting and amenorrhoea. Then, at about the twelfth week of gestation, there is a little vaginal haemorrhage, which soon clears up and which is succeeded by a period of further amenorrhoea. There is, however, no continued enlargement of the breasts, no enlargement of the abdomen, and the symptoms of pregnancy gradually subside. Usually, after several weeks and perhaps after several months, a brown discharge develops, and eventually the uterus contracts and expels the ovum, which usually takes the form of a carneous mole. The diagnosis of missed abortion may present difficulties. For example, a woman may miscarry early in pregnancy and then conceive immediately afterwards, so that when examined about eight weeks after the miscarriage the uterus is found to be slightly enlarged. If the history of the miscarriage is indefinite the case may be regarded as one of missed abortion, and if the uterus is then evacuated a normal pregnancy may be removed.

The treatment of missed abortion depends to some degree upon the inclination of the patient. In missed abortion the ovum will come away of its own accord in due course. Some women may be content to wait for the spontaneous evacuation of the uterus, but, as a general rule, patients insist upon the uterus being emptied as soon as possible. The technique of evacuation of the uterus will be described in detail below. In some patients with a carneous mole, a straightforward evacuation of the uterus can be performed by dilatation and curettage, provided that the danger of severe haemorrhage is not forgotten and the possibility of afibrinogenaemia is remembered. Provided that there is no urgency, an effective evacuation can quite often be achieved by the use of an oxytocic drip—Syntocinon, 2·5 units to the pint of normal saline, given intravenously. If not immediately effective the dose can be stepped up until massive, as much as 100 units per litre having been used. Equally massive doses of oestrogen were at one time advocated to prime the myometrium but this line of treatment is now outmoded.

Placental Polypi

Placental polypi tend to develop after miscarriage rather than delivery at term, and they cause extremely severe uterine bleeding. Clinically a history is obtained of a recent miscarriage, which is followed within a few weeks by a profuse and prolonged haemorrhage. The uterus is found to be slightly enlarged and perhaps the os is a little dilated. The uterus should be explored by currettage after preliminary dilatation of the cervix, when the polypus can be removed without difficulty. Histologically the polypus consists of degenerate, so-called ghost, chorionic villi surrounded by blood clot. The differential diagnosis is from chorion epithelioma, so that all material removed must be carefully examined microscopically to exclude this possibility.

Evacuation of the Uterus

The operation of evacuation of the uterus is simple to perform if the technique is correct, but it is not uncommon for serious mistakes to be made.

The patient should be anaesthetised and placed in the lithotomy position. The vulva, having been previously shaved, is cleaned with antiseptic solution. The sterile towels are applied and the bladder carefully emptied by catheter. The operation should be performed with the full ritual of asepsis. A bimanual examination is then made to determine the position of the uterus and the degree of dilatation of the cervix. When the cervix admits one finger, either the whole hand or half hand is introduced into the vagina and the index finger passed into the uterus. The external hand presses down the fundus of the uterus, and in this way the index finger of the right hand can reach it internally. It is impossible for the operator to reach the fundus of the uterus with his index finger if only two fingers are inserted into the vagina. It is essential that either the hand or half hand should be introduced into the vagina before the index finger is passed into the uterus. The index finger now sweeps round the wall of the uterus and separates the retained products from their attachment to the uterine wall. When the cervix will not admit a finger a suitable speculum is introduced to expose the cervix and as the cervix is very liable to tear two volsellum forceps are placed on the anterior lip and the cervix is drawn down. The cervix is then dilated to a size of Hegar proportionate to the duration of the pregnancy and a pair of ovum forceps is next introduced into the cavity of the uterus and removes the retained products. In order to ensure complete evacuation the uterus should finally be thoroughly and gently curetted with a large sharp curette which is safer, curiously enough, than the blunt instrument since its very danger demands the utmost gentleness and it is of course more effective in removing tenacious portions of placenta. The authors have now abandoned the use of the hot (105°F.) intra-uterine douche as a relic of the pre-chemotherapeutic era. A hot douche was supposed to control haemorrhage and wash out potential sources of sepsis. Its former recommendation can be better achieved by the complete evacuation of the uterus and, once a uterus is empty, it no longer bleeds. Sepsis, if present or likely, is better and more effectively controlled by chemotherapy. Oxytocic drugs such as ergometrine mgm. 0·5, or Syntocinon 5 units, may be given intramuscularly if there is any residual haemorrhage or if the uterus does not contract satisfactorily.

Although the operation can be performed easily and rapidly in the majority of cases, errors in technique may lead to serious complications.

Complications

Shock. If a cervix is rapidly dilated with dilators and if the patient is already anaemic, profound shock may follow the operation. It should be regarded as an error of judgment to evacuate immediately the uterus of a woman who is already suffering from severe haemorrhagic shock. In such cases the evacuation of the uterus should always be preceded by blood transfusion and the usual methods of resuscitation.

One cause of otherwise inexplicable shock after abortion is the possible infection with one of the Clostridia. A persistently low blood pressure, otherwise inexplicable and one which obstinately refuses to rise in spite of adequate transfusion or one not necessarily associated with severe haemorrhage, should always suggest the possibility of clostridial infection when occurring after an abortion, especially if there has been some criminal interference.

Haemorrhage. It is not uncommon for severe bleeding to develop from the uterus as soon as retained products have been removed. Haemorrhage of this kind is most frequent in septic cases. Treatment consists of intravenous injection of ergometrine, 0·5 mg., or Syntocinon 5 units by intramuscular or intravenous injection. In intractable cases the uterus should be plugged with sterile gauze wrung out in Hibitane but only after all precautions have been taken to ensure its complete evacuation. The gauze should be removed within twelve hours, otherwise it may lead to severe infection of the uterus. If severe bleeding occurs during the performance of the operation of evacuation the uterus can be bimanually compressed as an emergency measure while ergometrine or syntometrine are given intravenously and transfusion is organised if not immediately available.

After evacuation of the uterus, it is usual for the uterine bleeding to clear up spontaneously within a few days. Persistent haemorrhage is most likely to be due either to the presence of some placental tissue inadvertently left in the uterus or to a low-grade infection.

Sepsis. It is not uncommon for saprophytic organisms to invade the uterus when a piece of placenta has been retained, and a moderate degree of pyrexia is, therefore, not unusual. In most cases, evacuation of the uterus is followed by a fall in temperature without further complications. In patients who are frankly septic on admission, with hectic fever, toxaemia, high white count, a purulent uterine discharge and lower abdominal tenderness, a high vaginal swab should be taken, cultured aerobically and anaerobically and the organisms typed for antibiotic sensitivity. A wide spectrum antibiotic is then given and the patient's condition should improve in twenty-four hours. The general condition and temperature chart will indicate if the infection is responding and, if not, the antibiotic may be changed according to the sensitivities of the organism as soon as the result is available. It is quite safe to evacuate the uterus surgically in a day or two. While awaiting the operation ergometrine can be given if haemorrhage occurs. The objection to this expectant method of treatment is that the infected retained products may lead to the development of salpingitis and tubovarian abscess. Such a risk is, however, very small with modern chemotherapy. The only real indication for immediate operation in septic abortion is severe and uncontrollable bleeding. Evacuation in these cases should be accompanied by large doses of the most likely antibiotic. It rarely happens that, in spite of intelligently applied chemotherapy, the patient fails to respond and the infecting organism proves resistant. Signs of lower abdominal peritonitis develop, the lower abdomen is distended with a localised ileus; vomiting, rapid pulse, lowered blood pressure and signs of generalised toxaemia become apparent. These symptoms and signs suggest a pelvic peritonitis which may occasionally become generalised; a localised pelvic peritonitis with pelvic abscess formation; pelvic cellulitis—more commonly associated with a broad ligament haematoma and infection from injury at operation or perforation in a criminal abortion, or an infection spreading from a post-abortional salpingitis or tubo ovarian abscess.

If the uterus is irrigated with fluid under high pressure, which is a method dear to the heart of the criminal abortionist, there is always a possibility of the douche solution passing along the Fallopian tubes into the peritoneal cavity and leading to pelvic peritonitis. Similarly, in septic abortion, the infection may spread upwards and involve the Fallopian tubes during the second week.

Thrombophlebitis. Thrombophlebitis of the pelvic veins and of the femoral and saphenous veins is one complication of septic abortion. If the thrombophlebitis is restricted to the veins of the leg the patient develops white-leg. Thrombophlebitis of the pelvic veins causes persistent pyrexia which may last for many weeks. Suppurative thrombophlebitis may lead to pyaemia, with metastatic infection in the lungs and other viscera. This type of infection is usually due to the anaerobic infection of some products of gestation and the responsible organism is frequently an anaerobic streptococcus. Hence the importance of culturing vaginal swabs both aerobically and anaerobically.

Injuries. *Lacerations of the Cervix.* If the cervix is rapidly dilated with Hegar's dilators the soft cervix may split, and if the laceration spreads outwards, the uterine vessels may be torn and the patient develop a haematoma of the parametrium. The haematoma usually becomes infected and causes a parametric effusion or abscess. The volsellum forceps can also produce quite severe cervical lacerations.

Perforation of the Uterus. The uterus may be perforated, especially if it is retroverted and its position has not been recognised or verified by a pre-operative vaginal examination. The instrument may be pushed through the wall of the uterus into the peritoneal cavity. As a result a pelvic peritonitis may occur, and many fatalities of abortion are caused in this way. Sometimes the small intestine becomes adherent to the laceration in the wall of the uterus, and as the result of the contractions of the myometrium the small intestine may become drawn into the uterus, and in due course may appear at the vulva. The uterus may also be perforated by a metal dilator when the cervix is dilated in the operation of evacuation of retained products. Such a uterus is soft, and the dilator is not held up by the usual resistance when it encounters the wall of the uterus, so that the dilator may be pushed in further and so perforate the myometrium. When the uterus is perforated in a clean case and provided the perforation is small, it is not always necessary to open the abdomen. The patient should be placed on a half-hourly pulse chart and carefully observed for signs of internal haemorrhage, infection or the prolapse of any of the abdominal contents into the uterine cavity. If the surgeon suspects any intra-abdominal damage he should open the abdomen at once. It is usually easy to repair the uterine rupture and hysterectomy will only rarely be necessary. The large and small bowel must be explored for damage systematically from stomach to rectum.

Septic Abortion

It has already been pointed out that the most severe types of septic abortion follow criminal procedures, when solutions and instruments are introduced into the cavity of the uterus without proper aseptic precautions being taken. The infecting organisms are E. Coli, haemolytic and non-haemolytic streptococci, staphylococcus aureus, anaerobic streptococci, gonococcus, pneumococcus and Cl. Welchii. Clostridial and haemolytic streptococcal infections are the most dangerous. The worst forms of septic abortion are those in which the uterus is perforated and an acute peritonitis results. Other forms of sepsis, such as parametritis, thrombophlebitis and white-leg, salpingitis and tubovarian abscess are seen in septic abortion. Septicaemia occasionally follows the evacuation of an infected uterus, and the most dangerous infecting organism is the Cl. Welchii. These complications are essentially similar to those found in puerperal sepsis and their treatment should be carried out along similar lines.

Bacteriaemic Shock is a severe complication of septic abortion in which organisms gain access to the blood stream, where they liberate endotoxins and cause an anaphylactic reaction. The responsible organism is often E. Coli. The patient is suddenly collapsed with hypotension often with preceding rigors. The immediate treatment is massive doses of broad spectrum antibiotics, large doses of hydrocortisone and blood transfusion while awaiting the sensitivity cultures of high vaginal swabs and blood cultures. If there is any evidence that the uterus is not completely evacuated it will usually be safe to explore the cavity in 24 hours if the patient responds to antibiotic treatment. If the question of criminal interference arises the possibility of perforation and peritonitis must be considered and here laparotomy may become urgent.

Anuria following Abortion. This form of renal failure is a rare but serious complication of abortion and resembles the anuria seen in severe cases of concealed accidental haemorrhage or symmetrical cortical necrosis of the kidneys. The history is usually that of a severe haemorrhage accompanying abortion or one in which criminal interference has been associated with infection—possibly by Cl. Welchii. The patient has possibly been shocked on admission and required blood transfusions before evacuation or spontaneous expulsion. Decreasing amounts of urine are passed and finally the catheter produces ½ oz. of albuminous bloodstained fluid or none. The blood urea shows a progressive rise.

Treatment is by Bull's regime—1,000 ml. of water with 600 g. of sugar given by an indwelling duodenal tube. This provides the patient with 2,500 calories of protein-free diet and spares the kidney of all unnecessary work until such time as it may spontaneously recover—usually within ten days. A daily check must be kept on the fluid and electrolyte balance and these adjusted accordingly. Acidosis must be counteracted by sodium bicarbonate and no potassium must be given.

If an indwelling duodenal tube is not tolerated (some patients persist in pulling it out) or if the hypertonic glucose causes nausea and vomiting, an alternative is to pass a catheter via the saphenous vein into the inferior vena cava. By this route, it is feasible to administer sufficient calories in hypertonic glucose solutions intravenously without causing thrombosis. Such treatment can be continued safely for many days—7 to 10, or more if necessary. If the patient does not respond to Bull's regime as shown by a rise of more than 50 mgm. of blood urea per 100 ml. in a day she should be transferred not later than the fourth day to a special renal unit where facilities are available for dialysis.

CRIMINAL ABORTION

Every doctor should be conversant with the wording of section 58 of the Offences Against the Person Act, 1861:—

"Every woman being with child who, with intent to procure her own miscarriage, shall unlawfully administer to herself any poison or other noxious thing, or shall unlawfully use any instrument or other means whatsoever with the like intent, and whosoever with intent to procure the miscarriage of any woman, whether she be or be not with child, shall unlawfully administer to her or cause to be taken by her any poison or other noxious thing, or shall unlawfully use any instrument or other means whatsoever with the like intent, shall be guilty of felony . . . and . . . . shall be liable to be kept in penal servitude for life . . . ."

Section 59 of the same Act is also of interest:—

"Whosoever shall unlawfully supply or procure any poison or other noxious thing, or any instrument or thing whatsoever knowing that the same is intended to be unlawfully used or employed with intent to procure the miscarriage of any woman whether she be or be not with child, shall be guilty of a misdemeanour, and . . . shall be liable . . . to be kept in penal servitude . . . ."

These sections of the 1861 Act remain in force today. The Abortion Act of 1967 creates exceptions to the above by absolving from guilt a practitioner who terminates a pregnancy in certain circumstances. The Act of 1967 creates the sole exceptions to the Act of 1861. This statement is unequivocal. The Abortion Act of 1967 came into operation on 27 April 1968 and applies to England, Wales and Scotland but not to Northern Ireland.

Medical Termination of Pregnancy (Abortion Act of 1967)

The circumstances in which an abortion may be carried out are as follows:

(i)   Two registered medical practitioners must form in good faith the opinion set out in the next succeeding paragraph and certify it in accordance with the regulations made under Section 2 of the Act.

Section 1 (1)

(ii) The opinion must be to one or more of the following effects:

(a) that the continuance of the pregnancy would involve risk to the life of the pregnant woman greater than if the pregnancy were terminated; or

Section 1 (1) (a)

(b) that it would involve risk of injury to the physical or mental health of the pregnant woman greater than if the pregnancy were terminated; or

Section 1 (1) (a)

(c) that it would involve risk of injury to the physical or mental health of any existing children of the pregnant woman's family greater than if the pregnancy were terminated; or

Section 1 (1) (a)

(d) that there is a substantial risk that if the child were born it would suffer from such physical or mental abnormalities as to be seriously handicapped.

Section 1 (1) (b)

Any treatment for the termination of pregnancy must be carried out in a National Health Service hospital or in a place approved for the purpose by the Minister of Health or by the Secretary of State for Scotland. For the purpose of this provision "treatment" does not include any examinations carried out to decide if termination would be lawful.

The fact of the termination must be notified in a prescribed form to the Chief Medical Officer of the Ministry of Health or to the Chief Medical Officer of the Scottish Home and Health Department.

Section 2 (1) (b)

Emergencies provide an exception to the above circumstances. An abortion may be performed by a practitioner if he is of the opinion, formed in good faith, that immediate termination is necessary to save the life or prevent grave and permanent injury to the physical and/or mental health of the patient. In such an emergency no second opinion is required by law nor is there any restriction on the place in which the abortion may be performed. Certification and notification are obligatory by law.

Conscientious Objection

The Abortion Act of 1967 states that no person shall be under any legal duty to participate in any treatment authorised by the Act to which he has a conscientious objection unless the treatment is necessary to save the life or prevent grave permanent injury to the physical or mental health of the patient. This paragraph applies to the practitioner requested to do an abortion, his assistants, anaesthetist and nursing staff, any of whom has the right to conscientious objection. Conscientious objection does not exonerate a practitioner from his general duty to his patient. He should refer the patient to another doctor if he thinks that apart from his personal conscientious objection it might be lawful to recommend or perform an abortion or if he feels that owing to his conscientious objection he is unable to form an opinion in good faith. In England and Wales a practitioner who has a conscientious objection must be prepared to prove it in any legal proceedings and this he would be able to do by a statement on oath in the witness box. This is unlikely to be unacceptable to the court.

Consent. The written consent of the patient must always be obtained. We have deliberately used the imperative must rather than the conditional should. The same applies to the husband. A difficulty might here arise if the pregnant woman consented and the husband refused. In this rare circumstance if the practitioner was genuinely convinced of a risk to life or health for his patient he should obtain further opinions from his senior colleagues and proceed according to his judgment and conscience. The courts would be very unlikely to uphold the husband's claim for loss of parenthood.

13*

If the patient is single no consent need be obtained from the putative father.

If the patient is an unmarried girl between the ages of 16—21 it is unnecessary in law to obtain the parents' consent, though the patient's permission should be sought to do this. If she refuses to give this consent her wishes should be respected.

If the patient is under 16 her parents should always be consulted even if the patient forbids it. The parents should give their consent in writing but their refusal should not be allowed to prevent a lawful termination. Conversely, if the parents of a girl demand abortion and the patient refuses, termination should never be carried out against her wishes.

Abortion on demand, apart from the circumstances defined in the Act, is not available under the Abortion Act of 1967.

The preceding paragraphs have been included in this edition in the hope that they will be of assistance to the student and practitioner. The Act is in its infancy. Time and the experience of the law courts will no doubt clarify or moderate what has been written.

Incidence of Criminal Abortion

No accurate figure can be given for the number of criminal abortions performed in this country and only a guess can be made from an appraisal of those cases which actually come before the police; these, however, represent a very small proportion of the total number of abortions performed. The Abortion Committee of 1939 reckoned that between 110,000 and 150,000 abortions took place annually, of which 40% were considered to be criminal. In 1968 there were 42 notified deaths due to abortion in England and Wales and a total of 41,496 abortions notified under the Abortion Act.

The infant loss is appalling and it must be remembered that a number of victims of the criminal abortionist die annually; here, again, it is difficult to collect accurate figures. No doctor likes to state on a death certificate that a young unmarried woman has died as a result of a criminal abortion.

The amateur or professional abortionist relies on three methods: (1) drugs, (2) syringing, and (3) instrumentation.

(1) **Drugs.** A number of drugs are sold to the public thinly disguised as female correctives which are really abortifacients. The most effective and safest are violent purgatives. Next come a number of drugs such as pennyroyal, juniper, turpentine, apiol and oil of savin. Apiol is a dangerous drug because it contains tricresyl phosphate. The most dangerous and effective drug is lead, which has been known and used for a number of years.* Lead can be procured as an oleate in diachylon lead plaster, from which it is possible to make pills with a powerful ecbolic action. The fact that the patient will almost certainly suffer from lead poisoning does not interest the person who traffics in these drugs. An increasingly popular, but happily, less well-known method, is to insert potassium permanganate crystals into the vagina. Whether this technique is effective as an abortifacient is questionable but it

* Emperor Shen Nung of China (2787–2696 B.C.) recorded in an ancient medical work, "Shen-Nung pen ts' ao ching," that the giving of Shuh yin (mercury) would produce abortion.

certainly achieves a very severe and deep burn of the vagina which, in process of healing, leads to an obliterative vaginitis with dense and permanent adhesion in the vault. This certainly ensures that the patient never needs an abortifacient in the future since it precludes any further interest in or possibility of coitus unless a reconstructive plastic operation is performed.

(2) **Syringing.** The popular instrument here is the Higginson syringe, which is readily obtainable. All sorts of solutions are used but most of them contain a strong antiseptic, and many of them soap. A popular solution is a mixture of green soap and lysol which will cause superficial necrosis of the endometrium and lead to a very nasty septic endometritis. One of the authors has recovered this solution from the peritoneal cavity when it was associated with considerable shock and signs of chemical peritonitis. The aim of the abortionist is to insert the nozzle of the syringe into the external os and to dislodge the ovum by syringing the intrauterine cavity under pressure. The risks of this procedure are almost unthinkable and, apart from perforation and damage to the uterus, the great danger is air embolism from bubbles under pressure being pumped into the lacerated venous sinuses of the uterine plexus.

(3) **Instrumentation.** The safest instrument is a gum elastic catheter, but it is, of course, difficult to sterilise. The variety of instruments used is legion: needles, knitting needles, crochet hooks, bent wire, pins, pencils and, in fact, anything which comes to the hand of a desperate woman. The popularity of slippery elm bark, which is inserted into the cervix in the form of a primitive tent, is well known, and this bark can be bought over the counter in less reputable purlieus of any city. The idea of instrumentation is to perforate the gestation sac, and in order to achieve this the abortionist may well, and frequently does, perforate the uterus. All instrumentation and syringing of the uterus is fraught with a very real danger of intrauterine and peritoneal sepsis. These abortions are performed by dirty women who either do not care or do not know about sepsis. The operative environment is equally septic and it is surprising that the death rate is as low as 0·4%.

Particular Dangers of Criminal Abortion

Vasovagal Shock. The instrumentation of the cervix in a nervous woman by an unskilled operator is particularly liable to produce vasovagal shock. The most important contributory cause is the lack of anaesthesia. The injection of hot or cold or of powerful corrosive fluid into the cavity of the uterus is another cause. Death occurs almost immediately and the abortionist dreads this catastrophe more than any other because he or she is landed with a corpse on the premises.

Air Embolism. This has already been mentioned as a particular danger of intrauterine syringing. Death occurs within ten minutes and the post-mortem should demonstrate air in the cerebral vessels, and sometimes a track of bubbles can be traced from the pelvic veins up the inferior vena cava into the heart and the coronary arteries. A similar risk arises in air insufflation of the Fallopian tubes in the investigation of infertility when atmospheric nitrogen and not carbon dioxide is used.

Injuries. **Perforation and Laceration by the various Instruments used.** The
vagina may be perforated, especially in the posterior fornix, although
damage can occur in any position and may involve the bladder and rectum.
The cervix may be torn with resultant damage to the uterine vessels, which
gives rise to a broad-ligament haematoma. Infection of such a haematoma is
extremely likely. The uterus may be perforated anywhere, but the commonest

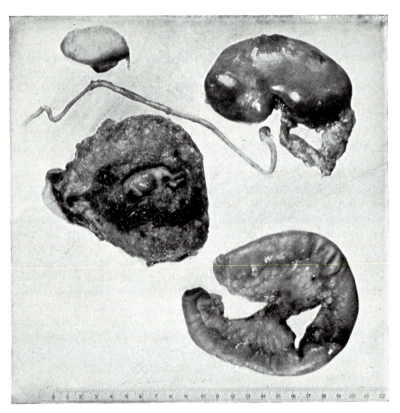

Fig. 190. Illustration showing damage caused by instrumental perforation
of the uterus during abortion. The right ovary and ureter were avulsed (top
left hand corner), necessitating a nephrectomy (top right hand corner). The
uterus was perforated from the internal os to the fundus (left centre.) A loop
of small bowel was torn from its mesentery, necessitating resection (bottom
right hand corner). The patient survived the ablation of the specimens
illustrated.

situation is into the pouch of Douglas. The retroverted gravid uterus provides
a particular danger in that the instrument goes straight through the anterior
wall into the uterovesical pouch. The great danger of perforation is, however,
that the bowel may be damaged by the perforating instrument or drawn down
and extruded through the hole in the uterus. Sometimes a whole coil of
bowel is found protruding from the vagina. If such a piece of bowel is not

detected at the time of the instrumentation, it will subsequently become gangrenous from interference with its blood supply and the patient is likely to succumb from pelvic peritonitis in which shock plays a large part. The more skilled professional abortionist who uses an ovum forceps is very liable, if the uterus is perforated, to catch a piece of bowel. Not only has the bowel been damaged but the right ureter has been avulsed (see Fig. 190).

Sepsis. Every criminal abortion should be considered to be potentially septic; the operator and the environment are dirty and the damage caused by the instrument provides an ideal culture medium for those organisms which must be introduced. Apart from septic endometritis, there is the risk of ascending salpingitis with pelvic peritonitis. A very lethal type of sepsis is that associated with Cl. Welchii.

Causes of Death in 100 Autopsies

In 100 cases dying of criminal abortion Keith Simpson reported the following causes of death:—

Sepsis	64
Air embolism	21
Vasovagal shock	11
Haemorrhage	2
Renal failure	2

It is interesting that haemorrhage is not a spectacular cause of death from criminal abortion, but it plays a secondary part in the deaths from sepsis.

It is a pious hope that the new Act of 1967 will considerably reduce the incidence of criminal abortion and thereby lessen its morbidity and mortality. But let it be clearly stated that legislation does not promise to put the criminal abortionist out of business.

16 Pathology of Pregnancy

Hydatidiform Mole and Chorion Epithelioma

In hydatidiform or vesicular mole, the chorionic villi are distended with fluid and form translucent vesicles varying in size from 2 to 25 mm. or bigger. In most cases the vesicular degeneration is spread uniformly throughout

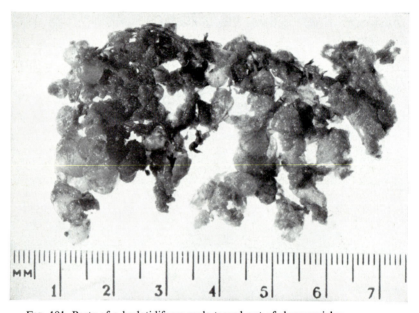

FIG. 191. Parts of a hydatidiform mole teased out of show vesicles.

the chorion, the amniotic cavity is obliterated or extremely difficult to identify, and the embryo and its umbilical cord disappear. The vesicles are usually covered with blood clot and fragments of decidua. The condition was recognised by Hippocrates and ably described by Smellie.

Morbid Anatomy

Simple benign hydatidiform mole. The vesicles vary in size. Usually about 6 mm. in diameter, they sometimes attain the size of a pigeon's egg, and are oval in shape. They develop only in the terminal branches of the chorionic villi, the main stalk always being unaffected. Vesicular degeneration is on

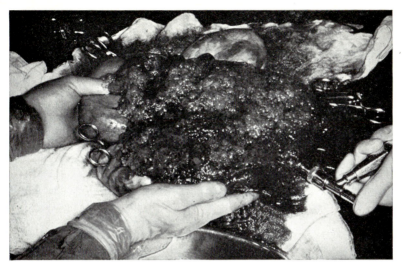

FIG. 192. Same patient as in Fig. 191, at operation. Mole being evacuated at anterior hysterotomy. Note the immense bulk of the mole and intervillous haemorrhage.

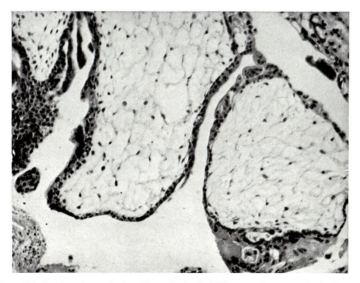

FIG. 193. Section through the villus of a hydatidiform mole. Note the hydropic connective tissue and the complete absence of all the vessels of the normal villus. The epithelium covering the villus shows proliferation of the cyto-trophoblast and Langhan's cells; though the histological appearance is sinister, the condition is benign.

rare occasions restricted to part of the placenta, the rest being normal in structure and function, so that the pregnancy may proceed to term. Whether these areas are a true example of hydatidiform mole or merely a cystic degeneration is debatable. In twin pregnancy the degeneration may be restricted to one ovum, the placenta and foetus of the second ovum developing normally. Vesicular degeneration may also arise in ectopic gestation (Figs. 191 and 192).

The histological appearances are difficult to interpret. Formerly it was believed that the vesicles were produced by a myxomatous degeneration of the chorionic villi, but as no mucin reaction is given by the contained fluid, it is now believed that the vesicular fluid is formed partly by degeneration of the stroma, and partly by secretion from the covering cells of the villi. It was shown by Marchand that the essential histological feature of hydatidiform mole was a proliferation of the epithelium covering the villi. This proliferation is irregularly distributed over the villi so that in some places the wall is thin and translucent, while in other areas a thick layer of epithelium can be detected with the naked eye. The proliferation of the epithelium leads to an appearance incapable of interpretation without some previous knowledge of the development of the trophoblast in the early human ovum. In the first few days of development of the human ovum the trophoblast becomes subdivided into cytotrophoblast and syncytiotrophoblast, the former eventually giving rise to Langhan's cells, the latter to the syncytium. In the earliest stage of development of the human ovum the cytotrophoblast proliferates far more than the syncytiotrophoblast. At this stage it is composed of large irregular nucleated cells which are matted together and show a tendency to be grouped into bunches. Many of the cells contain vacuoles, and large clear spaces are frequently seen between individual cells. In hydatidiform mole, masses of cells, similar in every way to the cytotrophoblast and plasmoditrophoblast of the early human ovum, are distributed irregularly over the vesicles, so that proliferation of both is a feature of hydatidiform mole.

The stroma of the villi is degenerate, and the cells which remain stain feebly and indistinctly. Another curious feature is that the blood vessels have disappeared from the affected villi. It is difficult to explain how vesicular fluid is produced, and a satisfactory solution has not yet been offered (see Fig. 193). The simple benign mole never invades the myometrium.

Invasive mole. Chorio-adenoma destruens. Some hydatidiform moles erode the wall of the uterus, burrow into the myometrium, and may even burst through the uterus into either the peritoneal cavity or the broad ligament, when dangerous internal haemorrhage may ensue.

To this type of mole the term invasive mole or chorio-adenoma destruens has been given. It should be emphasised that, though behaving as locally malignant, the invasive mole does not kill by distant metastasis and, therefore, cannot be considered to be a cancer. It is a characteristic of all trophoblast to invade maternal tissues and even a histologically normal placenta can go too far, e.g. placenta accreta or increta in which the normal villi penetrate into the myometrium beyond the basal layer of the decidua. It is moreover quite common to find fragments of trophoblastic tissue in the post-mortem lung where the patient has died from causes quite unconnected with hydatidiform mole or chorion epithelioma. It is not surprising that the proliferated trophoblast seen in a hydatidiform mole has enhanced powers of invasion. The relative proportion of invasive moles to the benign non-invasive variety is in the region of 1:12. An invasive mole is very likely to be mistaken for a chorion epithelioma but there is one distinguishing criterion. An invasive mole will show evidence of chorionic villi whereas in a chorion epithelioma all evidence of villous formation is lost.

The true malignant chorion epithelioma will be discussed later. Here all traces of villi are absent and this is diagnostic.

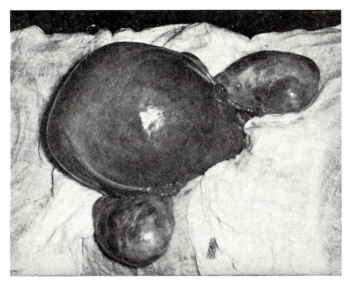

Fig. 194. Same patient as illustrated in Figs. 191 and 192, photographed at laparotomy before the uterus was opened. Note the bilateral enlargement of the ovaries by compound granulosa lutein cysts.

Ovarian changes. It is common for cysts to be present in the ovaries in cases of both hydatidiform mole and chorion epithelioma. These are bilateral and as many as fifteen or twenty, of about 25 mm. in diameter, may be found in the same ovary. Cysts up to a diameter of 10 cm. have been described but larger are exceptional. The surface of the ovary is smooth and free of adhesions but a bossy appearance is produced by the cystic projections into the peritoneal cavity (Figs. 194 and 195). The cysts are thin-walled, with smooth inner surfaces, and contain a clear fluid tinged with yellow. Frequently fibrinous material is found in the cavity after the fluid has been drained away. Yellow material can often be seen in the wall. The cysts seem to be of a similar type both with hydatidiform mole and chorion epithelioma. It has been shown recently that the cysts are granulosa lutein in type, that is to say, they show luteinisation of both the granulosa and theca interna layers of the follicle.

Luteinisation of the granulosa layer is better marked than that of the theca interna, and the lutein cells attain the size of those found in the corpus luteum of pregnancy. The lutein cells are, however, slightly different from the lutein cells of the corpus luteum of pregnancy, for they are never conjoined nor do they contain colloid droplets. Granulosa lutein cysts of this kind are found in 59% of cases of hydatidiform mole and in 9·4% of cases of chorion epithelioma. In hydatidiform mole they rapidly retrogress after the expulsion of the mole. Slow retrogression or persistence of the cysts cannot be regarded as indicative of the development of chorion epithelioma. Much more important in detecting early stages of chorion epithelioma is the persistence of a positive pregnancy test in the urine. One feature of benign mole

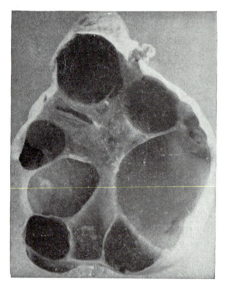

Fig. 195. The ovary from a case of hydatidiform mole. The ovary is studded with small granulosa lutein cysts.

and benign invasive mole which deserves mention is the reported presence of "benign" metastases in the lung. These have now been reliably reported by almost every authority on this subject. These so-called metastases may cause haemoptysis and cast a shadow on the X-ray. They naturally suggest chorion epithelioma but, provided the histological picture of the primary lesion shows the presence of chorionic villi, which are never seen in chorion epithelioma, the prognosis is good and in time the lung lesion will regress radiologically and the symptoms disappear. The incidence of pulmonary lesions in benign mole is 5 to 10%. Their spontaneous regression explains many remarkable cures of misdiagnosed chorion epithelioma.

Aetiology. There is some significant relationship between the incidence of hydatidiform mole and the parity of the patient, since it is commoner in multiparae.

The majority arise between the ages of 30 and 40, although the condition is not uncommon between 20 and 30 and seen occasionally in patients of menopausal and even post-menopausal age. The incidence of hydatidiform mole depends upon the criteria of the observer. The complete hydropic degeneration of the whole placenta is rare, perhaps 1:2000 pregnancies, whereas some degree of partial hydatidiform degeneration is much commoner and can be seen on histological examination of abortion specimens. If the products of gestation in all cases of spontaneous abortion were carefully examined histologically, Hertig and Edmonds claim that 40% would show some degree of vesicular degeneration. In other words hydatidiform degeneration is a far commoner cause of spontaneous abortion than is generally recognised. The finding of areas of vesicular degeneration in a placenta does not alone justify a diagnosis of hydatidiform mole unless associated with a pregnancy test positive in high dilution. Such vesicular changes without a strongly positive quantitative pregnancy test should be regarded as simply degenerative and of no significance.

Its geographical distribution is most interesting. It is more frequent in the Philippines, Hong Kong and Australia (1:820 normal pregnancies).

Little is known of the aetiology of hydatidiform mole. The association of lutein cysts of the ovaries and vesicular degeneration of the chorion has led to almost every theoretical possibility being explored. The primary fault almost certainly lies with the ovum itself for the vesicular degeneration may be limited to the chorion of one ovum of a twin pregnancy. The hydatids may be restricted to a localised area of chorion. In 1913, Aschner showed that the injection of placental extracts into female animals led to the formation of cysts in the ovaries which were similar to those found with hydatidiform mole. The ovarian changes are indeed almost identical with those found with a positive pregnancy test. The modern view of the formation of the ovarian cysts is that they are caused by placental gonadotropin being present in excess in the maternal circulation. This view is corroborated by assay of the gonadotropin content of the urine in hydatidiform mole pregnancy. The pregnancy test is strongly positive and it is usual for more than 200,000 units per litre to be found in the urine of women suffering from hydatidiform mole. This concentration falls, however, if the mole degenerates and is retained *in utero*.

Symptoms and Diagnosis. Hydatidiform mole usually leads to abortion between the fourth and sixth months of pregnancy, although very rarely the mole may be retained *in utero*, like a carneous mole, until term. In approximately half the cases, the abortion is spontaneous and medical treatment is not required. The diagnosis of hydatidiform mole may offer a difficult clinical problem, for it is generally agreed that such a pregnancy should be terminated at once and an inaccurate diagnosis may lead to interference with a normal pregnancy.

The most important symptom is vaginal bleeding, which takes the form of irregular small haemorrhages, often combined with a watery dirty coloured discharge, and, on rare occasions, with the passage of the characteristic vesicles. The haemorrhage usually starts during the second month of pregnancy, and recurs irregularly until the time of abortion when severe bleeding may develop.

Symptoms of pre-eclamptic toxaemia are frequent with hydatidiform mole and occur in half the cases. The patient feels ill throughout the pregnancy and suffers from headaches and malaise. Excessive vomiting is not uncommon, the blood pressure may be raised, and the feet may become oedematous. There is often some degree of albuminuria and casts may be found in the urine. The uterus is usually larger than would be expected from the calculated stage of gestation and has a peculiar doughy consistence. A foetus cannot be outlined, the foetal heart cannot be heard, nor can a foetus be detected on X-ray examination. Too much reliance should not be placed on a negative X-ray. A poor film, an inexperienced radiographer, movement, and gas in the colon can all explain a negative X-ray. A uterus containing a twin pregnancy is clinically large enough to be expected to give a picture of foetal bones, though in actual fact the twin foetuses may be too small to show in the photograph. Similarly, there is no history of quickening. In some cases the cystic ovaries can be palpated in Douglas's pouch, and it is well known that one or other ovary may undergo torsion during the pregnancy. A recent refinement in the diagnosis is the use of ultra-sound or sonar which though accurate is not likely to be readily available for some years to come.

The diagnosis is usually extremely difficult until vesicles have been discharged through the cervix. Threatened abortion, hydramnios, mistaken dates, twins, must all be considered in the differential diagnosis. The most important points in the establishment of a diagnosis are a strongly positive pregnancy test of the urine, the absence of foetal parts in an X-ray examination, a typical tracing by ultrasonic sounding (Sonar) and the presence of palpable ovarian cysts in the pouch of Douglas. A word of warning, however, should be given about the interpretation of the pregnancy test. There is normally a peak output of urinary Gonadotropin at the second month of pregnancy, which may give a positive reaction in dilutions up to 1:50 or even 1:100. In multiple pregnancy the urinary Gonadotropin titre is also raised. These two conditions, however, never give a positive test in dilutions of 1:200 which can be considered diagnostic of hydatidiform mole or chorion epithelioma.

Treatment. In half the cases the abortion is spontaneous, but there is always a tendency for the abortion to be accompanied by severe uterine bleeding. This suggests the retention of portions of the mole and it is wise to perform a dilatation and curettage on all spontaneously expelled moles after a week, whether the patient is bleeding or not.

A different problem is presented by the woman whose persistent bleeding and physical signs have led to a firm diagnosis of hydatidiform mole and in whom the uterus makes no attempt to expel its contents. The evacuation of the uterus can here be assisted by an oxytocin drip, as already described for carneous mole, gradually increasing the dosage until 50—100 units per litre are used. When abortion occurs this is followed by dilatation of the cervix and evacuation of any remaining contents. It is not uncommon, however, for severe haemorrhage to accompany the abortion if these methods have been adopted. There is therefore a tendency at the present day to prefer to evacuate the uterus by abdominal hysterotomy, if the case is clean. The abdominal operation allows the uterus to be emptied completely and there is little danger of severe uterine bleeding. Ergometrine can be given intravenously during the operation, when necessary. Further, the perforating type of hydatidiform mole can be recognised if the abdomen is opened, when hysterectomy should be performed. Chorion epithelioma is more likely to develop after hydatidiform mole in patients over the age of 40, so that with multiparae, approaching menopausal age, there is much to be said for removing the uterus as a general rule. The ovaries even if cystic should be conserved, as the cysts will regress spontaneously.

The four great complications of hydatidiform mole are haemorrhage, sepsis, perforation and the development of chorion epithelioma. Very severe uterine bleeding may accompany the abortion of a hydatidiform mole and repeated blood transfusions may be necessary. The haemorrhage should be controlled so far as possible by the administration of ergometrine. It is in this patient that digital exploration is dangerous in that it causes further and often alarming haemorrhage and there is, during the evacuation of the uterus by finger, ovum forceps or curette, a risk of perforation. This risk is naturally much increased if the mole is of the invasive (chorio-adenoma destruens) variety. As a rule, the moles which bleed most are seen when the uterus is over twelve weeks in size. In ordinary abortions after twelve weeks, haemorrhage and retention of the placenta is often a feature. It is suggested, therefore, that heavy bleeding with a retained or incompletely evacuated mole after the third month is best treated by transfusion and anterior abdominal hysterotomy.

Persistent uterine haemorrhage following the abortion of the hydatidiform mole is a common complication. The haemorrhage may be profuse and may last for several weeks after the abortion. In some cases the haemorrhage is caused by the retention of small fragments of the mole, in others by a septic puerperal endometritis, and rarely by the development of a chorion epithelioma. The correct treatment is to perform a dilatation and curettage and completely to empty the uterus. Once empty, the uterus should involute and all loss should cease. A pregnancy test should be taken at one- or two-monthly intervals and it may be six months or longer before it becomes negative when undiluted. This persistently positive pregnancy test causes anxiety to the attendant but, provided that the uterus is involuted, that all abnormal uterine bleeding has ceased and that the pregnancy test is not or does not become positive when diluted, a staunchly conservative attitude should be maintained in a young woman anxious to have children.

Sepsis is a common complication of hydatidiform mole, particularly if digital evacuation of the uterus has been carried out. It is not infrequent for patients to run temperatures of 103° and 104° F. immediately after the abortion, and for the lochia to be purulent and offensive. As a result of sepsis and the frequently associated anaemia, patients are often dangerously ill after the operation. Treatment consists in blood transfusion, the administration of ergometrine and antibiotics. Under modern treatment the mortality rate of hydatidiform mole should not exceed 1%.

All patients who have had a hydatidiform mole should be kept under careful observation for two years. Two per cent of Brews' 100 patients with hydatidiform mole subsequently developed chorion epithelioma. The earlier the diagnosis of chorion epithelioma is established the better are the results of treatment. As already stated, the most reliable method of detecting the development of chorion epithelioma is by the pregnancy test of the urine. The pregnancy test should be performed at monthly intervals for the first six months after the expulsion or removal of the mole. The result of the tests will be one of the following:

(a)   It becomes almost immediately negative and remains so over the period of observation, when taken at intervals up to two years.

(b)   It remains positive undiluted but negative diluted 1:10. This positive undiluted reading, as already stated, is not the signal for panic but the indication for close observation at monthly intervals provided that all other signs are favourable, e.g. no bleeding, normal pelvic examination and the return of normal menstruation.

(c)   A negative test becomes positive again.

(d)   A test positive in undiluted urine but negative in diluted becomes positive in diluted urine, possibly 1:100 ot 1:200. Both these two findings are so sinister that only one interpretation can be placed upon them—a diagnosis of chorion-epithelioma, provided that in (c) where a negative test becomes positive, a new normal pregnancy has not occurred. This is a well known trap for the unwary and can be evaded by repeating the test in dilution. Here a normal pregnancy will be negative in diluted urine whereas a chorion-epithelioma should be positive at the second test in diluted urine.

Persistent uterine bleeding after the evacuation of a mole always calls for a diagnostic curettage and the present authors strongly recommend that all moles should have a curettage one week after their spontaneous expulsion. The histological examination of the curettings may be suggestive of chorion epithelioma. Curettage does not, however, diagnose chorion epithelioma that is situated in the myometrium but, taken in conjunction with the pregnancy test, provides useful and suggestive evidence.

Another useful safeguard is to take a radiograph of the lungs. Not all shadows are diagnostic of chorion epithelioma but once diagnosed all shadows call for repeat serial chest X-rays. In any case of a suspicious chest shadow it is also a wise precaution to administer methotrexate (see under chorion epithelioma).

CHORION EPITHELIOMA

Chorion epithelioma, one of the most malignant growths arising in the body, is of some historical interest, for its pathology was indeterminate until recently. In woman the growth follows upon pregnancy, and the recognised figures of the incidence show that 50% of cases follow hydatidiform mole, 25% follow abortion, 20% follow normal labour, while 5% follow extraute-rine pregnancy. In a recently reported and fully authenticated instance, a chorion epithelioma occurred in a woman of 59 years of age, three and a half years after a radiation menopause, whose last pregnancy was nineteen years previously. Whatever the explanation, this patient does illustrate the long

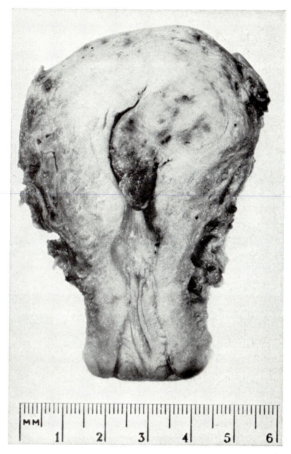

FIG. 196. Chorion epithelioma of the uterus. The tumour has infiltrated the myometrium and presents as a polypoid excrescence into the cavity of the uterus. It is therefore readily diagnosed on exploratory curettage.

period that may elapse between pregnancy and the development of the chorion epithelioma. It is of interest to note that a number of cases have been des-cribed in which multiple metastases, histologically conforming to chorion epithelioma, have been found but no primary growth has been identified in the uterus. Somewhat similar growths arise in men from primary growths of the testicle, which are probably teratoid in type, and in such cases the preg-

nancy test of the urine is positive. Chorion epithelioma should be regarded
as a rare tumour, and although the majority are recorded the total number
known is not large. The incidence in the U.K. is probably of the order of 1
in 100,000 pregnancies and at least ten times commoner in South East
Asia.

Morbid Anatomy

To the naked eye the growth appears as a solid purple friable mass. The
majority of primary growths arise in the body of the uterus and develop
first within the endometrium. In such cases the growth projects into the

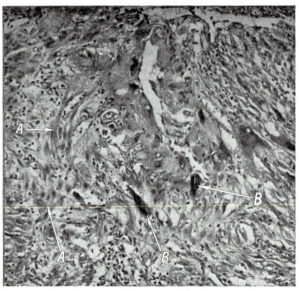

Fig. 197. Invasion of the myometrium by trophoblast in chorion epithelioma.
The section lay deep in the myometrium. Note the cytotrophoblast (A) and
dark syncytial cells (B). ($\times$ 145.)

cavity of the uterus, quickly ulcerates and causes a blood-stained discharge,
which later becomes offensive and purulent, as the growth becomes infected
and necrotic. There may be periodic severe floodings of bright red blood.
Growths of this kind superficially resemble placental polypi, but chorion
epithelioma always infiltrates the wall of the uterus, while a placental polypus
is clearly demarcated from the myometrium and can be easily detached from
it. Chorion epithelioma does not necessarily develop primarily in the endometrium, and it is not uncommon for the growth to start in the myometrium in the deeper tissues of the uterine wall. Such growths do not cause
uterine bleeding in the early stages of their development, nor can they be
detected by examination of endometrium removed by curetting. Primary
chorion epithelioma of the uterus may erode through into the peritoneal
cavity or into the broad ligaments and cause profuse bleeding, or it may

cause enlargement of the uterus to such a degree that the fundus of the uterus reaches upwards to the level of the umbilicus. Metastases form early and dissemination usually occurs by way of the blood stream. Metastases which can be detected easily are those found in the lower third of the vagina and at the vulva. Such metastases form purple haemorrhagic projections either into the vagina or around the vaginal orifice. Their appearance is characteristic and pathognomonic of chorion epithelioma. These metastases are interesting pathologically, for they are comparable to the vaginal metastases sometimes

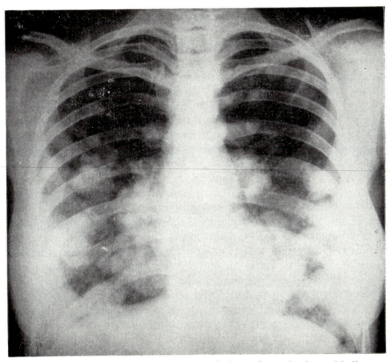

FIG. 198. Multiple cannon-ball metastases in lungs from chorion epithelioma. (With acknowledgement to Mr. R. Watson.)

found with carcinoma of the body of the uterus and malignant ovarian tumours. Such metastases are produced by retrograde spread along the venous channels of the vaginal plexuses of veins. The general metastases probably develop early, the growth disseminating by way of the blood stream. Multiple metastases may form in the lungs and cause haemoptysis (see Fig. 198). Deposits are frequently found in the kidneys, brain, spleen, and liver, but when the dissemination is widespread almost any organ may be affected and large emboli may get held up in the large arteries of the systemic circulation. In advanced cases, the parametrium may be extensively infiltrated with growth. Invasion of the ovaries is usually by way of the blood stream. Ovarian cysts of the granulosa lutein type are found in 9·4 % of cases.

The histological appearances are very typical. Syncytium, cytotrophoblast and degenerate red blood corpuscles constitute the growth. The cells are actively growing, and show such malignant characters as a typical mitotic division. In some areas the cells are translucent or vacuolated and may resemble decidual cells. No relics of chorionic villi can be detected, the growth consisting solely of embryonic syncytium, cytotrophoblast, and degenerate blood corpuscles. This absence of villi must be stressed as a differentially diagnostic feature which separates the malignant chorion epithelioma from the benign but invasive mole in which villi are demonstrable. The primitive infiltrating properties of the embryonic cytotrophoblast are retained in chorion epithelioma, so that vessels are eroded and local haemorrhages are produced, which cause the typical macroscopical appearances. As a result of erosion of vessels the growth penetrates into the systemic blood stream, so that generalised metastases are apt to develop early (see Fig. 198).

It should be remembered that the infiltrative faculty of chorionic tissue may be present in a penetrating but otherwise benign hydatidiform mole, and it may be extremely difficult or even impossible to decide on histological evidence alone whether the chorionic tissue of a penetrating hydatidiform mole has passed from the phase of local invasion only to the phase of true malignancy, capable of distant metastases, which is the characteristic of chorion epithelioma. Recognisable chorionic villi, when seen in the section, provide some reassurance to the histologist that the condition is probably benign. It has been cynically remarked that, if the patient lives, she had an invasive mole and, if she dies, a chorion epithelioma.

There is clinical evidence that metastases may retrogress after the removal of the primary growth. The clinical evidence is convincing, although no satisfactory scientific explanation can be offered. It is well known, however, that with benign hydatidiform mole, syncytium may be demonstrated in the capillaries of the pulmonary circulation. It is possible that the body tissues are capable of disintegrating these trophoblastic fragments by the formation of lysins, provided that the fragments are not produced continuously and in excess from a primary growth. In some instances, however, the blood deported trophoblast retains its erosive activity and, having gained lodgement in its new situation, e.g. the vascular bed of the lung, its erosive power opens up further blood vessels and a haemorrhagic reaction results. The X-ray picture presents these haemorrhagic shadows as metastases while, in actual reality, they are only zones of haemorrhage such as occur in the Fallopian tube from trophoblastic erosion. As such innocent tumours, they naturally disappear in due course irrespective of what treatment has been given to the patient. It must be remembered that vaginal nodules resembling the metastases of chorion epithelioma can occur with benign hydatidiform moles and even normal pregnancy according to Magnus Haines. This concept of benign trophoblastic embolism must considerably influence our thinking on the question of spontaneous regression of so-called malignant metastases in chorion epithelioma. In chorion epithelioma, as with hydatidiform mole, a strongly positive pregnancy test is given by the urine.

Symptoms and Signs. Persistent or irregular uterine haemorrhage following an abortion, particularly if a hydatidiform mole has been passed, should always cause chorion epithelioma to be suspected. In all suspected cases a pregnancy test of the urine should be made. Further, the characteristic metastases in the lower part of the vagina may also help in establishing the diagnosis. In obscure cases biopsy of the vaginal tumour is of great importance. The brain is sometimes the site of a metastatic deposit and in these cases the patient may present the signs of a rapidly enlarging cerebral tumour. The examination of scrapings from the cavity of the uterus, though perhaps the most convincing method of establishing the diagnosis, is open to the objection that curetting may cause further dissemination of the growth by opening up fresh venous channels. Moreover, curetting of the uterus will not dislodge fragments from a primary deep-seated growth in the myometrium. It should also be remembered that chorion epithelioma is more malignant in patients over the age of 40 than in younger women. In consequence there would be less hesitation in removing the uterus after the expulsion of a hydatidiform mole without preliminary curettage in a patient of this age.

Treatment. In early cases, most gynaecologists favour total hysterectomy. Even if repeated curettage is negative while the pregnancy test remains positive or becomes positive in high dilution, this is the treatment of choice. If the patient is young, the ovaries may be left, for ovarian metastases are rare with chorion epithelioma. The availability of chemotherapy has profoundly altered the prognosis of all cases of chorion epithelioma. The most effective agent is the folic acid inhibitor 4-amino-N^{10}-methyl-pteroylglutamic acid, methotrexate. Used alone or combined with hysterectomy, as it always should be, it has raised the five-year survival rate in this lethal disease to 50%. Even when metastases are present the five-year survival rate is only slightly less. Like all cytotoxic drugs methotrexate is toxic to bone marrow and a dangerous leucopenia may result, so that frequent white and platelet counts are necessary. A type of aplastic anaemia may also occur requiring transfusion. The accepted limit for treatment is a leucocyte count of 2000. The patient looks and feels ill and is particularly susceptible to any infection, so that she may need antibiotic protection. Loss of appetite and weight, gastro-intestinal disturbance and diarrhoea and a particularly severe, painful stomatitis are all features of the treatment. When these have been overcome the unkindest and most resented blow is the loss of hair. This is fortunately transient in nearly all patients.

The dose of methotrexate is 10–30 mgm. in aqueous solution by intramuscular injection daily for five days. This course of treatment is repeated until complete regression of the primary tumour and all metastases is achieved. It may take ten courses to effect this, but the average is usually four. When toxic reactions appear the interval between courses is spaced so as to allow the side effects to subside, which usually takes a fortnight.

If no response is obtained with methotrexate it is advisable to change to vincaleukoblastine 3–6 mgm. twice daily for three days administered by intravenous drip.

In the treatment of this rare disease there is much to be said for transferring the patient to a hospital where the staff have a special interest and special facilities in the supervision and care of these patients.

17 Pathology of Pregnancy

Ectopic Gestation

The fertilised ovum is normally implanted in the upper part of the body of the uterus. Fertilisation usually takes place in the Fallopian tube, the ovum being subsequently transported by contractions of the tube into the cavity of the uterus, aided by the fluid current imparted from the ciliated epithelium. This short journey probably occupies 6-7 days and during this critical period the developing ovum is nourished temporarily by the cells of the surrounding and still present corona radiata and by the secretion of special cells in the lining epithelium of the tube. In pathological circumstances the ovum may become implanted in situations other than the endometrium of the uterine body, the subsequent gestation being called ectopic. In the majority of such gestations the ovum is implanted in the Fallopian tube. More rarely, the ectopic gestation may be uterine, implantation occurring either in the interstitial portion of the tube or in an ill-developed cornu of a bicornuate uterus. The ovum may be implanted in the ovary leading to ovarian pregnancy, or, in very rare instances, ectopic pregnancy may be primary in the peritoneal cavity. The types of ectopic gestation can therefore be summarised under the following heads:—

Extrauterine { *Tubal.*
Ovarian.
Primary abdominal.

Uterine { *Interstitial pregnancy.*
Pregnancy in an accessory cornu.

Incidence. This is hard to assess accurately since many ectopic pregnancies are never diagnosed, as the ovum dies and forms a mole which is slowly absorbed. Probably an incidence of one ectopic to five hundred normal pregnancies is reasonable for the U.K. though it is far commoner in the West Indies, owing to the greater frequency of endosalpingitis there.

Aetiology. Ectopic gestation is determined by faulty implantation and the cause may be either in the ovum itself or in the maternal structures. The commonest cause of ectopic gestation is undoubtedly previous inflammation of the uterine adnexa. In catarrhal salpingitis and other forms of endosalpingitis the epithelial cells of the plicae become desquamated into the lumen of the tube, and in the process of healing, adjacent plicae adhere and form blind alleys in the tube, in which a migrating ovum may be held up in its passage towards the uterus. In addition to the formation of adhesions in the lumen of the tube, the ciliated cells are destroyed by the desquamative process and the ciliary propulsion of the ovum is lost, certainly to a considerable extent. At operation for ectopic gestation, it is common to find membranous adhesions around the unaffected Fallopian tube, and there may be difficulty because of adhesions in delivering the tubal gestation from the pelvis. These peritubal adhesions restrict the peristaltic movements of the Fallopian tube and provide a further factor of inadequate transportation. It is also well known clinically that ectopic gestation often arises in women who have been infertile for several years, and if a careful history is taken, some record may be obtained either of previous salpingitis or salpingitis following septic abortion or puerperal sepsis. Ectopic gestation is much more frequent in densely populated areas and in seaport towns, and its incidence was high during the post-war era.

The primary infection may be gonococcal, post-abortional, puerperal or secondary to an extra-genital pelvic infection or operation, notably appendicitis. Tuberculosis of the genital tract must not be forgotten and if conception is successful in the treated tuberculous patient there is always a high incidence of ectopic tubal gestation.

Although previous inflammatory lesions of the uterine adnexa are responsible for the majority of ectopic gestations, other causes must be recognised. Among them are congenital defects of the Fallopian tube, such as accessory ostia, congenital diverticula, partial stenosis and hypoplasia. In addition, the ovum may migrate transperitoneally from the ovary of one side to the Fallopian tube of the other, and become implanted ectopically in the Fallopian tube. This migration may be a relatively common cause, for it is not unusual to find the corpus luteum of pregnancy in one ovary with an ectopic gestation in the opposite Fallopian tube. Ectopic gestation has also been attributed to such pelvic abnormalities as fundal myomata and adenomyoma of the Fallopian tube, and operations for ventrosuspension of the uterus in which the round ligament has been reefed or shortened near the isthmus of the tube. In all these conditions the lumen of the tube is presumably obstructed by the extraneous factor, or an associated inflammatory reaction.

In some ectopic gestations it is probable that the ovum itself is at fault. It is possible, theoretically, that a rapid development of the trophoblast might lead to early implantation in the Fallopian tube, just as late implantation, owing to slow development of the trophoblast, could lead to placenta praevia. Such a hypothesis explains those examples of ectopic gestation in which there is no evidence of maternal abnormality.

In most ectopic gestations the cause can be attributed to previous inflammation of the Fallopian tube, which is, in most instances, an endosalpingitis. Extraneous causes of salpingitis, however, such as appendicitis and pelvic abscess which primarily do not affect the tube, can involve it in adhesions which limit its mobility and impair its peristalsis. Hence the greater frequency of right-sided ectopic gestation due to appendicitis.

Pathological Anatomy

Tubal Pregnancy. In tubal pregnancy the most frequent implantation site is the ampulla, perhaps because the plicae are most numerous in this situation, so that previous salpingitis is more likely to produce crypts here than else-where along the Fallopian tube. The ampulla is also the site of fertilisation of the ovum in the first instance. The attachment of the ovum must necessarily be eccentric, and much depends, so far as the patient is concerned, upon whether the ovum is primarily attached on the cranial or caudal side of the tube, for the placenta becomes differentiated adjacent to the side of implanta-tion. If attached cranially, the trophoblast may eventually erode through the peritoneal surface of the tube and lead to intraperitoneal haemorrhage, while with a caudal attachment, erosion of the trophoblast, though usually

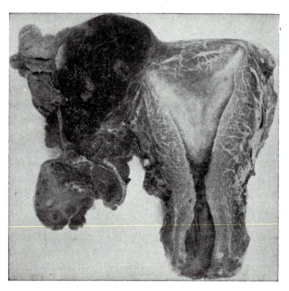

FIG. 199. Ectopic gestation. The uterus lies to the right. The gestation sac full of blood formed in the istlimic portion of the Fallopian tube. The ovary lies below the gestation sac.

causing haemorrhage into the lumen of the tube, may lead to the formation of a broad ligament haematoma (Fig. 199). The chances are about 20 to 1 against the broad ligament position.

The decidual reaction of the tissues of the plicae of the tube is both scanty and incomplete. There is therefore an inadequate barrier of decidual cells to limit the erosion of the trophoblast. In an intrauterine pregnancy the thickness of the decidua never allows the trophoblast to penetrate the myo-metrium except in the rare instance of placenta accreta, and the invasive hydatidiform mole (chorioadenoma destruens) described in the previous chapter. Moreover, the muscle wall of the tube is thin, and there is therefore little resistance to the eroding action of the trophoblast of the embedded ovum. Just as in normal intrauterine pregnancy maternal vessels are opened up by the developing trophoblast, so with ectopic gestation maternal vessels are eroded. With ectopic gestation fairly large vessels lie in close proximity to the developing ovum and larger haemorrhages are more apt to occur than with intrauterine pregnancy. The subsequent progress of tubal pregnancy may be considered under the headings **Haemorrhage** and **Fate of the Ovum.**

Ovarian Pregnancy. A small number of ovarian pregnancies have now been recorded, but it is exceptional for the specimens to show the exact relations of the ovum to the ovarian tissues. In most cases the ovum is fertilised before it is shed from the follicle, so that the site of implantation is the cavity of the corpus luteum of pregnancy. Ovarian pregnancies are always associated with a large haematoma surrounding the ovum. Decidual reaction in the ovary is relatively scanty except on the surface of the cortex. As a result, ovarian pregnancy produces the appearance of a large ovarian haematoma, foetal and trophoblastic tissues being identified histologically, so that the diagnosis is only established after microscopical examination.

Certain criteria must be fulfilled before diagnosing a primary ovarian pregnancy:

(i)   Both tubes must be anatomically normal at laparotomy so that all possibility of a primary tubal ectopic gestation with secondary ovarian implantation can be excluded.

(ii) The gestation sac must occupy the ovary in depth—not just be superficially adherent to it.

(iii) The wall of the gestation sac should consist of recognisable ovarian elements on histological examination, i.e. the gestation sac has expanded the ovary all around it.

(iv) The gestation sac should be attached to the uterus by the ovarian ligament and to the pelvic wall by the ovario-pelvic ligament.

Many so-called ovarian pregnancies are, in reality, corpus luteum haematomata, follicular or other ovarian cysts into which haemorrhage has occurred, associated with an extrauterine gestation aborted from the abdominal ostium and lying adjacent to the ovarian haematoma. Histological examination of such lesions fails to reveal chorionic villi in the depth of the ovary.

Primary Abdominal Pregnancy. This condition is so rare that it probably does not exist, and little is known of the method of implantation. It is possible that the ovum is implanted in areas of ectopic decidua.

Interstitial Pregnancy. Interstitial pregnancy is a very rare form of ectopic gestation, the ovum being implanted in the interstitial portion of the tube. Usually a muscular septum intervenes between the gestation sac and the cavity of the uterus, and the ovum gradually erodes through to the peritoneal surface of the uterus. Interstitial pregnancy usually terminates by rupture into the peritoneal cavity during the third month of pregnancy, but during the period of gestation the distension of the muscle wall of the uterus causes severe abdominal pain, and the tenderness found during bimanual examination of the uterus may lead to the uterus being removed through the mistaken diagnosis of a degenerate myoma (see Fig. 200).

Pregnancy in an Accessory Cornu. The fate of a pregnancy in a duplicated uterus depends upon the degree of development of the cornu. In uterus didelphys, or when both cornua are well developed, pregnancy usually proceeds normally to term, and parturition may be normal. If the cornu is ill-developed, the muscle wall becomes thinned out and may rupture during the pregnancy. This complication usually develops during the fourth month and causes extremely severe internal bleeding. At operation the type of gestation is recognised from the position of attachment of the round ligament, which

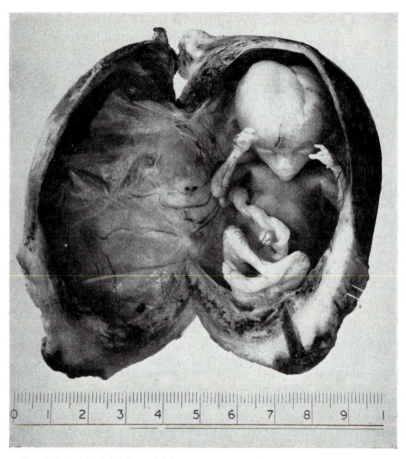

FIG. 200. A 16 weeks' interstitial pregnancy. The placenta is seen at the lower pole, where the gestation sac and surrounding myometrium were locally excised with conservation of the rest of the uterus.

passes from the lateral end of the gestation sac to the internal abdominal ring, whereas in an ectopic pregnancy in the isthmic part of the tube the round ligament lies internal to the gestation sac. Pregnancy in an accessory cornu has been recorded when the corpus luteum was present in the opposite ovary, with the accessory cornu shut off from the cavity of the uterus. This rarity is explained by transperitoneal migration of the fertilised ovum.

Multiple Pregnancy and Ectopic Gestation. The association of multiple pregnancy with ectopic gestation is not uncommon. A tubal gestation is occasionally a twin pregnancy, and one instance of quintuplets in a tubal pregnancy has been recorded. Coincident intrauterine and extrauterine gestations have also been described and authentic cases of bilateral tubal pregnancy have been recorded. It is not unusual, however, in cases of ectopic gestation for the opposite Fallopian tube to be distended with blood by regurgitation from the cavity of the uterus into the tube, the abdominal ostium of which is closed by adhesions from previous salpingitis. The diagnosis of bilateral tubal pregnancy must not be made, therefore, unless chorionic villi can be demonstrated in both tubes. The importance of examining both tubes when operating on a case of ectopic gestation must be emphasised.

Another important feature of tubal gestation is the frequency with which a subsequent ectopic gestation develops in the opposite tube. If a woman conceives after having had an extra-uterine gestation, the chances are 1 in 7 that she will have another in the other tube.

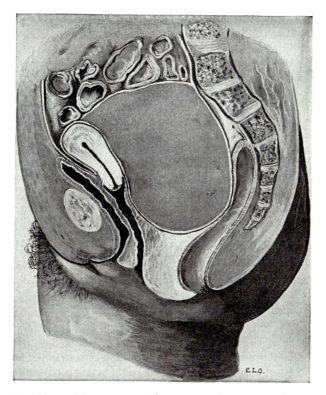

Fig. 201. A large pelvic haematocele from a case of a ruptured tubal gestation. Note how the swelling pushes the uterus forwards, and how retention of urine may develop from elongation of the urethra. Note the close relation to the rectum. (After Stoeckel.)

Haemorrhage

In favourable cases the haemorrhage takes the form of an ooze into the lumen of the tube. If the haemorrhage is slight, blood clots around the trophoblast, dislodging the ovum from its attachment and produces a **tubal mole.** This situation is exactly comparable to the missed abortion of the intra-uterine pregnancy and the term **carneous mole of the tube** is accurate and descriptive. The size of the mole depends partly on the extent of the haemorrhage, and partly upon the stage of pregnancy when the ovum is dislodged, so that a tubal mole may vary from the size of a cherry to a swelling 4 in. in diameter, in which case the tube wall is greatly thinned out. A tubal mole

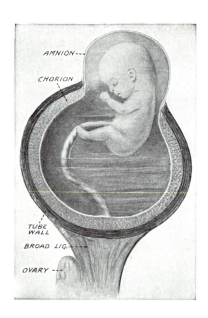

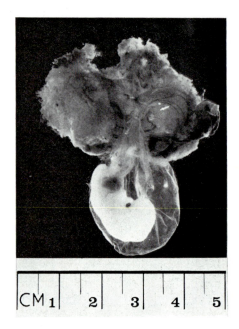

Fig. 202. Tubal rupture with intact gestation sac—a rare event. Compare with Fig. 203.

Fig. 203. Actual specimen removed at operation, illustrating the exact situation of Fig. 202.

may remain within the tube, or it may be expelled by contractions of the plain muscle through the abdominal ostium into the peritoneal cavity—**tubal abortion.** Sometimes the mole is only partly aborted and remains lodged in the abdominal ostium—rather like a cervical abortion in an intrauterine pregnancy. If the haemorrhage into the lumen of the tube is more severe, fluid blood may be discharged through the abdominal ostium, where it may form a clot around the fimbriated extremity of the tube—**peritubal haematocele.** If the haemorrhage is still more profuse, the blood discharged through the abdominal ostium may collect in the pouch of Douglas before clotting, and cause a **pelvic haematocele** (Fig. 201). Pelvic haematocele is also produced in cases of tubal rupture, when the ovum erodes through the wall of the tube and

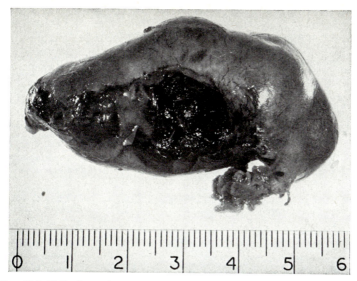

FIG. 204. Fallopian tube containing ectopic gestation on point of rupture, removed intact at operation. In the lower half of the picture, the point of erosion is shown by blood clot.

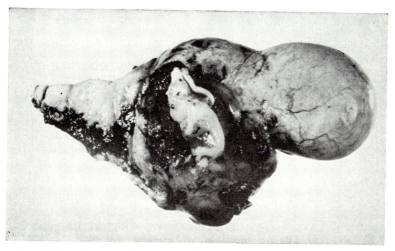

FIG. 205. Ruptured tubal pregnancy. Note the foetus surrounded by a haematoma being extruded through the wall of the distended tube.

blood is discharged directly into the peritoneal cavity. Indeed, pelvic haematocele is invariably produced when a tubal gestation gives rise to severe intraperitoneal bleeding. Peritubal haematocele, on the other hand, is relatively uncommon. It sometimes gives difficulty in diagnosis, Since, if the clot is well organised, it may not be easy to distinguish between a haematocele and a myoma attached to the cornu of the uterus. If of long duration, a pelvic haematocele may even become calcified. The types of haemorrhage just described result from bleeding into the lumen of the tube, and are sometimes referred to under the term **internal tubal haemorrhage.** The worst forms of haemorrhage, however, result from erosion of the trophoblast through the muscle wall of the Fallopian tube. The decidual reaction in the Fallopian tube is scanty, and as the ovum enlarges the tube becomes distended and the muscle wall is thinned out, so that the trophoblast of the ovum may erode through all the layers of the tube causing **tubal rupture** (See Figs. 202–206).

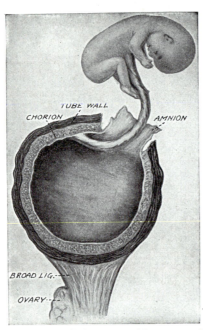

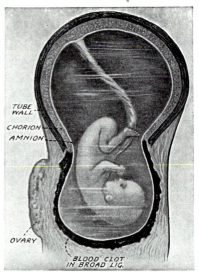

FIG. 206. Tubal rupture with rupture of gestation sac—the commoner event.

FIG. 207. Intraligamentary rupture of tube. Gestation sac intact.

Usually the peritoneal surface of the tube is involved, but on rare occasions the extraperitoneal portion of the tube is eroded, so that blood is discharged into the broad ligament, causing a **broad ligament haematoma** (see Figs. 207–208). With intraperitoneal bleeding, if the haemorrhage is scanty, blood may clot around the eroded area of the tube and form a **paratubal haematocele,** but this is rare. Usually intraperitoneal haemorrhage resulting from tubal rupture is severe, so that **diffuse intraperitoneal bleeding** takes place, and the patient's life is endangered from internal haemorrhage. The most dangerous type of ectopic gestation is when diffuse intraperitoneal bleeding follows tubal rupture. In the rare event when the tube is eroded into the broad ligament, a broad ligament haematoma forms, which may strip up the peritoneum and extend upwards above the pelvic brim.

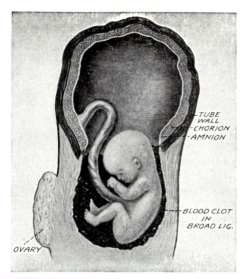

Fig. 208. Same as Fig. 207, but with the gestation sac ruptured.

Fate of the Ovum

In the majority of cases the haemorrhages which are produced around the ovum separate the chorionic villi from their attachment, so that the ovum is forcibly dislodged either into the lumen of the tube, or, in cases of tubal rupture, into the peritoneal cavity. In other cases, the ovum, though not completely dislodged from the tube, may be separated to a degree sufficient to deprive it of its nutrition, so that it dies and forms a tubal mole.

On rare occasions the dislodgment may be partial with incomplete separation of the trophoblast, so that the ovum continues to develop. Two types can be recognised. In the first group, the trophoblast is attached to the caudal aspect of the tube, adjacent to the broad ligament, so that the ovum grows cranially. In almost all cases the cranial surface of the gestation sac bursts through the tube, at first becoming surrounded by blood clot, and later forming adhesions to the omentum and intestine. In the second group, the attachment of the trophoblast is to the cranial aspect of the tube, and the ovum grows downwards in the broad ligament. Such a gestation is sometimes referred to as *secondary abdominal, or broad ligament*, pregnancy. The subsequent fate of such secondary pregnancies is variable. There is always a danger of further internal haemorrhage from erosion of maternal vessels or the trophoblast may become detached and the foetus deprived of its nutrition, so that the ovum dies. In other cases the pregnancy may proceed to term, when the patient experiences a spurious labour, during which there is again further risk of severe internal bleeding. If the patient survives these complications, the foetus dies and may remain inside the abdomen for many years, undergoing mummification and calcification, and become a **lithopaedion.**

A lithopaedion may be retained for many years; more than fifty years without complications having been recorded. In other cases the gestation sac may adhere to the abdominal wall or bowel and become infected, so that pieces of lithopaedion are periodically discharged in the stools.

The foetuses of secondary abdominal pregnancies are very often mal-developed, a fact which may be attributed to the disturbances to their nutrition and the pressures to which they are subjected in the early stages of development.

Secondary abdominal pregnancy and lithopaedion formation should, however, be regarded as extremely rare sequelae of ectopic gestation.

Symptoms and Diagnosis

The clinical picture in ectopic gestation varies with the pathological anatomy. With tubal rupture the picture is one of an abdominal catastrophe associated with internal bleeding, and such cases are of the greatest urgency. This is the so-called acute ectopic gestation. With tubal mole, and peri- and paratubal haematoceles, the urgency is not so great, and the patient complains of abdominal pain and irregular vaginal bleeding. This is the less urgent and dramatic situation and is sometimes called the chronic ectopic gestation. It is commoner than the acute variety. We would prefer the term subacute to chronic since the subacute may well be promoted into the acute, e.g. by vaginal examination (*vide infra*).

Symptoms. *History of Pregnancy.* In typical ectopic gestation the patient gives a history of a missed period, and states that between six and eight weeks from the first day of the last period vaginal bleeding has developed. If amenorrhoea has lasted for six weeks or more, the symptoms of early pregnancy, such as morning vomiting, frequency of micturition, tenderness and fullness of the breasts may be noted. Such symptoms, however, are not always present if the ectopic gestation ruptures in the early weeks. In many cases of ectopic gestation a history of amenorrhoea cannot be obtained. Probably the gestation sac is dislodged soon after implantation, the hormonal influences of pregnancy are disturbed, and the uterine decidua is shed early. With secondary abdominal pregnancy, amenorrhoea may continue until the ovum dies or the pregnancy reaches term.

Pain. The most constant feature of all ectopic gestations is the development of abdominal pain. The pain is always severe, much more so than with any form of abortion of an intrauterine pregnancy. The most severe pain is that of tubal rupture, when the wall of the Fallopian tube bursts and a large quantity of blood is rapidly discharged into the peritoneal cavity. In tubal mole, tubal abortion, and tubal erosion, the pain is sometimes colicky, and always severe, so that the patient has to stop her work. There is usually nausea, vomiting, and sometimes syncope. It must be emphasised that ectopic gestation always causes severe abdominal pain, comparable to that of appendicitis, while with tubal rupture associated with diffuse intraperitoneal bleeding, the pain, the collapse, and the shock are comparable to those found with a perforated gastric ulcer. The diagnosis of ectopic gestation, in which localised haematomata are formed, often presents an extremely difficult clinical problem, and a careful interrogation of the patient as to the severity and situation of the pain is always necessary.

An interesting type of pain occurs if the internal haemorrhage has been severe enough to flood the upper peritoneal cavity and irritate the under surface of the diaphragm. In these patients pain is referred via the phrenic nerve to the region of the shoulder and will be diagnosed by the patient as rheumatic. Shoulder pain is strongly suggestive of the severe internal bleeding of an extrauterine gestation.

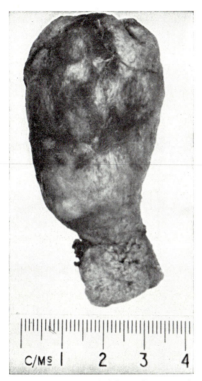

FIG. 209. Complete decidual cast extruded from the uterus in a patient operated on for ectopic gestation.

Vaginal Bleeding. The vaginal bleeding in ectopic gestation is of a peculiar type, for it consists either of dark altered and fluid blood, or of dark coagulated material. Severe vaginal bleeding is hardly ever seen, and it is very exceptional for clots to be passed. One important feature of this loss is that it is continuous without intermission. The vaginal haemorrhage originates in the endometrium of the uterus, although some of the blood may be discharged from the Fallopian tube through the uterus into the vagina. With ectopic gestation, the endometrium of the uterus hypertrophies and becomes converted into a decidua, which is macroscopically and histologically identical with the decidua of early pregnancy. When the ovum dies, following its dis-

lodgment by haemorrhage, the fall in chorionic gonadotropin level causes diminution in secretion of luteinising hormone with a resulting atrophy of the
corpus luteum and consequent fall in progesterone level. This causes retro-
gressive changes in the endometrium which at first take the form of haemorrhage into the spongy layer. It should be emphasised that uterine bleeding is a
sign of the death of the ovum. Sometimes the whole of the uterine decidua
separates from the uterus and is discharged as a **decidual cast** of the uterine
cavity into the vagina (Fig. 209). Decidual casts have smooth glistening inner
surfaces, the maternal surface being shaggy. The passage of a decidual cast is
pathognomonic of ectopic gestation. Histological examination of a decidual
cast demonstrates the presence of decidual cells and hypertrophied glands,
chorionic villi being absent. A cast of this kind may be confused with the
chorion of an intrauterine pregnancy. The diagnosis must be made with
precision, otherwise the presence of an ectopic gestation may be overlooked.
If there is any doubt about the diagnosis, the material should be examined
histologically. If chorionic villi are present the pregnancy must have been
intrauterine. When the endometrium disintegrates, without exfoliation of
its superficial layers to produce a cast, the altered blood is discharged from
the uterus and in many ways resembles the menstrual discharge. One of the
great characteristics of the vaginal bleeding in ectopic gestation is that it is
prolonged and continuous. Indeed, if a woman notices vaginal bleeding
some time after a period is due, and if this bleeding persists, ectopic gestation
should be suspected. It is not unusual to see patients in whom the haemorrhage has lasted for as long as two or three months, whose main complaint
is persistent bleeding, and for whom the abdominal pain was shortlived and
almost forgotten.

Women suspected of having ectopic gestation should be carefully inter-
rogated as to whether solid material has been discharged from the uterus.
One of the difficulties in the diagnosis of ectopic gestation is to distinguish
between pyosalpinx following septic abortion and ectopic gestation. Women
often attempt to conceal that they have aborted, particularly if the abortion
has been procured illegally.

If an ectopic gestation ruptures, and a large quantity of blood is rapidly
discharged into the peritoneal cavity, the woman immediately becomes
collapsed and shocked. Such patients are usually desperately ill, with subnormal temperature, rapid pulse and very low blood pressure. They usually
give a clear-cut history of a missed period and of violent abdominal pain
at the time of the collapse and shock. One of the most striking features of
patients with severe internal haemorrhage is the clear-headedness they
display. Although desperately ill and shocked, they may still ask intelligent
questions about their condition and take an active interest in the preparations
made for operation. The vaginal bleeding may develop subsequent to the
abdominal pain and shock.

Physical Signs. The physical signs vary according to whether the patient is
suffering from acute intraperitoneal haemorrhage or whether local haematomata have been formed in the pelvis.

With Diffuse Internal Bleeding. The appearance of the patient is characteristic. She has a real pallor, easily distinguishable from the greyness of shock, and the two other symptoms of internal haemorrhage, restlessness and air-hunger, may both be present. Superimposed upon the features of internal haemorrhage are those of collapse and shock, so that the patient is cold, the skin is clammy, the temperature subnormal, and the pulse thin and running. The degree of anaemia can be roughly determined by inspecting the conjunctivea, the tongue and the lobe of the ear. Examination of the breasts shows a mild degree of mammary activity, such as dilated veins on the surface, and hypertrophy of the lobules; clear secretion may be expressed. The breast signs are important, but they may not be detected without great experience. The abdomen is usually slightly distended and movements may be impaired. The distension is not due to the free intraperitoneal blood but to an associated localised ileus of the gut. This can be demonstrated in a plain X-ray of the abdomen and is a very important sign. On palpation there is extreme local tenderness in the hypogastrium, but rigidity is never well marked. Signs of free fluid in the abdomen are usually indefinite, even if large quantities of blood are present within the abdominal cavity. On vaginal examination the cervix is found softened, but blue discoloration of the vagina is usually absent at this early stage of gestation. In most cases there is some degree of uterine bleeding, although this may not develop until some hours after rupture. The abdominal tenderness may prevent an accurate bimanual examination of the uterus, but if the uterus can be felt it is found to be slightly enlarged and softened. In typical cases of tubal rupture with diffuse intra-peritoneal bleeding, it is exceptional to find clearly defined swellings in the pelvis apart from the uterus. Usually only a tender resistance in Douglas's pouch can be felt. In other cases, however, when the ovum still remains in the Fallopian tube, a firm rounded swelling can be palpated in this situation. Bimanual manipulation of the uterus almost always causes pain.

The differential diagnosis of tubal rupture with diffuse intraperitoneal bleeding must be made from such intra-abdominal catastrophes as perforated gastric or duodenal ulcer, perforated appendix with general peritonitis, perforated gall-bladder, or such rare conditions as ruptured spleen and acute pancreatitis. The main points in establishing the diagnosis are the history of a missed period, the signs of activity in the breasts, and the evidence of internal bleeding. The short history, combined with subnormal temperature and shock, serve to exclude appendicitis and inflammatory lesions within the abdominal cavity.

The diagnosis may be much more difficult with ruptured secondary abdominal pregnancy, as the differential diagnosis of ruptured uterus and concealed accidental haemorrhage has to be considered.

Localised Intraperitoneal Haemorrhage. In this condition although there may be some degree of constitutional disturbance as a result of the local intraperitoneal bleeding, the dominant features are recurrent abdominal pain and vaginal bleeding. Examination of the patient may show some degree of anaemia. The pulse rate is raised in proportion to the severity of the bleeding, but it is exceptional for the temperature to be raised more than 99·4°. The absence of severe pyrexia may be of some service in distinguishing between ectopic gestation and pyosalpinx. The breasts may show signs of early activity. On examination of the abdomen, tenderness in one or other iliac fossa is invariable, and sometimes the haematoma can be palpated, arising from the pelvis as a tender, firm swelling. Distension and rigidity are not characteristic of localised pelvic haematomata.

The most important physical signs, however, are found on vaginal examination, for an accurate bimanual examination is usually possible. The peculiar uterine haemorrhage can be recognised; the cervix is found to be softened and the uterus slightly enlarged. The other physical signs vary with the type of case. With pelvic haematocele an irregular swelling can be felt through the posterior fornix in the pouch of Douglas. It has a peculiar consistence, which is almost pathognomonic, for it has no definite outline, is neither fluid nor solid, and its consistence varies in different areas. Occasionally the haematoma is extremely tender. It pushes the uterus forwards and upwards, and on rare occasions produces retention of urine. Very occasionally it may extend upwards into the abdomen and be palpable on abdominal examination. Tubal mole and the haematosalpinx of intratubal haemorrhage form retort-shaped swellings which are tense, firm, and smooth, and which push the uterus to the opposite side of the pelvis. Peritubal haematoceles form firm hard swellings which may be mistaken for subperitoneal myomata. Firmness, tenderness, and smoothness are characteristic of the localised haematomata of this form of ectopic gestation. There is one real danger of vaginal examination which should be emphasised. It is possible to disturb a quiescent ectopic which has stopped bleeding and to cause a further severe haemorrhage. For this reason if an ectopic gestation is strongly suspected the vaginal examination should be postponed until the patient is in the theatre and all preparations for immediate operation have been made. The authors can well recall instances where vaginal examination was responsible for causing a further severe internal haemorrhage.

Differential Diagnosis. With physical signs of this kind there is often great difficulty in distinguishing between ectopic gestation and pyosalpinx. With pyosalpinx the temperature is raised, and there may be a history of gonorrhoea or septic abortion. A difficulty in establishing the diagnosis is that with pyosalpinx continuous vaginal bleeding is not uncommon, and if the pyosalpinx results from a septic abortion there may be a history of a missed period. Similarly, difficulty may be experienced in distinguishing between a pelvic haematocele and a pelvic abscess. A leucocyte count may be of some help in establishing the diagnosis, though it is raised moderately in ectopic gestation, and a pregnancy test may be of service.

A retroverted gravid uterus is sometimes confused with the pelvic haematocele of an ectopic gestation, as, vaginal bleeding may develop as a symptom of threatened abortion and the body of the uterus may be thought to be a pelvic haematocele. With pelvic haematocele the uterus can be palpated separate from the swelling in the pouch of Douglas, whereas in cases of retroverted gravid uterus the body of the uterus cannot be identified separate from the swelling in Douglas's pouch. Moreover, with a retroverted gravid uterus the anterior vaginal wall is stretched, the cervix points either downwards and forwards, or directly forwards, and the swelling in Douglas's pouch is smooth and soft, with clearly defined margins. With pelvic haematocele, the cervix points directly downwards, although it may be displaced forwards and upwards. The two conditions are easily distinguished if the two possibilities are borne in mind and the patient examined with proper care. Aspiration of the pouch of Douglas through the upper part of the posterior vaginal wall (see p. 129) is a possible but little used method of establishing the diagnosis of a pelvic haematocele.

Other gynaecological conditions which may be confused with ectopic gestation are endometriosis and, rarely, a small twisted ovarian cyst, as in both these conditions there may be some disturbance of menstruation. The early stages of an abortion in early intrauterine pregnancy, associated with a subperitoneal fibroid, may give a picture closely resembling that of ectopic gestation. Similarly, a threatened abortion associated with a corpus luteum cyst may be hard to distinguish from ectopic gestation. It has already been emphasised, however, that with ectopic gestation extremely severe abdominal pain is the rule, and such severe pain is not to be expected during the abortion of an intrauterine pregnancy. There are a number of conditions which give rise to slight or moderate intraperitoneal haemorrhages and which, therefore, give signs very suggestive of an ectopic pregnancy. These patients present with acute abdominal pain of sudden onset, may be collapsed with a rapid pulse and have acute lower abdominal tenderness and rigidity. The causative pathology is usually some bleeding into or from a ruptured follicle or follicular cyst or corpus luteum haematoma, the so-called ovarian apoplexy. Sometimes an endometriomatous cyst ruptures or leaks giving similar signs. Even on bimanual pelvic examination under anaesthetic, it is not always possible to make the diagnosis. These patients are most often admitted as surgical emergencies under general surgeons and frequently are given a preliminary diagnosis of acute appendicitis. The true state of affairs is then revealed by laparotomy.

Diagnostic investigations. In the treatment of acute ectopic gestation where the patient is obviously ill from severe internal bleeding, there is no time and no need for any investigation other than blood grouping, cross-matching and immediate laparotomy. The situation is, however, quite different when dealing with the subacute variety such as pelvic haematocele or a tubal mole in which internal bleeding is, at most, only moderate and localised. The differential diagnosis here is most frequently one of pelvic inflammatory disease in which the treatment is primarily conservative. Certain investigations may help to solve this type of problem:

(i) *Examination under anaesthesia* with one important proviso—that the surgeon is prepared then and there to proceed to laparotomy. The present authors know of half a dozen occasions where examination caused sudden and dangerous bleeding in which the patient's condition immediately deteriorated.

(ii) *Diagnostic curettage:* This is helpful if chorionic villi can be found in the curettings and rules out extra-uterine pregnancy—unless an extra-uterine pregnancy were to co-exist with an intra-uterine abortion—

a very rare but not unknown event. The finding of decidual reaction without villi is again suggestive of ectopic gestation.

(iii) *Aspiration of Douglas's pouch* is helpful if free blood is obtained but the method depends on a large element of luck.

(iv) *Culdoscopy*, not yet popular in this country, can be most helpful; it requires a special instrument, some technical skill and experience and, therefore, has a limited application.

(v) *Peritoneoscopy* is probably a safer and more informative method of diagnosis and though not yet commonly available will in future be more widely used in the obscure and difficult case.

(vi) *Pregnancy tests* are not much help in ectopic gestation and are, in fact, often confusing. A pregnancy test becomes negative soon after the trophoblast dies or is dislodged by bleeding, e.g. in pelvic haematocele, tubal mole or tubal abortion.

The diagnosis of ectopic gestation often presents great difficulty and it is usually missed because ectopic gestation is not suspected. Women, who during the child-bearing period of life complain of severe pain in the lower abdomen associated with continuous vaginal bleeding, should be suspected of ectopic gestation. It is far better to treat pyosalpinx by abdominal operation than to treat an ectopic gestation conservatively with antibiotics.

Treatment. All patients with ectopic gestation must be operated upon when the diagnosis has been made. Treatment consists in abdominal operation, but the technique differs according to whether the case is associated with diffuse intraperitoneal bleeding, or whether the haemorrhages are localised in the pelvis.

It is very exceptional for the diagnosis of ectopic gestation to be made before rupture or the development of some form of pelvic haematoma. Such cases should be treated by excision of the affected Fallopian tube.

With diffuse intraperitoneal bleeding immediate operation is necessary. Although such patients may be desperately ill the operative results are extremely good. It is probable that a great deal of the shock and collapse from which these patients suffer is caused by the blood which is pent up in the peritoneal cavity. Patients improve as soon as the peritoneal cavity is opened and the blood evacuated. Pre-operative treatment should be of the simplest, but care must be taken to shave the pubic hair and disinfect the abdominal wall. The patient should be blood grouped and Rhesus typed and blood cross matched for transfusion while she is being prepared for operation, but only if her condition warrants the delay inherent in the grouping and cross matching. In the desperately ill patient it is essential to operate first and transfuse as soon as blood is available, relying on oxygen and plasma as a stop gap. The abdomen is opened by a midline subumbilical incision, with the patient flat. A hand is passed down the pelvis, the affected Fallopian tube drawn out of the wound, clamps placed on the mesosalpinx and the tube excised. The pedicles are tied with catgut and the stump is allowed to fall back into the pelvis. With tubal rupture, owing to adhesions around the tube, there may be difficulty in delivering the Fallopian tube from the wound, and in some cases, where adhesions are present, it may be necessary to remove the ovary as well. Another difficulty is that the opposite Fallopian tube may be converted into a haematosalpinx, and the operator may have to spend some time in deciding which of the tubes contains the ectopic gestation. Blood clot and as much blood as is possible are removed from the peritoneal cavity. Finally, the abdominal wound is sutured in layers in the ordinary way. The operation can be performed quite quickly, within a few minutes. It should always be undertaken, however desperate the patient's condition may be. The patients improve as soon as the peritoneal cavity is opened and very little anaesthetic is required to allow this to be done. There is, therefore little risk of the patient dying under anaesthesia. The patient is treated by blood transfusion as soon as this can be safely started. Recovery is usually rapid and uneventful. Some degree of pyrexia is almost the rule during the first week after operation, probably because of the absorption of blood from the peritoneal cavity.

In the other forms of ectopic gestation there is not the same urgency and a patient can be prepared in the routine way for an abdominal operation. The earlier the patient is operated upon, however, the better, as there is always a risk of a living ovum causing tubal rupture with diffuse intra-peritoneal bleeding. Moreover, longstanding blood clot in the peritoneal cavity may be difficult to remove because it becomes adherent to adjacent structures. The risk of a haematocele becoming infected is extremely small. The principles of treatment are, as with a ruptured ectopic gestation with diffuse intraperitoneal bleeding, to remove the affected tube and blood clot. We do not consider it justifiable to remove the ectopic gestation sac by enucleating it from the tube by salpingostomy and conserving the affected tube. The primary cause of the original ectopic gestation is thereby preserved for a future repetition of the same trouble and this provides an unjustifiable risk to the patient. Tubal moles, peritubal and paratubal haematoceles, are easily delivered from the pelvis, and the affected tube can usually be removed without difficulty. In such cases, however, the ovary may be firmly adherent to the tube, and it may not be possible to excise the tube without removing the ovary as well. Old-standing pelvic haematoceles may be difficult to remove because of adhesions, and great care must be taken to avoid damage to the intestine, with resultant infection and peritonitis.

The treatment of secondary abdominal pregnancy is to perform a laparotomy as soon as the diagnosis is made, as there is an ever present risk of a serious internal haemorrhage endangering the life of the mother. No useful purpose is served in thinking of the foetus, since malformations are common and few children survive. If the ovum has died and been retained for any length of time, the gestation sac should be removed entire. There may be difficulty, however, in separating the placenta from its attachment to the abdominal viscera.

If the foetus is alive, although its removal from the gestation sac can be accomplished without difficulty, the separation of the placenta may lead to extremely severe haemorrhage, which may be uncontrollable. If, therefore, the attachment of the placenta is such that large vessels will be opened up if it is removed, it is better to leave the placenta within the abdomen to undergo slow absorption. The abdomen should not be drained. The absorption of a placenta in the pelvis may take eighteen months to two years, and a small symptomless residual induration may persist in the pelvis for several years.

18 Disorders of Menstruation

In healthy women menstruation begins at about the age of 12–14 years and persists throughout the child-bearing period of life, with a rhythm of twenty-eight days and a duration of between three to five days. It is common, however, for departures from this normal sequence to be seen in women who have no disturbance in health. Puberty may be delayed in girls who pursue strenuous activities, and with the peasant girls of the Balkan States the onset of menstruation is often delayed until the age of 20. The cycle of twenty-eight days is by no means invariable in healthy women, as frequently there is a variation of one or two days from the twenty-eight-day cycle. Minor variations from what is regarded as the physiological menstrual cycle should not therefore be regarded as pathological.

Disorders of menstruation are, however, extremely common and account for the complaints of a large proportion of gynaecological patients. Such menstrual disturbances are symptomatic and often the primary cause is indeterminate. It is customary, therefore, to group the cases symptomatically, and although this method of classification is theoretically unsound, it is the most practical that is possible from the clinical point of view.

PRECOCIOUS MENSTRUATION

If menstruation starts before the child reaches the age of 10 the condition is referred to as **precocious menstruation.** In precocious puberty, early menstruation may occur in addition to the development of secondary sex characters. In clinical practice it is first necessary to establish that the haemorrhage is true menstruation and not bleeding caused by injuries, scratching or foreign bodies inserted in the vagina.

Most examples of precocious menstruation and precocious puberty are constitutional without evidence of any primary fault. It is suggested as an explanation that the pituitary, ovaries and adrenals are prematurely adolescent. These premature precocious menstrual cycles are not necessarily anovular, as the well authenticated Peruvian case proves. The mother, when delivered, was a child aged less than six years. Certain pathological conditions may stimulate the ovaries to premature activity. For example, granulosa cell tumours, thecomata and some teratomata cause hypertrophy of the breast and irregular uterine bleeding. These patients do not ovulate or genuinely menstruate and their behaviour is comparable to that of the post-menopausal woman who is found to have an oestrogenic ovarian tumour. Similar but less striking effects are produced by oestrogen therapy in children, as is given, for example, in the treatment of vulvo-vaginitis. Very rarely, disorders of the pituitary and diseases of the midbrain and hypothalamus may induce premature menstruation. One interesting but rare condition which affects the pituitary is Albright's syndrome where there is a polyostosis fibrous dysplasia, fragilitas ossium with spontaneous multiple bone fractures and large coppery areas of skin pigmentation. The bone lesion at the base of the skull distorts the sella turcica and pituitary fossa and it is this which is thought to cause the menstrual precocity. In such cases the sex characters are isosexual and feminine, but the adrenogenital syndrome sometimes develops in young girls to produce masculine or heterosexual characters.

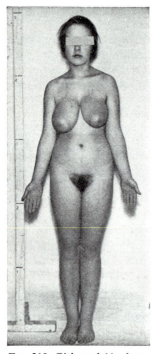

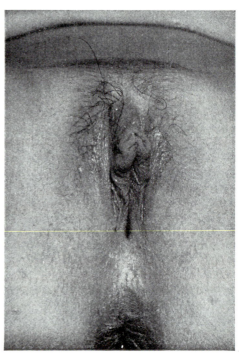

FIG. 210. Girl aged 11, showing precocious puberty. Note well-marked breast development and adult pubic hair growth.

FIG. 211. The vulva of a girl aged 7, showing precocious growth of pubic hair and hypertrophy of labia minora.

Diagnosis and Treatment of Precocious Menstruation. It is important to segregate these young patients into their correct clinical group.

(a) *Genuine precocious menstruation:* These girls have cyclical uterine bleeding, well-marked secondary sexual characteristics such as pubic and axillary hair, well-developed breasts and, if curetted, will show a mature endometrium possibly with secretory changes. No treatment except observation is indicated for these (Figs. 210 and 211).

(b) *Non-cyclical bleeding:* Some enlargement of breasts but no other secondary sexual characteristics suggests an oestrogenic ovarian tumour and this should be excluded by pelvic examination under anaesthesia. Curettage will probably show cystic glandular hyperplasia.

(c) *Neurological signs suggestive of a pituitary or hypothalamic disturbance,* associated with premature puberty. These patients present a primary neurological problem and should be transferred for expert investigation.

(d) *Occasional vaginal bleeding* in which no general or endocrine disturbance can be found and secondary sexual characteristics are absent. In these patients a foreign body in the vagina is a likely possibility and should be excluded by examination under anaesthesia and an X-ray.

(e) *Heterosexual precocity* is androgenic in origin and suggests adrenal cortical hyperplasia or adreno-genital syndrome. These patients show virilising signs and do not bleed from the uterus.

AMENORRHOEA

Amenorrhoea is a frequent symptom complained of by patients and its investigation demands careful examination combined with a wide knowledge of endocrinology. The cause of the amenorrhoea may be easy to detect but if obscure a complete investigation requires hormone assays which are not always available even in large hospitals. Furthermore, although great progress has been made in the identification of the different causes of amenorrhoea, only very recently has progress been made in their treatment.

It has been customary to classify amenorrhoea into **physiological** and **pathological** forms. Pathological types are usually subdivided into **primary amenorrhoea,** when the patient has never menstruated, and **secondary amenorrhoea** which develops after the patient has had normal menstrual function. In clinical practice, many patients suffer from delayed onset of puberty, and it is perhaps for this reason that much attention has been paid to the group referred to as primary amenorrhoea. A more modern system of classification is suggested below.

Classification of Amenorrhoea

PHYSIOLOGICAL: Prepubertal.
Pregnancy.
Lactation.
Post-menopausal.

PATHOLOGICAL, PRIMARY AMENORRHOEA:

(a) Congenital obstructive defects in the lower genital tract, e.g. non-canalisation of cervix, vagina or imperforate hymen leading to cryptomenorrhoea. This is not actual primary amenorrhoea since the patient is menstruating without visible loss.

(b) Congenital absence or gross hypoplasia of the uterus.

(c) Congenital aplasia of the ovaries—Turner's syndrome.

(d) Intersexualism—such as pseudohermaphroditism (Chapter 6).

(e) Hypopituitary dwarfism.

(f) Hypothyroid cretinism.

PATHOLOGICAL, SECONDARY AMENORRHOEA:

(a) Acquired obstruction in the lower genital tract—operative injury, chemical burns, leading to cervical and very rarely vaginal stenosis.

(b) Hysterectomy.

(c)   (i) Destruction of both ovaries by disease (very rare), radiation or removal by operation.

    (ii) Primary ovarian failure—Hypohormonal amenorrhoea.

    (iii) Hyperhormonal amenorrhoea—the early phase of metropathia and sometimes due to therapeutic use of hormones.

    (iv) Stein-Leventhal syndrome. Hyperthecosis ovarii.

    (v) Masculinising tumours of the ovary—Arrhenoblastoma, Hilus cell tumours, Masculinising luteoma, Adrenal-like tumours.

(d) Diseases and disorders affecting the pituitary:

    (i) Psychogenic from the higher centres via the thalamus and hypothalamus. Anorexia nervosa. Pituitary shock.

    (ii) Basophil adenoma—Cushing's disease.

    (iii) Acidophil tumours—producing gigantism and acromegaly.

    (iv) Pituitary failure due to chromophobe adenoma, cysts, Simmond's disease and post-partum pituitary necrosis (Sheehan's syndrome).

    (v) Suppression of F. S. H. by persistence of luteotropic hormone—Chiari Frommel syndrome.

(e) Adrenal cortical hyperplasia (adreno-genital syndrome), adrenal cortical tumours and adrenal failure (Addison's disease).

(f) Thyroid: Hyperthyroid states and the late stages of hypothyroidism.

(g) Diabetes mellitus.

(h) Severe debilitating general diseases.

(i) Nutritional.

(j) Amenorrhoea due to chromosomal anomalies.

Physiological Amenorrhoea. Menstruation is restricted to the child-bearing period of life, so that a girl does not menstruate before puberty, and the periods stop at the menopause. During pregnancy and lactation amenorrhoea is to be anticipated, although some women have regular slight haemorrhages in the early months of pregnancy, and many women menstruate even though they are feeding their children. All cases of amenorrhoea must be investigated with exceptional care to exclude pregnancy. Pregnancy is by far the commonest cause of amenorrhoea and it must be definitely excluded before any other diagnosis can be made. Menopausal cases sometimes present difficulty, as the onset of the menopause may be early, and great difficulty may be experienced in elucidating the cause. Sometimes women get an obsession that they are pregnant and may develop the clinical condition of **pseudocyesis.**

Pathological Amenorrhoea. As many of the pathological causes of primary and secondary amenorrhoea overlap, no attempt has been made in the text to follow the classification exactly as given above and the subsequent remarks are intended as an expansion and explanation of some of the causes of amenorrhoea.

Cryptomenorrhoea

Cryptomenorrhoea may be either congenital or acquired.

(1) **Congenital.** The causes of this have already been mentioned, and the failure of complete canalisation of the lower end of the Müllerian duct in the region of the sinovaginal bulbs discussed. This leads to one variety of so-called imperforate hymen. Very rarely there is a congenital atresia of the cervical canal.

Clinically the patients are normally young girls in their early teens who suffer from cyclical monthly pain without the discharge of the ordinary menstrual bleeding. The amount of retained blood may eventually reach as much as 5 pints, and an abdomino-pelvic tumour is produced which is palpable and visible on abdominal examination. Even with large tumours this retained blood is accommodated in the vagina since the cervix and uterus offer considerable resistance to distension. In long standing cases a haemato-metra, and later a haematosalpinx may develop. Such advanced cases are, however, rarely met with now as the condition is well recognised and treated before this stage. In spite of the distension of the tubes and uterus, relief of the vaginal pressure usually results in complete involution, and pregnancy has been reported by Searle and others after conservative treatment—namely, incision of the membrane. The contents of a haematocolpos are always sterile and only become infected after drainage. With modern chemo-therapy this risk should be minimal if certain precautions are taken. No vaginal examination should be made after operation for several weeks and no drainage tubes should be employed. Sometimes these patients present themselves with retention of urine as the primary symptom, and after the bladder has been emptied by catheter the abdomino-pelvic tumour is obvious and the bulging vaginal membrane gives the clue to the true state of affairs. The dark blue or purple colour of this membrane is due to the retained blood. Gentle pressure on the abdominal tumour will transmit a thrill to the vaginal membrane and cause it to bulge more distinctly (see Fig. 78). Sometimes it is possible to feel the uterus sitting on top of the cystic tumour. The differential diagnosis is from pregnancy.

More rarely, congenital cryptomenorrhoea results from a failure of canali-sation of the entire vagina, though the uterus and Fallopian tubes develop normally. In these cases haematometra and haematosalpinx form as soon as menstruation is established. In such cases the abdomen is first explored to confirm the nature of the tumour and the uterine cavity is opened and drained. An artificial vagina is then constructed with a Thiersch skin graft from the thigh surrounding a plastic mould which has a central canal. Before closing the uterus, an opening is made through the cervix into the new vaginal cavity so that menstrual bleeding can take place through the canal in the mould whilst the graft is taking. Successful pregnancy has been reported following this type of operation. Congenital absence of the uterus, tubes and vagina is more common than a failure of canalisation alone. In these cases there can,

DISORDERS OF MENSTRUATION

of course, be no expectation of menstruation or pregnancy, but many women with this defect of the entire Müllerian system retain all their other isosexual feminine characteristics and desire marriage. In these circumstances the construction of an artificial vagina is necessary and results usually in satisfactory intercourse. After full investigation of the urinary tract to exclude any congenital urological abnormalities, such as single pelvic kidney, which commonly accompany absence of the uterus and which may hazard the operation, a cavity is made between urethra and rectum up to the level of the rectovesical pouch of peritoneum. A polythene sponge mould is then covered with a single Thiersch graft taken from the inner aspect of the thigh and inserted into the cavity. After four months the mould is removed and an adequate vaginal cavity remains. An alternative operation described by Williams involves suturing the labia minora together in the midline to form a cul-de-sac ending at the fourchette. This simple operation provides an "artificial vagina" which functions quite satisfactorily.

(2) **Acquired.** All operations on the cervix, especially amputation and trachelorrhaphy, are liable to be followed by stenosis. Cauterisation by the actual cautery or diathermy, or even chemicals such as zinc chloride and carbolic, can also cause cervical occlusion. Radium treatment for benign and malignant conditions is also responsible for a number of cases and even a too vigorous curettage has been reported to result in cervical obstruction. If all these operations are preceded by a thorough cervical dilatation the risk of occlusion is small. At the end of such operations it is a wise precaution to pass a sound to ensure an unobstructed passage in the cervical canal.

Developmental and acquired defects of the upper genital tract

Sometimes the uterus fails to develop, but more frequently the uterus is ill-developed and of the foetal or infantile type, with its endometrium— if present at all—unaffected by ovarian stimulation. Failure of the ovaries to develop is exceptionally rare. In most cases of this group the patient presents herself for examination because of a delayed onset of puberty. The investigation demands a general examination of the patient to determine the degree of development of the secondary sex characters, combined with a pelvic examination—preferably with the patient anaesthetised. Many cases of primary amenorrhoea belong to this group. Amenorrhoea may be the result of surgical removal of the uterus, though the patient may not appreciate the exact nature of the operation. The cervical canal may very rarely become stenosed as a result of lacerations in a difficult delivery.

Disorders of the Ovaries

Very rarely the ovaries fail to develop. A large number of cases of amenorrhoea are due to hypofunction of the ovaries which, as the result of endocrine investigations, can be shown to be a primary ovarian deficiency. Many patients with delayed onset of puberty belong to this group, as do many with a precocious menopause. In *Turner's syndrome* there is a primary ovarian aplasia, and the patient has a short stature, congenital webbing of the neck and well-marked cubitus valgus. The breasts are hypoplastic and the secondary sexual characteristics poorly developed. The excretion of gonadotropins in the urine is excessive, which distinguishes the case from pituitary infantilism, when gonadotropins cannot be identified in the urine. The patients have amenorrhoea and a limited growth of axillary and pubic hair. Turner's syndrome is one example of a chromosomal abnormality, sex chromosome monosomy X O and it should more accurately be classified under chromosomal anomalies (see below).

Amenorrhoea also follows the surgical removal of both ovaries, and when the ovaries are inhibited with X-rays or radium to create an artificial menopause or to treat pelvic malignant disease. Inflammations of the ovaries do not cause amenorrhoea except in advanced tuberculosis when the whole of both ovaries may be destroyed. Tumours of the ovary rarely produce amenorrhoea except in the case of advanced bilateral ovarian carcinomata.

The virilising ovarian tumours, namely, the arrhenoblastoma, the Hilus cell tumour and the masculinising luteoma which are described in more detail on page 747, also cause amenorrhoea. There is also a very rare suprarenal tumour of the ovary which is a virilising tumour and which produces amenorrhoea. This tumour is of great interest because it causes signs both of Cushing's syndrome and of the adrenogenital syndrome.

The *Stein-Leventhal syndrome* is a rare but important cause of secondary amenorrhoea in young women. These patients are infertile, often obese, hirsute and frequently have hypoplasia of the breasts. On pelvic examination, both ovaries are enlarged to two or three times their normal size and, at laparotomy, show a firm, rubbery consistence. Oestrogen, gonadotropin and 17-ketosteroid excretion levels are normal and the latter point differentiates the Stein-Leventhal from the adreno-genital syndrome. At operation, multiple cysts are found in the ovaries and, on histological examination, a thick layer of theca cells surrounds the cysts. The endometrium is oestrogenic and there is no secretory change. It is suggested that the hyperthecosis is androgen-producing.

Bilateral wedge resection of the ovaries is said to restore normal menstruation in nearly all patients and fertility in 80%. These figures are probably somewhat optimistic. The scientific basis of this operation is difficult to explain but its efficacy is unquestioned (see page 708).

Clomiphene is the drug of choice in patients suffering from polycystic ovaries, or Stein-Leventhal syndrome. It is of the utmost importance, however, that patients should be properly and adequately investigated before commencing treatment with Clomiphene, the dosage of which is 50–100 mg. daily for five days each month for six months. The routine administration of Clomiphene to any patient with amenorrhoea who is thought to have enlarged ovaries is to be deplored.

Diseases of the Pituitary

It is difficult to separate the hypothalamus from the pituitary, and these two structures should be considered in association.

The sensitivity of the hypothalamus to higher cortical influence is well known and amenorrhoea of hypothalamic type is seen in emotional and depressive states and as a result of shock, stress and fear. Certain organic lesions occurring in the brain may affect the hypothalamus, such as a cerebral tumour, encephalitis, meningitis; and a fractured base of the skull may involve the region of the pituitary fossa. These lesions are all rare causes of amenorrhoea.

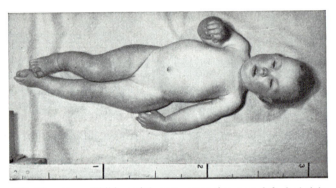

Fig. 212. Gigantism. Child aged 1 year, measuring over 3 ft. in height.

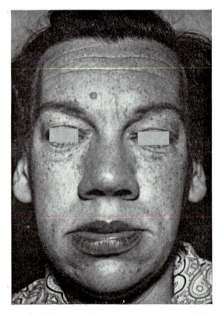

Fig. 213. Acromegaly. Note the broad enlargement of the nose and coarse facies.

Acidophil cell tumour of the pituitary produces an excess of somatotropic hormone. If this operates before epiphyseal closure, *gigantism* results (Fig. 212); if after, acromegaly. In the early stages there is no alteration in the

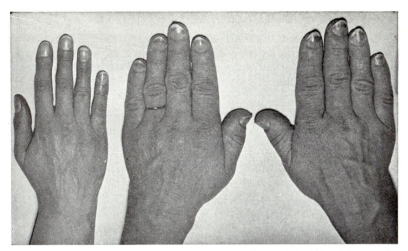

FIG. 214. Acromegaly. Hands from the same patient as Fig. 213, with control on the left.

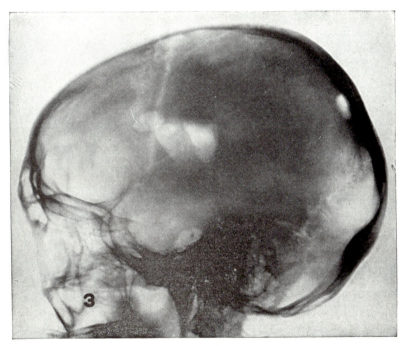

FIG. 215. X-ray of pituitary fossa, showing extreme bony expansion due to pituitary tumour.

menstrual functions, but when the tumour infiltrates into and destroys the basophil cells the patient develops amenorrhoea (Figs. 213, 214 and 215).

Fröhlich's syndrome consists of lethargy, obesity, genital hypoplasia and amenorrhoea. In the Laurence-Moon-Biedl syndrome polydactyly, retinitis pigmentosa and mental deficiency are additional features to the dystrophia adiposo-genitalis (see Fig. 216).

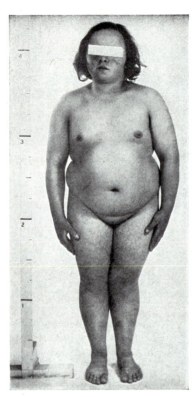

FIG. 216. Fröhlich's syndrome.

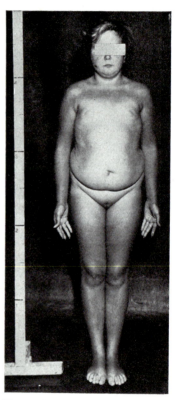

FIG. 217. Pituitary infantilism—patient aged 17. Note obesity, aplasia of breasts, absence of pubic hair and short stature.

Pituitary infantilism is a condition of retarded sexual and physical development (Lorain's syndrome) (Fig. 217) and is sometimes associated with the presence of progeria or premature ageing. Pituitary dwarfs are deficient in growth factor but gonadotropic functions are normal.

Simmond's disease or pituitary cachexia is the corollary of an arterial thrombosis of the pituitary following haemorrhage and shock of obstetric origin. In the fully developed case all pituitary function is depressed so that the syndrome consists of frigidity, amenorrhoea and loss of thyrotropic hormone. The patient is lethargic and poikilothermic. The blood sugar is lowered. In some cases there is not loss of weight and no wasting, though this feature is often included in the syndrome. Axillary and pubic hair is lost and the uterus on bimanual examination is hypoplastic. Skin pigmentation is also deficient, but the patient will often show areas of erythema *ab igne* where in an attempt to keep warm she has burned her legs in front of the fire. This condition, when following a post-partum haemorrhage, is often called Sheehan's syndrome.

Cushing's disease must be distinguished from Cushing's syndrome. Cushing's disease is due perhaps to a basophil adenoma of the anterior pituitary which leads to hyperfunction of the suprarenal cortex. The main symptoms and signs are those due to a disorder of the suprarenal which are now referred to under the term Cushing's syndrome. This condition is described below. An interesting example of pituitary dysfunction leading to amenorrhoea is the Chiari-Frommel syndrome. Amenorrhoea, persistent galactorrhoea, obesity and headache occur after delivery. F.S.H. excretion is diminished while luteotropic hormone is increased, leading to continued lactogenic stimulation. The occasional finding of expansion of the pituitary fossa on X-ray suggests an acidophil adenoma as a possible cause and this may later lead to narrowing of the visual fields.

Disorders of the Adrenal Gland

In *Addison's disease* the hormones secreted by the suprarenal cortex are greatly reduced and in due course are not produced at all. The 17-ketosteroid excretion is reduced to a minimum. The late phases of the disease are associated with weakness, gastro-intestinal upset, emaciation, pigmentation, lowered blood pressure and basal metabolic rate, genital atrophy and amenorrhoea.

Tumours of the adrenal cortex lead to an excessive production of the suprarenal hormones so that the 17-ketosteroids excreted in the urine may be raised from the normal limit of about 15 mg. to as much as 300 mg. in twenty-four hours.

Cushing's syndrome is usually associated with a tumour or with hyperplasia of the suprarenal cortex, as a result of which the corticosteroid hormones are produced in excess. An abnormal amount of protein is converted into carbohydrate so that the patients have thin skins with well-marked striae and the skin bruises easily. The muscles show weakness. Osteoporosis can usually be demonstrated and patients may develop an insulin resistant diabetes, polycythaemia, hypertension and amenorrhoea. Hirsutism and the virilising sign of hypertrophy of the clitoris, though often present, are not invariable. Obesity is usually well marked (Figs. 218 and 219).

In the *adrenogenital syndrome*, which is quite distinct from Cushing's syndrome, the suprarenal androgenic hormone is produced in excess, either through hyperplasia or tumour formation. Cases are seen both in juveniles and in adults. There is well-marked hirsutism, the voice becomes deep and sometimes there is loss of hair on the head. Acne may develop on the face, and the musculature of the body increases to become masculine in type. The clitoris hypertrophies. 17-ketosteroid excretion in the urine is greatly increased. Amenorrhoea is invariable, and the uterus and breasts atrophy.

Diseases of the Thyroid

In cretinism and childhood myxoedema the child sometimes suffers from amenorrhoea. In many cases, the onset of menstruation is delayed, and when

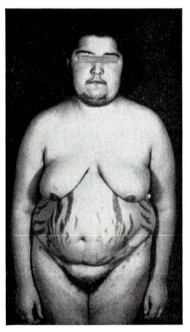

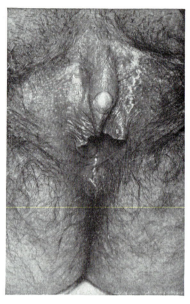

Fig. 218. Cushing's syndrome. Note hirsutism of face, obesity and striae.

Fig. 219. Vulva from patient with Cushing's syndrome showing hypertrophy of clitoris.

menstruation does occur it is irregular and scanty (Fig. 220). In adult myxoedema the patient may suffer from amenorrhoea but many patients suffer from menorrhagia, particularly if the myxoedema is post-operative (Fig. 221). In severe hyperthyroidism menstruation is suppressed, scanty, or irregular.

Diabetes Mellitus

In adolescence, diabetes is associated with amenorrhoea and genital hypoplasia in a large number of patients—perhaps as many as 50%. Unless diagnosed and controlled early, the amenorrhoea may persist and permanent infertility result.

Amenorrhoea due to General Diseases

Most patients of this group are under the care of general physicians, and the gynaecologist is called in to determine the cause of associated amenorrhoea. Carcinoma, severe anaemias, and advanced tuberculosis sometimes cause amenorrhoea. In mental disease, amenorrhoea is common. In gynaecological practice these cases are of no great importance, for the amenorrhoea is always overshadowed by the severity of the primary disease.

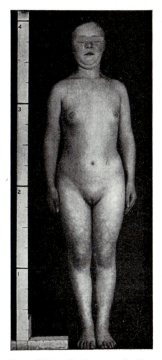

FIG. 220. Cretin, aged 20. Note the facies, aplasia of the breasts and absence of pubic hair.

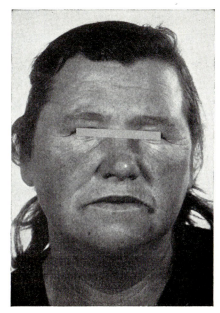

FIG. 221. Myxoedema. Note stolid facies and loss of eyebrow hair.

Malnutrition

Malnutrition is an important cause of amenorrhoea, as the World Wars have shown, and was very noticeable in nurses interned in the Far East. *Anorexia nervosa* provides a good example of nutritional and psychosomatic amenorrhoea. This syndrome is associated with extreme emaciation and distaste for food; the blood pressure is low and the fractional test meal shows achlorhydria. Muscular weakness and atrophy, genital atrophy and lowered basal metabolic rate are features. Amenorrhoea appears early, often before the emaciation is fully developed, and persists after the patient has been restored to a normal diet (Fig. 222).

Change in environment, and climate or altitude especially if associated with stress, often produces amenorrhoea in young students, nurses and country girls who seek employment in sedentary urban jobs. It was commonly seen in the women's Services in the last war.

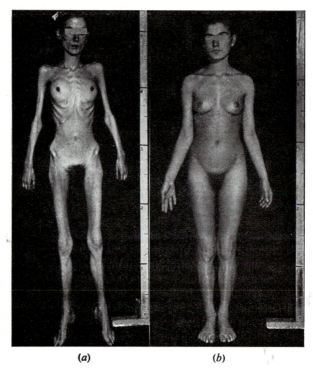

(a)   (b)

FIG. 222. (a) Anorexia nervosa; (b) the same patient after six weeks' treatment.

Amenorrhoea Due to Chromosomal Anomalies

(1) Sex chromosome monosomy (X O) has already been mentioned under Turner's syndrome. Such patients are obviously amenorrhoeic.

(2) There are two well known varieties of sex chromosome trisomy, one of which is associated with amenorrhoea:

(a) Kleinefelter's syndrome XXY in which the phenotype is male. In spite of the gynaecomastia the patient is unlikely to be wrongly sexed though the buccal smear will be chromatin positive.

(b) The super female (trisomy X or XXX) is known to be associated with secondary amenorrhoea in certain instances, although this chromosomal anomaly can be found in otherwise normal parous females.

There is no doubt that chromosome studies will play a much more important part in the future investigation of unexplained problems of amenorrhoea and infertility. Jacobs in 1961 found abnormal chromosomes in 22%

of 68 patients referred to a gynaecologist complaining of primary amenorrhoea.

Investigation and Diagnosis

A thorough general examination of the patient should first be made and the presence of systemic disease excluded. Hyperthyroidism and hypothyroidism should be excluded, and if necessary the basal metabolic rate should be estimated. Absence of secondary sex characters and failure of axillary and pubic hair to develop is suggestive either of pituitary infantilism or Turner's syndrome. Hirsutism, associated with amenorrhoea, suggests an adrenogenital syndrome or a virilising ovarian tumour. The degree of development of hair on the body, however, varies enormously, even in healthy individuals, and many women with well-marked hirsutism are otherwise perfectly healthy. Adiposity without striae and hirsutism suggests a Fröhlich type of syndrome, whereas adiposity associated with striae is indicative of Cushing's syndrome. The next step is to make a pelvic examination either vaginally or rectally. It may be necessary to make this examination with the patient anaesthetised. The state of the vulva and vagina should be noted, as the development of these organs provides a reliable index of ovarian function. Poorly developed labia and a thin, glazed vaginal epithelium with absence of rugae suggest ovarian subfunction. Such abnormalities as imperforate hymen, stenosis of the vagina and stenosis of the cervix can be recognised. Similarly, the size of the uterus determined if necessary by the passage of a sound and any abnormality in the size of the ovaries can be detected. A simple clinical investigation of this kind combined with knowledge of the possible diseases which cause amenorrhoea should enable the diagnosis to be made with a moderate degree of precision.

Further investigations should be undertaken:—

(*a*) **Radiological examination of the chest** will exclude pulmonary tuberculosis and should always be performed in cases of amenorrhoea.

(*b*) **An X-ray of the pituitary fossa** is usually taken, but the findings are nearly always negative.

(*c*) **A glucose tolerance test** is performed.

(*d*) **Protein Bound Iodine Test** and I.[131] uptake should be estimated in every case of suspected thyroid dysfunction. These are low in cases of hypothyroidism secondary to pituitary dysfunction.

(*e*) **Blood cholesterol estimations.** Deviation from the normal reading of 180—250 mg. per cent. suggests thyroid dysfunction.

(*f*) **Water excretion tests and sodium and potassium estimations** may be helpful in cases of adrenal cortical dysfunction.

(*g*) **A diagnostic curettage** may be combined with the examination under anaesthesia. This will give some idea of the response of the endometrium to ovarian activity, e.g. absence of any curettings suggests ovarian subfunction. Genital tuberculosis may be unsuspectedly diagnosed in this way.

(*h*) **Hystero-salpingography** may furnish evidence of genital hypoplasia where ordinary clinical methods are not conclusive.

(*i*) **Vaginal smears** provide a further method of assaying ovarian function—

evidence of good oestrogen function being shown by well-keratinised epithelial cells with small dark-staining nuclei. The cytoplasm is essentially eosinophilic.

(*j*) **Hormonal Assays.** The value of these is limited by the fact that only a few large laboratories are prepared to undertake them, and there is little standardisation of the results obtained by different workers. Urinary gonadotropin is increased in pregnancy, and to a lesser extent at the menopause, and in some cases of primary ovarian failure; it is reduced in cases of pituitary failure such as Simmond's disease.

Oestrogen excretion in the urine is increased in pregnancy and with feminising tumours, and reduced in case of primary ovarian failure, at the menopause and with virilising tumours of the adrenal and ovary, and in Cushing's syndrome. Pregnandiol excretion roughly follows the behaviour of urinary oestrogen and is especially raised in pregnancy.

17-*Ketosteroids*. The average range of excretion is 5—15 mg. in the twenty-four hours, and this may be increased to 50—100 mg. and over in virilising states, such as adrenal cortical over-activity or tumour—adrenogenital syndrome. In pituitary basophilism and arrhenoblastoma it is increased to a lesser extent.

Follicle stimulating hormone levels will be low in pituitary failure and normal in ovarian or uterine deficiency.

(*k*) **The response of the endometrium** to synthetic oestrogen—ethinyl oestradiol 0·05 mg. or stilboestrol 1 mg. *twice* daily for twenty-one days—can be tested. If oestrogen withdrawal bleeding does not occur after one or two trials the endometrium can be considered to be refractory.

(*l*) **Culdoscopy or peritoneoscopy** is particularly useful in the diagnosis of the Stein-Leventhal syndrome.

(*m*) **X-ray gynaecography** using the peritoneal insufflation of carbon dioxide can be similarly employed to demonstrate the Stein-Leventhal ovary, though it is not as conclusive as culdoscopy or peritoneoscopy.

The treatment of amenorrhoea with drugs which induce ovulation is described on page 482.

INFREQUENT AND SCANTY MENSTRUATION

The Greek prefix *hypo* suggests subnormality. Unfortunately, most authors use the term hypomenorrhoea both to describe a menstrual loss less than normal and, also, a cycle less frequent than normal so that the terms hypomenorrhoea and oligomenorrhoea have become synonymous and meaningless. It is, therefore, more precise to use the terms *scanty menstruation* or subnormal menstrual loss to describe a period that is regular but small. When the intermenstrual interval is increased and the cycle is abnormally lengthened, the term *infrequent menstruation* is accurate and descriptive.

INFREQUENT MENSTRUATION

In this condition, the intermenstrual cycle is prolonged beyond the normal twenty-eight days. Some women have a perfectly normal cycle at thirty-five days and, for them, no pathological interpretation is necessary since their fertility is unimpaired. Genuinely infrequent menstruation should only be diagnosed when the cycle is quite erratic or unduly prolonged, sometimes to three or four months or even longer. It is most frequently seen at the menarche and at the menopause and can be regarded as a form of modified amenorrhoea. It is not, however, incompatible with a normal reproductive capacity within the limits of its own infrequent ovulation. In the pathological variety of this condition, the causes and findings on clinical and special investigation resemble those of amenorrhoea and the patient is, therefore, often obese, hirsute, has poorly developed secondary sexual characteristics and hypoplasia of the genitalia. In this variety, the most usual and constant finding is one of ovarian subfunction. As a rule, these patients require no treatment apart from diet and reassurance.

SCANTY MENSTRUATION

In some patients menstruation only lasts one to two days and the loss may be so small as merely to require the changing of one or two diapers. Scanty menstruation which occurs regularly is not necessarily pathological since its regularity at least presupposes a normal pituitary ovarian cycle, nor are these patients necessarily infertile. If, therefore, the secondary sexual characteristics are normal and there is no sign of any general or local disease, the condition can be dismissed by reassurance and without any treatment. If, however, scanty menstruation is accompanied by infrequency of the periods, it suggests a primary or secondary ovarian subfunction, depending on whether the patient has always had scanty and infrequent periods or whether, having previously menstruated regularly and in normal amount, her recent menstrual behaviour has become erratic and the loss small or negligible. These symptoms suggest an ovarian failure and a premature menopause. The investigation and treatment is the same as for primary or secondary amenorrhoea. These patients and their relatives are always obsessed with the sinister import of deficient or irregular menstruation. To the lay mind these symptoms suggest grave constitutional, local and sometimes mental disease. In fact, an anxiety neurosis can easily be engendered. It is, therefore, of first importance that they be assured on this point to their complete satisfaction.

PREMENSTRUAL TENSION

Many women experience premenstrual symptoms seven to ten days before the onset of bleeding; irritability, lassitude, malaise, headache, gastro-intestinal upsets such as colon spasm and constipation, frequency of micturition, and a feeling of fullness in the breasts, abdomen, face and feet. In patients with introspective tendencies all these symptoms become exaggerated and form a well-marked psychosomatic disorder. In some cases there is demonstrable water retention and a weight gain of between 2 or 3 lb. up to 10 lb. can be measured; this is accompanied by actual oedema of the legs and is especially marked in those patients who have had a previous phlebo-thrombosis. The breast symptoms are particularly marked and give rise to a feeling of fullness, weight and tenderness. The breast on examination feels hard and lumpy and is tender to the examining hand. Some patients suffer from a type of migraine which is most noticeable in the premenstrual phase and disappears with pregnancy.

The aetiology of this syndrome is obscure and it has been suggested that the constant factor is an increase in the extracellular water throughout the body, possibly due to excessive oestrogen production, or to some cyclical disturbance of adrenal cortical function. Oestrogen is recognised to produce water and sodium retention, e.g. when given in large doses for carcinoma of the prostate, but this theory is criticised on the grounds that it is not seen in cases of excessive oestrogen production such as granulosa cell tumours and metropathia haemorrhagica. Adrenal cortical steroids, and possibly progesterone, may have a similar effect on water retention, so that it is not necessarily oestrogen that is at fault. Progestogen containing-contraceptive pills are notorious promoters of water retention.

The treatment of the condition therefore depends on the elimination of excessive extracellular fluid by a limited water intake and a salt-free diet for the ten days preceding menstruation. Saline purgatives, ammonium chloride and more powerful diuretics such as chlorthiazide in a single daily dose of 250 mg. or more from the onset of the symptoms until menstruation is established have been used with success. Other workers claim that large doses of progesterone have a beneficial effect, and in certain cases methyl testosterone 10 mg. daily in the last half of the cycle has proved useful. This therapy is difficult to explain scientifically since it is directly contradictory to the above-mentioned theory of water retention. For the congestion of the breasts adequate support is essential, and fluid restriction and elimination is probably the best treatment. For menstrual migraine ergotamine tartrate in fairly large doses by mouth up to a total maximum of 10 mg. is the most effective, but this dose must not be exceeded because of the dangers of peripheral vascular spasm, an ever-present danger with all the alkaloids of ergot.

It should be mentioned here that certain patients suffer from acne on the body and face and other mild skin eruptions in association with menstruation. The treatment of these conditions is unsatisfactory. The main importance of the premenstrual tension is psychosomatic. It often affects the highly strung, introspective and neurotic woman. The discomfort of headache and mastalgia becomes exaggerated into an obsession of serious nervous disease or cancer. The patient becomes short-tempered and is difficult to live with so that matrimonial and family harmony is disturbed. For the potential suicide, this time of extreme depression can be an actual danger. It has even been stated that the female crime rate rises in the premenstrual phase of the cycle. In treating the syndrome, much patience and reassurance is needed. In some, amphetamine in small doses and, in others, phenobarbitone will be needed; therapeutic experiment will usually decide the proper drug. Hysterectomy or an artificially induced menopause is not to be recommended though the patient may earnestly request it.

DYSMENORRHOEA

Dysmenorrhoea, or painful menstruation, is one of the most frequent of gynaecological complaints, and there is reason to believe that its incidence becomes higher with the degree of civilisation of the community. Severe dysmenorrhoea is most prevalent in young single women leading sedentary lives, and its frequency has some economic importance, for the patients are often incapacitated from work for one or more days during each period. Although dysmenorrhoea should not be regarded as a serious affection, its treatment is of great importance to the practising physician in view of the interruption in the patient's economic and social life, not to mention the important psychological effects.

The usual method of classifying the different types of dysmenorrhoea is to identify three groups:—

> Congestive.
> Spasmodic.
> Membranous.

Congestive Dysmenorrhoea. This takes the form of premenstrual pain situated either in the back or lower abdomen, occurring between three and five days and sometimes even longer before the onset of menstruation; it is always relieved by the menstrual flow. Congestive dysmenorrhoea should in the first instance be regarded as a concomitant symptom of pelvic disease, and if the typical history is obtained some pelvic abnormality may well be found. Inflammatory diseases such as salpingo-oöphoritis, parametritis and pelvic adhesions almost always produce the symptoms of congestive dysmenorrhoea, probably because the ovaries are hyperaemic and covered by adhesions from the inflammatory lesions so that they become tense during the premenstrual phase of the menstrual cycle. Congestive dysmenorrhoea is a common symptom of certain myomata, of chocolate cysts of the ovaries, of adenomyomata and acquired retroversion of the uterus. Not all patients, however, who suffer from congestive dysmenorrhoea have an organic basis to account for their pain. The premenstrual congestion or tension syndrome is one good example of this. In others, quite a large number, the pain or discomfort is referred to one or other iliac fossa, usually the left, and it is accompanied by an alteration in bowel habit, usually constipation, with some flatulent distension of the upper colon. The basis here is a colon spasm and the descending colon can be palpated as a tender, obviously spastic, segment. Barium enema confirms this finding. Quite strong aperients are taken in the mistaken idea that purgation will relieve the spasm whereas, in practice, it aggravates it. The real cause of the condition is a sympathetic parasympathetic imbalance, influenced by the cyclical changes in the adjacent genital tract. The correct treatment is diet and the avoidance of excess carbohydrate and strong purgatives, and some antispasmodic drug that acts on the bowel such as Buscopan or Probanthine. Exercise is important for these patients since they are usually sedentary office workers.

Spasmodic Dysmenorrhoea. The majority of cases of dysmenorrhoea fall into this group, and it is probable that nearly 50% of the adult female population suffer at some time from varying degrees of this symptom, though less than 10% will seek medical advice. With congestive dysmenorrhoea the symptom is masked by others which are more prominent in the disease.

For example, with inflammatory pelvic lesions discharge, abdominal pain, and menorrhagia are more dominating symptoms than congestive dysmenorrhoea. It can, therefore, be taken as a principle that if a patient's main complaint is dysmenorrhoea, the dysmenorrhoea is most likely to be of the spasmodic type. The typical patient's history is very characteristic. The pain develops on the first day of the menstrual period, when excruciating pain is experienced which lasts for a relatively short time, perhaps for half an hour to an hour. This very severe pain is intermittent and spasmodic, and may cause faintness, collapse, vomiting or nausea. A mild degree of shock may follow upon a very severe attack. The severe attack of pain is followed by a similar but less pronounced type of pain, felt in the lower abdomen and pelvis, and often down the antero-medial area of the thighs. Such pain persists for not usually more than 12 hours.

It is important to realise that there is much variation in the type of pain experienced by patients with spasmodic dysmenorrhoea. Sometimes considerable discomfort starts on the day before the menstrual flow and may persist after the actual severe pain has lessened for more than 12—24 hours. Similarly, premenstrual pain may be complained of, either in the back or lower abdomen, which leads up to the excruciating pain felt on the first day of the period. It is wrong, however, to regard such cases as being of the congestive dysmenorrhoea type. They represent variations of spasmodic dysmenorrhoea. The severity of the pain varies greatly. Sometimes it is extremely severe, causing well-marked shock and incapacitating the woman from her employment. The best method of determining the severity of the pain is to enquire into the symptoms of faintness, vomiting, and the degree to which the patient is incapacitated.

In true spasmodic dysmenorrhoea, the condition does not become established until two or three years after the menarche (that is, the severe pain of dysmenorrhoea) though there may be a degree of discomfort associated with earlier periods. There is a well-defined group of patients where menstruation is painless until about the age of 18 or 19, when very severe pain develops. The significance of these cases is great, since it is known that the monthly loss during the first few years of menstruation is often due simply to oestrogen withdrawal, the cycles being anovulatory. It will be shown later that suppression of ovulation by oestrogens can be used to produce a painless period. It can therefore be concluded that in these cases the dysmenorrhoea is coincident with ovulatory cycles, and it is the secretion and withdrawal of progesterone that is responsible for the pain. Probably the most severe forms are seen in patients between the ages of 19 and 21. It is rare to encounter severe spasmodic dysmenorrhoea in women over the age of 35. For some reason dysmenorrhoea becomes less severe about that time, and it is exceptional for the excruciating pain to persist after that age, although the less severe pain lasting during the first day of the period usually persists until the woman approaches menopausal age.

Spasmodic dysmenorrhoea is usually cured by pregnancy, and exceptions to this rule are infrequent. A woman who has only one child is more likely to develop a recurrence of spasmodic dysmenorrhoea than a woman who gives birth to several children. Dysmenorrhoea is often cured by marriage, and almost all married women will say that they have not suffered so much from dysmenorrhoea since their marriage. It is, however, much too optimistic to advise a patient that she is certain to be free of dysmenorrhoea if she marries or if she has a baby and, in fact, this dangerous advice of therapeutic marriage should never be given if only out of consideration for the unfortunate male victim of the treatment.

Some degree of menstrual irregularity is not uncommon with spasmodic dysmenorrhoea. Sometimes the onset of puberty is delayed, and the menstrual cycle is a little irregular. In spasmodic dysmenorrhoea the amount lost during each period is less than the average, and not infrequently patients give a history that the severe pain is relieved by the passage of a clot. It is interesting that patients who are sterile do not usually give a history of spasmodic dysmenorrhoea. It should be noted that anovular cycles are painless.

Aetiology

The exact aetiology of spasmodic dysmenorrhoea is unknown. Some light has been shed, however, on the responsibility of progesterone secretion and withdrawal for spasmodic dysmenorrhoea in ovulatory cycles. Under the influence of progesterone and its withdrawal, uterine contractions of considerable intensity occur, and at the peak of these contractions the intrauterine pressure has been shown to exceed the systolic blood pressure, so that uterine ischaemia results (Moir). It is customary to group the causes into (1) Disorders of Structure, and (2) Disorders of Function.

Disorders of Structure. *Uterine Hypoplasia* has, in the past, been given pride of place as a causative factor. The condition is rare and usually associated with ovarian deficiency and amenorrhoea when it does exist. As a clinical entity, it has been grossly exaggerated if it exists at all in the normally menstruating patient. Similarly, the congenital acutely anteflexed or cochleate uterus and the congenitally retroverted uterus have been unfairly regarded as a cause of dysmenorrhoea. There is no observed or scientific evidence to support the hypoplasia theory. In fact, the only time a uterus is hypoplastic is at the menarche and at this time menstruation is usually painless.

Maldevelopment. If the uterus is bi-cornuate or septate, or if an accessory cornu is present, severe spasmodic dysmenorrhoea is fairly frequent.

Disorders of Function. (1) *Deficient Polarity.* When the body of the uterus contracts the cervix normally dilates, and, conversely, when the cervix is forcibly dilated, as for example as a result of introduction of dilators into the cervical canal, the body of the uterus contracts. The term polarity is applied to this coordinate association between contractions of the body of the uterus and dilatation of the cervix. It has been suggested that the polarity of the uterus is disturbed with spasmodic dysmenorrhoea, so that there is difficulty in the discharge of menstrual blood through the cervix.

It seems to be well established that all cycles with concomitant dysmenorrhoea are ovulatory, while with non-ovulatory cycles the period is painless, so that, if the theory of deficient polarity is accepted, progesterone must in some way influence neuro-muscular incoordination.

(2) *Inadequate liquefaction of the menstrual clot*. It has been somewhat fancifully suggested that deficiency of thrombolysin causes failure of menstrual clots to become liquefied, and that the consequent passage of these clots through the cervical canal causes menstrual pain. Others maintain that the enzyme normally secreted by the endometrium during menstruation is deficient, so that the endometrium is discharged into the cavity of the uterus in the form of shreds or, in cases of membranous dysmenorrhoea, as membranes or even as casts of the endometrium. It is true that with membranous dysmenorrhoea such casts are characteristically discharged. The pain is caused by distension of the uterus, either with menstrual blood or perhaps by large haemorrhages into the endometrium. The pain should therefore be regarded as uterine. If a patient has a fibroid polypus which is in process of extrusion through the cervical canal, a type of uterine colic may develop. This somewhat resembles the painful contractions of labour or abortion. It is questionable, however, if the small clots of menstruation can evoke this violent, colicky reaction and so explain the pain of dysmenorrhoea.

(3) *The Ischaemic Theory*. This explains spasmodic dysmenorrhoea as being a painful cramp due to myometrial ischaemia resulting from spasm somewhat similar to the cramps associated with vascular spasm or occlusion in other parts of the body, e.g. Buerger's disease or myocardial insufficiency. In other words it is a myometrial angina. The main basis of this hypothetical explanation is that spasmodic dysmenorrhoea is cured by childbirth which improves the blood supply of the myometrium and incidentally dilates the cervix, usually permanently. The histology of the myometrium of the multiparous uterus which shows considerable vascular degeneration and occlusion certainly does not support the ischaemic theory, since no grand multipara ever had spasmodic dysmenorrhoea.

(4) *Hormonal Imbalance Theory*. It can be reasonably accepted that only ovular menstruation is painful since, if an anovulatory period is produced by inhibiting the F.S.H. of the anterior pituitary with oestrogen, previously painful periods are painless. This painlessness of the periods lasts as long as the treatment is continued and the dysmenorrhoea recurs on cessation of oestrogen administration. It can be proved that the bleeding is anovulatory by taking an endometrial biopsy just before or at the time of bleeding when no secretory change is found in the endometrium on histological examination. Conversely, if a patient with spasmodic dysmenorrhoea is curetted in the premenstrual phase, secretory endometrium is always found. It can be logically deduced that progesterone is in some way responsible for the pain of dysmenorrhoea and it is suggested that this hormone enhances the force of myometrial contraction so that it reaches the threshold level of conscious pain. Tocometric studies of the uterine contractions at the late progestational phase support this theory as the amplitude of uterine contractions is demonstrably increased.

(5) *Psychosomatic Overlay*. The importance of the psychological aspect of dysmenorrhoea cannot be over-estimated. Misdirected parental influence, supplied by a mother or other female relative who is, herself, a sufferer from dysmenorrhoea, tends inevitably to condition the child to the acceptance and

association of pain with menstruation. The taboo of uncleanliness inherited from Mosaic tradition and the restriction of social and physical activity tend to confer an idea of ill-health upon a natural and physiological process. A feeling of shame and disgust soon encroaches upon the youthful and susceptible mind. The common appellation of "the curse" is a typical example of this attitude. Two types of personality particularly prone to dysmenorrhoea will serve as examples: (i) The Atalanta or tomboy personality—slightly virile, sport-loving, superficially matter-of-fact or even aggressive, resenting the process of menstruation as a bore, a nuisance and an enforced limitation of physical activities, inclined to frigidity and certainly not yet interested in the opposite sex. (ii) The immature, shy, self-conscious, parent-fixed, unself-reliant, spoiled and ready to use menstruation as an escape from unpleasant school or other duties. In this second personality group, menstruation provides a wonderful opportunity for blackmailing parents, teachers and employers into a sympathy that is both comforting and comfortable. "The poor child does suffer so with her unwell times" that she must go and lie down with a hot water bottle; school is quite out of the question, the office must be telephoned at once, aspirin procured and the doctor sent for to provide the necessary certificate. The least discomfort becomes an intolerable pain and solicitous relatives propagate the vicious syndrome. In these girls with a large functional overlay, psychological rehabilitation is all-important in the treatment of this dysmenorrhoea.

Diagnosis

It has already been emphasised that spasmodic dysmenorrhoea not infrequently departs from the classical type. Severe dysmenorrhoea occurring either during or about the time of a period in young women should be regarded as spasmodic. A rectal examination should be made to determine that the genital tract is anatomically normal and in order to reassure the patient and her mother that there is definitely no physical abnormality. A vaginal examination should be limited to those in whom it is feasible and acceptable.

Treatment

It has already been stated that dysmenorrhoea is almost invariably improved after marriage and it is usually cured by childbirth. Vaginal operations upon the uterus and cervix should be avoided so far as possible in young girls, for after such operations the patients may develop introspection about their pelvic organs. It follows that treatment in young women should be directed along general lines, and every effort should be made to treat the patient symptomatically rather than to adopt operative measures. Of course there are exceptions. With very severe pain the incapacity may be so great that operations are justified even in young patients, but such cases are very rare. Much help can be given by a sensible and sympathetic attitude on the part of the practitioner and his convincing assurance that, on pelvic examination, there is no anatomical abnormality. Many of these young patients have a lurking fear that they are abnormal, and they cannot or should not marry, and that, if they do, they will be sterile. On all these points verbal contra-diction is necessary.

General treatment is of great importance. Open-air exercise, games and gymnastic exercises should be encouraged. Constipation should be treated by simple laxatives and anaemia, if it should be present, which is very rare, treated with iron. It is always difficult to suggest means whereby the patient's attention is diverted from her menstrual functions, but much can be done by a sensible mother.

In addition to the general treatment other methods are necessary during the attack of acute pain. Aspirin, phenacetin and codeine are the most valuable drugs to give during the pain. While it is necessary to use large doses at the onset of the severe pain, it is obvious that repeated medication with drugs of this kind, except during the maximum intensity of the pain, is both unnecessary and dangerous. The most remarkable results are perhaps obtained by the injection of atropine at the onset of the severe pain, but the method cannot be widely employed in practice because the medical attendant cannot be available at a moment's notice. The administration of belladonna before and during the menstrual period does not give good results. Atropine or buscopan given by mouth in tablet form is occasionally of some value.

In practice it is found that the results obtained from a particular drug are less pronounced with succeeding menstrual periods and it is necessary to change the analgesic every few months. Other drugs, in addition to those already mentioned, are frequently employed, particularly the different members of the barbiturate group, and the medical practitioner will usually find that there is a well-marked idiosyncrasy with each particular patient. Morphia and pethidine are always to be avoided, however severe the case, because of the risk of the development of addiction. A popular remedy is alcohol, in the form of gin or whisky, and hot baths are sometimes of service. With young people the principle of treatment is to employ these temporary palliative measures until the patient is of marriageable age. A 10 mg. dose of amphetamine sulphate (benzedrine) given at the onset of menstruation will benefit roughly half the patients suffering from dysmenorrhoea, and the same dose can be repeated in four hours. It is, however, a drug to be used with the utmost caution, since it is habit producing and may lead to addiction.

It is well known that if sufficient oestrogens are given to a patient during the first half of the menstrual cycle, ovulation is inhibited so that the succeed-ing menstrual period is painless because it belongs to a non-ovulatory cycle. The principle of treatment is to give the correct dose of stilboestrol or other synthetic oestrogen during three weeks commencing with the fifth day of men-struation. The first difficulty is to find the correct dose sufficient to inhibit ovulation. The exact dose required depends upon the individual patient and can be determined only by trial. 1 mg. of stilboestrol three times a day should produce an anovular period in over 90% of patients. Treatment should be started on the fifth day of the cycle and must be continued for twenty-one days. The production of anovular cycles is not to be continued indefinitely but is useful for some special occasions, e.g. an important engagement.

Similar results can be achieved by the cyclical use of the contraceptive pill, although some patients will resist this treatment.

The ordinary synthetic oestrogens are only effective for producing ano-vulatory and painless cycles in over 90% of patients. More potent drugs have recently been introduced of which Enavid is one example. It is a synthetic steroid consisting of nor-ethynodrel (17α-ethinyl-17 hydroxy-5(10)-oestren-3-one) with 1·5% of ethinyloestradiol 3 methyl ether. Its oestrogenic activity is equivalent to that of oestrone but the drug is essentially a potent, orally active progestational steroid. It is a most effective inhibitor of ovulation, and withdrawal bleeding is a less troublesome complication than with the syn-thetic oestrogens. The dosage is one 10 mg. tablet daily from the 5th to the 24th day of the cycle for three cycles. Surprisingly, 68% of patients have been reported as free from pain six months after cessation of treatment and this can be attributed to the psychological benefit of having controlled the pain during treatment, since subsequent cycles are ovulatory and potentially painful.

In older patients, women above the age of 20, operative treatment is some-times indicated.

Dilatation of the Cervix. Dilatation should be performed under anaesthesia, with the patient lying in the lithotomy position. The patient is prepared in the ordinary way for a vaginal operation. The vagina is swabbed out and a Sims' speculum introduced. The cervix is drawn down by means of a volsellum forceps attached to the anterior lip of the cervix. The cervix is again swabbed. A uterine sound is now passed into the cervical canal. If the os is narrow, difficulty may be experienced in passing the sound. In such cases it is necessary to pass a small blunt-pointed probe or a very small Hegar dilator to find the direction of the uterine canal. The cervix is then dilated slowly with metal Hegar dilators. The dilatation must be performed slowly as far as a No. 10-12 Hegar or Fenton dilator. If force is used, the cervix may split or the dilator may be pushed through the posterior surface of the uterus into the peritoneal cavity. If the cervix is split there is immediate severe haemorrhage, and if the laceration spreads laterally it may injure the uterine artery and a large broad ligament haematoma may result, which may in some cases burrow upwards into the perinephric region. If the cervix is damaged during the dilatation a lacerated cervix, with ectropion, chronic cervicitis, and discharge, may be the end-result of the operation and incompetence of the internal cervical os is an additional recently recognised hazard. Perforation of the uterus with a dilator is the result of carelessness and bad technique. Fortunately there is little risk of peritonitis if the case is clean, and it is not necessary to perform a laparo-tomy. The patient, however, should be watched carefully during the next few days to ensure that peritonitis is not developing. In practice it will be found that the dilatation of the cervix is relatively simple until a dilator of about size No. 10 Hegar is introduced. A No. 11 dilator is introduced only with difficulty, and during its passage the cervical tissues will usually be felt to tear. If the introduction is performed slowly and carefully no harm will result. It is unnecessary to keep the patient in bed after the operation and she should be discharged from hospital the next day. Dilatation of the cervix should not be regarded as a certain cure of dysmenorrhoea, and it is important to indicate the doubtful prognosis to the patient's relatives when the operation is advised. Even when the operation is performed carefully, permanent cure is obtained in about 25% of cases. Most patients are much better for about six months after the operation, when the pain may recur with modified severity. In the remainder little or no benefit is experienced from the operation. It is difficult to understand why dilatation of the cervix should cure the pain in spasmodic dysmenorrhoea. It is obvious that a clear passageway through the uterus to the vagina will allow the menstrual discharge to drain more efficiently than when the cervical canal is small and this may eliminate uterine spasm. It is also possible that the dilatation disrupts the circum-cervical nerve plexus and thus blocks the afferent pathway for pain. These rather specious theories are purely hypothetical.

If, after dilatation of the cervix, pain is relieved temporarily but recurs in six to twelve months, it is sometimes justifiable to repeat the operation as the second dilatation sometimes controls the pain.

Other Operations. As the operation of dilatation of the cervix is only rarely a satisfactory method of treatment various other operations have been suggested.

Presacral sympathectomy in the treatment of spasmodic dysmenorrhoea has been occasionally advocated and employed, though all gynaecologists will agree that it is only justifiable after all other methods, including one or two dilatations, have failed. It should be reserved for those patients who are genuinely anxious to overcome their disability and in whom the dysmenor-rhoea is a serious menace to their health and employment. The neurotic and introspective are never candidates for this operation. The abdomen is opened by a low transverse incision (Pfannenstiel) with the patient lying in the Trendelenberg position. Retractors are inserted into the wound and the intestines packed away upwards and the bifurcation of the aorta exposed. The peritoneum is incised below the bifurcation and the sympathetic nerve ganglia and nerve fibres are excised by dissecting the large vessels clear of fat and connective tissue, until the periosteum of the lumbar vertebrae is quite clean. Care must be taken not to injure the ureters, inferior mesenteric artery and the median sacral vessels. Dramatic cures are sometimes obtained by this operation, but it is clearly a severe procedure which should be adopted only in intractable cases when other methods have failed. The operation has no effect upon subsequent childbirth except to render the first stage of labour painless, if the operation has been complete. When assessing the results from surgery in a disease which has a large functional overlay it is wise to give some of the credit to the applied psychotherapy rather than all of it to the operative procedure. Hence the very limited application of all surgical treatment in this disorder.

Hysterectomy may sometimes be necessary in older patients and certainly never before the middle thirties, but only as a last expedient and after the significance of the removal of the uterus has been clearly explained to the patient. The possibility of adenomyosis interna is the most plausible and reasonable indication for hysterectomy. It must be clearly understood that adenomyosis interna is not a cause of spasmodic but congestive dysmenorr-hoea. Hysterectomy is, therefore, almost never indicated for spasmodic dysmenorrhoea per se but only when a congestive element has appeared in later life in a patient previously suffering from the spasmodic variety. This combination of spasmodic and congestive is occasionally seen in the 30–40 year age group when the congestive moiety tends to overshadow the spas-modic.

Membranous Dysmenorrhoea

Membranous dysmenorrhoea should be regarded as an extreme form of spasmodic dysmenorrhoea. It is fortunately extremely rare, said to run in families and to recur after pregnancy. The dysmenorrhoea is accompanied by the passage of membranes which may take the form of casts of the uterine cavity. Microscopically the casts have the structure of the endometrium during menstruation, except that the disintegrative processes are ill-defined. It is most likely that the tryptic ferment secreted by the endometrium in normal menstruation is deficient. Small membranes may, however, be passed during menstruation by patients who are free from dysmenorrhoea. Inflam-matory infiltration of the tissues of the casts is unknown and there is no reason to suspect that the condition is caused by a chronic inflammation of the uterus. The treatment of membranous dysmenorrhoea should follow the same lines as those recommended for spasmodic dysmenorrhoea but the prognosis is even worse.

Ovarian Dysmenorrhoea

The late O'Donel Browne has drawn attention to the possible part played by the ovary in menstrual pain, and he concluded that in over half the cases of dysmenorrhoea the ovary was at fault. In ovarian dysmenorrhoea the pain is felt for two or three days before menstruation in one or both lower quad-rants in the areas innervated by the tenth thoracic to the first lumbar seg-ments. Browne advised ovarian sympathectomy, which should be combined with presacral neurectomy. The operation is extremely simple and consists in clamping and transecting the infundibulo-pelvic ligament. Infertility does not result and the only adverse effect is a temporary menorrhagia due to a sympathetic release of the ovary. This symptom lasts from three to six months. Browne claimed a far higher cure rate for dysmenorrhoea by this method than by simple presacral neurectomy. The cases in which this operation is indicated are very few, and it should be reserved only for those patients in which the clinical examination strongly suggests that the pain is of ovarian origin. This operation and that of presacral neurectomy can have no good effect upon the distant manifestations of dysmenorrhoea, such as headache and gastrointestinal upset. After its performance the patient may lose her lower abdominal pain but will still experience, often in a greater degree, her other symptoms. Patients who display a large functional overlay in their dysmenorrhoea provide absolute contraindication to any form of surgical operation. This last point should be once more strongly emphasised.

15*

Gastrointestinal Symptoms associated with Dysmenorrhoea

Gastrointestinal upset associated with dysmenorrhoea has already been mentioned, and the anorexia and vomiting seen in a severe attack are well recognised. The close relationship of the autonomic nerve supply of the lower bowel and the genital tract is significant, and an example of this is the time-honoured use of purgation and enemata in the medical induction of labour. Many women associate menstruation with disordered bowel function, such as flatulence and constipation, and in some there is actual pain referable to the sigmoid colon, which is spastic, and to the caecum. For this reason many an innocent appendix is removed, and by the same token many a left appendage has been sacrificed on the assumption that the left-sided colonic pain is due to a diseased ovary. Spastic colon is now realised to be largely a functional disorder and the abuse of purgatives tends only to exaggerate this condition. Anti-spasmodics and not purgatives should be exhibited, and a drug such as probanthine is far more efficacious than a cathartic, which only tends to increase the irritability of the bowel. Proper diet and simple psychotherapy are important adjuvants in the treatment of this essentially functional aspect of dysmenorrhoea.

Orthopaedic Aspects of Dysmenorrhoea

A number of patients similarly complain of backache before and during the menstrual periods, and, while it is tempting to explain this on a purely hormonal basis due to the relaxant effects of progesterone on smooth muscle and ligaments in general, it is always wise to exclude an orthopaedic lesion by X-ray examination of the spine and sacro-iliac joints.

The old adage that if a woman complains of backache there is usually something wrong with her back holds good, and it is bad practice to blame the uterus for her symptom. In some cases fibrositis, sacro-iliac strain or a prolapsed disc will be discovered on careful investigation, and relief of these conditions by an orthopaedic surgeon will do much to improve her dysmenorrhoea.

MITTELSCHMERZ

Painful ovulation is characterised by a consciousness of abdominal discomfort which recurs at a regular time in succeeding or intermediate menstrual cycles—usually about the fourteenth day. The pain varies from a mild discomfort to an acute abdominal crisis of short duration, rarely more and usually less than twelve hours. If associated with ovulation spotting due to oestrogen withdrawal bleeding, the diagnosis is usually obvious but many women are subjected to an unnecessary laparotomy on a diagnosis of acute appendicitis. A careful history of the timing of the pain is the most useful help to the correct diagnosis and, once this is confidently made, no treatment, apart from explanation and reassurance is needed.

MENORRHAGIA

In menorrhagia the menstrual cycle is unaltered but the duration and quantity of the menstrual loss are increased. It is important to emphasise that the menstrual cycle is unaltered, as excessive bleeding associated with an irregular cycle should not be regarded as menorrhagia. Menorrhagia is essentially a symptom and not in itself a disease. The underlying cause may be difficult to detect. The causes can be divided into: (a) those due to some general cause; (b) those which are local in the pelvis; (c) those caused by endocrine disorders.

(a) *General Diseases causing Menorrhagia.* Contrary to time honoured teaching, heart disease and hypertension do not themselves cause menorrhagia and, in fact, only those blood dyscrasias which are associated with a deficiency of haemostasis can affect the menstrual loss, such as thrombocytopenic purpura. Severe anaemia, whether cause or effect, is often associated with menorrhagia and its correction alone may well lead to control of the uterine symptom.

Psychological disorders, emotional upset, matrimonial disharmony and anxiety states are undoubtedly important factors in this as in any disorder of menstruation. Prolongation of the menstrual loss provides a specious excuse for avoidance of a sexual relationship which has become tedious or distasteful. In a patient who dreads a pregnancy for any reason, it is one method of escape from the risk of matrimonial duties.

(b) *Local Causes.* In a large number of cases menorrhagia is caused by local disease in the pelvis. Myomata afford the best example and menorrhagia can be regarded as their most characteristic symptom. Endometrial polypi, apart from myomatous polypi, are often found when performing a diagnostic curettage in the investigation of an obscure menorrhagia. Pelvic inflammation such as salpingo-oöphoritis, by inducing hyperaemia, also leads to menorrhagia. Similarly the first menstrual periods after abortion and childbirth may be excessive because the uterus is enlarged and imperfectly involuted. In retroversion the periods may be excessive. With chocolate cysts of the ovaries menorrhagia is sometimes a symptom, perhaps because of the ovarian hyperaemia induced by the presence of the chocolate cysts. But it should be remembered that a hormonal disturbance is probably associated with the incidence of these cysts in the ovaries. Apart from endometriosis, ovarian tumours, unless oestrogenic such as granulosa cell tumours, do not cause menorrhagia. In certain cases of menorrhagia pelvic examination demonstrates symmetrical enlargement of the uterus which resembles that associated with a ten-weeks pregnancy. When such a uterus is removed the myohyperplasia of the muscle is obvious. In the past such terms as metritis, fibrosis uteri and chronic subinvolution have been used to describe it. The modern view is that the myohyperplasia is due to excessive *oestrogen stimulation.*

(c) *Endocrine Disturbances.* Menorrhagia is a frequent symptom of endocrine disease. In hyperthyroidism menorrhagia is occasionally seen in the early stages, but in advanced cases patients usually have amenorrhoea. The converse holds for hypothyroidism, although in cretinism the patient may have amenorrhoea. In myxoedema, particularly in women over the age of 40, menorrhagia is not uncommon. Similarly, in the early stages of acromegaly menorrhagia may be complained of, while with advanced cases the patient develops amenorrhoea.

Apart from an excess of naturally occurring oestrogen the therapeutic use of the synthetic product should be mentioned. Many patients, for example those attending the dermatologist, are prescribed oestrogen for the relief of non-gynaecological conditions and often over long periods and in fairly substantial dosage. Practitioners are also sometimes too ready to prescribe this therapy for menopausal symptoms. The resulting menorrhagia in both these instances can be classed as iatrogenic.

(d) The intrauterine contraceptive device has provided a recent aetiological factor. In quite a large proportion of women using the device the first few periods after insertion are excessive and in some determine the abandonment of this method of contraception.

DYSFUNCTIONAL UTERINE BLEEDING

In a large number of patients menorrhagia is not associated with any structural abnormality in the pelvis or evidence either of general disease or endocrine disorder. If on clinical bimanual examination the uterus and appendages are found to be normal, the term dysfunctional uterine bleeding is used. This term should be reserved for those patients in whom not only is pelvic examination normal but in whom there is no other demonstrable extra-genital cause for the bleeding. In past years it was customary to attribute menorrhagia to abnormalities of the myometrium, such as chronic inflammation and subinvolution. The modern tendency is to regard such cases as being caused by ovarian dysfunction. In many cases of menorrhagia no abnormality and no abnormal physical signs can be detected except that the uterus is symmetrically enlarged. In a multigravida who has borne many children, as a result of the deposition of elastic tissue in the uterus after each delivery, the uterus is hard and firm and the vessels stand out prominently when the myometrium is incised. Originally this was attributed to chronic metritis but when histological studies excluded the presence of inflammatory lesions, the enlargement of the uterus was regarded as being caused by subinvolution. It is now believed that the aetiology is purely hormonal and that the hypertrophy and hyperplasia of the myometrium are induced by a high titre of oestrogen in the circulating blood. Contradictory opinions are held of the precise endocrine disturbances which lead to myohyperplasia and its consequent menorrhagia. It will be pointed out later in this chapter that menorrhagia is the main symptom in some cases of metropathia haemorrhagica, when no corpus luteum is produced in the ovaries.

If a diagnostic curettage is performed on certain patients suffering from menorrhagia immediately before a period or during a period, the histological features of incomplete progestational change may be seen. The glands are not fully ripened, the epithelium being immature for the time of the cycle and the stroma does not show the decidua-like oedema of the late secretory phase. This picture is called *irregular ripening* of the endometrium. It suggests a deficiency of corpus luteum function.

In other patients the exact opposite obtains. A curettage performed after menstruation shows not simply follicular or oestrogenic endometrium but a persistence of secretory changes, usually with a patchy distribution. This condition has been called *irregular shedding* of the endometrium and suggests a persistence or over-activity of corpus luteum function.

In 1,000 patients investigated by diagnostic curettage for dysfunctional bleeding in the absence of any pelvic pathology, Sutherland and Bruce reported as follows:

Normal endometrium	54·7%
Hyperplastic endometrium	26·5%
Irregular ripening	2·6%
Irregular shedding	1·3%
Atrophic endometrium	1·0%
"Chronic endometritis"	11·0%
Uterine polypi	1·1%
Tuberculosis	1·0%
Malignancy	0·8%
	100.0

Menorrhagia of this type is frequent at puberty and at the time of the menopause.

A further 1,000 patients were similarly investigated by curettage but in these there were gross pelvic disease, as follows:

Fibroids	830
Pelvic inflammatory disease	168
Adenomyosis of uterus	35
External endometriosis	26
Ovarian tumour	19

(Discrepancy in total due to some patients having two lesions)

In these, the endometrial histology was as follows:

Normal endometrium	648
Hyperplasia	195
Atrophy	49
Chronic endometritis	40
Malignant disease	23
Uterine polypus	18
Irregular ripening	18
Irregular shedding	0
Tuberculosis	9
	1,000

From a study of this very large series of patients with menorrhagia, certain facts emerge:

(1) Roughly 60% have a normal endometrium.

(2) Roughly 20–25% show some endometrial hyperplasia.

(3) Irregular ripening and irregular shedding are rare disorders.

(4) Tuberculosis and malignancy must always be excluded.

The finding of chronic endometritis is more a histological entity than a pathological state denoting true uterine infection.

Diagnosis

The patient must be investigated carefully to find the cause of the symptom.

(1) A history of the onset, duration and amount of bleeding; its character and cyclical features.

(2) A full general examination, with special reference to thyroid dysfunction and including a full blood count, is followed by a bimanual pelvic examination.

(3) A diagnostic curettage, primarily to obtain material for histology rather than as a curative measure.

(4) If no satisfactory explanation is forthcoming and the menorrhagia persists, a hysterosalpingogram may reveal some intra-uterine cause such as a fibroid polypus which has been missed.

Treatment

Under this heading only menorrhagia without an obvious primary cause will be dealt with.

Treatment depends on several factors:

(1) The age of the patient, her fertility and her desire for children. Under forty, treatment is essentially conservative.

(2) The degree of anaemia and its control by iron. If uncontrolled, except by transfusion, conservatism gives way to more radical surgery.

(3) The response to curettage, which is performed primarily as an aid to diagnosis, may be therapeutically beneficial. There is no scientific explanation why curettage should benefit dysfunctional bleeding, though occasionally it does. Curettage should, therefore, precede hysterectomy in almost every instance.

Conservative Treatment. *General.* In any patient suffering from severe dysfunctional bleeding, some degree of anaemia is to be expected. It is wise to ask for a full blood count and not only the estimation of the haemoglobin. Oral iron should be given and the response to it checked by serial blood counts. If the response is unsatisfactory due to iron intolerance or failure of the patient to utilise it, the therapy must be varied until the anaemia is fully controlled and corrected. Of all the drugs available in the pharmacopoeia, iron is the most reliable and effective. Rest, sedatives and reassurance must not be neglected and, during a severe bout of bleeding, it may be necessary to confine the patient to bed. The use of ergot is essentially unscientific in this type of bleeding and plays little or no part in the general treatment.

Hormone Therapy. (1) *Oestrogen:* The aim of treatment here is to raise the blood oestrogen level to the super-threshold for bleeding so that to achieve this a large initial dosage is necessary. This means 5 mg. of stilboestrol t.d.s., or ethinyl oestradiol, 0·25 mg. t.d.s. As much as 50 mg. a day of stilboestrol have been given. This high dosage must be maintained until bleeding is controlled which should occur in 3 to 5 days. Having achieved temporary haemostasis, it is now necessary to avoid oestrogen withdrawal bleeding which may be as severe as the original haemorrhage. It is, therefore, necessary to continue an artificial cycle at a fairly high level of blood oestrogen by maintaining the oestrogen dosage at 5 mg. daily for twenty-one days. During the last ten days of this artificial cycle, 10 mg. of oral progestational steroid are given. At the conclusion of treatment, progesterone withdrawal bleeding occurs after 48 hours and it is hoped a more normal period, although artificially induced, will result. The treatment is continued for the next three to six months, after which the patient is kept under observation. The treatment is permanently successful in a modest number of patients and more so in the adolescent than the adult.

The criticism of the treatment is that it is tedious and time-consuming and involves frequent medical supervision. It must not be forgotten when assessing the effect of therapy that at least some of the successes would have occurred spontaneously without treatment since dysfunctional bleeding is notoriously capricious in its behaviour.

(2) The newer orally active progestational steroids, such as nor-ethynodrel, nor-ethisterone or lynestrenol can be used as an alternative and these certainly have the great advantage of convenience. A high initial dose of 10 to 30 mg. a day should arrest bleeding in 24-48 hours, after which 5 mg. a day for twenty days is given. Withdrawal bleeding occurs two to five days after cessation of treatment and a normal loss is to be expected. A second course of 5 mg. daily is given from day 5 for twenty days, after which anovular menstruation should again occur by withdrawal bleeding two to five days after stopping the drug. This treatment can be continued for three to six months and should then be suspended to observe the patient. The side-effect of this drug is gastro-intestinal upset, nausea and vomiting; this is more likely in the larger dosage and may prove troublesome. To some extent the side-effects can be minimised by giving the drug at night on retiring to bed.

Testosterone. It has in the past been fashionable to use small doses of testosterone in the treatment of dysfunctional uterine bleeding. The reason given was that testosterone was supposed to enhance the action of oestrogen. There are many proprietary tablets on the market containing a mixture of oestrogen and testosterone. The administration of testosterone for dysfunctional uterine haemorrhage or uterine haemorrhage of any kind is not recommended and should not be used.

Radiotherapy. The action of X-rays and of radium upon the ovaries is to inhibit ovarian function so that follicles fail to ripen and ovulation is inhibited. With castration doses of X-rays or radium, menstruation ceases after two months. If bleeding continues after this hysterectomy is always indicated on the assumption that a carcinoma of the corpus may have been missed or at best that there is some organic local cause for the bleeding. The patient subsequently develops menopausal symptoms, which are usually severe in women between the ages of 30 and 45. These radiotherapy methods of treatment are of most service in the treatment of menorrhagia in women approaching menopausal age. In young women they should be avoided, because of the destructive effect of the radiations upon the ovaries. Most authorities do not now advise the creation of an artificial menopause by radium or radiation in women under 40, and the modern tendency is to advance the age limit to 45 and beyond.

The technique employed in creating an artificial menopause by radiotherapy will be described in detail in Chapter 26. The advantages of the method are a negligible mortality, a short stay in hospital and a high degree of efficiency. It has, however, certain disadvantages.

(1) An anaesthetic is essential in order to perform preliminary curettage.

(2) Unsuspected pelvic pathology, such as small myomata, endometriosis and pelvic inflammatory disease, may be missed which could be discovered and eradicated by operation.

(3) Radiation injuries to the bladder and rectum may rarely result.

(4) The incidence of carcinoma of the corpus after radiation is said to be 0·3%–1.4%, so that any persistence or recurrence of bleeding calls for a hysterectomy as already stated.

(5) The symptoms of a radiation menopause may be very severe.

(6) There is a danger of foetal malformation should pregnancy result when radiation has been employed in women who are still in the child-bearing period of life. For this reason its use should be reserved for patients of menopausal age, and the so-called substerilisation dose advocated by some authors in the treatment of menorrhagia in younger women is never considered justifiable.

Operation—Curettage. There is no scientific reason why curettage should ever benefit a patient with dysfunctional bleeding. Removal of the surface of the target organ cannot influence a disorder of pituitary-ovarian origin. The operation should, therefore, never be regarded as therapeutic except in so far as it influences the psychosomatic element of this essentially functional disease.

Curettage is, however, an essential diagnostic feature of all dysfunctional bleeding and, in a fortunate few, it will remove a possible organic cause such as an endometrial polypus. As a diagnostic step, it must never be neglected and a number of patients will be cured by curettage alone, however unscientific this beneficial result may be. It is particularly important in the diagnosis of unsuspected genital tract tuberculosis and, in the older patient, of endometrial cancer.

In some cases of severe menorrhagia the patient should be treated by hysterectomy. Hysterectomy is a major procedure, and the patient must be considered very carefully before the operation is advised. If hysterectomy is performed the ovaries should be conserved, for if they are removed an artificial menopause is created and the patient would have been treated just as efficiently by radiation methods, without the inconvenience of an abdominal operation.

it is therefore important to emphasise the necessity of leaving the ovaries intact. The argument that the ovaries should be removed whenever the operation of hysterectomy is performed is fallacious, for there is no increased tendency for the ovaries to develop ovarian tumours after excision of the uterus. Moreover, the removal of the ovaries is of comparable importance to the removal of both testicles in the male, an operation which no surgeon will undertake unless the testicles are the seat of either tuberculous or malignant disease. Nevertheless, at the present day there is some discussion as to whether the ovaries atrophy after total hysterectomy, and some gynae-cologists maintain that severe menopausal symptoms follow total hysterec-tomy even when the ovaries are retained. These views are not in accordance with the clinical and laboratory experience of Wilfred Shaw and the present authors and will no longer bear critical examination.

It has been argued that bilateral oöphorectomy is an insurance policy against the subsequent development of ovarian cancer following conserva-tion. In our own practice the risk of this is of the order of between 1:1000—1:2000. There is a small but significant risk of increased coronary and cerebral thrombosis in those patients in whom both ovaries have been removed.

The decision as to whether hysterectomy should be performed in cases of menorrhagia depends upon the features of each individual case. If the woman has acquired a severe degree of anaemia and her general health is impaired by the menorrhagia, drastic treatment is justified. Similarly, if the woman has children and has no desire for further offspring, there would be more inclination towards hysterectomy than in the case of a recently married woman. Features of this kind must all be taken into account before deciding upon hysterectomy. If a woman is a good subject for operation, total hysterectomy has a low mortality of the order of less than 0.2% in good hands. With anaemic women preliminary blood transfusion must be performed where the level of haemoglobin is 70% (10.1 Gm) or less.

The above outline of the available methods of treatment in cases of menorrhagia shows that each individual must be treated on her merits and not according to a fixed plan. With girls and young women, conservative treatment must be pressed to the utmost and every effort should be made to spare the patient from hysterectomy. With older patients one would be more inclined to advise hysterectomy for intractable bleeding, while with women approaching the age of the menopause the creation of an artificial meno-pause by radiotherapy is an alternative method of treatment.

POLYMENORRHOEA

In polymenorrhoea, or epimenorrhoea, the menstrual cycle is reduced from the normal of twenty-eight days to a cycle of two to three weeks and remains constant at that frequency. Women with polymenorrhoea therefore men-struate more frequently than normal women, and the frequent menstruation is usually associated with excessive bleeding, which is prolonged. This com-bination of menorrhagia with epimenorrhoea is termed **epi-menorrhagia.** Polymenorrhoea is a common symptom in gynaecological practice. Little is known of the exact aetiology, but it is established that ovarian function is increased so that ovulation occurs more frequently than normally, and that it is the maturation of the Graafian follicle which is accelerated, since the active life of the corpus luteum has been shown to remain constant at about fourteen days. This opinion is not accepted either by Rock or by Neuweiler who maintain that the cycles in cases of polymenorrhoea are sometimes anovulatory. It is not uncommon to find several corpora lutea of corresponding age if the ovaries are examined. The ovaries are often hyperaemic and contain blood follicles, and it is extremely common for the myometrium of the uterus to be thickened through myohyperplasia. The endometrium is sometimes found to be thicker than normal without polypoidal excrescences. In other cases the endometrium is of normal thickness without hypertrophy or hyperplasia. The cause of the ovarian over-activity does not necessarily lie in the ovaries themselves, and it is more than probable that disorders of the anterior lobe of the pituitary are responsible for many cases of polymenorrhoea. Most types of polymenorrhoea are now grouped together under the heading "Dysfunctional Uterine Haemorrhage."

Clinical Aspect. Polymenorrhoea is characteristically seen at the time of the menarche and the menopause, and for the first few periods after a recent confinement. It is at these times that the pituitary ovarian relationship is disturbed. Certain local conditions in the pelvis which congest the ovaries are probably causative, such as salpingo-oöphoritis, chronic pelvic inflammatory disease, occasionally endometriosis and the presence of fibroids. The symptom of polymenorrhoea is usually seen in certain definite clinical groups of patients. One of the most frequent groups is where polymenorrhoea develops after pregnancy. This can be explained by supposing that the increase in function of the anterior lobe of the pituitary which develops normally during pregnancy subsequently persists, so that the anterior pituitary gonadotropic hormones stimulate the ovaries to frequent ovulation with resultant frequent menstruation. This has been called pituitary subinvolution. This suggestion is purely hypothetical, for there is little direct evidence that this is the case. Postpartum polymenorrhoea rarely leads to anaemia, although the woman naturally complains of the discomfort of frequent menstruation.

Polymenorrhoea is also a recognised symptom of salpingo-oöphoritis, when it is perhaps induced because the inflamed ovaries ovulate more frequently. There is some evidence also that the frequency of menstruation varies not only according to race but also with latitude, so that a woman is likely to menstruate more frequently if she migrates to tropical climes. Polymenorrhoea is also a symptom with chocolate cysts of the ovaries and uterine myomata. In the case of chocolate cysts of the ovaries, there is reason to believe that ovarian function is increased, polymenorrhoea being regarded as the natural sequel. With uterine myomata polymenorrhoea should be regarded as a coincident complication, for although the ovaries are typically hyperaemic in cases of uterine myomata, polymenorrhoea is by no means an invariable symptom. It should be emphasised that it is not the presence of the fibroids which causes the polymenorrhoea but the hyperaemia of the ovaries resulting from an increased vascular supply.

Polymenorrhoea may arise at any age during the child-bearing period of life without localising physical signs in the pelvis. It is a frequent symptom in women of menopausal age. In fact, one of the common forms of menstrual irregularity in women over the age of 40 is polymenorrhoea. In such cases the myometrium of the uterus is hyperplastic. The syndrome of polymenorrhoea associated with a bulky uterus in a woman of the age of about 45 is well recognised. It has already been emphasised that in these patients the ovaries are found to contain more than one corpus luteum, together with haemorrhagic follicles. It is difficult on theoretical grounds to postulate that the cause of polymenorrhoea lies in the uterus itself, for there is no evidence that any abnormality of the uterus can disturb the rhythm of the menstrual cycle. It is therefore difficult to believe that local treatment applied to the uterus, such as, for example, curettage, can be of service in the treatment of polymenorrhoea.

Diagnosis and Treatment. The diagnosis and treatment of polymenorrhoea depend upon the principles already outlined in the section on menorrhagia. These two conditions are in many ways comparable and should be regarded from the same point of view. So far as treatment is concerned, exactly the same lines should be followed as when dealing with menorrhagia. As yet, there is no specific drug or hormone capable of altering the rhythm of the menstrual cycle, although menstruation can be temporarily inhibited or postponed by oestrogen or orally active progestational steroids. Cyclical hormone therapy can be employed to restrict the amount of blood lost during each period. Many women are content to suffer the inconvenience of frequent menstruation so long as they escape the effects of anaemia.

METRORRHAGIA

Metrorrhagia should be defined as irregular, acyclical bleeding from the uterus. The bleeding may be intermittent or continuous. It is not infrequently superimposed upon a normal, regular menstrual cycle. The addition of acyclical bleeding to normal menstruation results in a pattern of haemorrhage from which it is difficult or impossible to distinguish the pathological bleeding from that of the normal period. Strictly speaking, metrorrhagia should be limited to uterine bleeding only but, in clinical practice, any bleeding from any part of the genital tract is labelled metrorrhagia. The importance of metrorrhagia as a primary symptom of genital tract neoplasm, often malignant, can never be over-emphasised. In almost all cases the cause of the metrorrhagia depends upon the presence of some local abnormality of the uterus which can be demonstrated by physical examination. Among the causes of metrorrhagia are carcinoma of the cervix and uterine body, submucous fibroids, uterine polypi, particularly mucous polypi of the cervix, vascular erosions, and, rarely, growths of the vagina and vulva.

In some cases of metrorrhagia the woman gives a history of regular intermenstrual bleeding on about the fourteenth day of the cycle, the haemorrhage lasting only for a short time and being of small amount. These haemorrhages are of some academic interest, for they are comparable to the prooestrus bleeding of animals and are caused by oozing of blood from the hyperaemic endometrium at the height of the proliferative stage of the menstrual cycle. The condition arises most frequently in women about the age of 35, and the blood losses are often combined with severe pain in the lower abdomen. Treatment is unsatisfactory and usually unnecessary. The bleeding seldom amounts to more than a spotting for a few hours to a day or so, and its physiological explanation as an oestrogen-withdrawal bleeding should satisfy most patients, and no treatment is otherwise indicated.

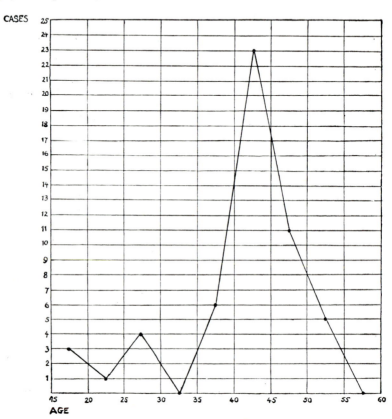

FIG. 223. The age-incidence of metropathia haemorrhagica. The maximum-age incidence is between 40 and 45, but a few cases are seen before the age of 20.

METROPATHIA HAEMORRHAGICA

Metropathia haemorrhagica should be regarded as a specialised form of dysfunctional uterine haemorrhage. Its characters are well defined and the condition is capable of accurate diagnosis. Consequently it is considered separately from the other forms of dysfunctional bleeding.

In this disease the endometrium of the uterus is thick and polypoidal, and one or other ovary contains a cystic follicle. The disease is most prevalent in women over the age of 40, the maximum incidence being between the ages of 40 and 45. Occasionally it develops in young girls under the age of 20, when by producing prolonged periods of uterine bleeding it may lead to a severe degree of anaemia. It is not uncommon between the ages of 45 and 55, and accounts for many cases of irregular and prolonged bleeding in women who have a delayed menopause. There is little evidence that parity is related to its incidence. Similarly, there is no evidence that it is determined by infection of the genital tract, and it develops very rarely in conjunction with uterine myomata (see Fig. 223).

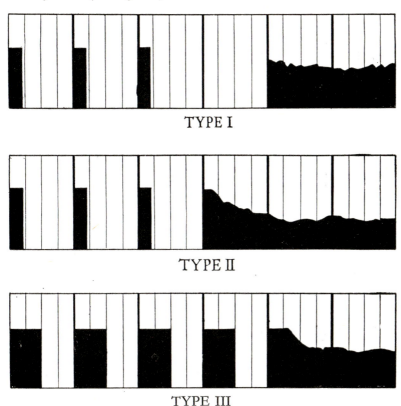

TYPE I

TYPE II

TYPE III

FIG. 224. The menstrual histories in cases of metropathia haemorrhagica. Continuous uterine bleeding is the most constant symptom, and most frequently this is preceded by amenorrhoea of about eight to ten weeks' duration. Sometimes the bleeding follows upon a normal period, while at other times the continuous bleeding may be preceded by menorrhagia.

The symptoms are very typical. The most common complaint is of continuous vaginal bleeding which may last for many weeks. In half the cases the continuous bleeding is preceded by a short period of amenorrhoea, an interval of about eight weeks elapsing between the last period and the onset of the continuous haemorrhage. The continuous bleeding is not usually particularly severe and is comparable to the normal menstrual discharge, consisting of dark fluid blood. It is exceptional for patients to have severe bleeding on any particular day, but the continuous drain of blood in due course produces a state of anaemia. There are sometimes departures from the typical history. The continuous bleeding may start at the time a period is expected, or it may be preceded by menorrhagia without any intervening period of amenorrhoea. The bleeding is always painless, since it is anovulatory (see Fig. 224).

The clinical history of metropathia is similar to that obtained with ectopic gestation and abortion, and these two conditions must always be borne in mind when the differential diagnosis is considered. The physical signs which

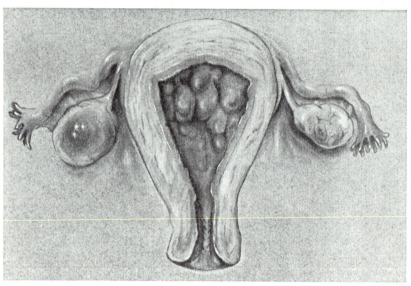

Fig. 225. Metropathia haemorrhagica. Note that the right ovary is cystic and that the endometrium shows diffuse poly, due to hyperplasia.

are usually obtained are those of a slight symmetrical enlargement of the uterus together with the presence of a cystic ovary. If care is taken over the history, it is fairly easy to diagnose the condition clinically.

Pathological Anatomy

The Uterus. There is a mild degree of myohyperplasia of the myometrium which causes the symmetrical enlargement of the uterus. The walls of the uterus may measure up to 25 mm. in cross-section. The endometrium is thick, haemorrhagic, and polypoidal, and thin, slender polypi project downwards towards the internal os. These features of the endometrium used to be called polypoidal endometritis (see Fig. 225). The endometrium has very characteristic features when examined under the microscope. In the first place, the endometrium shows the characteristics of a cystic glandular hyperplasia. Many of the glands show cystic dilatation, and the larger cysts can be identified with the naked eye (see Fig. 226).

The second characteristic is the absence of secretory hypertrophy, so that corkscrew-shaped glands are never seen.

Thirdly, areas of necrosis are scattered over the superficial layers of the endometrium and the histological features in these necrotic areas correspond with those found in the menstruating endometrium. The histological picture of the endometrium is that of an abnormal hyperplastic endometrium which is menstruating continuously without signs of secretory hypertrophy (see Fig. 227). Some degree of adenomyosis is frequently found in these cases.

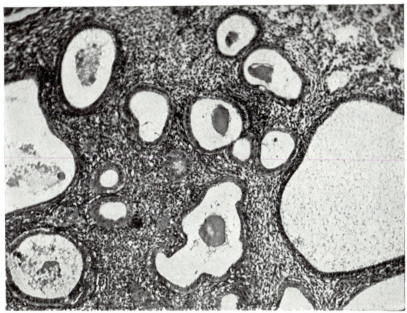

FIG. 226. Cystic glandular hyperplasia of the endometrium in metropathia haemorrhagica. ($\times$ 85.)

Ovaries. One or other ovary always contains a cyst which is seldom more than 5 cm. in diameter. The opposite ovary is often atrophic. Recent corpora lutea are never found in the ovaries. The cyst has the characters of a cystic ripening follicle, but it is not uncommon for both the granulosa and theca interna cells to show some degree of luteinisation. The ovarian changes indicate, therefore, that ovulation and corpus luteum formation are inhibited, and that for some reason or other a Graafian follicle becomes cystic (see Fig. 228).

The disease shows an association between ovarian dysfunction and an abnormal condition of the endometrium. The endometrium can be regarded as menstruating continuously, but little is known of the factors which determine the failure of corpus luteum formation.

Treatment. The principles of treatment correspond to those which have been outlined in the section on menorrhagia, except that for no clear reason curettage of the uterus cures a certain percentage of cases. It is important that curettage should be performed carefully and as much as possible of the endometrium scraped away. The most difficult patients are young women in their twenties, in whom pronounced anaemia may be produced by the continuous bleeding. If conservative methods of treatment have failed it may be necessary to perform hysterectomy as a last resort. Most patients respond to hormone therapy but for those over the age of 40 who fail to respond to a

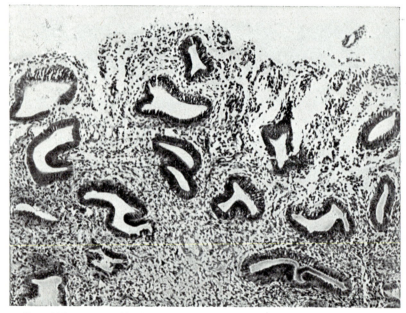

FIG. 227. Metropathia haemorrhagica. Endometrium showing superficial necrosis. This necrosis resembles that seen on the first day of menstruation. The glands, however, do not show any secretory change. ($\times$ 110.)

reasonable trial of hormone treatment then hysterectomy with ovarian conservation is the treatment of choice. If hysterectomy is contraindicated the production of an artificial menopause by radium or deep X-ray therapy is an effective alternative for patients of menopausal age. Operations of ovarian cystectomy or wedge resection of the ovaries do not help the underlying condition and are not indicated.

The treatment of metropathia by progesterone is most effective and important. The dose of orally active progestogen varies according to the age of the patient, the amount of bleeding and the time in the cycle at which treatment commences. Nor-ethynodrel, nor-ethisterone and lynestrenol are the progestogens most commonly used. Continuous or heavy bleeding is treated by giving 5—10 mg. three times daily until bleeding ceases, which usually occurs within 48 hours, and is followed by a maintenance dose of 5—10 mg.

daily until a period is desired. Bleeding commences approximately 48 hours after stopping treatment. During the maintenance treatment, which is usually continued for about 20 days, the patient's haemoglobin is checked and anaemia is corrected. Having treated the acute episode, assuming that diagnostic curettage has been performed previously to exclude other intrauterine pathology, intermittent therapy is commenced for either 10 or 21 days in each cycle.

Ten-day treatment consists of 5 mg. daily for 10 days starting on the seventeenth day of the cycle. This will be followed by a regular period on the twenty-eighth day. This scheme is satisfactory more especially for those patients who do not wish to take "the pill" or who have side-effects therefrom. This particular schedule is also of value in those patients who wish to become pregnant.

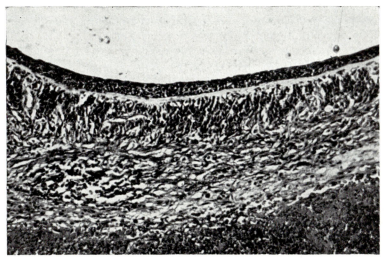

FIG. 228. The wall of the ovarian cyst in metropathia haemorrhagica. The appearances are those of a ripening follicle. (× 180.)

Twenty-one day treatment consists of 1—5 mg. daily for 21 days and is most easily given in the form of a combined type of contraceptive pill. This treatment is most efficient especially in the younger patient.

Treatment by either the ten-day or twenty-one day schedule should not be continued indefinitely in the patient with established metropathia because the disease is self limiting. If treatment is stopped after one year many patients will revert to a normal menstrual rhythm, whilst others will require progestogen until they become menopausal. As stated above, hysterectomy is indicated when or if hormone treatment fails or in those who become intolerant to progestogen.

Puberty menorrhagia is a temporary phenomenon associated with anovular cycles and may become so severe as to warrant hormone treatment. In the acute episode a dose of 5—10 mg. per day is given for seven days. This controls the bleeding and a further but normal period follows 2—3 days after cessation of treatment. If further haemorrhage occurs the course may be repeated. Occasionally haemorrhage is so severe that 5—10 mg must be given daily for 21 days for three cycles, after which a normal ovulatory cycle is usually established.

Oestrogen is very efficient in stopping the haemorrhage of metropathia by forcing the oestrogen level above the so-called threshold level. Stilboestrol 1 mg. is given hourly until bleeding ceases, after which a maintenance dose of 1 mg. three times daily will prevent further bleeding for several weeks. Patients should be warned that nausea or even vomiting may occur when they are taking 1 mg. every hour and these side-effects may interrupt treatment before bleeding has actually ceased. In patients, however, who do develop these side-effects bleeding is usually rapidly controlled by the dosage already given. A five-day course of progestogen 5 mg. daily must be given before stopping the oestrogen therapy in order to obtain a secretory endometrium which will shed easily and produce a normal and not unduly heavy loss. Cyclic oestrogen-progestogen therapy may be continued for several months if desired.

Androgens have been extensively used in the treatment of metropathia. They should be avoided because of their virilising activity. Combinations of progestogen-androgen and oestrogen-androgen are commercially produced but these have no special virtue and are also better avoided.

Clomiphene 50—100 mg. daily for five days is the drug of choice for metropathia haemorrhagica, especially in the young (puberty) age group and in those under 40. This is particularly applicable to those who are wishing to become pregnant, because Clomiphene acts by inducing ovulation, after which the metropathic syndrome cannot continue. Clomiphene must not be given until the patient has been fully investigated and then only when under expert supervision, because although ovarian hyperstimulation syndrome can occur it is unlikely to do so at the dose suggested and even if it does occur it will only be the mild variety (p. 482).

Adenomatous Polypus of the Endometrium of the Body

This form of polypus should not be regarded as a new growth and in fact the term adenomatous is illogical since the polypus is really a localised area of hyperplasia. Unfortunately common usage condones the retention of this misnomer. A better term would be localised polyposis of the endometrium in contradistinction from the generalised polyposis of metropathia. The polypus takes the form of an area of true hyperplasia of the endometrium of the body of the uterus. It is possible that when the endometrium is thickened through simple hyperplasia, as in cases of myomata, small areas may project into the cavity of the uterus and as a result of uterine contractions become extruded into the cavity and form a polypus. Adenomatous polypi of this kind are met with most frequently in association with myomata, but they also develop without obvious cause. They are covered with cubical epithelium and contain glands of a type similar to those of the endometrium of the body, although the glands do not necessarily undergo secretory hypertrophy during the menstrual cycle. It is rare for adenomatous polypi of the endometrium of the body to produce localising symptoms in women during the child-bearing period of life, but when arising after the menopause they may cause post-menopausal bleeding. If the polypi cause irregular uterine bleeding the uterus must be curetted. It is not always easy to remove polypi of this kind by simple curettage and occasionally it is found necessary to perform hysterectomy to ensure that the cause of the bleeding is not carcinoma of the endometrium of the body. It should be noted that occasionally an endo-metrial polypus may become malignant and for this reason all polypi re-moved by curettage should be carefully examined histologically.

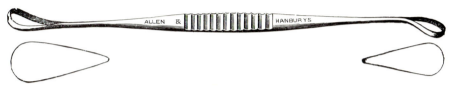

Fig. 229. A curette.

Diffuse polyposis of the endometrium is quite commonly seen in the cystic glandular hyperplasia of metropathia haemorrhagica when it can be re-garded as the response of the endometrium to a hyperoestrogenic state.

Adenomyomatous polypi of the uterus resemble adenomatous polypi except that they contain plain muscle tissue in the stroma. They are usually associated with adenomyosis of the uterus. The symptoms, diagnosis and treatment correspond to what has been described with adenomatous polypi.

19 Hormone Therapy in Gynaecology

The administration of the sex hormones plays an important part in modern gynaecological therapeutics. Many of the sex hormones have been isolated in a state of purity and some of them have been synthesised and are now available in dosages which can be controlled with precision. It is important that the practitioner should have some knowledge of the indications for the use of these substances in clinical gynaecology.

Unfortunately, the indications for treatment are not always well defined, nor is it always possible to gauge the correct dosage except by trial in the individual patient. There is no simple method of determining the concentration of oestrogen, progestogen, or the anterior pituitary sex hormones either in the blood or in the urine excreted. The laboratories which undertake these investigations are few, the techniques are exacting and expensive. Moreover, the physiology of the sexual functions is highly complex with many of the other ductless glands inter-related in function. Disorders of menstruation and of the sexual functions are not always easy to diagnose with precision on clinical grounds. Another difficulty is that many of the gynaecological disorders which respond to hormone therapy also tend to undergo spontaneous remission. It is not, therefore, always correct to maintain that improvement results from treatment, since it may have been spontaneous. Another mistake which is often made is to postulate that most functional gynaecological disorders respond to hormone treatment. Experience shows that this is far from being the case and the treatment of menorrhagia and dysmenorrhoea by hormone therapy should never be undertaken with optimism. The first essential is to be exact in diagnosis and it is doubtful if a high standard can be achieved without a precise knowledge of sexual physiology and pathology. The second essential is to select cases for treatment on a scientific basis. Unless there are rational indications for hormone therapy it is doubtful if this form of treatment should be employed.

Clinical Use of Oestrogen

Oestrogens are one of the naturally occurring sex hormones, being produced by the ovary, the adrenal gland and, during pregnancy, by the placenta. The actual oestrogen produced by these organs is oestradiol which they synthesise from cholesterol. The actual pathway of synthesis undoubtedly varies and the figure on page 477 indicates the most likely routes whereby cholesterol is converted into progesterone, testosterone and oestradiol. Oestradiol is metabolised in the liver to form oestrone and oestriol, both of which are only very mildly oestrogenic and both of which are amongst the oestrogens excreted in the urine. Oestriol excretion in the urine during 24 hours can be used in certain circumstances, especially in pregnancy, as an indication of the oestrogen production.

Types of Oestrogen

Oestrogens in clinical use may be either (1) synthetic or (ii) natural. *The synthetic oestrogens* stilboestrol, hexoestrol, dienoestrol, chlorotrianisene are biologically active and are excreted without modification. synthetic adaptations of oestrogen such as ethinyl-oestradiol and ethinyl-oestradiol 3-methyl ether (known as Mestranol) are metabolised by the body. *Natural oestrogens* are obtained from animal sources such as pregnant mares' urine. The modern tendency is to use the synthetic oestrogens in preference to the natural oestrogens, since the therapeutic results are equally effective, the assay and therefore the dosage is accurate and the preparations available are much cheaper. The synthetic oestrogens can be given by mouth although in susceptible patients they produce nausea, headache and malaise. Many women will tolerate a dose as great as 5 mg. of stilboestrol three times a day, and this is particularly true of puerperal patients. On the other hand, many women are subjected to great inconvenience, even by such small doses as 2 mg. of stilboestrol once a day. The synthetic oestrogen should be given to such patients parenterally, when it will usually be found that the subjective symptoms are less. Although there is some experimental evidence that synthetic oestrogens are carcinogenic, it is highly improbable that such an effect can be obtained with the relatively small doses which are used therapeutically. Most clinicians, however, would withhold oestrogen from a patient who has been treated by surgery or radiation for a carcinoma of the breast or genital tract.

Comparison of Potency of the Various Preparations Available
Synthetic Oestrogens

(a) Ethinyl oestradiol, available in 0·01, 0·02, 0·05, 0·1, 0·5 and 1·0 mg. tablets is twenty times as potent as stilboestrol.

(b) Mestranol, available in 0·05 mg. tablets is ten times as powerful as stilboestrol.

(c) *Stilboestrol,* available in 0·1, 0·5, 1·0 and 5·0 mg. tablets. This is probably the cheapest effective oral oestrogen available.

(d) *Dienoestrol,* available in 0·1, 0·3, 1·0 and 5·0 mg. tablets. The potency is one-quarter that of stilboestrol.

(e) *Hexoestrol,* available in 0·5, 1·0 and 5·0 mg. tablets and ampoules of 15 mg. for injection. The potency is one-tenth that of stilboestrol.

Dienoestrol and hexoestrol are seldom indicated in preference to stilboestrol and are then used on the assumption that they are less toxic in their side effects, such as gastro-intestinal upset, headache and water retention. This is largely due to their reduced potency and stilboestrol in smaller dosage would be equally less toxic.

Naturally Occurring Oestrogens. These, as stated above, are oestradiol, oestrone and oestriol and are to be found in the blood and the urine especially during pregnancy as well as in the placenta. They are also present in the ovary, in the corpus luteum and in the fluid of a Graafian follicle as well as in the fluid contained in a follicular cyst. Naturally occurring oestrogen is usually produced as oestradiol and is metabolised to oestrone and oestriol, in which form it is excreted via the urine and the faeces. Naturally occurring oestrogen is marketed in the form of water soluble conjugated oestrogens prepared from pregnant mares' serum as Premarin, in tablets containing 0·625 mg. and 1·25 mg., and is used mostly in the treatment of menopausal and postmenopausal states. They are also prepared as benzoate or propionate esters in oil to prolong their absorption time. These are given by injection as they are not absorbed if given orally. Oestradiol benzoate or dipropionate is the most widely used. 10,000 units is equivalent to 1·0 mg. Oestradiol benzoate is available in 1·0, 2·0 and 5·0 mg. ampoules, it is given by intramuscular injection two or three times a week in 5·0 mg. doses which are roughly equivalent to 1·0 mg. of stilboestrol three times a day by mouth. It is, therefore, no more effective, more expensive and far more time and trouble consuming.

Locally applied creams or ointments, usually containing natural oestrone, are available. Oestrone ointment contains 0·1 mg. (1,000 international units) per gram.

Oestrogen-containing Pessaries. There are many commercial varieties of oestrogen pessary, mostly containing oestrone, dienoestrol or stilboestrol in various dosage.

Oestrogen pessaries, creams and ointments have really no virtue over oral oestrogen. Only a fraction of the total drug is absorbed and utilised (perhaps one-tenth) and it is doubtful if it is utilised locally where it is intended. It is more probable that it is absorbed into the blood stream and, if so, this is a very circuitous route of administering a drug.

Pellets Designed for Slow Absorption and Long Action. These are available in 25, 50 and 100 mg. sizes. Their main indication is where hysterectomy and bilateral salpingo-oophorectomy has been performed in a woman before the menopause, or where menopausal symptoms develop after hysterectomy. The insertion of 50—100 mg. under the rectus sheath at the end of the operation should ensure freedom from flushes for about one year, after which a further pellet can be inserted. This therapy is contra-indicated unless a hysterectomy has been performed since severe uterine bleeding may result. The authors have on three occasions been obliged to perform a hysterectomy for oestrogen implant bleeding.

Fat Soluble Oestrogens. Chlorotrianisene is given by mouth and is stored in the fat depots, from which it is gradually released over the following 100 days. Its rate of release, however, is unpredictable and uncertain and at present there is little to recommend its use in preference to other simpler active oestrogens.

Summary. Stilboestrol and ethinyl oestradiol are effective when given orally and are inexpensive. Provided the dosage is kept to the lowest effective level, gastro-intestinal upset and headache should not occur in more than 10% of patients. If severe and disturbing, intramuscular injection or local application provides an alternative route of treatment.

Effects of Oestrogen Therapy

The theoretical basis for the administration of oestrogens is that the hormones stimulate the myometrium to hypertrophy and the endometrium also becomes hyperplastic so that withdrawal bleeding may occur when treatment is discontinued. Moreover the endometrium must be primed with oestrogen before progesterone is capable of producing secretory hypertrophy or withdrawal bleeding. The vagina becomes more cornified and probably the cornification involves the inner surfaces of the labia minora and labia majora as well. The effect of oestrogens on the body is obscure, but it is established that the treatment of Turner's syndrome with oestrogens is followed by hypertrophy of the breasts and the development of hair in the axillae and on the mons. In addition, oestrogens react upon the anterior lobe of the pituitary. In the first place they inhibit the activities of the anterior pituitary, such as the production of prolactin, the follicle stimulating hormone, and stimulate the production of luteinising hormone. In this way the inhibition of ovulation and suppression of lactation can be explained. Non-synthetic oestrogens are metabolised in the liver and in the presence of liver damage they may be excreted unchanged. There is some evidence that continued administration of oestrogen in high dosage may cause further injury to the already damaged liver.

Sensitivity to Oestrogen. The sensitivity of the female to oestrogen varies throughout her life. The newborn child has been subjected to a fairly high oestrogen level and may respond to its withdrawal by menstruation in the female and gynaecomastia in the male, both of which are of temporary duration. After this, however, the female infant is very sensitive to oestrogen and the minutest of dosages will be sufficient to produce a clinical response. A dose of stilboestrol 0·05 mg. daily will produce clinical changes in a young baby. Sexual development at puberty, however, requires a dose of 0·5 mg. daily, whilst suppression of ovulation during the reproductive period of life needs a dose of 2 mg. daily. The dose required to produce a clinical response during pregnancy and lactation is correspondingly increased, and as much as 10 mg. daily may be required to suppress lactation. The sensitivity of the body is again increased at the menopause and in the postmenopausal state 0·5 mg. daily will usually produce an adequate response. In the very elderly a dose of 0·1 mg. of stilboestrol will often be effective.

Dangers of Oestrogen Therapy. Every drug has its dangers, especially if it is misused and oestrogen is no exception. Oestrogens alter the clotting mechanism and are undoubtedly a factor in causing intravascular venous thrombosis and therefore leading to thrombo-embolic disease and cerebral thrombosis. They do not, however, predispose to coronary arterial thrombosis. In large doses they certainly lead to electrolyte storage with subsequent fluid retention and weight gain.

Indications for Oestrogen Therapy

Amenorrhoea. In this condition, whether primary or secondary, the causative factor is either (i) inadequate stimulation of the ovary by the pituitary gonadotropin, in other words a primary pituitary inadequacy or a pituitary failure, or (ii) a failure of the ovary to respond to pituitary stimulation, possibly because the pituitary stimulus itself is inadequate, or because the ovary is refractory or incapable of response, or (iii) very rarely the target organ is incapable, usually because of gross maldevelopment, of responding to ovarian stimulation.

If oestrogen therapy is to be used in the treatment of amenorrhoea, the clinician should realise exactly what he is doing and what he is capable of doing.

(A) In amenorrhoea due to pituitary inadequacy or failure—usually a primary amenorrhoea—he is dealing with a lack of gonadotropic F.S.H., in other words a state of anovulation. Here the exhibition of oestrogen is merely a test of sensitivity for the endometrium.

1·0 mg. of stilboestrol or 0·05 mg. of ethinyl oestradiol, given three times a day for twenty-one days and then discontinued, should produce withdrawal bleeding. This treatment can be repeated for two or three artificial anovulatory cycles. The bleeding produced is not menstruation and, though comforting to the patient and reassuring to the mother, it has not established nor is it likely ever to establish a normal rhythm of ovulatory menstruation. It is no more than a test of endometrial susceptibility to oestrogen stimulation.

The more elaborate methods of adding progesterone to the oestrogen starting on the eleventh day of oestrogen therapy and continuing for ten days will produce a secretory type of endometrium and thus ensure a reduction in total blood flow as well as a shorter period of withdrawal bleeding.

(B) In secondary amenorrhoea due to temporary ovarian failure and probably due to temporary pituitary failure, the production of cyclical artificial oestrogen withdrawal cycles may be sufficient to reactivate a deranged or suspended pituitary ovarian function. The exhibition of oestrogen provides a mechanism of pituitary shock or recoil as a result of which the pituitary may be stimulated once more to provide a threshold level of F.S.H. In the pursuit of this happy achievement, the use of oestrogen has some value but, when it does occur, the clinician should not congratulate himself too much on the efficacy of his treatment but realise that spontaneous correction might well have occurred without any treatment at all.

(C) To test the response of the target organ. In certain patients the endometrium may be completely absent or incapable of response to the stimulation of oestrogen. This failure of response indicates the futility of any endocrine therapy directed to initiate cyclical bleeding.

Oestrogen Deficiency States

Menopausal symptoms. Many menopausal symptoms are relieved by the administration of oestrogen. The symptom most responsive to this treatment is the hot flush and it is this symptom which provides the commonest indication for treatment. Other symptoms, however, such as sweating, depression and mild gastro-intestinal symptoms will respond to oestrogen. It is important to keep the dose of oestrogen to the minimum effective range and never to continue treatment for more than one month. It is difficult to judge the correct dose. One method is to give the patient a single dose of stilboestrol 1·0 mg. or its equivalent and let her assess the response, which is confirmed by repeating the dose after a gap of seven days. She then takes that amount which will control her flushes without eliminating them entirely. Treatment may be repeated after a month's interval in which no oestrogen is given but it is inadvisable to continue this therapy indefinitely in spite of the patient's requests and although this type of dose schedule will seldom cause any trouble there is always the danger of any oestrogen therapy in that it may induce withdrawal bleeding, especially if the dosage is large. The practitioner is then in a dilemma: he feels confident that the bleeding is due to oestrogen but at the back of his mind there lurks the grim possibility that a carcinoma of the endometrium may have developed. For this reason many unnecessary curettages must be performed.

Menopausal symptoms are sometimes severe after hysterectomy where bilateral salpingo-oophorectomy has been performed. Where the indication for the operation is malignant disease of the genital tract, or when a patient has suffered from carcinoma of the breast, it is not justifiable to use oestrogen in the relief of the menopausal symptoms. Nor is it considered advisable in endometriosis since there is a real danger of stimulating extra-genital foci of endometriosis such as may be present in the bowel or elsewhere. Apart from these two contra-indications, the insertion of oestrogen by intramuscular or subfascial implantation (50–100 mg.) will provide a depot sufficient to last for a year, after which the pellets can be renewed, under local anaesthesia, if required. This is an effective and trouble-free method of treatment in most patients but should always be reserved for those in whom a hysterectomy has been performed, otherwise very troublesome and uncontrollable uterine bleeding may result. Implants, however, have little advantage over oral medication, the dose of which can be accurately assessed and varied if and as required.

The modern concept of *feminine forever* is based on the cyclical administration of oestrogen to menopausal women in order to "preserve their youth" or to prevent them "growing old". It is supposed to prevent all the degenerative changes that occur during and after the menopause and obviously has many attractions to sensitive ladies of menopausal age who imagine that they are going to degenerate into sexless old women within a few years. Oestrogen does of course prevent the postmenopausal degenerative changes which are caused by oestrogen lack, but most authorities doubt if this is sufficient indication for continuous oestrogen medication, when occasional intermittent therapy will prevent or cure these changes. Oestrogen in the form of conjugated urinary oestrogens (Premarin 0·625 mg. or 1·25 mg.) is given cyclically for twenty one days each month. It may or may not be combined with small doses of progesterone to ensure shorter withdrawal bleeding. This treatment is continued indefinitely, with bleeding occurring each month until the patient decides to give it up or until she has irregular or continuous bleeding resulting from continuous over-stimulation of her endometrium. If these symptoms occur then diagnostic curettage must be performed.

The cyclical administration of oestrogen to menopausal patients is potentially dangerous. It may stimulate endometrial carcinoma, certainly causes endometrial hyperplasia, maintains endometriosis in its active form and frequently terminates in curettage or hysterectomy for continuous or heavy bleeding. All menopausal and postmenopausal patients should be gynaecologically examined annually and a cervical smear taken. If the clinical examination or the smear show any degenerative changes that may cause symptoms these should be treated by a short course of oestrogen such as stilboestrol 0·5 mg. daily for two weeks and repeated in six months. Local senile or degenerative changes in the vagina can be treated by inserting oestrogen creams or pessaries nightly for two or three weeks.

The activity of oestrogen is potentiated by the administration of testosterone. Many preparations are available containing a mixture of oestrogen and testosterone, some of which have a recommended dose as high as 20 mg. of testosterone daily. As some patients continue to take oestrogen for their menopausal symptoms for many months or even years the potential dangers of testosterone, especially hirsutism, are a very real problem. Testosterone should not be administered to menopausal women except in very special circumstances.

Development of Secondary Sexual Characteristics. Oestrogen is of some value in developing the hypoplastic breast in patients suffering from ovarian deficiency, e.g. Turner's syndrome. It increases areolar pigmentation and effects a certain temporary degree of mammary hyperplasia, which can be considerably increased if a small amount of progesterone is added. Much of this regresses on cessation of treatment. The same effect occurs in the male breast but the dosage must be larger.

Oestrogen is mainly responsible for the development of all secondary sex characteristics and may be used in patients suffering from vulval hypoplasia to effect some development of the vulva and also of the vagina. Oestrogen has also been used to effect development in the so-called infantile or hypoplastic uterus. It is doubtful if very much enlargement does occur as a result of oestrogen stimulation and even more doubtful if such benefit is permanent.

Vulvovaginitis and Vaginitis. Good results are obtained with small doses of oral oestrogens in the treatment of vulvovaginitis in children. In adults the oestrogen may be given in the form of a vaginal pessary, or it may be given by mouth.

The same principles hold good in the treatment of some forms of vaginitis in adults and certain types of postmenopausal vaginitis respond particularly well. The treatment may be either local with the use of oestrogen creams, such as stilboestrol cream 1% or dienoestrol cream 0·01%. This local treatment can be combined with the oral administration of oestrogen in relatively small doses. It is customary in the treatment of refractory vaginal infections to administer oestrogens in the hope that the increased cornification of the vagina will make the vagina become more resistant to infection. Small doses should be used similar to those advised for menopausal cases, otherwise severe uterine bleeding may result. It should be emphasised that the aim of treatment is to discover the minimum effective dose that will relieve symptoms and not to exceed this.

Oestrogens increase the vascularity of the vagina, the cornification of its epithelium and therefore the acidity of the vagina and thereby help it to resist infection and also aid it to heal more rapidly. It is for these reasons that it is given in vulvovaginitis of children, in chronic vaginitis of adults and in postmenopausal vaginitis. It is also given to help healing of the decubitus ulcer in patients with severe degrees of prolapse and the healing of pessary ulcers or other traumatic lesions of the vagina. It is often given pre-operatively to patients in the postmenopausal age group who are awaiting repair of vaginal wall prolapse. In these patients it results in thickening of the vaginal epithelium and more rapid healing but carries the disadvantage of increased vascularity.

Oestrogen is also of value in the postmenopausal patient who complains of vulvitis secondary to atrophic change, infection or trauma. It should not be given to patients suffering from carcinoma of the vulva, leukoplakia or lichen sclerosus.

Oestrogens in Pregnancy. Oestrogens may be used as a test of pregnancy. Stilboestrol 0·5 mg. (or its equivalent) given daily for three days, especially if combined with progesterone, will produce withdrawal bleeding within three days in the non-pregnant state, but will not do so during pregnancy. These hormones given in this dosage during early pregnancy will not harm the pregnancy or the foetus.

Oestrogens have been used for many years for the treatment of recurrent or threatened abortion in the hope that they might improve placentation. It is doubtful if they have any beneficial effect.

Oestrogens have also been used to "prime" the uterus prior to the induction of labour, but there is no evidence that they have this effect.

Suppression of Lactation. It is established that oestrogens inhibit the secretion of the follicle stimulating hormone, and it is well known clinically that the lactogenic hormone, which is possibly identical with luteotropin (L.T.H.), is also inhibited, although the exact method of inhibition is not yet finally settled. Synthetic oestrogens are widely used to suppress lactation when breast feeding is contra-indicated, and when mammary distension must be relieved after the delivery of a stillborn child. A single intramuscular dose of 15 mg. of hexoestrol dipropionate is usually effective if given early before lactation has become well established. If inhibition is not affected the dose may be repeated. Oral oestrogen, such as ethinyl oestradiol is equally effective provided that the gastro-intestinal side effects are not distressing with the fairly high dosage necessary to suppress the anterior pituitary. Small doses of orally effective oestrogen, such as ethinyl oestradiol 0·05 mg. may be given even after the onset of lactation to control and diminish breast engorgement.

Dysmenorrhoea, Ovulation Pain and Contraception. In the treatment of dysmenorrhoea, oestrogen can only be effective in one way, by the inhibition of ovulation. To achieve this 0·1 mg. of ethinyl oestradiol or mestranol 0·1 mg. should be given daily from the fourth day of the cycle for at least twenty-one days. The dose of oestrogen may be halved if progesterone is added each day. Obviously only spasmodic dysmenorrhoea, due to painful ovulatory menstruation, can be expected to benefit by being converted into a painless anovulatory menstruation. As a therapeutic test for the true nature of the pain and as a confirmation that it is due to a painful ovulatory menstruation, the use of oestrogen is valuable since it is ineffective in all other types of dysmenorrhoea.

It is obvious that the easiest and most convenient method of suppressing ovulation is by means of one of the contraceptive pills, either the combined or sequential variety. These will also control pain at ovulation and ovulation bleeding, as well as controlling conception. These are dealt with further in Chapter 18.

Dysfunctional Uterine Haemorrhage. In dysfunctional uterine bleeding, it is usually possible to stop the haemorrhage by raising the blood level of oestrogen to super-threshold level. Massive dosage—5 mg. of stilboestrol or 0·25 mg. of ethinyl oestradiol every two hours—is given to achieve a quick rise and with this dosage the bleeding should be controlled in twenty-four hours or less. As soon as bleeding ceases, a maintenance dose of oestrogen, sufficient to keep the blood oestrogen at super-threshold level, is continued. 5 mg. of stilboestrol daily should suffice and this is continued for twenty-one days after which it is stopped. In two to five days, oestrogen withdrawal bleeding occurs after which a similar course of oestrogen is given. This type of therapy is useful as a temporary measure to tide the patient over a critical period of bleeding, pending admission to hospital. It is always liable, on cessation, to lead to severe haemorrhage due either to oestrogen withdrawal bleeding or oestrogen hyperplasia of the endometrium unless progesterone is added for a few days before stopping treatment.

Associated Diseases. Dermatologists frequently use oestrogen-containing creams for the treatment of skin conditions. They may be of considerable value in some conditions in the postmenopausal patient and also in children, and occasionally in the adolescent, but are of doubtful value during reproductive life. Many atrophic conditions which occur in the elderly, such as atrophic rhinitis and atrophic skeletal changes, may respond rapidly to oestrogen. The value of oestrogen in the treatment of carcinoma of the prostate in the male is well known.

PROGESTOGENS

Production. Endogenous progesterone is produced in the corpus luteum of the ovary. Very little progesterone is produced in the first half or proliferative phase of the menstrual cycle; production commences with the formation of the corpus luteum immediately after ovulation and rises to a peak on the 23rd day of the cycle which it maintains until the 26th day, after which the level falls to almost zero at the onset of menstruation. Progesterone is metabolised in the liver and excreted in the urine as sodium pregnanediol glycuronide and is recoverable as such for assay in the secretory phase of the menstrual cycle.

Actions of Progestogens. These are also discussed on page 82 and may briefly be summarised here.

Endometrium. Progestogens cause secretory hypertrophy and decidual formation if the endometrium has been previously primed with oestrogen.

Pregnancy. Progestogen firstly from the corpus luteum and later from the placenta is essential for the continuation of pregnancy.

Uterus. Progestogens cause myohyperplasia of the uterus. They increase the strength but diminish the frequency of uterine contractions.

Fallopian Tube. Progestogens cause hyperplasia of the muscular lining of the Fallopian tube and make peristaltic contractions more powerful as well as increasing the secretion of the tubal mucous membrane.

Cervix. Progestogens cause some hypertrophy of the cervix and make the cervical mucus more viscous.

Vagina. During early pregnancy the vagina becomes violet coloured due to venous congestion. The epithelial cells fail to mature and cornify. They are classically basophilic with fairly large nucleii and folded edges.

Breasts. Progestogens, with oestrogen, cause breast hypertrophy. They increase acinar epithelial growth.

Pituitary. The exact action of progestogens on the pituitary is not known. Progestogens may inhibit the production of follicle stimulating hormone, and thus suppress ovulation. A certain percentage of most progestogens is metabolised to oestrogen and it may well be that the oestrogen so produced is responsible for inhibiting pituitary activity.

Fluid Retention. Progestogens cause water and sodium retention and become a contributory factor in premenstrual tension and weight gain.

Smooth Muscle. Progestogens relax smooth muscle, although the exact mode of action is not known.

Thermogenic. Progestogens raise the body temperature by up to 0·5°C.

Anabolic Effect. Progestogens exert an anabolic effect and this partly accounts for some of the weight gain which may follow their administration.

Libido. Diminution of libido infrequently occurs.

Virilisation. Whilst part of administered progestogen is metabolised to oestrogen, it is also partly metabolised to testosterone and if therefore administered to a patient during pregnancy can have a virilising effect upon a female foetus.

Source of Progestogens

The diagram below indicates the relationship between progestogens and testosterone, and also shows their relationship to oestrogen. Progesterone is the naturally occurring progestogen. Numerous synthetic progestogens have been

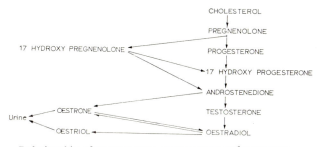

Relationship of progestogens, testosterone and oestrogen.

discovered and some of them are marketed. They are either derivatives of testosterone such as ethisterone or 19 nor-steroids, such as nor-ethisterone, or derivatives of progesterone such as 17αhydroxy progesterone caproate.

The synthetic progestogens vary considerably in the details of their effect upon the body. This is because they are partly metabolised into testosterone and oestrogen and the percentage so metabolised with each progestogen varies, as also does their anabolic effect and their action on electrolyte balance. Broadly speaking the general effect of synthetic progestogens is twenty-five times more powerful than ethisterone.

Dangers. There are few dangers attached to the administration of progestogens in small or reasonable doses. Larger doses, however, may cause side effects such as weight gain, nausea, vomiting, headache, fluid retention and oedema. Some progestogens may also cause hirsutism and skin pigmentation. Virilisation may occur in the female foetus if they are administered during pregnancy, with the exception of 17αhydroxy progesterone caproate which does not cause virilisation. Progestogens cause an increase in the coagulability of blood and there is an increasing amount of evidence that they, or their oestrogen metabolites, do predispose to intravascular clotting with the resulting deep venous thrombosis and thrombo-embolic disease.

Treatment

1. *Oral Administration.* All synthetic progestogens may be given by mouth with the exception of 17αhydroxy progesterone caproate, which has to be given by injection. Ethisterone is absorbed from the mouth but is destroyed by gastric acid and is therefore given as linguets. Their effect lasts for approximately three days.

2. *Systemic Administration.*

(i) Injection. 17αhydroxy progesterone caproate is given by deep intramuscular injections at a dose varying from 125 mg. to 500 mg. It does not cause masculinisation of the female foetus and is therefore the progesterone of choice during pregnancy. Its effect lasts about seven days.

(ii) Implants. Progesterone subfascial implants varying from 50–200 mg. are occasionally used. They take up to three months to absorb.

Local Applications. There is no evidence that local applications of progesterone have any beneficial effect.

Indications for Treatment

(1) *Inhibition of Ovulation.* All the active synthetic progestogens certainly inhibit ovulation but it is not known whether this is a direct action of progesterone itself or of its oestrogen metabolites. Apart from the dangers referred to above there do not appear to be any disadvantages in the suppression of ovulation by progestogens. There is no evidence that they affect eventual fertility or that they have any deleterious action upon the ripe ova or subsequent offspring.

Ovulation Pain. If ovulation is suppressed obviously ovulation pain will also be relieved

Ovulation Bleeding. If ovulation is suppressed ovulation bleeding from the endometrium will not occur. Ovulation pain and bleeding should, however, only be treated after it has been carefully explained to the patient that both these phenomena are a manifestation of a normal physiological process and that they are in no way pathological.

(2) *Contraception*. Contraception by the use of oral progestogens is well known. The majority of oral contraceptives contain some added oestrogen (see Chapter 14) since progestogen alone is not so efficient at suppressing ovulation as a combination of oestrogen and progestogen. The continuous administration of low dose progestogen (chlormadinone 0·5 mg. daily) is a reasonably effective contraceptive agent which acts by increasing the viscosity of the cervical mucus and so creating a barrier to sperm penetration. Ovulation may be suppressed by this dose in about 50% of patients. Chlormadinone has recently been withdrawn from the British market because it may cause breast tumours in some animals.

(3) *Spasmodic Dysmenorrhoea*. Since oral progestogens will suppress ovulation they will also give relief from spasmodic dysmenorrhoea by converting painful ovulatory cycles into painless anovulatory bleeding.

(4) *Premenstrual Tension*. Premenstrual tension which results from the retention of fluid secondary to the high level of hormones in the immediate premenstrual phase does sometimes respond to the administration of exogenous progestogen.

(5) *Metropathia Haemorrhagica*. True metropathia haemorrhagica which has been histologically proven will nearly always respond to the administration of cyclic progestogen.

(6) *Dysfunctional Bleeding*. Dysfunctional uterine haemorrhage which is not caused by metropathia haemorrhagica will frequently improve on cyclic progestogen therapy. The duration and the amount of loss will be reduced in the majority of instances but the results obtained will not be so dramatic as with metropathia haemorrhagica itself. Curettage must always be performed in order to exclude intrauterine pathology and to confirm the diagnosis prior to progestogen therapy.

(7) *Puberty Menorrhagia* can be similarly controlled by short courses of progestogen as described on page 453. In severe instances it may be necessary to give two or three months' complete cyclic treatment until ovulation is established.

(8) *Pregnancy Test*. Progestogen may be used with oestrogen in the diagnosis of pregnancy since administration of an oestrogen-progestogen mixture for two or three days will induce uterine bleeding in the non-pregnant state, whereas it will fail to do so during pregnancy (see page 475).

(9) *Amenorrhoea*. Progestogen is frequently administered alone in both primary and secondary amenorrhoea to test for the presence of circulating oestrogen since the endometrium will not bleed unless it has been previously primed with oestrogen. If it is desired to produce withdrawal bleeding then usually progesterone is combined with oestrogen in cyclical therapy.

(10) *Pituitary Rebound*. Several cycles of an oestrogen-progestogen mixture are occasionally given to patients suffering from anovulatory cycles in the

hope that this may induce ovulation following the withdrawal of the pro-gestogen. There is a certain amount of clinical evidence to support the view that this does occur but statistical proof is lacking.

(11) *Control of the Menstrual Cycle.* Women occasionally request help because their menstrual period is to occur on a date which may cause them some embarrassment. This request may come from younger patients with severe dysmenorrhoea and examination commitments, patients who have theatrical or athletic commitments, patients who have particularly arduous social engagements or who have to undertake tiring journeys, as well as the wedding which has to be arranged at an inappropriate time for reasons beyond the patient's control. Using a synthetic oestrogen-progestogen com-bination it is comparatively easy to advance menstruation or to postpone it indefinitely, but before doing so it is advisable to discuss the disadvantages of so doing with the patient. It may subsequently take one or two months for the menstrual cycle to return to its normal rhythm. It requires a fairly large dose to ensure success and it is possible that the patient may experience side effects greater than the disadvantages of the period which she wishes to avoid. In order to bring the period forward it is necessary to start an oestrogen-progestogen mixture on the fourth or fifth day of the menstrual cycle. Ethinyl oestradiol 0·05 and nor-ethisterone 5 mg. given daily for 14 days will produce a period on the twentieth day, but to ensure that there is no further bleeding a further course of ethinyl oestradiol 0·05 mg. together with nor-ethisterone 5 mg. should be given daily from the fourth to the twenty-fourth day or until such time as the patient is prepared to have the next period. In order to postpone menstruation a similar dose (ethinyl oestradiol 0·05 mg. together with nor-ethisterone 5 mg., or mestranol 0·05 mg. together with nor-ethynodrel 5 mg.) should be given daily starting at least seven days before the expected period and continuing until such time as the patient wishes to have her period.

(12) *Infertility.* Since one of the causes of infertility may be irregular or inadequate ripening of the endometrium, progestogens are sometimes given in the second half of the menstrual cycle to ensure a good secretory endo-metrial response. Although frequently used it is difficult to prove that this particular form of treatment is of any real benefit.

(13) *Abortion.* The use of progesterone in the treatment of threatened or habitual abortion has been discussed on page 376. Some indication of the progesterone response of the body may be obtained by the examination of vaginal smears, and if these show a deficient progesterone response it seems logical to administer progestogen in the form of 17αhydroxyprogesterone caproate by intramuscular injection 250 mg. weekly and to increase this dose until a satisfactory progesterone response has been obtained on the vaginal smear. Many authorities consider that this form of treatment is of no actual benefit to the patient or to her pregnancy but is only of psychological advantage and fairly expensive psychological treatment at best. Whilst the value of these injections remains unproved the clinical impression is that they are of benefit to the patient.

(14) *Endometriosis.* The control of endometriosis by non-surgical treatment

and the administration of progestogen is well recognised. This may be performed by creating a state of pseudo-pregnancy by the administration of oral progestogen over a long period, or by the administration of cyclical progestogen as described on page 704.

(15) *Carcinoma of the Body of the Uterus.* The continuous administration of progestogens in the treatment of endometriosis causes a regression of the endometrium within the uterus and of the ectopic endometrium. It seems a natural progression from this to treat endometrial carcinoma by large doses of progestogen. It has been shown that large doses of progestogen (17α-hydroxyprogesterone caproate 1 Gm or more weekly) will sometimes control endometrial carcinoma and its metastases for a varying time.

Treatment of Amenorrhoea

Considerable judgment is required in treating amenorrhoea. Many girls are brought by their mothers to the doctor because they have not started menstruation at the age their parent expects. The lay mind regards retardation of menstrual function in a very sinister light. In actual fact the age of the onset of menstruation is extremely variable, and many women of proved subsequent fertility do not start to menstruate before 18 or 20 years of age, or even later. No harm can result in delaying treatment in such patients, nor is the beneficial result of subsequent treatment in any way prejudiced. Fussy investigation and tedious and complicated treatment is far more likely to upset the delicate mechanism of menstruation, and all that these patients require is a general and pelvic clinical examination and sensible reassurance that all is normal and that there is no evidence of any organic disease. In many cases spontaneous cure will ultimately result. Furthermore, in those patients who have undergone a premature menopause or who are suffering from severe genital hypoplasia the production of false periods by cyclical oestrogen withdrawal bleeding is unlikely to be of any genuine benefit and is scientifically pointless.

The amenorrhoea resulting from pelvic surgery and therapy will not be considered. Pituitary and suprarenal diseases are outside the province of gynaecologists. Cryptomenorrhoea can be dealt with surgically. Virilising tumours of the ovary must be removed. In clinical practice the types of case which are dealt with by gynaecologists are hypothalamic amenorrhoea, ovarian aplasia, and ovarian hypofunction. In the hypothalamic cases psychotherapy is of the greatest importance. The patient should be removed from worries, anxieties and overwork. Environmental changes and malnutrition must be corrected. Many patients associate amenorrhoea with insanity and still believe that suppressed menstruation affects the brain. Open-air exercise and interests should be encouraged, and a holiday in a warm climate is often of the greatest help in these cases. Even a change of employment can be helpful.

Amenorrhoea is often associated with obesity, and the reduction of weight following strict diet, with limited salt and water intake, is frequently accompanied by a spontaneous cure of the amenorrhoea. The scientific explanation of this improvement is unconvincing, but in all cases of obesity dietetic

16*

restriction is well worth a trial. In such cases and where there is evidence of hypothyroidism the addition of thyroid may be helpful.

The specific hormone therapy is dealt with more fully below. The exhibition of oestrogen followed by progestogen in cyclical dose patterns designed to mimic the natural phases of menstruation is of some value primarily as a test of the responsiveness of the endometrium. The production of cyclical bleeding is certainly reassuring to the patient and may be beneficial where the psychosomatic factor plays a part in the causation of the amenorrhoea. In a few patients it may be actually curative, at least temporarily, in restarting the normal pituitary ovarian cycle.

Where underdevelopment of the secondary sexual characteristics is a sign of ovarian insufficiency, the exhibition of oestrogen in large doses over a long period may be successful in achieving a more feminine contour. This is of cosmetic and psychological benefit to the patient.

Apart from the removal of virilising tumours of the ovary and adrenal cortex, surgery plays no part in the treatment of amenorrhoea with one notable exception. This is the operation of wedge resection of the ovaries in the Stein-Leventhal syndrome, itself a relatively rare condition.

The prognosis in cases of amenorrhoea can be summarised as follows.

Primary amenorrhoea is rarely cured except in young girls with a delayed menarche. Primary amenorrhoea is not, however, always a bar to conception and women over 20 are seen in whom pregnancy has occurred without any preceding menstruation. In cases of secondary amenorrhoea the prognosis depends largely upon the duration of the symptom. The longer it has lasted the more gloomy the outlook becomes. Provided, however, that gross abnormalities can be excluded a number of patients will undergo a spontaneous cure, so that the claims of individual lines of treatment should always be regarded with some suspicion.

The isolation of active human pituitary follicle stimulating hormone by Gemzell in Sweden in 1958 has altered the whole outlook in the treatment of amenorrhoea due to pituitary ovarian dysfunction. The use of Clomiphene followed in 1961. Out of 51 patients with functional secondary amenorrhoea Clomiphene therapy achieved conception in 9. These recent advances are in their infancy, the availability of therapy is limited and the dosage not yet standardised. They promise, however, to be of immeasurable value in the future.

Treatment of amenorrhoea by the use of drugs which induce ovulation

Various compounds are now available which can be used for the induction of ovulation in the human:

(1) *Heterologous gonadotropins.** These preparations are mostly extracted from pregnant mares' serum but are occasionally made from sheep pituitary. Their dominant effect is follicle stimulating but they also have some luteinising activity. Their prolonged use in the human unfortunately occasionally results in anti-hormone production antagonistic to human gonadotropins.

(2) *Homologous gonadotropins.* Human Chorionic Gonadotropin (H.C.G.)

* See footnote p. 76

is a glycoprotein with a predominantly luteinising action which will not itself induce either follicular maturation or ovulation but is capable of provoking ovulation after F.S.H. has been given to induce follicular maturation. H.C.G. is at present the preparation of choice as a luteinising agent.

(3) *Human pituitary gonadotropin* (H.P.G.) commonly known as follicle stimulating hormone (F.S.H.). This is prepared from human pituitary extract, contains a mixture of follicle stimulating hormone and luteinising hormone. Although it is a combination of F.S.H. and L.H. it is certainly capable of inducing follicle maturation. The supply is very restricted owing to the limited number of human pituitaries available.

(4) *Human menopausal gonadotropin* (H.M.G.). Human menopausal gonadotropin contains both F.S.H. and L.H. These gonadotropins in predictable potency can be extracted from the urine. They contain more F.S.H. than L.H. and in fact the amount of L.H. is seldom sufficient to induce maturation without the addition of H.C.G. Pergonal and Humegon are preparations of F.S.H. and L.H. obtained from human menopausal urine. It is usual to express its potency in terms of the number of international units of F.S.H. and L.H. per ml.

(5) *Clomiphene* (*Clomid*). Clomiphene is not a steroid. It is both oestrogenic and anti-oestrogenic. It is capable of inducing ovulation but its exact mechanism of action is not known. It is considered that it may increase the excretion of F.S.H. from the pituitary by blocking the pituitary uptake of oestrogen. It may also have a direct depressive action on the synthesis of oestrogen in the ovary itself.

It is of the utmost importance that any patient who is to be considered for treatment by any of the drugs which induce ovulation should be extensively and fully investigated whether the amenorrhoea be primary or secondary in origin. A detailed history must be taken, full examination performed, X-ray examination of the skull and pituitary fossa, full blood count and complete examination of the urine, urine estimations of 17-ketosteroid, 17-hydroxysteroid and urinary oestrogen excretion patterns. Chromosomal studies whilst not being essential are of benefit. The F.S.H. levels should be estimated. Three main groups of patients will be demarcated by these investigations in whom it is reasonable to consider the induction of ovulation: **firstly** those with primary amenorrhoea having a normal chromosomal pattern and a normal genital tract. It is important to differentiate between true gonadal agenesis and hypoplastic ovaries. **Secondly** a number of patients who ovulate only two or three times each year and are thereby relatively infertile. **Thirdly** a group of apparently normal women who do not ovulate, may be suffering from either premature menopause, hyperthecosis syndrome, metropathia haemorrhagica, occasional anovulatory cycles or current anovulatory cycles. Shearman has described the standardised gonadotropin stimulation test which will differentiate these groups. Urinary oestrogen excretion levels are measured to form a baseline. The patient is then given 1,000 units of H.C.G. daily for three days, followed by F.S.H. (Pergonal 225 I.U.) by injection daily for three days. Urinary oestrones are estimated for eight days and four distinct patterns emerge:

(1) Patients in whom the urinary oestrone is unaltered (less than 5 micrograms per 24 hours). These patients are suffering from gonadal agenesis or premature menopause.

(2) Patients with hyperthecosis ovarii. Oestrone excretion rate rises to 50 or 100 micrograms per 24 hours and is usually accompanied by palpable ovarian enlargement.

(3) Patients with metropathia haemorrhagica. These patients have a relatively high base level of urinary oestrone which is not altered by administration of H.C.G.

(4) Patients with persistent anovulatory menstruation or hypogonadism have a base level of urinary oestrone of less than 5 micrograms per 24 hours. This level rises to 10 or even 15 micrograms following stimulation.

Patients with Stein-Leventhal syndrome respond well to surgery if they are properly selected. They also respond well to Clomiphene, but the good result only lasts so long as treatment continues. There is a possible danger that these patients may develop hyperstimulation syndrome.

Patients with metropathia haemorrhagica respond well to Clomiphene. Patients with irregular ovulation will usually respond satisfactorily to Clomiphene. Patients with hypogonadism respond reasonably well to Clomiphene with about 30% success and these patients should be treated initially with Clomiphene, reserving gonadotropin for the treatment of those in whom Clomiphene fails.

Human gonadotropins. Human gonadotropins (F.S.H. and L.H.) are identical whether the source be urine or pituitary. In theory F.S.H. is given in order to induce follicular maturation and this is followed by H.C.G. to provoke ovulation. This sounds simple but in practice it proves extremely difficult because of the varying sensitivity of patients to gonadotropins and a dose which will fail to stimulate a ripening follicle in one patient may be sufficient to produce gross ovarian enlargement or multiple pregnancy in another (Townsend). The great dangers of treatment lie in over-stimulation with the resulting incidence of multiple births and also in the development of the hyperstimulation syndrome.

The hyperstimulation syndrome can be extremely dangerous and can be divided into three categories:

(1) Mild hyperstimulation which is reflected only in laboratory findings and there are no abnormal symptoms.

(2) Moderate hyperstimulation in which there is ovarian enlargement, lower abdominal pain, nausea and occasional ascites.

(3) Severe hyperstimulation in which there is gross ovarian enlargement, abdominal pain, vomiting, ascites, occasionally ovarian necrosis, intra-peritoneal haemorrhage and possibly major thrombo-embolic episodes.

It will be seen from the description of hyperstimulation syndrome that this must be avoided at all costs and dosage schedules have been carefully designed in order to avoid this complication. It is essential to predetermine an individual patient's sensitivity. This is determined by daily estimations of ovarian size, cervical mucus, vaginal smears and urinary oestrogen excretions following an initial dose of F.S.H. A single dose of F.S.H. is given every three weeks and is increased by 50% each time until a positive response is obtained. When a positive response has occurred a single dose of H.C.G. 24,000 I.U. is given on the tenth day after the injection of F.S.H. The results of treatment by gonadotropins, as measured by a pregnancy rate, vary according to the care with which the patients are selected and with which their treatment is arranged and controlled. A success of 50% can confidently be expected in cases which are well chosen and well controlled.

Clomiphene does not suffer from the disadvantage of severe hyperstimulation syndrome, although some ovarian over-stimulation does occur. The side effects are trivial, mainly sensations of heat and sweating, frequency of micturition, occasional blurring of vision, sometimes some loss of hair which is reversible. The initial course of Clomiphene is 50 mg. daily for five days and if menstruation does not occur within 35 days this dose is increased to 100 mg. daily for five days, thence to 150 mg. daily for five days, if menstruation still fails to occur. The patient should be seen and examined every two weeks to see if ovarian enlargement has occurred and, if so, treatment should be suspended until the ovaries have returned to their former size. Clomiphene is the drug of choice in patients with metropathia haemorrhagica whose main complaint is infertility rather than haemorrhage. Clomiphene is certainly as effective as surgery in patients with Stein-Leventhal syndrome but is only effective so long as treatment is continued, whereas an adequately performed wedge resection may well provide permanent relief from the symptoms. It is the drug of choice in those patients who suffer from infrequent ovulation and are thereby infertile and is the correct initial treatment in those patients suffering from anovulatory cycles of unknown origin. Clomiphene may also be successful in some cases of hypogonadism.

Treatment by gonadotropins should be reserved for those patients in whom Clomiphene treatment has failed. No patient should be treated by Clomiphene unless the doctor in charge of the patient has facilities for adequate investigation and is prepared to see the patient at frequent intervals, and no patient should be treated by gonadotropin therapy unless full and adequate facilities are available for supervising the treatment as outlined above.

It is essential that the cause of anovulation should be determined before attempts are made to induce ovulation by drug therapy. The diagnosis frequently requires extensive and exhaustive investigation. The results obtained by the correct treatment in the individually supervised patient are good. The inherent dangers in the use of gonadotropins may gradually lessen in the future as they are gradually better understood. Hyperstimulation with its attending risks will continue to be a dangerous problem. Because Clomiphene is relatively free from side effects the tendency to use it without proper supervision and control must be resisted.

Finally in relation to induction of ovulation the doctor must remember that he is treating a patient who with her husband must be continuously consulted and informed of the details of both the investigations and the treatment, together with the risks that the latter entail, for without the dedicated co-operation of the patient and her husband induction of ovulation can neither be properly organised or supervised.

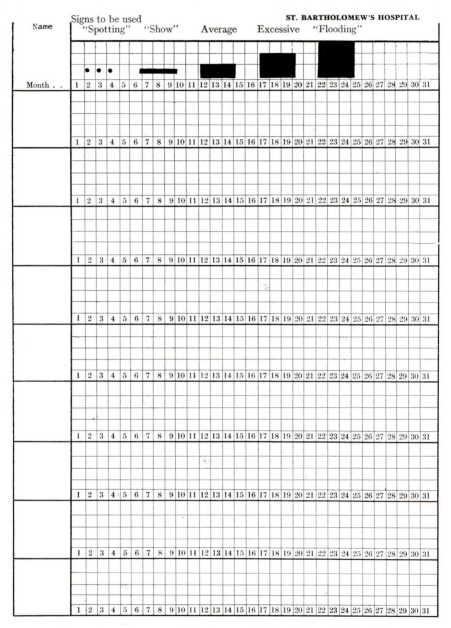

The pattern of menstrual chart in use at St. Bartholomew's Hospital.

Androgens in Clinical Practice

In the recent past, androgens have been used in the control of dysfunctional bleeding, dysmenorrhoea and for severe menopausal symptoms. They have also been employed in the treatment of the premenstrual congestion syndrome. Their place in modern practice has been steadily usurped by the newer oral progestogen and, with the possible exception of endometriosis they now play little or no part in gynaecological therapy. They, therefore, merit only perfunctory mention in this chapter.

Endometriosis. Androgens (testosterone) depress the activity of ectopic endometrium and may therefore be used as a diagnostic test for the presence of endometriosis as a cause of pelvic pain and a differential diagnosis from pelvic infection. Testosterone 10 mg. is given twice daily for three weeks and this dose will frequently result in considerable improvement of symptoms if the patient is suffering from endometriosis but will not cause any improvement in a patient suffering from pelvic infection. It must be stressed, however, that this does not cure endometriosis but only provides temporary relief in a few instances. It must not exceed the schedule detailed nor may it be repeated in less than six months.

Some of the synthetic progestogens are partly metabolised into testosterone so that occasionally patients will in fact complain of androgenisation even of minor degree, secondary to the administration of some of these progestogens. For this reason it may be worth recounting the androgenising symptoms which may occur. They are: amenorrhoea; change of hair distribution with hirsutism of the upper lip, chin, chest; male hair distribution on the lower abdomen, hair on the extensor surfaces of the arms and legs and hair on the back; dorsal acne; clitoral hypertrophy; breast atrophy; changes of body contour and fat distribution; and alteration of the voice.

Far too much androgen is administered to far too many unsuspecting women by means of its inclusion in commercial preparations. Testosterone should never be administered to a female patient without telling her of its possible consequences. The authors do not recommend the use of testosterone in gynaecology, with the possible exception of its use as a diagnostic test for endometriosis.

20 Inflammations of the Uterus

Acute inflammations of the uterus are usually the result of either septic abortion, puerperal sepsis or acute gonorrhoea. Chronic inflammation of the body of the uterus, apart from tuberculosis, is rare in the reproductive period. The exfoliation of the endometrium provides a natural scavenging effect which deters any endometrial infection from becoming established. Chronic inflammation of the cervix and particularly of the racemose glands of the cervical canal are common, because the epithelial crypts provide an ideal nidus for organisms. Once established in these glands, infection is difficult to eradicate.

Acute Endometritis

It has already been stated that acute endometritis is caused by septic abortion, puerperal sepsis and acute gonorrhoea. In all three conditions, the other clinical features tend to overshadow the inflammation of the endometrium of the uterus. From the purely pathological aspect, however, in septic abortion and puerperal sepsis the acute inflammation of the endometrium is the essential feature. In acute gonorrhoea, infection of the endometrium is probably common, but causes relatively few symptoms and is overshadowed by the more acute cervicitis, urethritis and salpingitis.

Acute endometritis may follow the introduction of tents, dilators and particularly radium tubes into the cavity of the uterus, when it gives rise to uterine bleeding and discharge. It is also a complication of any foreign body such as the Gräfenberg ring, the wishbone and collar-stud pessary. The modern intra-uterine contraceptive devices must be added to this list of foreign bodies.

The clinical features of septic abortion and puerperal fever, viz., high fever and purulent vaginal discharge, are well known. The uterus is tender and because of the recent pregnancy, is larger than normal. The histological appearances of the lining of the uterus are those to be expected in acute inflammation. The endometrium is hyperaemic with a multitude of dilated capillaries and small interstitial haemorrhages. The stroma is oedematous and infiltrated with leucocytes and plasma cells and the leucocytic infiltration is often considerable. In septic abortion and puerperal sepsis the infective processes involve the myometrium to a variable degree so that the myometrium is oedematous and infiltrated with small round cells.

In gonococcal endometritis the infiltration with round cells is scattered irregularly over the endometrium, and there is little evidence of any involvement of the myometrium. The intense hyperaemia of the inflamed endometrium causes an oozing of the blood into the cavity of the uterus and continuous bleeding. Clinically, the development of uterine bleeding is a characteristic sign of gonococcal infection of the endometrium.

The acute endometritis of puerperal sepsis and septic abortion is dealt with in text-books of obstetrics. In gynaecological practice, acute endometritis is not often seen. The two examples which are encountered with any frequency are acute gonococcal endometritis and the acute endometritis caused by the application of radium to the uterus. Conservative measures are always employed. In gonorrhoea, the essential treatment is the administration of chemotherapy. Intrauterine medication with antiseptics is unnecessary and may do more harm than good. The patient should always be watched carefully, as salpingitis may develop from the upward spread of the infection to the Fallopian tubes. In most cases of acute endometritis, the bloodstained discharge from the uterus clears up spontaneously after a few weeks. Menstrual periods which occur during or after acute endometritis are usually excessive.

Except for the acute endometritis of septic abortion and puerperal sepsis, acute endometritis should not be regarded as a serious disease. Unless it is infected by virulent organisms such as the clostridia, the endometrium seems capable of dealing with infections by its own resistance, partly because the products of infection can drain away from the uterus through the cervical canal, but mainly because the superficial layers of the endometrium are shed by menstruation.

Chronic Endometritis

Chronic endometritis is relatively uncommon. Some degree of chronic infection of the endometrium accompanies any persistent source of infection in the uterus such as infected myomatous polypi, carcinoma of the cervix and body of the uterus, any foreign body such as the modern intrauterine contraceptive device is liable to cause a low grade chronic endometritis. Tuberculous endometritis has already been mentioned (page 260).

Pyometra, which is usually met with in elderly women, is one of the best recognised forms of chronic endometritis. The clinical term, senile endometritis, suggests a chronic infection of the endometrium, usually low-grade, and only demonstrable histologically. In practice, it is almost synonymous with pyometra and can be conveniently regarded as an intermittent pyometra. Pyometra is caused by a stenosis of the cervical canal either from a carcinoma of the cervix, as the result of operation on the cervix such as amputation, as the result of radiation, or lastly by post-menopausal involution of the uterus which leads to the cervical canal becoming blocked in the region of the internal os. Apart from these obstructive lesions it is a very common associate with carcinoma of the endometrium. The pent-up discharges from the glands of the endometrium collect in the uterine cavity and become infected, the infection probably reaching the body of the uterus by upward spread from the vagina. In fact, senile vaginitis and senile endometritis often co-exist. Later, as a result of the infection, the endometrium becomes converted into granulation tissue which discharges pus into the uterus to produce a pyometra. Pyometra of accessory cornua of the uterus has already been described in

Chapter 5 in the section dealing with Malformations of the Uterus (see page 156).

In chronic endometritis, the histological appearances of the endometrium are as follows: The stroma is infiltrated with leucocytes and plasma cells, and the capillaries are dilated. Granulation tissue is found in cases of pyometra and in the vicinity of degenerate malignant growths. Squamous metaplasia of the epithelium is often seen. The essential symptom of chronic endometritis is bloodstained purulent discharge, but this symptom is characteristic of all the conditions leading to the development of chronic endometritis.

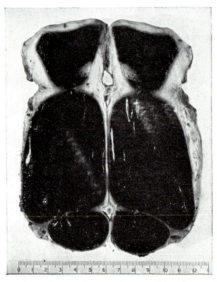

Fig. 230. An unusual specimen of pyometra resulting from adhesive vaginitis following a prolapse operation. The photo shows three loculi; the upper is a true pyometra involving the body of the uterus; the middle locule consists of the grossly expanded cervix and the lower small locule represents the vaginal vault.

It follows that the symptoms of chronic endometritis are overshadowed by those of the primary cause. The diagnosis is often missed and only made when the cervix is dilated as a preliminary to diagnostic curettage performed to exclude a uterine cancer. The passage of sound or dilator releases a flow of pus which is often blood-stained. Sometimes the uterus is enlarged, tense and tender on bimanual examination and the signs may be associated with fever, leucocytosis and some lower abdominal pain. When a known cancer of the cervix is accompanied by such a slightly enlarged and locally tender uterus with fever the most likely diagnosis is pyometra.

The **treatment of pyometra** consists in dilating the cervix carefully under anaesthesia by means of metal dilators and taking a swab for culture and sensitivity test. If there is any suspicion of carcinoma either of the body of the uterus or cervical canal gentle curetting must be performed. A smal rubber drainage tube should then be placed in the cervical canal and retained in position with a suture of thin catgut through the cervix. Manipulations of this kind in a case of pyometra must always be performed with gentleness and care, because of the risk of perforating the uterus and spreading infection to the peritoneal cavity. The myometrium is notably friable and easily breached in carcinoma of the endometrium without a pyometra and doubly so when the two conditions coexist.

The main principle in the treatment of pyometra is to exclude a cancer of the endocervix or uterine corpus which is significantly associated with this condition. It is, essential, therefore, to perform a thorough endocervical biopsy by curettage and, in addition, a thorough endometrial curettage. Owing to the very real danger of perforation, this curettage may have to be postponed for ten to fourteen days after the initial drainage of the pyometra but it must never be neglected. If a carcinoma of the endocervix is found, the patient is treated by Wertheim's hysterectomy or radium but neither of these must be considered until the pyometra has been drained and the infection controlled by antibiotics. If an endometrial carcinoma is discovered, a Wertheim's hysterectomy is performed with the same reservations. One of the present authors has recently seen a well established carcinoma of the endometrium which presented as a pyometra and in which two careful and conscientious curettages completely missed the growth. Other writers have concurred in this observation. The frequent coincidence of carcinoma of the uterus and pyometra provides a strong argument for treating many of these patients by total hysterectomy and bilateral salpingo-oophorectomy, even if the curettage is negative. It has even been suggested by Jeffcoate that pyometra is a precancerous lesion. It is, however, more likely that it is a post-cancerous condition and, therefore, merits radical surgery.

Metritis

Acute Metritis. Some degree of inflammation of the myometrium accompanies the acute endometritis of puerperal sepsis and septic abortion. In severe cases of uterine sepsis a well-marked metritis, with leucocytic infiltration and oedema may develop. Very rarely interstitial abscesses may form in the myometrium. In severe streptococcal and clostridial infections the organisms may penetrate through the wall of the uterus into the parametrium and peritoneal cavity. It is probable that the acute metritis accompanying puerperal sepsis clears up completely and leaves no permanent damage to the myometrium. Histological examination of the myometrium in these patients fails to demonstrate evidence of chronic inflammation, once the primary inflammation has subsided.

Chronic Metritis. Pathologically, there is little, if any, evidence that a chronic inflammation of the myometrium, apart from the very rare tuberculous forms, is ever seen. The term chronic metritis was originally used for a clinical group of cases in which the dominant symptoms were irregular and profuse haemorrhage, back-ache, and discharge. The uterus was often found to be bulky, and not infrequently its consistence was firmer than normal. It has been shown, however, that the elastic tissue content of the uterus is increased after each pregnancy and that the normal result of pregnancy is a deposition of elastic tissue around the arteries and veins of the myometrium which accounts for the greater bulk and firmness of the multiparous uterus. The increase in the amount of elastic tissue is to be regarded as a physiological process, and not due to subinvolution. It is not uncommon to find a large deposition of elastic tissue in the uterus of a multipara without the patient having had any gynaecological symptoms whatsoever.

The involution of the vessels of the puerperal uterus is a highly complex process. The lumen of the vessel is reduced by proliferation of the subendo-thelial tissues. In the media of the vessel the muscle cells undergo granular

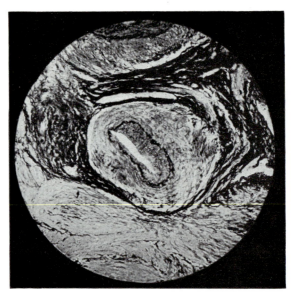

FIG. 231. An artery in the wall of a multiparous uterus. The black areas illustrate the distribution of elastic tissue. Elastic tissue has been deposited plentifully around the veins.

atrophy, and in the sinuses and veins there is well-marked hyaline degenera-tion. At a later stage in the process of involution elastic tissue is deposited in the adventitia and the hyaline tissue is absorbed. The internal elastic lamina becomes thicker and is often laminated (see Fig. 231).

The cases which were formerly described under the term chronic metritis are now regarded as being due in the main to ovarian disturbances and are exemplified by metropathia haemorrhagica, and the other types of irregular haemorrhage described on page 460. There is very little pathological evidence that either a chronic inflammation, a fibrosis of the myometrium, arterio-sclerosis of the uterine vessels, or delayed subinvolution are processes res-ponsible for the causation of the symptoms of this group. It is much more scientific and much more serviceable clinically to classify these patients according to the scheme outlined in Chapter 18.

It should also be remembered that some degree of chronic myometritis is associated with chronic inflammations of the pelvis, such as adnexal inflammation, parametritis, pyometra, and degenerate new growths of the uterus. But in all such patients the chronic myometritis is of secondary importance compared with the primary cause.

Cervicitis

Acute Cervicitis. In septic abortion, puerperal sepsis and gonorrhoea, the cervix is acutely inflamed. When the cervix is examined through a vaginal speculum it is seen to be reddened, swollen with oedema, and muco-pus can be seen to be discharged through the cervical canal. Not uncommonly tenderness is elicited by palpation of the cervix. In acute gonococcal cervicitis there is often a little backache and a feeling of fullness in the lower abdomen, which may be due to the acute inflammation of the cervix, but is more likely to be caused by the coincident parametritis. In acute cervicitis, just as with acute endometritis, the symptoms and clinical course are overshadowed by those of the associated lesions of the disease. For example, in septic abortion and puerperal sepsis acute cervicitis is of less importance than endometritis with its risk of septicaemia, salpingitis, and peritonitis. Similarly, in acute gonorrhoea the acute inflammation of the cervix is apt to be regarded as only one of the associated lesions of the acute attack. Treatment of acute gonococcal cervicitis has already been described (see page 244).

Chronic Cervicitis. Chronic inflammation of the cervix is very common and will be seen to some extent in four out of five women attending for any gynaecological reason. The inflammation of the cervix is brought about by infection during abortion or childbirth, and this method of infection accounts for the majority of cases. Lacerations of the cervix during childbirth usually lead to some degree of chronic cervicitis. And if the wound of the cervix does not heal cleanly by first intention there is tendency for the edges of the laceration to become everted. In this way the cervical canal is made more patent and organisms can more easily ascend from the vagina and infect the cervical canal. Instrumentation may also lead to chronic cervicitis, particularly if the cervix is dilated rapidly with metal dilators and is split.

Acute infections of the cervix tend to persist as chronic infections. The mucous membrane of the cervical canal is rugose and the cervical glands are racemose in type, so that if organisms penetrate into the depth of the glands they are difficult to eradicate by local treatment to the cervical canal. Moreover, the mucous membrane of the cervix is not exfoliated during menstruation, and there is no natural method of overcoming the infection such as is seen in the case of the endometrium of the body of the uterus. Chronic cervicitis therefore represents a form of focal sepsis. It causes vaginal discharge and, in some cases at least, infertility. The general effect of chronic cervicitis is important, as the latent infection may be responsible for metastatic infections such as arthritis, in addition to inducing a feeling of constitutional ill-health.

Chronic cervicitis is associated with the presence of an erosion, but it is impossible to subdivide a superficial lesion of the portio vaginalis from the deeper seated extensions to the endocervical canal and its glands. In fact, endocervicitis is an invariable concomitant of all superficial lesions. This has an important bearing on treatment (see later).

Erosion of the Cervix

The name "erosion" is time-honoured but unfortunate since it suggests that the cervix has been eroded by some ulcerative process whereas, in fact,

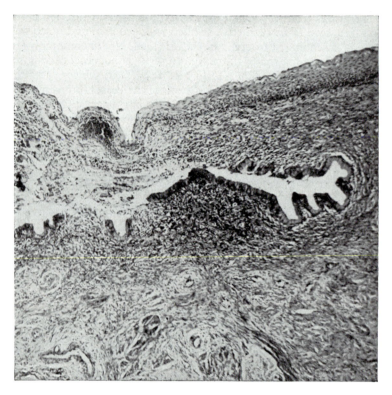

FIG. 232. The margin of an erosion. Note the squamous epithelium on the right terminating in an area of granulation tissue with destruction of a gland. (× 75.)

an erosion is never ulcerated unless it is malignant when it ceases to be an erosion. It is questionable if an erosion is of even inflammatory origin and many are congenital. Students, therefore, are confused by the term erosion and it is only in deference to custom and teaching that it is included in this chapter on inflammatory diseases of the uterus.

Erosion of the cervix can be demonstrated only by inspection, as small erosions cannot be detected by palpation. An erosion takes the form of a reddened area around the external os. Most commonly the reddened area is slightly raised above the level of the squamous epithelium of the vaginal portion of the cervix and is smooth and glistening. In such cases the erosion is covered by columnar epithelium similar to that lining the cervical canal, and the mucous membrane of the cervical canal is continuous with the columnar epithelium of the erosion. If the erosion is extensive, the covering epithelium may be thrown into folds when the erosion is described as papillary in type. In another form of erosion small follicles, or cysts, can be seen in the

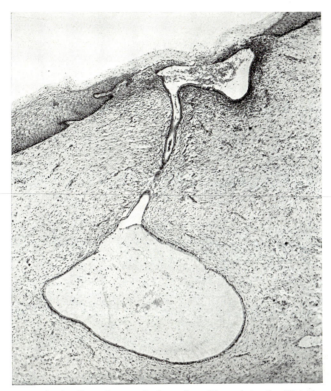

FIG. 233. The healing of a cervical erosion. There is early dilatation of a cervical gland due to obstruction of its duct by regenerating squamous epithelium at its mouth. Note also the flattening of the glandular epithelium by intra-cystic pressure. Such a dilated gland becomes a Nabothian follicle. (× 56).

vicinity of the external os, the follicles being covered either by thin squamous epithelium or lying beneath an erosion of the papillary type.

So-called "Congenital" Erosion. Some erosions are congenital. During intrauterine life the vagina and the vaginal portion of the cervix are lined by transitional epithelium, and this epithelium extends into the cervical canal until the sixth month. Towards the end of intrauterine life, columnar epithelium grows down from the cervical canal, and in one-third of all newborn female children extends to some degree over the vaginal portion of the cervix. This condition persists for only a few days until the level of oestrogen from the mother falls and the "congenital" erosion heals spontaneously. The real "congenital" erosion occurs or reappears under the influence of oestrogen at puberty and may then persist into adult life. A simple erosion is an oestrogen-dependent condition; apart from birth it does not occur before puberty or in the postmenopausal state.

The pathology of erosions of the cervix offers an extremely difficult problem, and opinion is divided as to the interpretation of the histological appearances. It has been computed that 85% of adult women, whether single or married, have some degree of erosion at the cervix.

Erosion associated with Chronic Cervicitis. In chronic cervicitis, pus and mucus are discharged from the cervical canal and bathe the posterior lip of the cervix if the uterus is retroverted, and the anterior lip if the uterus is

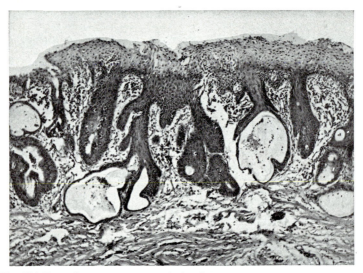

Fig. 234. Extensive squamous metaplasia of the cervix. Note how the squamous cells apparently "invade" the endocervical glands. This condition is not malignant.

anteverted. The discharge is alkaline and tends to produce maceration of the squamous epithelium. In chronic cervicitis the stroma of the cervix is oedematous and the resistance of the individual squamous cells around the external os reduced, so that after a time these desquamate and leave a raw red area denuded of epithelium around the external os. This represents the first stage in the development of an erosion (Fig. 232). Microscopical examination shows that the tissues beneath the raw area are infiltrated with round cells and plasma cells. There is, however, no destruction of tissue, so that the appearances are not those of an ulcer. In the process of healing, columnar epithelium from the cervical canal grows over and covers the denuded area, so that macroscopically the red area is covered by smooth glistening translucent epithelium. The affected area around the external os is a **simple flat erosion.** After a variable interval, the squamous epithelium of the vaginal portion of the cervix replaces the columnar epithelium of the erosion, the squamous epithelium growing under the columnar epithelium and gradually pushing it away, until finally the squamous epithelium has completely grown over the eroded area. Unless the chronic cervicitis has been cured in the meantime, the process is repeated: in other words, chronic cervicitis leads to recurrent erosions of the cervix. One important feature of this squamous epithelial activity is that sometimes the glands themselves exhibit downgrowths of squamous epithelium. This ectopic squamous downgrowth is called epidermidisation. Its importance lies in the fact that, to the untutored eye, it looks like an epidermoid carcinoma which has invaded the glands. The condition is neither malignant nor pre-malignant (Fig. 234).

Papillary erosion is produced by columns of cervical stroma growing into the erosion from above, so that the surface of the erosion becomes ridged and furrowed. In this way false glands are formed which may penetrate into the cervical stroma. The papillary effect is merely the result of local proliferation. A **follicular or cystic erosion** is produced by the squamous epithelium occluding the mouths of these glands, as it replaces the columnar epithelium of the erosion during the stage of healing. The blocked glands become distended with secretion and form the small cysts which can be seen with the naked eye, the so-called Nabothian follicles (see Fig. 233).

The description given above explains the types of erosion associated with chronic endocervicitis, although in the opinion of some authorities this inflammatory aetiology is denied.

Erosion due to Hyperplasia of the Mucous Membrane of the Cervix. Because the inflammatory theory in the genesis of erosions has been regarded as untenable, it has been suggested that one explanation is hyperplasia of the columnar epithelium of the cervical canal, which grows down to extend over the vaginal portion of the cervix, just as it does in the latter months of intrauterine life. One possible cause of this columnar epithelial hyperplasia is an ovarian hormonal imbalance. The protagonists of this theory point out that simple erosions, apart from congenital, are only seen during the years of ovarian activity and that they do not occur after the menopause, and that they are commonly seen in pregnancy and tend spontaneously to regress in the puerperium. During pregnancy, oestrogen and progesterone are certainly produced in very large quantities. Oestrogen is probably the hormone responsible for the erosion but as yet the hormonal basis has not been conclusively proved. The interpretation of the histological appearances of an erosion may be difficult. If a patient has leucorrhoea, an adenomatous erosion caused by hyperplasia may become infected by micro-organisms from the vagina. This type of erosion may then be regarded as being due to chronic cervicitis. It is difficult to believe that all erosions are caused by chronic cervicitis, for then one would have to assume that 85% of women have suffered from chronic inflammation of the cervix, which is highly improbable. Moreover, in large papillary erosions there may be no inflammatory reaction in the erosion itself, nor microscopical evidence of cervicitis on examination of the cervix. On the other hand, proliferation of the mucous membrane of the cervical canal occurs frequently, and it is in this way that mucous polypi of the cervix are produced. It is extremely probable that the majority of erosions of the cervix of the papillary glandular type are caused by hyperplasia

Hyperplasia of the mucous membrane of the cervix is manifested, not only by the development of mucous polypi and glandular erosions, but by a condition of adenofibrosis in which a multitude of Nabothian follicles form in the tissues lining the cervical canal. Little is known of the aetiology of these hyperplastic conditions of the cervix; they are not associated with hyperplasia of the endometrium of the body of the uterus.

So far as erosions of the cervix are concerned, papillary and glandular erosions are mainly due to hyperplasia. Simple flat erosions, particularly when the squamous epithelium has desquamated, are possibly the end result of chronic cervicitis. Whether the erosion is caused by chronic cervicitis, or whether it is due to hyperplasia of the mucous membrane of the cervical canal, the essential feature in almost all cases is the downgrowth of columnar epithelium to replace squamous epithelium in the vicinity of the external os. The hyperplastic erosions lead to an increased mucus discharge from the cervix, but the discharge is composed mainly of clear mucous. Nevertheless, the patient complains of the discharge, so that it is justifiable clinically to treat the cervix itself. It has already been emphasised that hyperplastic erosions may become infected by the vaginal bacteria, because the columnar epithelium has less resistance than the squamous epithelium which normally covers the vaginal portion of the cervix.

Ectropion

A cervix which has been badly lacerated during childbirth frequently shows the condition of ectropion, which results, as in the case of the badly burned eyelid, from the contraction of scar tissue, which tends to evert the endo-cervical canal, the lining mucosa of which is now exposed. Ectropion can be detected by digital examination, as the external os is patulous, so that the lower part of the cervical canal, and very frequently the longitudinal columns which lie in the mid-line, both anteriorly and posteriorly, can be felt with the examining finger. Chronic cervicitis usually accompanies ectropion, and the main symptom is vaginal discharge, which is mucopurulent.

Symptoms of Chronic Cervicitis and Erosion of the Cervix. The main symptom of cervicitis and erosion is vaginal discharge, which is commonly mucous and if infected mucopurulent. If hypertrophic the erosion may cause post-coital spotting and similarly it may ooze a little blood if swabbed vigorously during examination. Erosions become very vascular during pregnancy, so that intermittent but slight vaginal bleeding is a frequent complaint. After the menopause, erosions regress, though this may take some time—occasionally a year or more. Any so-called erosion arising *de novo* after the menopause is most suspicious of being an early neoplasm. Chronic endo-cervicitis has been wrongfully cited as one cause of infertility. This proposition is untenable because many fertile multiparae have a well-marked endo-cervicitis and it should therefore be discarded. Symptoms such as backache and vague abdominal pain may be attributed to chronic cervicitis in a small percentage of cases. In a few instances chronic cervicitis is associated with a chronic parametritis and this is especially likely if the cervicitis is the result of a severe obstetric injury. In these patients a deep dyspareunia will be complained of and the chronic cervicitis and erosion will be blamed unfairly for it, whereas it is the parametritis which is really responsible.

Bladder symptoms are not infrequent with chronic cervicitis and erosion and it has been suggested that the cervical infection spreads into the bladder to cause a trigonitis, with a resulting irritability of bladder function and increased frequency of micturition. There is certainly a free lymphatic anastomosis between these two organs but whether the infection can spread from the cervix to the bladder in this way is not proven. Some congestion of the trigone is, however, reasonable and the bladder symptoms frequently improve when the cervicitis is corrected surgically.

Diagnosis. Chronic cervicitis and erosion can be detected with accuracy only by speculum examination of the cervix. Clinically, for the recognition of chronic cervicitis, a discharge of mucus and pus from the cervical canal must be present. A profuse discharge of clear mucus from the cervix is not evidence of chronic cervicitis, but is indicative of a hyperplastic condition of the cervical mucosa. In chronic cervicitis, the cervix is hard and firm and often somewhat hypertrophied, and appears more vascular than normal when examined with a speculum. Care must be taken to distinguish between a vaginitis involving the vaginal portion of the cervix and a true endocervicitis, for it is not uncommon, in some forms of vaginitis, e.g. trichomoniasis, for small red areas to be distributed over the vaginal portion of the cervix.

A typical erosion is soft to touch with a tendency to bleed easily and gives to the examining gloved finger a peculiar velvety feeling. If the erosion is covered by columnar epithelium the surface is smooth and glistening and bright red in colour. It must be distinguished from an early carcinoma of the cervix, and if there is any doubt a biopsy must be performed. A carcinoma of the cervix is indurated, friable, usually ulcerated, and bleeds very easily (Chapter 24, page 620).

A primary sore of the cervix may be difficult to distinguish from either an erosion or an early carcinoma, as its characters are intermediate between those of these two conditions. It should always be borne in mind if a red area is found on the cervix which is vascular, denuded of epithelium, yet without excavation of the cervical tissues. Tuberculosis of the cervix is a rare disease which may be difficult to distinguish from carcinoma of the cervix, but with advanced tuberculosis, caseous material can be seen in the deeper part of the ulceration. A method of distinguishing between carcinoma of the cervix and erosion has been described by Schiller. The cervix is painted with Lugol's solution and examined through a speculum. In early carcinoma of the cervix the malignant cells do not assume the brown stain with iodine and the cervix appears to be stippled with small grey areas. In erosions, the columnar epithelium does not take up the iodine and the eroded area appears bright red. Colposcopic examination of the cervix is another useful method of establishing the true nature of an erosion (see page 137). It is now our practice to screen all erosions by cytological smears taken from the vaginal pool and by scrape surface biopsy of the portio vaginalis with an Ayre's speculum. Both cytology and colposcopy should be employed in the differential diagnosis of all pathological conditions of the cervix as part of the diagnostic routine.

Even under the microscope, there may be great difficulty in distinguishing between an early carcinoma and an erosion, for with healing erosions the squamous epithelium often grows deeply along the glands into the tissues of the cervix. Also, there is frequently some degree of hyperkeratosis which may cause difficulty. A skilled pathologist alone can give an opinion in difficult cases of this kind.

CERVICAL POLYPI

Mucous Polypi

Although cervical polypi are sometimes of undecided aetiology, their frequent association with chronic inflammatory disease of the cervix justifies their inclusion in this chapter. Mucous polypi arise from the mucous membrane of the cervical canal. They form swellings about the size of a pea, and, in rare cases, may become as much as $\frac{3}{4}$ in. in diameter. To the naked eye a mucous polypus is a red vascular swelling which bleeds easily on touch and is covered by smooth glistening epithelium bathed in clear mucus. The polypus is pedunculated, the pedicle being attached to the upper part of the mucous membrane of the cervical canal. The swellings are soft, smooth and slippery to the touch. It is not uncommon for the polypi to be multiple, so that two or three may be seen in the neighbourhood of the external os.

Mucous polypi cause an increased vaginal discharge, and as they bleed easily the patient may complain of irregular bleeding particularly after coitus. Except for these two symptoms, mucous polypi cause little inconvenience. In most cases the polypi can be detected by palpation, but small sessile polypi can be detected only with precision by speculum examination. In any case, a speculum must be passed before the diagnosis of mucous polypus can be made with accuracy.

Histologically the polypi have a typical appearance. The surface epithelium is of the high columnar type similar to that of the cervical canal. Glands are found in the stroma of the polypus and the glands tend to be racemose in type, similar to those found in the cervical canal, and are lined by tall columnar epithelium. The stroma is always extremely vascular, containing a large number of dilated capillaries with some degree of round-celled infiltration near the lower pole of the polypus. One of the most constant features of mucous polypi of the cervix is that the surface epithelium in the region of the lower pole shows well-marked squamous metaplasia, and the squamous epithelium may penetrate into the depths of the glands (see Fig. 235).

The aetiology of mucous polypi of the cervix is unknown. The polypi certainly cannot be regarded as neoplasms nor do they arise as the result of cervicitis, although these are frequently seen in association with erosions of the cervix. They should be regarded as being produced by hyperplasia of the mucous membrane of the cervical canal which becomes thrown into folds and finally one of the folds, projecting into the cervical canal, assumes the characteristics of a polypus. There is some relation between the development of glandular erosions and the development of mucous polypi of the cervix.

Mucous polypi usually occur in women during the child-bearing period of life, but they develop also in women of menopausal age, and are occasionally seen in women past the menopause.

Polypi used to be treated by out-patient avulsion by torsion and no anaesthetic was needed for this. If avulsion is to be employed, a speculum

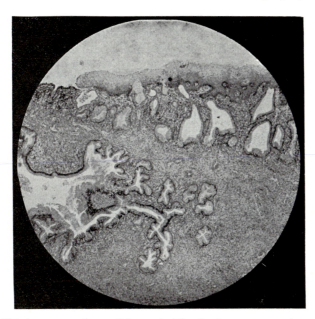

FIG. 235. A mucous polypus of the cervix. The glands are racemose in type and the stroma is infiltrated with round cells. Above and to the right there is squamous metaplasia of the surface epithelium. The appearances are not unlike those of the cervical mucous membrane.

is passed into the vagina to expose the cervix. The polypus is grasped with forceps and twisted off. The polypus should always be sent for microscopic examination as in a very small proportion malignant changes may be seen. It should be remembered, however, that fresh mucous polypi may develop at a later date. The diagnosis of mucous polypi is made without difficulty, for the appearances are characteristic and the absence of induration excludes the presence of carcinoma. Myomatous polypi are firm and spherical, paler in colour than a mucous polypus and of a larger diameter.

If a mucous polypus persists for any length of time it becomes covered completely with squamous epithelium from metaplasia of its surface columnar epithelium. Finally the polypus hangs down into the vagina and is covered by firm pale squamous epithelium. This form of polypus is sometimes referred to as a fibro-adenomatous polypus of the cervix, which is a pathological misnomer as the condition is one of localised hyperplasia and not neoplastic. The mouths of the glands may be occluded as the result of squamous epithelium growing over them, so that the glands become distension cysts containing pent-up secretion. Occasionally, from fusion of adjacent retention cysts, the polypus is found to contain a single large cyst filled with mucus. A polypus of this kind may develop a long pedicle and may actually appear at the vulva. The treatment of such a polypus is removal by torsion of the pedicle. We question the rectitude of this time honoured and popular procedure as it does not effectively eradicate the stalk from which a recurrent polypus tends to arise. A preferable attitude is that all polypi should be removed under a general anaesthetic so that the uterine cavity can be explored and curetted. By this means any tendency to haemorrhage can be controlled by diathermy coagulation of the base of the polypus. In this way an unsuspected endocervical polypus not visible to the examiner on ordinary speculum examination is disclosed and effectively dealt with as is also any endometrial polypus which may rarely be coincident. Curettage is without question obligatory if the polypus is the alleged cause of postmenopausal bleeding, since it can perfectly well mask the more sinister implication of an intra-uterine malignancy. It is perhaps a wise precaution to treat all patients with a large vascular polypus as in-patients and to remove such polypi under an anaesthetic. In addition, out-patient avulsion is sometimes, though rarely, followed by a severe reactionary haemorrhage.

Myomatous Polypus

The characters, symptoms and treatment of this type of uterine polypus will be described in Chapter 23.

Treatment of Chronic Cervicitis

The application of antiseptics to the cervical canal seldom, if ever, results in permanent cure of chronic cervicitis, for the infection is deep-seated in the cervical glands and the antiseptics do not penetrate so far. The treatment of chronic cervicitis and glandular erosions of the cervix is diathermy cauterisation or cauterisation with an electric cautery. The tissues of the cervix are coagulated, the columnar epithelium is destroyed and the raw area left on the vaginal portion of the cervix is subsequently covered by squamous epithelium. In the cervical canal, diathermy coagulation destroys all infection lying in the depths of the racemose glands and in due course healthy epithelium grows down from the upper part of the cervical canal to cover the raw area. The most modern method is to carry out **conisation** and a diathermy needle or loop with the instrument set at 5 cutting is used to cut through the cervical tissues and to remove a cone-shaped piece of tissue. The cone includes all the racemose glands of the endocervical mucous membrane together with the eroded area on the vaginal portion of the cervix. Any bleeding vessels are coagulated with the diathermy button. The results of treatment are so good that the operation of trachelorrhaphy is rarely indicated at the present day. There is, however, some risk of secondary haemorrhage, so that the operation of conisation should only be performed on an in-patient. Secondary haemorrhage is invariably due to infection, which may be prevented by giving systemic and local antibiotics for fourteen days after conisation. It is wise to detain these patients for a sufficient stay in hospital to ensure against a secondary haemorrhage and to warn them to return at once if there is any bleeding. Coitus is interdicted for six to eight weeks, by which time the cervical wound has firmly healed. Douching with can and tube, using a solution of isotonic bicarbonate or normal saline, may be carried out by the patient in her home morning and evening until all discharge has ceased. The results of this operation are excellent, and if the cervix is dilated thoroughly before conisation no stenosis should result. If pregnancy occurs after conisation, no dystocia should be expected and normal delivery is the rule. One

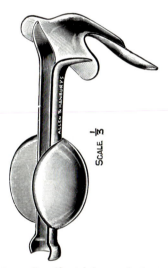

Fig. 236. Auvard's self-retaining vaginal retractor.

word of warning should, however, be given about diathermy conisation in young women who are likely to become pregnant after the operation. In these patients, the conisation should not be deep or radical as the liability to abortion is thereby increased. Deep conisation should be reserved for the older patient whose desire for further children has been satisfied.

Operative treatment of chronic cervicitis aims at excising as much as possible of the infected tissues. It should be emphasised that the operation about to be described has, as a result of the introduction and popularity of the operation of conisation, a very limited indication. There are very few cases of endocervicitis and erosion, ectropion and laceration which cannot now be cured by conisation.

The results of surgical treatment of chronic cervicitis are good, but if much of the cervix is removed or if thick scar tissue forms in the cervix, subsequent parturition may be difficult even to the extent of indicating delivery by Caesarean section. A high amputation undoubtedly results in an incompetent cervix which is a potent cause of middle trimester abortion. This operation, therefore, is to be studiously avoided. The indications for surgical treatment in chronic cervicitis are therefore very limited. If the cervix is badly lacerated with ectropion, the operation of trachelorrhaphy, which consists of repair, is sometimes indicated as an alternative to diathermy conisation, where it is felt that a plastic operation is likely to increase the chances of future pregnancy, when this is especially desired.

Technique of Trachelorrhaphy. The patient is prepared for operation in the usual way, and vaginal douches are given during the twenty-four hours before operation. The patient is anaesthetised and placed in the lithotomy position. A speculum is placed in the vagina (Fig. 236) and a lateral retractor, such as Jayle's, introduced to expose the cervix. The cervix is pulled down with two volsellum forceps, one on the anterior lip and the other on the posterior lip. The cervix is now dilated with Hegar's dilators to No. 10. The edges of the laceration are excised so that skin and a small amount of mucous membrane are removed. The raw areas are then approximated by interrupted No. 1 chromic catgut or nylon sutures. This operation should not be performed in the presence of sepsis or where the laceration is complicated by an erosion.

Haemorrhage is easily controlled by the sutures, which may be removed on the twelfth day if unabsorbable. The patient is given sulphonamide pessaries (1 nocte) to insert high in the vagina for two weeks in order to prevent infection and therefore diminish the risk of a secondary haemorrhage. The cervix will be healed in one month. The patient should be warned about the presence of bloody or purulent discharge for two or three weeks after the operation.

Small granulations may develop at the site of the sutures after the operation and these should be treated by electric cautery.

In conclusion we very rarely perform this and similar plastic operations on the cervix owing to the efficacy of the simpler procedure of diathermy conisation, which has now almost entirely superseded this more complicated surgical technique. The surgical treatment of chronic endocervicitis and erosion is therefore almost entirely of historical interest.

21 Prolapse

The normal position of the uterus is one of anteversion and anteflexion, with the body of the uterus tilted forwards so that it lies almost horizontally when a woman assumes the erect posture. Normally, when a woman strains there is no descent either of the vaginal walls or of the uterus. In prolapse, straining causes protrusion of the vaginal walls at the vaginal orifice, while in severe cases the cervix of the uterus may be pushed down to the level of the vulva. In extreme cases the whole uterus and the whole of both vaginal walls may be extruded from the vagina.

Prolapse is a common complaint, and severe degrees are most often seen in women of menopausal age who have borne children. The inconvenience of the prolapse is accompanied by micturition symptoms, by low mid sacral backache, and by a sense of weakness and insecurity in the region of the perineum. The causation of prolapse is difficult to understand without a knowledge of the anatomy of the pelvic floor and of the ligamentary supports of the uterus and vagina. Moreover, the treatment of prolapse must be based upon attempts to restore the normal anatomical relations.

ANATOMY OF THE PELVIC FLOOR

The pelvic floor consists of the two levator ani muscles. When examined from above, after the removal of the pelvic viscera, the upper surfaces of the levator ani muscles are seen to be covered by a dense layer of pelvic fascia. In the midline, the pelvic floor is pierced by the urethra, the vagina and the rectum. The levator ani muscle consists of three parts, the pubococcygeus, the iliococcygeus, and the ischiococcygeus. The **ischiococcygeus** muscle—the coccygeus muscle of the anatomists—arises from the spine of the ischium and spreads out in a fan-shaped manner backwards and upwards to be inserted into the front of the coccyx. The **iliococcygeus** arises from the "white line" on the lateral wall of the pelvis, directly from the pelvic fascia, and passes backwards and inwards, to be inserted partly into the tip of the coccyx and also into the ano-coccygeal raphe, which passes from the rectum to the tip of the coccyx. The **pubococcygeus** muscle is the most important of the three. It arises from the back of the pubic ramus and passes backwards to be inserted, partly into the tip of the coccyx, and partly into the raphe which passes between the rectum and the coccyx. Some of the inner fibres of the **pubococcygeus** (the puborectalis muscle) decussate behind the rectum at the level at which the rectum turns sharply backwards to form the anal canal. These fibres act as a sling to the rectum and probably have some sphincteric action. The innermost fibres of the pubococcygeus muscle are the most important of all, for they fuse with the plain muscle and fascia of the vagina and decussate between the vagina and the rectum. These decussating fibres are of the utmost importance in gynaecology. Normally, they cause the opening in the pelvic floor to be divided into two parts: one in front, called the **hiatus urogenitalis,** through which passes the urethra and the vagina, the other posteriorly, through which passes the rectum, the **hiatus rectalis.** It is clear that

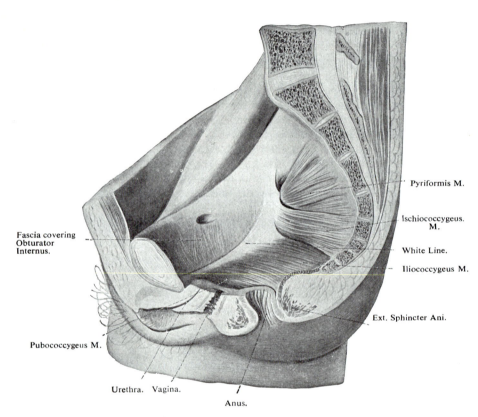

FIG. 237. The pelvic floor. A median sagittal section through the pelvis. (Veit-Stoeckel.)

if these decussating fibres are well developed and intact, the hiatus urogenitalis is small. On the other hand, if the fibres have been torn during childbirth the hiatus urogenitalis becomes wide and patulous, with an increased tendency for the vagina and uterus to prolapse through the pelvic floor. In the surgical treatment of prolapse, the operation of perineorrhaphy, which is commonly performed whatever other plastic operations may be done as well, depends essentially upon suturing together the pubococcygeus muscle between the vagina and the rectum, and reducing the dimensions of the hiatus urogenitalis (Fig. 237).

The Muscles of the Perineum. Although the pelvic floor consists mainly of the muscles of the levator ani group, the muscles of the perineum offer some support. In anatomical descriptions the superficial layer of perineal muscles consists of the bulbospongiosus and the superficial transverse muscle of the perineum, both of which pass to the central point of the perineum. The ischiocavernosus belongs to the same plane. Deep to the superficial muscles lies the urogenital diaphragm of dense fascia which is not so well developed as in the male. Between the layers of the triangular ligaments lie the

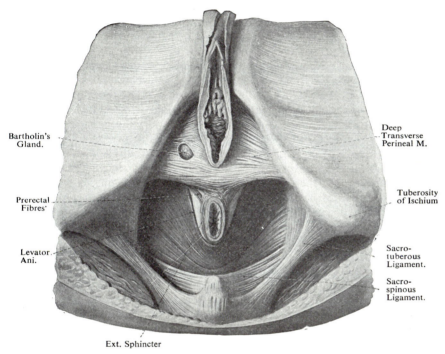

Fig. 238. The urogenital diaphragm seen after the removal of the superficial muscles of the perineum. (Veit-Stoeckel.)

deep transverse muscles of the perineum, which pass transversely to the central point of the perineum. On the whole, relatively little muscle tissue is contained in these two planes of muscles, and the fibrous tissue of the urogenital diaphragm lacks the firmness and strength of the urogenital diaphragm of the male perineum (see Fig. 238).

The Perineal Body. The perineal body consists of the tissue intervening between the posterior vaginal wall and the anterior wall of the anal canal. The perineal body is roughly pyramidal in shape, the apex corresponding to the point where the anterior wall of the rectum turns backwards and downwards to become the anterior wall of the anal canal. The perineal body, when dissected from below, contains the superficial muscles of the perineum, the central point of the perineum, with its dense fascial and tendinous tissue, both layers of the triangular ligaments enclosing the deep transverse muscles of the perineum, while above on a more cranial plane lie the fibres of the pubococcygeus which decussate between the vagina and rectum.

In gynaecological examination of patients with prolapse the pelvic floor should always be palpated. Two fingers are inserted into the vagina, the thumb placed externally over the perineum and the amount of intervening tissue together with the tone of the muscle determined. The pubococcygeus is easily palpated by flexing the fingers laterally in the vagina above the level of the muscle and pressing the muscle downwards towards the thumb placed over the labium majus. This examination indicates the horizontal level of the muscles of the pelvic floor. Anteriorly near the urethra the pubococcygeus lies only a little above the level of the external meatus. Further back the anterior vaginal wall is found to lie well above the level of the cranial surface of the pubococcygeus, and it is difficult to believe that the muscles of the pelvic floor can directly support the anterior vaginal wall. On the other hand, the posterior vaginal wall is more directly supported by the levator ani muscles, for the decussating fibres extend upwards to a level of about one-third of the length of the posterior vaginal wall. Although the direction of the vagina is upwards and backwards, the vagina is always inclined at an acute angle with respect to the pelvic floor, so that the levator muscles cannot, on anatomical grounds, be regarded as affording a direct support. Moreover, the cervix and uterus, which lie on a still higher plane, are not directly supported by the pelvic floor but by the condensed endopelvic fascia of the cardinal (Mackenrodt) and uterosacral ligaments.

In spite of the above considerations, injury to the muscles of the pelvic floor and laxity of the individual muscles are undoubtedly important factors in the causation of prolapse. Both factors, injury and atony, cause the hiatus urogenitalis to become patulous, so that protrusion of the vagina or uterus through the hiatus can more easily occur.

The Ligamentary Supports of the Uterus and Vagina. There is no reason to believe that the round ligaments support the uterus, since they are never found tense and stretched at operation, and from their direction they can be of little service except to maintain anteversion. They are in fact atavistic structures. The broad ligament, consisting of thin sheets of peritoneum, serves no purpose in the support of the uterus.

It will be remembered that the pelvic cellular tissue is the loose tissue intervening between the peritoneum above and the pelvic fascia which covers the upper surfaces of the levator ani muscles below. The term **pelvic fascia** is restricted to the dense fascial tissues which cover the levator ani and obturator internus muscles. All the organs in the pelvis, namely the vaginia uterus, bladder and rectum, are surrounded by layers of condensed pelvc, cellular tissue, and these condensed layers form what is called the **endopelvic fascia.** The endopelvic fascia is essentially derived from the pelvic cellular tissue. Its function is to support the pelvic organs, yet at the same time it must be capable of stretching as the organs distend. Each organ has its own specialised layer of fascia, and each layer contains a considerable amount of plain muscle tissue. Condensations of the endopelvic fascia pass from the pelvic organs to the walls of the pelvis and fix and support these organs.

The endopelvic fascia has a basal portion, or ground bundle which lies on the upper surface of the levator ani muscles on each side of the midline and is attached to the back of the pubic bones. Posteriorly, the ground bundle terminates in a dense band of tissue which passes from the lateral aspect of the

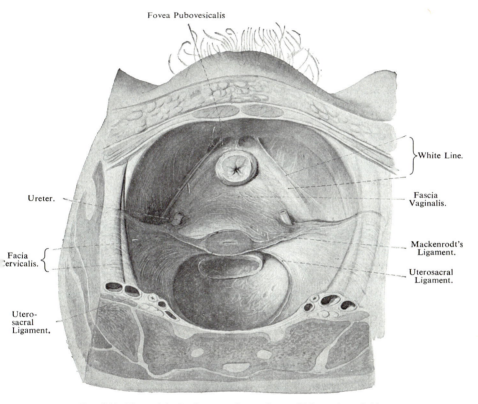

Fovea Pubovesicalis

White Line.

Ureter.

Fascia Vaginalis.

Facia Cervicalis.

Mackenrodt's Ligament.

Uterosacral Ligament.

Utero-sacral Ligament.

FIG. 239. The pelvic fascias seen from above. (Peham-Amreich).

upper part of the vagina and cervix outwards to the pelvic wall. This condensation is known as **Mackenrodt's ligament** or the **cardinal ligament of the uterus** or the **transverse cervical ligament.** Extending upwards from the ground bundle are septa of endopelvic fascia which pass to the bladder, the vagina and the rectum, and the blood vessels pass to the different organs in these septa.

Mackenrodt's ligament lies below the level of the uterine vessels and passes out in a fan-shaped manner towards the pelvic wall. It consists of cellular tissue with a little plain muscle, and contains sympathetic nerve fibres, lymphatics and veins. The posterior part of the fan-shaped condensation passes upwards, lateral to the rectum, to gain insertion on to the sacrum, and is termed the **uterosacral ligament.** It is important to remember, however, that Mackenrodt's ligament and the uterosacral ligament arise mainly from the lateral aspect of the vagina rather than from the cervix or the uterus. Normally, these condensations of the pelvic cellular tissue, which are perhaps best referred to under the term **retinaculum uteri,** afford the main support of the uterus and the upper part of the lateral vaginal wall. These condensations not only fix the uterus and upper part of the vagina to the lateral walls of the pelvis, but also fix them to the bladder and to the pelvic fascia covering the upper surface of the levator ani muscle. None of these supports is peritoneal. The uterosacral ligaments, although following the direction of the uterosacral folds of peritoneum, lie well below the horizontal level of these peritoneal folds (see Fig. 239.)

In order fully to understand the importance of Mackenrodt's ligament, the reader should refer back to Fig. 22 on page 33. This diagram shows that there are three parts to Mackenrodt's ligament:

(1) The lateral, transverse cervical or cardinal ligament which passes from the cervix and upper vagina to the lateral pelvic wall. This is the textbook Mackenrodt's ligament which has received the homage and publicity of all writers.

(2) A posterior prolongation of the same structure from the cervix and upper vagina round the rectum to the sacrum—the uterosacral ligament, less publicised but equally important with Mackenrodt's ligament in the support of the uterus and vaginal vault.

(3) An anterior prolongation from the cervix under the bladder to the back of the symphysis—the pubo-cervical ligament particularly important in the support of the bladder.

All these three parts are really one and the same structure anatomically, morphologically and functionally. They all arise from one common origin from the cervix and upper vagina. They form a three-spoked *triradiate ligament* and, though given different names, they are really a single unit. This hammock-like arrangement of condensed endopelvic fascia is the cardinal support of the uterus and, when intact, is the most important support of the uterus against vertical descent. The structure is, therefore, rightly named the cardinal ligament but it is more than a lateral support as taught by tradition—it is an anterior support under the bladder (pubo-cervical fascia) and a posterior (uterosacral) support round the rectum. The truth of the above statement will forcibly strike the operator who performs a Wertheim's hysterectomy, since is it impossible to free the cervix and upper vagina until all three spokes of this triradiate structure have been transected. Merely cutting the lateral part of Mackenrodt's ligament does not free the uterus and this liberation can only be achieved by cutting the anterior and posterior prolongations in addition.

The supports of the anterior vaginal wall are quite different from those already mentioned, and are also extremely difficult to understand. The vagina and the bladder are each surrounded by a layer of endopelvic fascia. The **vaginal fascia** is normally well developed, containing plain muscle tissue.

The **vesical fascia,** on the other hand, is much thinner and of less importance. Normally, a plane of cleavage, the **vesicovaginal space,** can be defined between the vaginal fascia and the vesical fascia in the region of the upper third of the anterior vaginal wall. In the lower part of the anterior vaginal wall the vesical and vaginal fascias fuse in the region of the internal urinary meatus. Along the line of fusion is a linear depression which is responsible for the

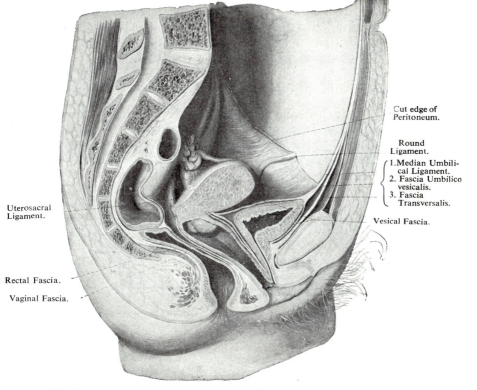

Cut edge of Peritoneum.

Round Ligament.

1. Median Umbilical Ligament.
2. Fascia Umbilico vesicalis.
3. Fascia Transversalis.

Vesical Fascia.

Uterosacral Ligament.

Rectal Fascia.

Vaginal Fascia.

Fig. 240. A median sagittal section through the female pelvis showing the connective tissue sheaths of the bladder, rectum and vagina. The vaginal fascia and the vesical fascia are separated by the vesicovaginal space. Below, the vaginal and vesical fascias fuse. Above, both fascias are adherent to the cervix. (Peham-Amreich.)

formation of the transverse vaginal sulcus (see page 6). The fused fascias extend downwards behind the urethra almost to the level of the external meatus and here form a well-defiend ligament known as the **posturethral ligament.** The ligament extends on each side to the pubic rami and forms a shelf of tissue composed almost entirely of plain muscle which supports the urethra. In the upper part of the anterior vaginal wall, the vesical fascia is continued on to the front of the cervix to form the **vesicocervical ligament.** Above the vesico-cervical ligament is a clear bloodless space known as the **vesicocervical space.**

A vesicouterine ligament passes from the front of the uterus to the fundus of the bladder above the level of the vesicocervical space (see Fig. 240).

Laterally, the endopelvic fascial layers extend downward as anterior prolongations of Mackenrodt's ligament. These fascial layers are easily recognised during the operation of anterior colporrhaphy. In this operation, after the vagina has been incised, the vaginal fascia is next exposed. After the vaginal fascia has been cut through, the vesicovaginal space is opened up, and if the cervix is pulled down, the vesicocervical ligament can be seen passing between the bladder and the front of the cervix of the uterus, and the ligament is always best developed laterally. These anatomical considerations show that the anterior vaginal wall is supported:—

(1) By the attachment of the vagina to the cervix of the uterus.

(2) Laterally, on each side the vesical and vaginal fascias fuse with the downward anterior prolongation of Mackenrodt's ligament—the so-called pubo-cervical ligament.

(3) The bladder itself directly holds up the anterior vaginal wall, and if the bladder is fixed firmly in position by its true ligaments to the back of the symphysis pubis and by the lateral ligaments which fix it to the anterior extension of Mackenrodt's ligament, the bladder of itself directly supports the anterior vaginal wall.

Supports of the Posterior Vaginal Wall. Prolapse of the posterior vaginal wall is rarely of the same degree as prolapse of the anterior vaginal wall, probably because the intra-abdominal pressure is directed more anteriorly than towards the pouch of Douglas. The uterosacral ligaments pass laterally from the upper part of the lateral walls of the vagina, and maintain the posterior vaginal wall in its position. Just as with the anterior vaginal wall, there is a vaginal fascial layer and also a layer of fascia covering the rectum, but the rectovaginal space is less dense and more extensive than the vesicovaginal space.

Aetiology of Prolapse

It is generally admitted that injury during childbirth is the most important aetiological factor, but insufficient emphasis has been given to the contribution of musculo-fascial atony which occurs at, and increases after, the menopause. With a complete perineal tear, even when the whole perineal body has been torn through, prolapse of the vaginal walls is almost unknown, so that injury of itself does not necessarily lead to prolapse of the vaginal walls or of the uterus. Probably a patient with a complete perineal tear exercises her levator muscles continuously, and to an extreme degree, in order to obtain some sphincteric control over the rectum, and in this way tones up not only the muscles of the pelvic floor but all the ligamentary supports in the pelvis.

It is well known clinically that most patients with prolapse are women of menopausal age, when, as a result of the menopause, the tissues become slack and there is less support for the vagina and uterus. Many women who develop minor degrees of prolapse immediately after childbirth have slack abdominal and pelvic muscles with lax vaginal walls and a retroverted uterus, yet if these women exercise their muscles and improve their general muscular tone, they can, to a considerable degree, control the prolapse. In other words, they neutralise the part played by musculo-fascial atony in the causation of prolapse, though it is impossible to modify the damage done by actual obstetric trauma. The rarity of prolapse in complete tear of the perineum, where the anatomical damage is severe, is explained by the compensatory hypertrophy of the levatores ani, constantly exercised to retain some control of the bowel.

The importance of these clinical observations is that they confirm the anatomical descriptions which have been given above. Prolapse of the uterus and the anterior vaginal wall is mainly due to laxity of the endopelvic fascial supports, resulting partly from asthenia and partly from stretching and injury during childbirth. The patient who complains of prolapse is the woman aged about 50, who has given birth to several children, or one who usually gives the history of a perineal tear or of a difficult confinement, or of the birth of large children. There are signs of an old tear of the perineum, the vaginal orifice is relaxed, the hiatus urogenitalis is patulous, and the paravaginal tissues are slack. In the typical case of prolapse, therefore, many causal factors can be demonstrated; only exceptionally can a single isolated cause of the prolapse be found.

Prolapse in young virgins is seen in cases of spina bifida occulta and split pelvis. It develops occasionally in virgins of menopausal age with extreme asthenia, when there is well-marked visceroptosis. The majority of patients, however, give a history of difficult delivery, although the symptoms may not become well marked until the woman reaches the age of the menopause. Amongst the predisposing abnormalities of childbirth, which tend to cause subsequent prolapse, are:—

The Application of Forceps before Full Dilatation of the Cervix. Traction on the forceps pulls down the cervix and stretches both Mackenrodt's ligaments and the uterosacral ligaments. If the ligaments are stretched to an extreme degree or are actually torn, however well the pelvic cellular tissue may involute after childbirth, it is unlikely that the ligaments will regain normal tone, so that the uterus with an abnormal degree of mobility tends to be pushed down into the vagina each time the patient strains. Precipitate labour produces a similar result.

Lacerations of the Perineal Body. When the perineal body is lacerated during childbirth, unless the torn and retracted muscles are brought into accurate apposition by immediate suturing, the hiatus urogenitalis will become patulous. A mistake which is frequently made is to omit examining the posterior vaginal wall for a laceration after delivery. Although neither fourchette nor the skin of the perineum may be torn, it is not uncommon for the lower third of the posterior vaginal wall to be lacerated during childbirth, and for the muscles of the perineal body to be severed and to retract laterally. Unless the practitioner investigates his patient for tears of this kind there will be a subsequent tendency to prolapse, although the perineal body is superficially intact.

The Passage of Large Children through the Birth Canal. This stretches the surrounding tissues, and if these tissues fail to involute normally and lose their tone, there will be a tendency for the vaginal walls to prolapse at a later date. This is especially applicable in the anaemic or obese patient or when severe haemorrhage has occurred.

Inadequate Puerperal Rehabilitation. In urban populations, the hospital maternity services provide 10 to 14 days of in-patient treatment after delivery, and there is now a constant and insistent demand for earlier discharge, often at 48 hours. During this brief 10-day lying-in period, physiotherapy and exercises are provided for the patients and they are encouraged to continue these excellent practices when they are discharged to their homes. It is extremely doubtful if one in a hundred ever perseveres with this beneficial

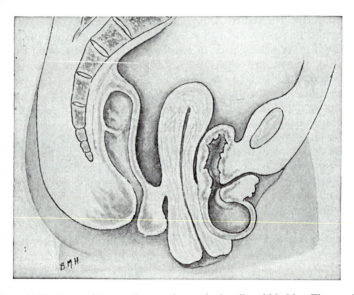

Fig. 241. Prolapse of the cervix, anterior vaginal wall and bladder. The cervix is elongated and hypertrophied. The anterior vaginal wall and bladder have prolapsed outside the vaginal orifice. The cervix is also prolapsed. In this case ligamentary supports hold up the body of the uterus. Note the almost vertical direction the uterosacral ligament must follow from the cervix to the junction of the 2nd-3rd sacral vertebra. Compare Fig. 243.

treatment, not because the patient is non-cooperative but simply because the all-absorbing burden of maternity precludes the luxury of rehabilitation. The strain of modern life, the pace of mere existence, the demands of domesticity all effectively compete with the proper performance of these simple exercises of prolapse prophylaxis. A physically fit subject before delivery soon degenerates into a state of general ill-health and muscular laxity. The posture and figure of these patients is the external evidence of their pelvic musculo-fascial inefficiency.

A Rapid Succession of Pregnancies. This tends to produce prolapse in the same way.

Asthenia and Visceroptosis. It is well established that asthenic patients are the most prone to develop prolapse. At the menopause and for some years afterwards the tissues in the pelvis lose their tone, and the uterus and vagina obtain an increased mobility, so that when the abdominal pressure is raised during coughing and straining there is a tendency for these structures to prolapse. Most patients with prolapse have a well-marked degree of visceroptosis and their abdominal musculature is poor.

Raised Intra-abdominal Pressure. Chronic bronchitis, large abdominal tumours, obesity and constipation tend to increase any degree of prolapse which may previously be present by raising the intra-abdominal pressure.

The Anatomy of Prolapse

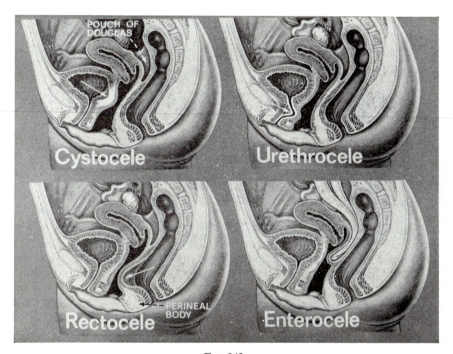

Fig. 242.

Classification of prolapse:—

Anterior vaginal wall:—

    Upper two-thirds—cystocele   } —Cystourethrocele
    Lower one-third—urethrocele }

Posterior vaginal wall:—

    Upper one-third—enterocele (Pouch of Douglas hernia).
    Lower two-thirds—rectocele.

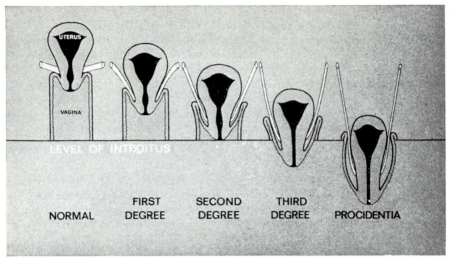

Fig. 243. Note the descent of the cervix which is accompanied by stretching of the ligaments and by supravaginal elongation of the cervix.

Uterine descent:

    1°—descent of the cervix in the vagina.
    2°—descent of the cervix to the introitus.
    3°—descent of the cervix outside the introitus.
    Procidentia—all of the uterus outside the introitus.

Cystocele. Prolapse of the anterior vaginal wall is, of all anatomical varieties, the most frequently encountered. When the patient strains, the upper part of the anterior vaginal wall descends, and in advanced cases may protrude outside the vaginal orifice. In such cases the vaginal and vesical fascias are thinned out and fail to support the bladder, so that the bladder prolapses with the anterior vaginal wall. This condition is termed cystocele. In mild cases the lower part of the anterior vaginal wall does not prolapse and the urethra is supported by the fascial tissues which intervene between the urethra and vagina, and which form the post-urethral ligament. In most cases of prolapse the submeatal sulcus and the transverse vaginal sulcus can be distinguished quite easily. It is customary to describe prolapse of the lower third of the anterior wall as **urethrocele.** It is important to distinguish urethrocele on clinical grounds because it is frequently associated with the symptom of imperfect control of micturition. Weakness and laxity of the posturethral ligament are responsible for most cases of urethrocele. In cystocele the anterior vaginal wall is stretched and thinned out except when the cystocele protrudes outside the vulva, when, owing to friction, the epithelium becomes thickened and hypertrophied.

    Although cystocele and urethrocele have been described separately, they are sometimes associated when the whole anterior vaginal wall protrudes from the urethral meatus to the cervix. This anatomical variety of prolapse is called cysto-urethrocele.

Prolapse of the Uterus. A mild degree of cystocele may be present without prolapse of the uterus. On the other hand, if the uterus prolapses, there is always some associated descent of the anterior vaginal wall. It is customary to describe three degrees of prolapse of the uterus. In the first, the cervix

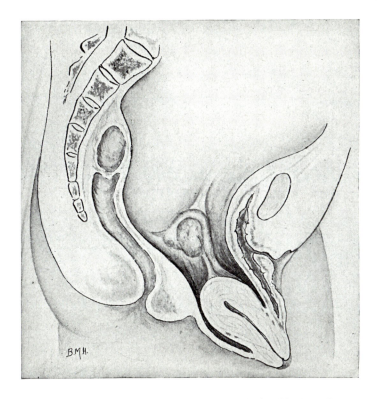

FIG. 244. Complete procidentia. Notice that the whole of both vaginal walls lie outside the vaginal orifice. The whole of the uterus also lies below this level. Clearly the ligamentary supports of the uterus must be greatly stretched to allow such a degree of prolapse. Compare Fig. 243.

descends into the vagina; in the second, the cervix descends to the level of the vulva, while in the third degree the cervix protrudes outside the vaginal orifice. In **complete procidentia,** the whole uterus protrudes outside the vulva, bringing with it both vaginal walls, and it may be possible to feel coils of small intestine in the pouch of Douglas outside the level of the vaginal orifice. If the uterus prolapses it is invariably found to be retroverted in the later stages of its descent. In most cases the vaginal portion of the cervix is hypertrophied, and in uterine prolapse of the third degree the epithelium covering the cervix is thickened and it is not uncommon for trophic ulcers to form both on the cervix and on the prolapsed anterior vaginal wall (see Figs. 241 to 247.)

In prolapse of the uterus, the supravaginal portion of the cervix is sometimes elongated. It is believed that supravaginal elongation of the cervix is caused by venous stasis induced by the descent of the cervix. It is also possible that the cranial part of Mackenrodt's ligament supports the upper part of the

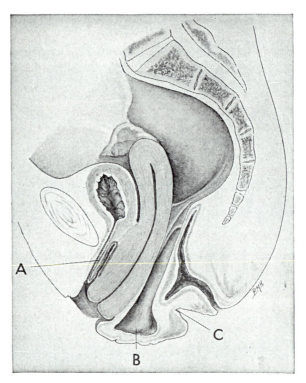

FIG. 245. Prolapse of the pouch of Douglas. The body of the uterus is supported by ligaments, but there is well-marked supravaginal elongation of the cervix. A indicates the position of the anterior fornix, B the pouch of Douglas prolapsed outside the vaginal orifice and C the junction of the posterior vaginal wall with the perineum.

cervix and that only the caudal portion of the retinaculum uteri is slackened. Supravaginal elongation of the cervix must be distinguished from congenital vaginal elongation, in which the fornices are deep and the elongation is restricted only to that portion of the cervix which projects into the vagina (see Figs. 241, 243, 245 and 247).

Prolapse of the Posterior Vaginal Wall. Prolapse of the posterior vaginal wall is not so frequent as cystocele. It is usually associated with severe injury to the perineal body. In **rectocele** the rectum protrudes with the posterior vaginal wall, and the tissues which normally intervene between the posterior vaginal wall and the rectum must have been torn by obstetrical injury, and the vagina and rectum must be adherent by scar tissue. One of the worst forms of prolapse occurs when the pouch of Douglas prolapses through the posterior fornix. In **prolapse of the pouch of Douglas** it is not uncommon for the upper part of the posterior vaginal wall to protrude outside the vulva and for coils of the intestine to be palpated in the prolapsed part. The term enterocele is used to describe this type of prolapse (see Figs. 242 and 245).

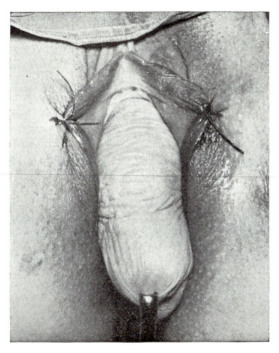

FIG. 246. Prolapse of the uterus at operation. The cervix has been drawn down, and the whole of the uterus can be pulled outside the vaginal orifice.

If a woman with prolapse is examined and asked to strain down, the usual sequence of events is for the anterior wall to protrude first, to be followed by the cervix, and then by the posterior vaginal wall.

Symptoms of Prolapse

In prolapse the patient complains of something descending in the vagina or of something protruding either at the vulva or externally. The prolapse is aggravated by straining and coughing, and by exercise. It is always most noticeable at the end of a hard day's work, whereas on rising the physical signs are naturally at their least obvious. Often the patient states that the prolapse reduces itself when she lies down. If there is a large prolapse, the external swelling may inconvenience the patient in walking and in carrying out her everyday duties. Even in mild degrees patients are conscious of a sense of weakness and of a lack of support around the perineum, and sensitive women may complain of this sense of weakness and the loss of confidence thereby induced before they are aware of anything prolapsing.

Prolapse has in the past been overrated as a cause of backache. It is true that towards the end of the day the patient may complain of a vague mid-sacral discomfort relieved by rest and recumbency. This symptom is most

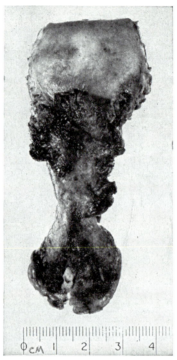

FIG. 247. Supravaginal elongation of the cervix from a vaginal hysterectomy specimen.

logically explained as a uterosacral strain. Too many backaches are, how-ever, incriminated against the obvious prolapse where in fact they are really of orthopaedic origin. After all the prolapse patient is of all women most likely to suffer from a coincident back lesion quite unconnected with her prolapse. Abdominal pain is never a predominant symptom, although some women suffer from what they describe as a bearing-down feeling above the pubes.

In most cases of prolapse there is some degree of vaginal discharge. The discharge may emanate from a chronically inflamed lacerated cervix, but usually it is caused by the relaxation of the vaginal orifice which allows foreign organisms to invade the vagina and produce a mild degree of vaginitis. A friction or decubitus ulcer is an obvious cause of discharge.

Some of the most important symptoms of prolapse are micturition disturbances. The most frequent is imperfect control of micturition, so that when the patient laughs or coughs or in any way raises the intra-abdominal pressure, urine dribbles from the urethra. This important symptom of stress incontinence must always be directly enquired into since many sensitive patients are ashamed of its presence and only point-blank inquisition in plain basic English will elicit it. This imperfect control of micturition is caused by a lack of support to the sphincter mechanism of the urethra. Frequency of micturition is also a common symptom, caused in some by chronic cystitis and in others by irritability of the bladder due to displacement. In severe degrees of cystocele patients frequently complain that they have difficulty in performing the act of micturition and that the more they strain the less easily can they pass urine. The explanation of this symptom is that when the intra-abdominal pressure is raised in straining, the bladder is pushed down in the cystocele so that most of the bladder lies below the level of the external meatus. Patients usually offer the information that they can only empty the bladder by pressing back the cystocele into the vagina with their fingers. Another symptom of this inadequate emptying of the bladder is that, as soon as micturition has been completed, the patient has a strong desire to pass urine again.

Rectal symptoms are less remarkable, although many women with prolapse are constipated. In rectocele patients may complain that they have difficulty in emptying the bowel, that having passed their initial motion they must return a second time to complete the evacuation. The explanation is simple—they have emptied the colon but only into the hypotonic pouch of their rectocele.

It is exceptional for prolapse to be associated with menstrual disturbances but slight haemorrhages from trophic ulcers developing over large prolapses may occur.

Investigation and Diagnosis

It is important to examine all patients with prolapse with care, because the treatment to be adopted is based upon the physical signs found. First, the vulva should be examined for evidence of old lacerations of the perineum, and inspection will show whether the vaginal orifice is relaxed. The patient is then asked to strain down, and partly by inspection, partly by palpation, the nature of the prolapse, whether of the anterior vaginal wall, or of the uterus, or of the posterior vaginal wall, is determined. It is important to know exactly which structures prolapse, whether there is a urethrocele, of which degree the prolapse of the uterus may be, whether there is a prolapse of the pouch of Douglas, and whether there is a rectocele. A rectocele can be accurately diagnosed only by rectal examination. The next step is to palpate the perineal body and the levator ani muscles to determine the muscle tone and the dimensions of the hiatus urogenitalis. Supravaginal elongation of the cervix is to be suspected if the uterus is found to be abnormally long when palpated bimanually, but the most reliable method is to pass a sound and find the length of the uterine cavity. The position of the uterus is then determined by bimanual examination and the cervix always examined with a speculum (see Fig. 248).

On the whole, there is not much difficulty in arriving at an exact diagnosis if the patient is examined thoroughly and systematically. Difficulty may be experienced in distinguishing between a cyst of the anterior vaginal wall and

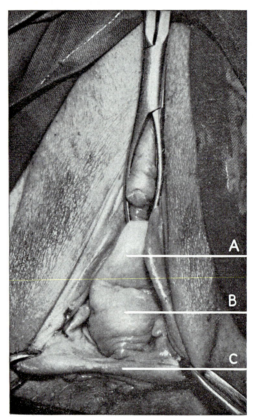

FIG. 248. Prolapse of the posterior vaginal wall at operation. The photograph illustrates A a hernia of Douglas's pouch, B a rectocele, together with C a weak perineal body.

a cystocele, but cysts of the anterior vaginal wall are usually tense with well-defined margins and cannot be reduced by pressure. Diverticula of the urethra are extremely rare, always small, and are situated low down in the anterior vaginal wall. Sometimes large tumours in the pouch of Douglas press down the posterior vaginal wall and cause a feeling of pressure and fullness in the pelvis, and unless the possibility of their presence is considered the practitioner may regard the case as one of prolapse. Myomatous polypi may present at the vulva, and unless the medical attendant examines the patient he may misdiagnose the myomatous polypus as being a simple prolapse. A bulky retroversion causes somewhat similar symptoms to those of prolapse, such as a feeling of fullness or of pressure in the vagina especially interpreted as a discomfort in the bowel due to the direct pressure of the uterine body on the anterior rectal wall.

Prophylaxis of Prolapse

Careful attention in the obstetric patient can do much to prevent a subsequent prolapse.

(1) Ante-natal hygiene and physiotherapy, relaxation exercises and due attention to weight gain and anaemia as well as to the fitness of the patient before delivery are important.

(2) The proper supervision and management of the second stage of labour:—

   (a) A generous episiotomy should be employed as a routine in all primigravidae and in all complicated labours, e.g. breech delivery.

   (b) Low forceps delivery should be more readily resorted to if there is any delay in the second stage.

   (c) Any posterior vaginal wall and perineal tear must be immediately and accurately sutured after delivery.

   (d) Postnatal exercises and physiotherapy are essential for every patient.

   (e) Early postnatal ambulation.

   (f) The provision of adequate rest for the first six months after delivery and the availability of home help for heavy domestic duties and in the assistance of the mother in the care of her baby so that she gets some rest and relaxation.

   (g) A reasonable interval between pregnancies so that too many children in too short an interval are avoided.

Treatment of Prolapse

One of the most important problems that a practitioner has to consider is the appropriate treatment to be advised in a case of prolapse arising in a young woman after childbirth. Some degree of relaxation of the vaginal orifice is a normal sequel to childbirth, and often there is some prolapse of the vaginal walls. Such patients are often fatigued by the strain of childbirth and lactation, and suffer from backache caused by muscle strain, weakness of the sacroiliac joints or some purely orthopaedic lesion such as a prolapsed intervertebral disc. It is a great mistake to advise immediate operative treatment in such cases. If an operation is performed for the relaxed vaginal orifice, for the prolapsed vaginal walls, and for the retrovertal uterus, there is always the possibility of a recurrence after a succeeding pregnancy. The next point which must be borne in mind is that such patients rapidly improve if well-directed conservative measures are adopted. The patient should be told that she must obtain the necessary amount of sleep and she should be freed as far as possible from anxieties. Abdominal exercises, massage and exercise of the muscles of the perineum should be advised, and the patient should be encouraged to take every opportunity to get out into the open air. Most patients of this kind suffer from leucorrhoea, which should be treated as already discussed in a previous chapter. Riding is the best exercise possible for the perineal muscles, for the levator ani muscle contracts in association with contraction of the adductor muscles of the thighs. This form of therapy is unfortunately available only to the more favoured class of our patients. Postnatal patients respond admirably to conservative measures if they are adopted early and the exercises carried out strenuously. It should be regarded as an error of judgment to advise operative treatment for the correction of a prolapse in a young woman within six months of childbirth.

On the other hand, moderately severe prolapse associated with the distressing symptoms of imperfect control of micturition is not uncommon in young women within a relatively short time of childbirth, when such conservative measures are ineffective. The question must be answered whether such women are to be treated by operation or whether they should be condemned to a pessary life. If an operation is performed there is always the possibility that a good operative result may be ruined by a subsequent childbirth. On the other hand, to be doomed to wear a pessary is an unpleasant

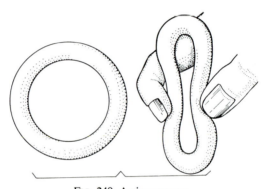

FIG. 249. A ring pessary.

prospect for any sensitive woman. With young women each case must be treated on its own merits. A well-marked cystocele or a badly torn perineum are real indications for operative treatment, and it should be remembered that succeeding labours are less likely to be so difficult and complicated as the first confinement. A carefully performed and accurately sutured episiotomy will do much to preserve the good results of a recent repair.

With women between the ages of 50 and 60, and these comprise the majority of patients with prolapse, operations should be advised unless there is some general contraindication such as severe cardiovascular disease, gross obesity or chronic bronchitis. Some women, however, prefer to wear a pessary rather than subject themselves to operative treatment.

In the case of some old women pessary treatment is to be preferred to operation if the patient is frail. On the other hand, prolapse in frail old women is apt to be of a severe degree, and quite often patients are unable to retain the usual forms of pessary.

Pessary Treatment of Prolapse. The use of a ring pessary is sometimes advised where operative treatment is contraindicated, though with modern anaesthesia and good pre-operative care such patients are few and decreasing. Age is no longer a contraindication to operation and many older patients tolerate operation better than their juniors, provided their general physical condition is good. A few patients will obstinately refuse operation, though if the reasons and risks are carefully explained to them their number is small.

It should be clearly understood that the pessary treatment of prolapse has certain limitations:

(1) It is never curative and can only be palliative.

(2) Unless the hygiene of the vagina is meticulous a vaginitis invariably results. Pessaries must be changed every three months and daily douching is essential.

(3) If the vaginal orifice is patulous the ring type of pessary cannot be retained.

(4) The wearing of a pessary in some women causes more discomfort than the prolapse.

(5) A pessary rarely, if ever, cures stress incontinence, which is therefore almost always an indication for operation.

(6) No young woman should be condemned to a pessary life.

Pessaries are made from some variety of polythene and the old rubber or vulcanite variety should be discarded as they were a potent cause of vaginitis. Vulcanite pessaries are somewhat rigid and, therefore difficult and painful to introduce. The present authors find both the virtues of compressibility and freedom from inflammatory reaction combined in the soft plastic polyvinyl chloride pessary and, if a pessary is to be used, this is the substance of choice. The ring pessaries are first compressed in the hand, having been previously softened in hot water, and introduced into the vagina in an anteroposterior sagittal plane, the perineum being pressed back to allow the pessary to pass into the vagina. The pessary is then rotated until it lies horizontally on the upper surfaces of the levator ani muscles. The diameter of the pessary is greater than the transverse diameter of the hiatus urogenitalis, and consequently the pessary is retained in the vagina. The pessary stretches the walls of the vagina and takes up the slack vaginal tissues, so that when the patient strains there is not only a feeling of support, but there is less slack vaginal tissue to protrude. Patients must be fitted with the correct size of pessary, and much experience is required before this can be judged. An accurately fitting pessary causes no discomfort and is an adequate method of treatment if the correct type of case is chosen. If the hiatus urogenitalis is widely patulous, or if there is extensive prolapse not only of the vaginal walls but of the uterus itself, then the pessary will not be retained. Pessaries should be changed at least every three months, and as they cause vaginal discharge the patient should be instructed to douche herself every day with plain warm water. If the uterus is retroverted and can be replaced, a Hodge pessary is to be preferred to a ring pessary, for cradle pessaries of this type help to keep the uterus back in its normal position of anteversion, in addition to stretching the vaginal walls (see Fig. 249).

In old patients with extensive prolapse, when a ring or cradle pessary cannot be retained, a Napier cup and stem pessary, preferably made of rubber, which is attached by tapes to a belt placed around the waist, is a useful method of treatment.

Innumerable forms of pessary have been introduced in past years, but few have advantages over the types described above. If a pessary is retained for a long time, it produces extensive vaginal discharge, and may cause ulceration of the vaginal walls, and the development of carcinoma in ulcers of this type is not unknown. It also tends with time to stretch the vagina so that progressively larger sizes have to be used in order to control the prolapse.

The Operative Treatment of Prolapse. The type of operation to be advised in a case of prolapse depends upon the individual features. There is no fixed routine and the operation decided upon is selected according to which structures prolapse. The operation of perineorrhaphy is, however, almost always performed, the object of the operation being to reduce the dimensions of the hiatus urogenitalis.

(1) For prolapse of the *anterior vaginal wall* some form of anterior colporrhaphy is performed. It cannot be emphasised too strongly that perineorrhaphy and anterior colporrhaphy are not operations for prolapse of the uterus. In such cases surgical treatment consists either in Fothergill's operation or Mayo's operation.

(2) For prolapse of the *posterior vaginal wall* perineorrhaphy is combined with a posterior colporrhaphy in the operation of colpoperineorrhaphy.

(3) The treatment of prolapse of the *pouch of Douglas* consists of an elaborate posterior colpoperineorrhaphy. The hernial sac is dissected clear and excised. The aperture through which the hernia protrudes is closed by suturing together the two uterosacral ligaments and by joining together the two levator ani muscles as far forwards as possible without reducing the size and length of the vagina.

(4) If the **vault prolapses,** i.e. there is actual uterine descent, the standard operation is the Manchester or Fothergill's—amputation of the cervix with shortening of Mackenrodt's ligament and re-suturing of these shortened structures into the anterior aspect of the uterus above the site of amputation. This effectively elevates the uterus and should antevert it and support the vaginal vault.

(5) If the **uterus is diseased** and presents symptoms inviting its removal, apart from the prolapse, vaginal hysterectomy and repair is the operation of choice.

The surgical treatment of prolapse can be summarised as follows:—

(1) *Vaginal prolapse—cystocele or rectocele or both* (without vault prolapse or uterine descent): Anterior and posterior colporrhaphy.

(2) *Vaginal prolapse with stress incontinence:* Anterior and posterior colporrhaphy with special reference to the suburethral and bladder neck buttressing by the pubo-cervical fascia in order to reconstitute the posterior urethro-vesical angle.

(3) *Hernia of the pouch of Douglas:* A specialised posterior colporrhaphy with special sutures introduced into the utero-sacral ligaments and the upper fibres of the pubo-rectalis fascia.

(4) *Vault prolapse or uterine descent:* Fothergill's (Manchester) operation.

(5) *Utero-vaginal prolapse associated with uterine symptoms* which of themselves warrant hysterectomy: Mayo's vaginal hysterectomy and repair.

Pre-operative Treatment for Vaginal Operations. The patient should be given antiseptic douches for some days before the operation and each evening the vagina should be packed with gauze soaked in flavine solution, strength one in a thousand. Another method is to pack the vagina with gauze impregnated with an antibiotic. The patient is given an aperient about midday on the day before operation and if necessary an enema the same evening. On the evening before the operation the vulva should be shaved or close clipped and

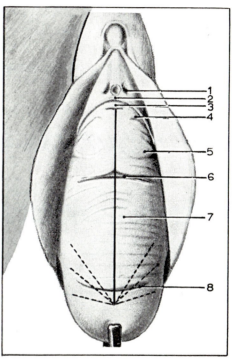

FIG. 250. The cervix has been drawn down. (1) Parameatal recess. (2) Hymen. (3) Submeatal sulcus. (4) Paraurethral recess. (5) Oblique vaginal fold. (6) Transverse sulcus of the anterior vaginal wall. (7) Arched rugae of the vaginal wall. (8) Bladder sulcus. The oblique lines indicate the direction of the incisions for different degrees of prolapse of the anterior vaginal wall, the uppermost being for slight degrees and the lowest for the most severe. (*Brit. med. J.*)

the patient given a bath. The patient should be catheterised in the theatre as the first step in the operation. Only in this way can the surgeon be sure of an empty bladder, which is an essential safeguard against the danger of its injury. The empty bladder has a thick wall resistant to trauma, the distended bladder's muscle is thin and much more easily damaged. The operation is performed with the patient lying in the lithotomy position under general anaesthesia.

Anterior Colporrhaphy

The indication for this operation is prolapse of the anterior vaginal wall. The bladder always comes down if the anterior vaginal wall prolapses and if the lower third of the anterior vaginal wall is involved the urethra will descend with it. The principles of the operation are to excise a piece of the anterior vaginal wall, to mobilise the bladder and push it upwards, and permanently to support the bladder by suturing together the fascial tissues which intervene between the vagina and bladder.

The posterior vaginal wall is retracted by an assistant holding a Sims' speculum. If the labia minora obtrude upon the operation field they should be sutured to the skin external to the labia majora by temporary sutures of

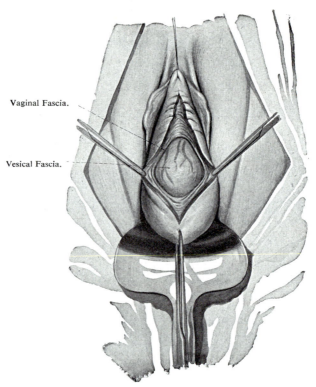

Vaginal Fascia.

Vesical Fascia.

FIG. 251. Anterior colporrhaphy. A midline incision is made and the vaginal wall and vaginal fascia are cut through. The vesico-vaginal space is opened up. The vesical fascia is recognised because of the dilated veins which ramify in its layer. (Peham-Amreich.)

catgut. The vaginal walls and cervix are now disinfected with an antiseptic solution such as flavine or chlorhexidine. The cervix is grasped with volsellum forceps and firmly brought down by an assistant. A longitudinal incision is made, extending from just below the urethral meatus to the point of junction of the vagina and cervix. Lateral incisions are now made from the cervical end of this incision. On each side an angular piece of tissue is enclosed by the incisions and the flap is now dissected clear from the subjacent tissues. The line of cleavage is the vesicovaginal space between the vaginal and vesical fascias. In this way the vaginal fascia is included in the lateral flap of tissue.

The flap can be dissected away easily provided the correct layer is reached. Unless this layer is found, the separation may be extremely difficult and if the dissection goes too deeply, there is a risk of injury to the bladder. Brisk haemorrhage indicates an incorrect plane of dissection (see Figs. 250–253), whereas the correct plane of cleavage is almost bloodless.

The next step is for the assistant to pull down the cervix firmly while the operator exposes the vesicocervical ligament as in Fig. 254. The ligament

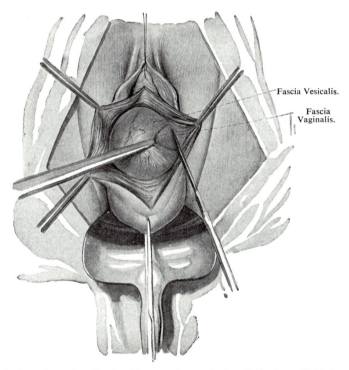

Fascia Vesicalis.

Fascia
Vaginalis.

Fig. 252. Anterior colporrhaphy. The anterior vaginal wall has been divided in the midline and the vaginal fascia has been cut through to open the vesico-vaginal space. The vesical fascia is recognised because conspicuous veins ramify in it. The illustration shows how the two fascias have to be separated from each other laterally with a scalpel. (Peham-Amreich.)

fixes the bladder to the front of the cervix. The ligament is divided with scissors, which mobilises the bladder so that it can now easily be pushed back with gauze. The separation of the bladder from the cervix is easy, provided that the correct layer of the vesicocervical space is reached. The lateral parts of the vesicovaginal ligament are sometimes firmly adherent and there may be brisk haemorrhage when the ligament is divided in this vicinity (Fig. 255). It is always advisable to secure any bleeding vessel by a suture ligature at this stage of the operation. The next step is to prevent the bladder from pro-lapsing again. A shelf of tissue to support the bladder is now formed as follows:

After the bladder has been freely mobilised and dislocated upwards from the cervix—the so-called advancement of the bladder—its lateral attachments to the vaginal flaps are carefully dissected in an outwards direction until the musculo-fascial tissues of the pubo-vesico-cervical ligament are reached. The inner aspect of this ligament fuses with the vesical fascia—hence the name pubo-vesico-cervical fascia. The whole purpose of the operation of anterior colporrhaphy is to coapt these two divaricated lateral structures by suture in the middle so that a stout musculo-fascial buttress is obtained from urethra to cervix. In a good subject this tissue is stout and well-developed, in an

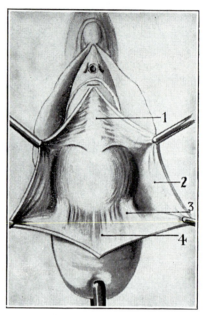

FIG. 253. The appearance after the dissection of the vaginal flaps. (1) Post-urethral ligament. The well-defined cranial border is emphasised. In the illustration the vesicovaginal space has been opened up, and the vaginal fascia (2) remains attached to the vaginal wall. (3) Bladder septum. (4) Vesico-cervical ligament. (*Brit. med. J.*)

asthenic and aged patient less so, but careful and thorough lateral dissection will always display it. A series of vertical mattress or Lembert sutures of 0 or 1 catgut are placed from the urethra to the cervix and, if stress incontinence is a symptom, special care is taken to obtain a good bite and a stout support under the bladder neck. When the urethra and bladder are thus well supported and firmly held upwards, the hiatus between the cervical ends of the pubocervical ligament is closed with sutures which include a bite of the cervix. These sutures somewhat elevate the cervix. The redundant vagina is now trimmed and closed by interrupted, and never continuous, sutures. A continuous suture shortens the vagina and causes dyspareunia.

In brief, anterior colporrhaphy, therefore, means dissection of the bladder from the cervix and anterior vaginal wall of sufficient degree to identify the pubo-cervico-vesical fascia so that this structure may be sewn together in the midline under the bladder to buttress it and the urethra, if there is stress incontinence, and thereby prevent the protrusion of the bladder and urethra. Failure to identify and suture the pubo-cervical fascia will give a poor result and certainly will not cure stress incontinence. The suture of the vaginal skin

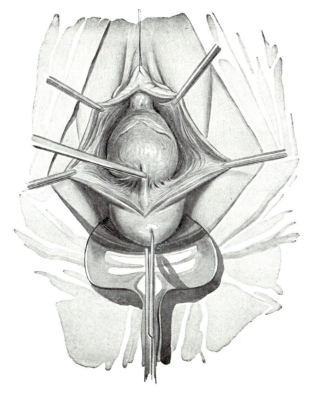

FIG. 254. Anterior colporrhaphy. After the bladder has been mobilised laterally the supravaginal septum which consists of the vesicocervical ligament is held up with forceps, divided, and then the bladder is retracted upwards. (Peham-Amreich.)

is purely cosmetic and haemostatic and plays no part whatever in the cure of anterior vaginal prolapse (Fig. 256).

Colpoperineorrhaphy. A pair of tissue forceps is placed on each side at the lower end of the labium minus, while a third pair of tissue forceps is attached to the posterior vaginal wall in the midline about one-third of the distance along the posterior vaginal wall. The triangular piece of vaginal wall enclosed by the three pairs of forceps is first removed. Some operators prefer to dissect away the flap from below, others from above. Extreme care must be taken in the removal of the flap because dense scar tissue may fix the vagina directly to the rectum, so that it is quite easy to injure the bowel. After the triangular flap has been removed the rectum should be pushed backwards and upwards with a finger placed in the middle of the wound. The internal margins of the levator ani muscles can then be identified. Deep sutures are passed through the two muscles so that after tying the sutures the two muscles come into apposition in the midline between the vagina and rectum. At least three such sutures should be passed. The remains of the transverse muscles of the perineum are then sutured together superficial to the levator ani muscle in a separate layer, and lastly the cut edges of the vagina are sutured together so that a longitudinal scar is produced. It is extremely important to obtain good

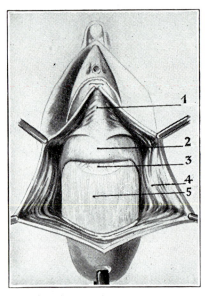

FIG. 255. The vesicocervical ligament has been divided, the bladder retracted upwards, and the vesicocervical space exposed. (1) Posturethral ligament. (2) Bladder. (3) Peritoneum of the uterovesical pouch. (4) Vaginal fascia. (5) Front of the cervix. (*Brit. med. J.*)

apposition, otherwise the wound will not heal cleanly. The amount of posterior vaginal wall that is removed depends upon the amount of its prolapse. With well-marked prolapse it may be necessary to extend the incision upwards as high as the pouch of Douglas. In the operation of colpoperineorrhaphy, there is a tendency for there to be fairly severe haemorrhage, and care must be taken either by ligature or by suturing to control the bleeding (see Figs. 257–259).

After the operations of anterior colporrhaphy, posterior colporrhaphy and perineorrhaphy the vagina should be packed tightly with dry sterile gauze for twenty-four hours, because there is always a tendency to reactionary haemorrhage. Tight packing of the vagina is the only reliable method for preventing this complication. If the vagina is properly packed a self-retaining catheter must always be inserted, as the patient is unable to pass her urine until the pack is removed. (Compare the retention of urine, which is often a feature of haemotocolpos where the retained blood acts in the same way as the vaginal pack).

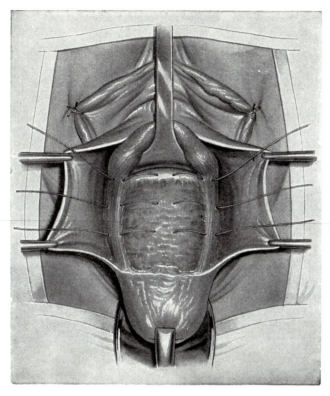

Fig. 256. The bladder is retracted upwards so that the lateral pillars of the pubo-cervical fascia can be sutured together in the region of the cervix. These sutures tend to elevate the cervix and antevert the uterus. (From Shaw's "Operative Gynaecology," 2nd ed., E. & S. Livingstone Ltd.)

Fothergill's (Manchester) Operation

This is now generally recognised to be the standard procedure for most cases of vaginal prolapse associated with uterine descent and is particularly indicated for those cases where the cervix lies at or below the level of the vaginal orifice. It is also indicated in those patients in whom the cervix is lacerated or infected as a result of childbirth.

In this operation an anterior colporrhaphy and colpoperineorrhaphy are combined with excision of the cervix. Moreover, after the cervix has been amputated, the slackness of Mackenrodt's ligaments is taken up by suturing the ligaments to the front of the uterus. Another important point in the technique is to cover the raw surfaces of the cut cervix with vaginal flaps.

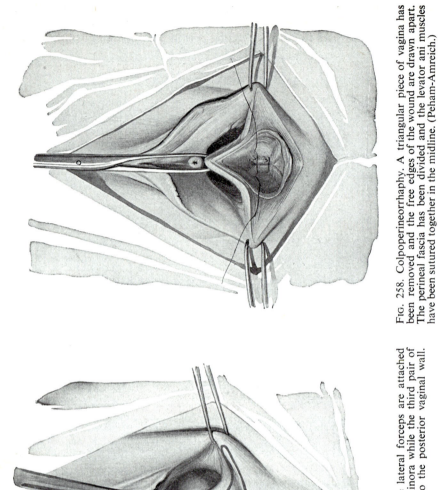

Fig. 258. Colpoperineorrhaphy. A triangular piece of vagina has been removed and the free edges of the wound are drawn apart. The perineal fascia has been divided and the levator ani muscles have been sutured together in the midline. (Peham-Amreich.)

Fig. 257. Colpoperineorrhaphy. The lateral forceps are attached to the posterior part of the labia minora while the third pair of forceps is attached in the midline to the posterior vaginal wall. (Peham-Amreich.)

The cervix is first dilated with Hegar's dilators, and the uterus should always be curetted to exclude endometrial disease. One important reason for a thorough dilatation of the cervix is to ensure adequate uterine drainage and the avoidance of cervical stenosis when the new external os heals. Failure to dilate could result in haematometra in a patient operated on before the menopause.

A triangular flap is now marked out in the vaginal walls. The apex of the triangle lies immediately below the urethral meatus while the base of the

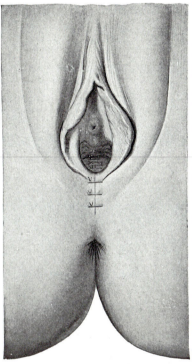

Fig. 259. The completion of the operation of colpoperineorrhaphy. (Peham-Amreich.)

triangle lies posterior to the cervix at about the level of the junction of the posterior vaginal wall with the cervix. The lateral angles of the triangle lie a short distance lateral to the cervix (see Fig. 260). The flap is marked out by incisions with a scalpel and the triangular piece of vaginal wall included in the incisions removed. Usually, the operator works from above downwards, starting near the urethra and working down towards the cervix. It is most important that the plane of cleavage is the vesicovaginal space. The cervix is now pulled down and the bladder mobilised as in the operation of anterior colporrhaphy as follows: The vesicocervical ligament is divided and the bladder pushed back. In this way, the anterior surface of the cervix is exposed.

The cervix is now pulled to one side and the parametrium of Mackenrodt's ligament exposed. A clamp is placed on the ligament and the ligament divided near the cervix. The same procedure is carried out on the opposite side. The cervix is now mobilised and it is amputated by cutting with a scalpel. The amputation stump of the cervix is drawn down with volsellum forceps. Haemorrhage from the cervix is controlled by haemostatic sutures and care must always be taken to ensure complete haemostasis. Any lateral vessels which bleed must be caught up with forceps and ligatured separately.

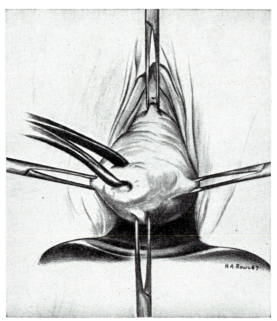

FIG. 260. Manchester operation with tenaculum forceps applied at Fothergill's four points. These points demarcate the area of vaginal skin to be excised.

Amputation of the cervix is notorious as a cause of secondary haemorrhage hence the importance of thorough haemostasis.

The next step is to shorten Mackenrodt's ligaments. This is performed by passing a suture through the lower part of the ligament lateral to the cervix, then passing the suture through the front of the uterus and then through Mackenrodt's ligament of the opposite side. When the suture is tied, the two ligaments are fixed together *in front of* the uterus and consequently shortened considerably (see Figs. 261–264.) The cut surface of the cervix is now covered with vaginal flaps.

The bladder is now dealt with just as in the operation of anterior colporrhaphy described on p. 530. The wound in the vagina is now closed by suturing the cut edges in the midline. A colpoperineorrhaphy is then performed in the usual way. Considerable judgment is required in assessing exactly how much

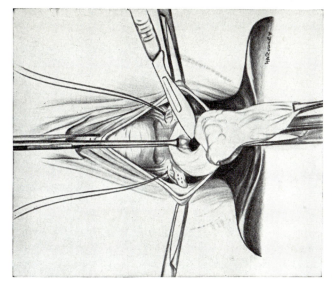

FIG. 262. Both Mackenrodt's ligaments have now been ligated and the cervix almost completely amputated. A volsellum is attached to the anterior lip of the cervix above the amputation.

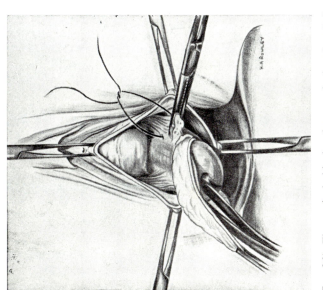

FIG. 261. The vaginal skin has been excised and pulled down over the cervix. Mackenrodt's ligaments have been clamped and cut and a suture ligature has been inserted in the left Mackenrodt's ligament. Note that the bladder has been freely mobilised and pushed well up out of danger.

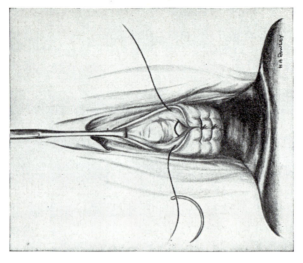

FIG. 264. The anterior vaginal wall is being closed. Note that the pubo-cervical fascia is carefully sutured under the vaginal skin.

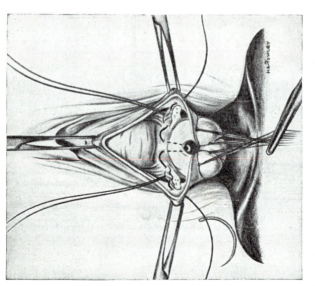

FIG. 263. A covering for the posterior lip of the cervix has been fashioned from the mobilised vaginal skin of the posterior fornix and this has been secured to the new cervix by deep sutures. Fothergill's stitch is illustrated and it should be noticed that it passes through vaginal skin in the region of Fothergill's lateral point, through Mackenrodt's ligament and through the anterior lip of the cervix into the cervical canal, and thence out the other side and through Mackenrodt's ligament and vaginal skin.

vagina should be removed. Over-zealous excision will result in obstructive dyspareunia, and it is therefore better to remove too little rather than too much. Any residual redundancy can be trimmed off as the operation proceeds, and a final calibre of two fingers should be aimed at by the operator. It is also important not to shorten the vagina unduly as this also results in dyspareunia, and an adequate vaginal length is one of the criteria of a properly performed Fothergill operation.

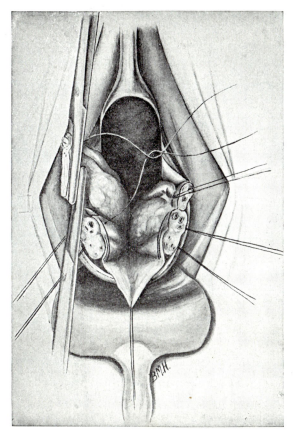

FIG. 265. Vaginal hysterectomy. The uterus has been removed and the pedicles are being ligatured.

Vaginal Hysterectomy for Prolapse. Although Fothergill's operation gives extremely good results in most cases, some surgeons regard it as insufficient for complete procidentia. The alternative operation for this form of prolapse consists in a vaginal hysterectomy, after which the cut edges of Mackenrodt's and the uterosacral ligaments, the broad ligaments, the round and ovarian ligaments, are sutured to the corresponding structures of the opposite side in the midline, to form a support for the bladder (see Figs. 265–267). Vaginal hysterectomy is also indicated in those cases of prolapse associated with uterine symptoms sufficient of themselves to warrant a hysterectomy.

The following technique is employed. The cervix is pulled down with volsellum forceps and a midline incision made extending from the urethral meatus anteriorly to the cervix below. By means of lateral incisions, two triangular flaps are marked out and then dissected away just as in the operation of anterior colporrhaphy. The vesicocervical ligament is divided and the

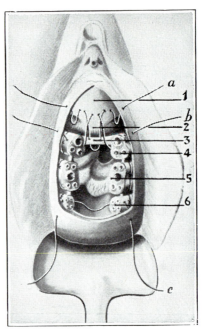

FIG. 266. Technique for the operation of vaginal hysterectomy for prolapse before suturing the pedicles together. (1) Posturethral ligament. (2) Bladder. (3) Peritoneum (diagrammatic). (4) The pedicle containing the round ligament, the ovarian ligament, and the Fallopian tube. (5) The pedicle containing the uterine vessels. (6) The pedicle containing the uterosacral ligament. (a) The suture is passed through the vaginal wall, then through the peritoneum covering the bladder, the procedure being repeated on the opposite side. (b) The suture is passed through the vaginal wall, the vaginal fascia, the first pedicle, and then through the posturethral ligament, the procedure being repeated on the opposite side. (c) The suture is passed through the vaginal wall and the uterosacral pedicle, and repeated on the opposite side. (Brit. med. J.)

bladder retracted upwards and held back by an assistant with a Sims' retractor. The lateral incisions are now carried around the cervix just as in Fothergill's operation. This incision enables the uterus to be pulled down still farther.

The uterovesical pouch of peritoneum is now identified as a convex fold of tissue and the pouch of peritoneum opened up with scissors. The incision in the uterovesical pouch is now extended laterally and the fundus of the uterus pulled through this opening either by hooking with a finger or with the help of volsellum forceps. In most cases, the uterus can be pulled down without difficulty. This is vaginal hysterectomy by anteversion.

The next step is to remove the uterus. Long curved clamps are used. The first clamp is placed immediately lateral to the uterus and includes the ovarian ligament, the Fallopian tube and the round ligament of one side and these structures are cut through with scissors on the uterine side of the clamp. Further clamps are placed over the broad ligament and uterine artery of that side and the tissues again cut on the uterine side of the clamp. A similar

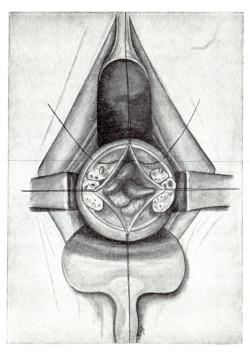

FIG. 267. Vaginal hysterectomy. The pedicles have been ligatured. The upper suture helps to hold back the bladder. The large peritoneal opening in this case is closed by a purse-string suture.

procedure is then followed on the opposite side so that the uterus is now attached only by Mackenrodt's ligaments, the uterosacral ligaments, and the posterior part of the vagina in the region of the pouch of Douglas. Each of these structures is now clamped separately and the uterus removed. The pedicles are now ligatured with strong catgut and then sutured to the corresponding pedicle of the opposite side in the midline. The next step is to fix this shelf of tissue below the bladder. A series of sutures are therefore passed through the pubo-cervical fascia of one side, through the tissues of the shelf, and then through the vaginal fascia of the other side. The peritoneal cavity is closed by including the peritoneum covering the bladder in the most anterior of these sutures, and the peritoneum covering the rectum in the most posterior of them. The cut edges of the vagina are now sutured together in the midline. Subsequently an extensive colpoperineorrhaphy is performed.

An alternative and probably more popular method of vaginal hysterectomy is to work from below upwards. As soon as the pouch of Douglas is opened the uterus is left undisturbed and not delivered by fundal traction as above described. First the uterosacral ligaments on each side are clamped and doubly ligated and cut, next by traction on the cervix the uterus is pulled down to expose the uterine vessels, which are clamped, cut and tied. This second manoeuvre is always made easier once the uterosacral ligaments have been cut as this step greatly increases the descent of the uterus. When the uterine vessels have been secured, cut and tied the uterus is only held by the ovarian and round ligaments which are clamped, cut and tied in their turn, but last, not, as in the previous description of vaginal hysterectomy by anteversion, first. A versatile operator will use both methods according to the variations of the individual case.

These are the main steps of the operation. One of the complications of the operation is that a hernia of the pouch of Douglas may develop at a later date. This complication is also seen after other operations for prolapse; even after Fothergill's operation. The great advantage of the vaginal hysterectomy technique is that steps can be taken during the operation to prevent this possibility (a) by removing the redundant peritoneum of Douglas' pouch, (b) by suturing together the uterosacral ligaments, and (c) by suturing the levator ani muscles together with stitches which include the uterosacral ligaments.

Le Fort's Operation. In this operation rectangular flaps are dissected away from the anterior and posterior vaginal walls and the raw surfaces sutured together so that the vagina is closed except for small channels on each side through which the normal uterine secretions can be discharged. In other words a single-barrelled organ is converted into a double-barrelled and it is the median septum thus artificially formed which prevents any future prolapse.

The operation is simple to perform provided that the flaps are marked out accurately. The operation is suitable for cases of procidentia in old women, and it gives good results. It is not, however, often performed as it has no advantages over the Fothergill operation or vaginal hysterectomy and repair, nor is it any quicker than its rivals when these are performed by expert hands.

After treatment of Vaginal Operations for Prolapse

The patient is nursed in any position she likes and is encouraged to move freely in bed. She is encouraged to sit out of bed in a chair on the second postoperative day unless there is some valid contraindication. Most patients have a great deal of pain from the perineal sutures, and sedative drugs should be given freely during the first three days after the operation. The bowels should be confined for at least three days after the operation. During the third day the patient should be given paraffin by mouth followed by an aperient on the night of the third day. If the bowels fail to act and are causing discomfort from flatulence glycerine suppositories are helpful. After plastic vaginal operations the vagina is packed tightly with gauze to prevent reactionary haemorrhage. The packing should be removed twenty-four hours after the operation. Patients often have difficulty in passing urine, particularly on the day following the operation. For this reason the usual practice is to introduce a self-retaining catheter into the bladder after the operation. The catheter can be kept in situ for at least a week without causing much discomfort. Catheterisation is particularly indicated in all vaginal operations for stress incontinence, as these patients are unlikely to pass urine spontaneously for some days—sometimes as long as a fortnight after operation. If a catheter is employed for either continuous or intermittent drainage it is wise to give prohylactic nitro-furantoin for one week while the catheter is in use. This prophylaxis will reduce the urinary infection rate from 80% to 10%.

Unless the wounds in the vagina heal cleanly a vaginal discharge develops towards the end of the first week after operation. In this event, the patient should be treated with vaginal irrigations of warm, weak antiseptic solutions, and it is best for a rubber catheter to be introduced into the vagina rather than a glass douche nozzle. The patient should be allowed to walk about the ward at the end of the first week, for it is important to exercise the abdominal and perineal muscles as early as possible. Much depends upon the skill of the operator for a good result to be obtained. Accurate apposition and the requisite amount of tension on the sutures are important factors. Of equal importance, perhaps, is the nursing care. The perineum should be kept clean and dry, being irrigated after micturition and defaecation with some antiseptic solution, and the wound itself then swabbed with flavine in spirit. If the wounds suppurate, plentiful irrigations with weak peroxide followed by saline should be given, and as soon as possible—usually five to seven days after operation—the patient should be given hot baths.

Chemotherapy is advisable in all instances of prolapse wound infection.

Complications of the Vaginal Operations for Prolapse

The most frequent complication is **retention of urine,** which may be caused by the gauze packing in the vagina or may be reflex from the trauma to the perineum. The use of a self-retaining catheter will overcome this complication.

Another common complication is **lower urinary tract infection** induced by injury to the bladder, and quite often the infection is severe. The use of an indwelling catheter or intermittent catheterisation also plays a part in urinary infection. It should be treated by prophylactic nitro-furantoin and if the urine culture shows an infection insensitive to this drug the appropriate chemotherapy should be substituted. Under this régime, extension of the infection of the upper urinary tract is almost never encountered. Urinary fistulae due to injury either to the ureters or bladder represent the results of bad technique and are extremely rare.

Haemorrhage. Reactionary haemorrhage is not uncommon after plastic operations on the vagina. Such operations are sometimes accompanied by fairly profuse haemorrhage, with the result that the patient's blood pressure falls towards the end of the operation. During recovery from the anaesthetic, when the blood pressure rises, vessels which have not been tied are apt to bleed fairly profusely. It is most important to pack the vagina tightly with sterile gauze soaked in chlorhexadine immediately after the operation, for this serves to control reactionary haemorrhage of this kind. If reactionary haemorrhage develops there is only one course to pursue. The patient must be anaesthetised, clots removed from the vagina, and the vagina sponged clean with swabs. No attempt should be made to open the wound and clamp bleeding points, but the vagina should be packed tightly with dry sterile gauze. The gauze can be removed almost painlessly without anaesthesia twenty-four hours later.

Secondary haemorrhage following plastic vaginal operations is more frequent than reactionary haemorrhage and is caused by sepsis. The principles of treatment are the same as those recommended for reactionary haemorrhage, the patient being anaesthetised, the vagina cleared of all blood and clot, and packed tightly with dry sterile gauze. Sometimes haemorrhage following plastic vaginal operations is severe and the patient has to be treated by blood transfusion. Moreover, with secondary haemorrhage it may be necessary to repack the vagina, for recurrent haemorrhage is quite likely to occur. If adequate packing of the vagina fails to control the bleeding the pack must be removed and the bleeding point found and ligated. This may involve a deep exploration of the operation site, and on rare occasions after vaginal hysterectomy it may be necessary to open the abdomen to ligature a pedicle which has retracted out of reach of the vaginal wound. A resuture of the vaginal wound is usually necessary as the manipulations involved in dealing with the bleeding vessel will usually have disrupted the vaginal suture line.

Suppuration in the Wound. Although the wounds in the vagina heal remarkably well if good apposition is obtained, there is a tendency for the vaginal and perineal wounds to break down and suppurate. Fortunately, the sepsis is usually superficial and gives rise only to a purulent offensive vaginal discharge which responds readily to vaginal irrigation with antiseptic solutions and the exhibition of the appropriate antibiotic. Severe pelvic cellulitis is not unknown, but is extremely rare. If the perineal wound breaks down and suppurates, it should be treated with copious irrigations and the patient should be given frequent hot baths during the second week after operation. Treatment with chemotherapy and antibiotics should follow the usual lines.

After vaginal hysterectomy a haematoma sometimes forms in the broad ligament causing a raised temperature and pulse rate and pain or discomfort in the pelvis. A vaginal examination will show that there is a brawny mass on one or other side of the vagina. This is sometimes better appreciated by rectal examination. The lower abdomen may be a little tender and there is some moderate rigidity. The bowel tends to be distended in the lower abdomen due to a localised paralytic ileus. Such a haematoma can readily become infected and give rise to one form of pelvic abscess. There is first a discharge of dark altered blood and clot and later a frankly purulent discharge which is dark and offensive. When such a haematoma becomes infected quite a high fever may result and there may be signs of pelvic peritonitis—with local ileus, local tenderness in the lower abdomen and pain. The treatment of the haematoma or abscess when found is to encourage vaginal drainage by passing a finger into the haematoma or abscess and by warm vaginal irrigation, followed by the installation of an ounce of glycerine into the vaginal vault. The organisms should be typed for sensitivity and the appropriate chemotherapy given. Any local pelvic peritonitis usually responds to chemotherapy without more elaborate treatment. Anaemia may need treatment by transfusion. Fortunately the condition rapidly subsides as a rule, although tubo-ovarian abscesses occasionally result and may need subsequent abdominal operation.

Visceral Injuries. The bladder may very rarely be torn or opened during a prolapse operation. This injury is usually recognised at once and if carefully repaired and treated by continuous urethral drainage should cause no trouble. A more serious injury is damage to the urethra which usually results from a too tight suturing of the suburethral fascia in the operation for stress incontinence. The urethra can also be damaged by inexpert catheterisation after operation. The result is a urethrovaginal fistula which will necessitate a difficult plastic operation three to six months later.

The ureters are very rarely damaged in prolapse operations, although cases have been recorded of their inclusion in an injudiciously placed Fothergill suture. They are also endangered by vaginal hysterectomy but surprisingly free from actual trauma.

The rectum is far more likely to be injured than the bladder, since the scarring of old perineal tears distorts the anatomy and obliterates the normal planes of cleavage at operation. If the rectum is torn or opened during the operation of posterior colpoperineorrhaphy it should be immediately sutured in the same way as a complete tear of the perineum occurring in childbirth. The bowels should be confined for five to seven days and chemotherapy employed. If the surgeon is in any doubt about the integrity of the rectum he should place a finger in the rectum and establish the true situation. As a rule the muscle of the bowel only is damaged and all that is needed is a few interrupted tacks of fine catgut to approximate the torn muscle. Rectovaginal fistulae very rarely result from prolapse operations.

Phlebothrombosis and Pulmonary Embolism. This complication, though rarer than after abdominal gynaecological operations, is none the less important in vaginal surgery. The patient usually exhibits a small fever with a slight rise of pulse rate and may notice some pain in the calf, knee or thigh. Examination shows tenderness in the muscles of the calf and often in the popliteal fossa. Anticoagulants should be given at once until all symptoms have subsided. Any pain in the chest or dyspnoea should be regarded as due to an infarct and confirmation of this obtained by chest X-ray twelve hours later. Chest symptoms suggestive of an infarct or embolus call for a continuation of anticoagulant therapy, and if the prothrombin level is maintained at 15%—25% most cases fortunately respond, though a fatal pulmonary embolism has twice resulted in the authors' experience after vaginal hysterectomy which was in every other way uncomplicated. A history of previous phlebothrombosis, e.g. after operation or confinement, calls for great caution and observation, and possibly prophylactic anticoagulant treatment. All prolapse

18*

patients should receive preoperative and postoperative physiotherapy and breathing exercises. They should be encouraged to get up as early as the vaginal wound permits, certainly by the fourth postoperative day, though actual ambulation cannot usually be undertaken before the seventh day.

Late Complications of Prolapse Operations

Recurrence. However technically good the operation and however expert the surgeon there will always be a small recurrence rate for repair operations. This is especially so where stress incontinence is a symptom or where the patient is a chronic bronchitic subject. Obesity, constipation and a job involving hard physical work are all unfavourable factors. It is important with such patients to provide adequate convalescence after operation. A particularly difficult complication to treat is the development of a hernia of Douglas' pouch following vaginal hysterectomy, and great care should be taken to minimise the chance of this by carefully suturing the uterosacral ligaments together at the original operation.

Dyspareunia has already been mentioned as the result of too wide an excision of the vagina, and in younger patients this complication can be very distressing. It is sometimes possible to dilate the vagina with graduated plastic dilators or to perform a small plastic enlargement of a too narrow introitus. The best treatment is to avoid the complication by correct operative technique.

Complications in Subsequent Pregnancy and Labour. In young women submitted to Fothergill's operation a high amputation of the cervix should not be performed, as this is liable to cause abortion from cervical incompetence or premature labour. Sometimes the scarring of the cervix resulting from this operation causes dystocia and necessitates delivery by Caesarean section. A properly performed repair operation is not, however, a bar to normal vaginal delivery provided a generous episiotomy is used, nor does the prolapse necessarily reappear as the result of delivery. In such patients, however, a readier resort to Caesarean section is more justifiable than in the normal woman.

22 Displacements

The usual position of the uterus in 80% of nulliparous women is one of anteversion and anteflexion, in which the uterine body is bent forwards at its junction with the cervix. The normal uterus in a normal pelvis is not a static organ and its position is naturally altered by the state of the bladder

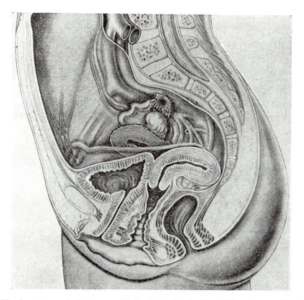

FIG. 268. A retroverted uterus. Note that the body of the uterus lies in the pouch of Douglas, and is also retroflexed as well as being retroverted. The cervix points downwards and forwards.

which, when full, displaces the uterus backwards. If the uterus lies anteverted and anteflexed, the external os is found, on vaginal examination, to be pointing downwards and backwards, and the anterior lip of the cervix is the first part of the uterus to be felt. The uterus may, however, lie so that the axis of the cervix is rotated backwards through an angle of 90 degrees, so that the external os points downwards and forwards, and the posterior lip is the first part of the cervix to be felt on vaginal examination. In such cases the cervical canal, when traced upwards, is directed upwards and backwards, and the uterus is described as being retroverted. In most cases of retroversion the uterus is also retroflexed, so that the body of the uterus is flexed backwards on the cervix. Version, therefore, refers to the direction of the cervical canal. whereas flexion refers to the inclination of the body of the uterus on the cervix. If the uterus is retroverted but anteflexed, it is customary to describe the uterus as lying far back in the pelvis, or retroposed, rather than to introduce the pedantic nomenclature of the "retroverted anteflexed uterus". In clinical practice, whether the uterus is retroverted or retroflexed, it is convenient to use the simple term retroversion for all positions in which the organ is not anteverted (Fig. 268).

It is difficult to explain why the uterus is usually anteflexed, because the round ligaments do not of themselves maintain the position of anteflexion. In fact, the position of anteflexion of the body on the cervix is largely inherent in the uterine myometrium since, if the organ is removed by hysterectomy, it is impossible in the normal organ forcibly to retroflex it and, if this is done, it immediately resumes the anteflexed position.

The significance of retroflexion and retroversion, whether these displacements are responsible for symptoms and whether treatment should be recommended to correct such displacements, offers one of the most difficult problems in the whole of gynaecology. Probably all gynaecologists will admit that the uterus may be retroflexed and retroverted without attendant symptoms, while they will also admit that some patients with retroflexion and retroversion, who have such symptoms as backache and dyspareunia, can be cured completely of these symptoms if the displacement of the uterus is corrected. The problem, therefore, is to determine which type of case causes symptoms which are amenable to treatment. From the clinical point of view it is best to group the patients into those in which the uterus is movable and replaceable and those in which the uterus is fixed in its retroverted position.

Mobile Retroversion

(a) The uterus is congenitally retroverted in 20% of patients, and it is not uncommon to find the uterus in the retroverted position without the patient complaining of gynaecological symptoms. The term congenital is somewhat inaccurate because the neonatal position of the uterine body in reference to the cervix is in a straight line and the position of anteversion or retroversion is only acquired later, probably at the time of puberty when the myometrium undergoes a hyperplasia under the influence of the ovarian oestrogen. It is retained because of its traditional status. A pelvic examination may be indicated because of leucorrhoea or dysmenorrhoea; if in such a case the uterus is found to be retroverted it does not conclusively follow that the backward displacement is responsible for the symptoms. Unfortunately some practitioners when finding a retroverted uterus immediately incriminate it as being the responsible factor in a host of symptoms quite unrelated to the so-called malposition. The retroversion provides a convenient label, which is all too readily acceptable to the relatives and the patient. This facile philosophy has nothing to recommend it.

(b) In asthenic subjects with visceroptosis the uterus is frequently found to be retroverted. In such patients the displacement should be regarded as being determined by an intrinsic fault in the myometrium. Most patients of this kind have no gynaecological symptoms, but some of them suffer from backache. It is unwise to consider that this backache is in any way due to the retroversion. If a woman complains of backache there is usually something wrong with her back and not her uterus.

(*c*) A large number of retroversions are seen in women after childbirth and can be regarded as comparable to those of the previous group. Indeed, by far the largest group of acquired retroversions arise in the puerperium. About 25 % of women have a retroverted uterus after their first confinement. This group includes about half the women who had congenital retroversion of the uterus before pregnancy, in the remainder of whom pregnancy results in correction of the displacement. It has been pointed out already, on page 523, that such displacements often right themselves spontaneously when the patient's muscle tone is improved by massage and exercises. This puerperal mobility of the uterus should be regarded as due to a temporary slackness in the endopelvic fascial supports associated with a physiological degree of subinvolution or pregnancy myohyperplasia. The incidence of puerperal retroversion largely depends upon the time that elapses after a confinement before the postnatal examination is made, and therefore, depends on the degree of involution. A retroversion at six weeks after confinement is more frequent than one at six months.

(*d*) It is well recognised that alteration in the position of the uterus occurs early in the development of uterine prolapse, so that the axis of the body follows the axis of the cervix into alignment with the vaginal canal.

(*e*) Sometimes the displacement of the uterus is caused by the presence of tumours such as myomata and ovarian cysts in the pelvis, which push the uterus backwards and by their presence cause retroversion.

Symptoms of Retroversion

Most textbooks give an impressive list of the symptoms caused by acquired retroversion and it is, therefore, necessary critically to examine this list before accepting its accuracy.

Symptoms referable to a Congestive State of the Uterus, associated with chronic subinvolution or myohyperplasia.

(1) *Congestive dysmenorrhoea.* This term is reasonably accurate and describes a type of premenstrual heaviness and discomfort in the pelvis which is gradually relieved by the establishment of menstruation. When removed at hysterectomy, this type of uterus is enlarged, perhaps to twice its normal size, and the myometrium is hyperplastic. This symptom is, therefore, genuine though seldom severe and in all fairness as much due to the myohyperplasia as to the retroversion.

(2) *A moderate degree of menorrhagia* is explicable on exactly the above lines and is characteristic of all types of myohyperplasia.

(3) *A congestive state of the cervix and endocervical glands* causes an increased secretion of mucus and gives rise to a non-purulent leucorrhoea. Again, if strict impartiality is to be observed the confinement which is blamed for the retroversion will also be responsible for the cervical trauma and subsequent endocervicitis.

(4) *A feeling of heaviness* felt in the middle of the sacrum and interpreted by the patient as a backache which it really is not.

It should be emphasised that these four symptoms will not be evident unless there is a demonstrable state of chronic subinvolution and myohyperplasia, and they are, therefore, not to be expected in a well involuted, normalsized retroverted uterus. Moreover, the leucorrhoea is only explicable by congestion if the cervix is healthy. The more normal explanation of the vaginal discharge is that it is due to a laceration, infection, erosion or ectropion acquired, at the same time as the retroversion, from childbirth injury. In this type of cervix, the discharge is more likely to be muco-purulent.

Similarly, the backache, so plausibly explained by the retroversion is just as and, in fact, more likely to be due to a pregnancy or puerperal back strain, to faulty posture or other orthopaedic causes.

Symptoms attributable to the Position of the Uterus. (1) *Dyspareunia.* Of all symptoms of retroversion this is the one which, in the authors' opinion, is indisputably genuine and attributable to the retroversion. The term collision dyspareunia is descriptive. When making a vaginal examination on these patients, the body of the retroverted uterus is tender on digital palpation and the patient may wince when it is even gently touched. But, more important is the prolapsed ovary which is often found in the pouch of Douglas, slightly enlarged, presumably congested and often exquisitely tender. These patients suffer from severe dyspareunia on full penetration and after coitus they may complain of an ache in the pelvis that persists for twelve to twentyfour hours, so that they volunteer that they feel internally bruised after coitus and come to dread the experience. As a result, they develop a protective frigidity and matrimonial disharmony or rupture may result.

(2) *Infertility.* It is a theoretical possibility that, in the retroverted uterus, the external os is not accessible to the spermatozoa in the seminal pool in the posterior fornix. This hypothesis is rather hard to believe when it is remembered that a woman can conceive without ever having been penetrated and with an intact hymen. There is, however, some logic in the idea because correction of the retroversion certainly does result in conception in a certain number of infertile women. It is suggested that the reasons for the success of this correction are not entirely referable to the cervix. For instance, correction will improve the congestive state of the uterus and very possibly eliminate the dyspareunia which may have well been a more important causative factor than the position of the cervix. Retroversion *per se* is not therefore regarded as a direct aetiological factor in infertility.

(3) *The responsibility of retroversion for abortion* has been greatly exaggerated. Apart from the rare incarceration of the retroverted, gravid uterus, it is not of itself likely to cause abortion. It must be remembered that at least one in five conceptions ends in abortion whatever the position of the uterus and the natural incidence of this mishap will, when found in a woman with retroversion, be quite wrongly attributed to the malposition. There are a few patients, however, who may have had two or more abortions, usually at about ten weeks, and who, apart from the retroversion, are completely normal. In such, the congestive state of the uterus may be contributive since its correction by pessary or operation often results in a successful **pregnancy.**

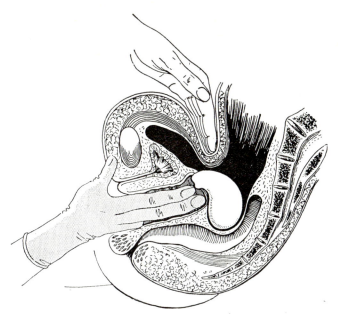

FIG. 269. Digital replacement of a retroverted uterus. The diagnosis is made with the help of two fingers placed in the posterior fornix. (After Neuweiler.)

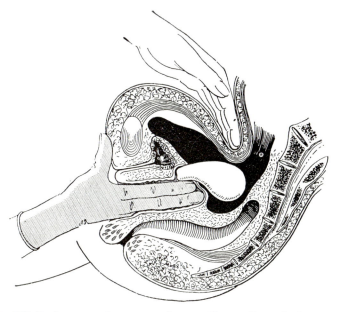

FIG. 270. Replacement of a retroverted uterus. The two fingers in the posterior fornix push the fundus of the uterus upwards and forwards. (After Neuweiler.)

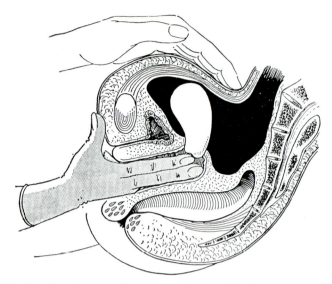

FIG. 271. Digital replacement of a retroverted uterus. The fingers placed on the abdomen by pressing the body of the uterus downwards, together with help from the internal fingers which push the cervix upwards, correct the displacement. (After Neuweiler.)

(4) *Retroverted Gravid Uterus with Retention of Urine.* This is a genuine symptom and needs no comment except that considering the number of pregnancies which occur in the retroverted organ it is an extremely rare event. Owing to its dramatic associations it has received a publicity quite undeserved by its rarity.

(5) A few intelligent patients will notice a sensation that something is displaced in the vagina and they naturally imagine that they are developing a prolapse. Some even complain of a feeling of something pressing on the bowel which, after defaecation, gives them a feeling that the motion is not completely evacuated. These rectal symptoms will be more accurately found if specifically enquired into by direct questioning.

In retroversion, as in many gynaecological conditions, the functional side of the problem must not be forgotten and undue credit must not be given to the simple correction of the malposition when the explanation of the improvement in the symptoms is as likely to be due to the psychological rehabilitation.

The question which must now be answered is whether a mobile retroflexion of the uterus of this type is responsible for gynaecological symptoms.

If the retroversion is mobile and the patient free of symptoms no treatment is necessary. If, on the other hand, the patient complains of infertility, dyspareunia or backache, and the uterus is found to be retroverted, the uterus should be replaced and kept in position with a Hodge pessary. If the symptoms persist after the uterus has been replaced by this relatively simple method, operative treatment for the retroversion is clearly unjustifiable, as the symptoms must necessarily be due to some other cause. This is known as the pessary test and is a valuable prognostic index in assessing the pros and cons of surgical treatment. The test can be carried a stage further by imposing a second period of trial when the retroflexion recurs, inserting on this occasion a simple ring pessary which does not correct the retroflexion. If relief of symptoms is maintained with the uterus retroflexed above the ring, then it can be fairly assumed that the patient has responded to a mechanical placebo and that her original symptoms were not in any way attributable to the retroversion.

The Technique of Replacement of the Retroverted Uterus. It is possible to replace a mobile retroversion bimanually, although much experience and skill are necessary. The patient should first lie in the left lateral position. Two fingers are placed in the posterior fornix of the vagina and should attempt to push up the body of the uterus, preferably a little to one side of the midline. The patient should then be turned on her back and the operator's left hand placed on the abdomen just below the level of the umbilicus. If the fingers of the left hand can be made to reach behind the uterus replacement is easy. The fingers in the vagina should now be placed in front of the cervix

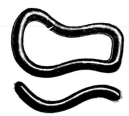

Fig. 272. A Hodge pessary.

and should push the vaginal portion of the cervix downwards and backwards, which will tend to make the uterus anteflexed. Some authorities recommend that the patient should be placed in the knee-elbow position while this is being done. When the fingers of the left hand have been made to reach behind the body of the uterus, the body should be pushed forwards and if possible, downwards to promote anteversion. Bimanual replacement of this kind is sometimes remarkably simple. At other times it is impossible, owing to the abdominal wall being fat, the abdominal muscles rigid, or the uterus being small (see Figs. 269–271).

In difficult cases it may be necessary to attach volsellum forceps to the anterior lip of the cervix before the uterus can be replaced. A Sims' speculum is introduced into the vagina and a pair of volsellum forceps attached to the anterior lip of the cervix. Traction is now applied to the volsellum forceps with the left hand and two fingers of the right hand are placed in the posterior fornix to push up the retroverted body of the uterus. After a time, the fingers of the right hand are withdrawn from the vagina and traction is made by means of the right hand on the volsellum forceps, the left hand being placed on the abdomen and an effort made to place the fingers of the left hand behind the uterus. The cervix should now be drawn downwards and pushed backwards, and in this way the fingers of the left hand may be insinuated

behind the body of the uterus. With the volsellum method the technique should
be performed very slowly and continuous traction made. In a nervous
patient an anaesthetic is necessary for this manoeuvre.

Pessary Treatment. After the uterus has been replaced a pessary should
be introduced into the vagina to maintain the uterus in its anteverted position.
The pessary should be made of plastic and the most frequently used is the
Hodge. In Hodge's pessary the upper and lower ends are approximately of
the same diameter, but the upper end is curved and the lower square. The
pessary lies above the level of the levator ani muscles and is supported by

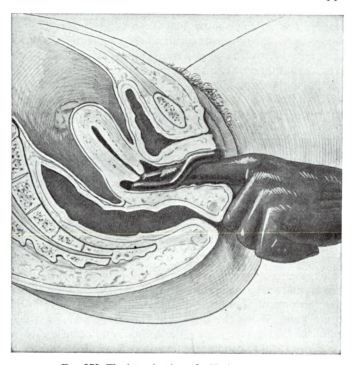

FIG. 273. The introduction of a Hodge pessary.

their most medial part, the pubococcygeus. Pessaries of this kind are almost
useless in the treatment of retroversion unless the uterus has first been anteverted. They are intended to maintain anteversion and prevent retroversion,
and not of themselves to cure retroversion. If a patient is using a Hodge
pessary of this type, she should douche herself as already described on p. 525
(see Figs. 272–274).

Fixed Retroversion

Fixed retroversion is much more important clinically than mobile retroversion. Most fixed retroversions result from salpingo-oöphoritis and pelvic
peritonitis, endometriosis or the presence of pelvic tumours. In salpingo-

oöphoritis the oedematous, distended Fallopian tubes prolapse behind the uterus, and, partly by their weight and partly through forming adhesions to the posterior surface of the pouch of Douglas, pull back the uterus and cause retroversion. In the process of healing, adhesions form which bind the uterus firmly in its retroverted position. Moreover, the ovaries are prolapsed behind the uterus and from the previous inflammation become tender and cause backache and dyspareunia. Fixed retroversion is also caused by chocolate cysts of the ovary and pelvic endometriosis, which fix the uterus by adhesions in a retroverted position. It must be understood, however, that fixed retroversion is a relative term, and pelvic tumours above and in

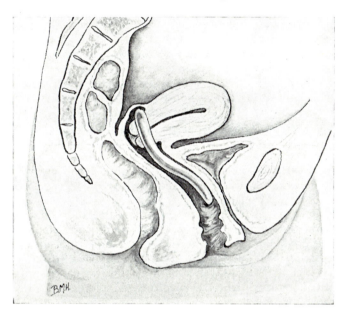

FIG. 274. A Hodge pessary in situ. The upper end lies in the posterior fornix while the lower part of the pessary is in contact with the anterior vaginal wall and is supported by the pubococcygeus muscle. Any tendency to retroflexion or retroversion is resisted by the upper end of the pessary.

front of the retroverted uterus may render it immobile. Mobile retroversion may seem to be fixed to a practitioner who is not experienced in gynaecological examinations.

Patients with fixed retroversions usually have gynaecological symptoms. Deep-seated dyspareunia is caused partly by the tender prolapsed ovaries and partly by adhesions in Douglas's pouch. Infertility is caused by adhesions around the Fallopian tubes. Backache can be explained by the tender ovaries, by chocolate cysts and by pelvic endometriosis in the uterosacral ligaments.

If a patient with such symptoms as infertility, dyspareunia, and backache is found to have a fixed retroversion and if induration or enlarged appendages are found in Douglas's pouch the symptoms can reasonably be attributed to one of the causes named above. Moreover, it is clear that attempts at replacement are almost certain to fail, and operative treatment is justifiable although something more than fixation of the uterus in an anteverted position will be necessary to cure the abnormalities of the appendages.

Indications for Operation for Retroversion

It should be clearly and unequivocally stated that the genuine indications for the surgical correction of a retroversion—unless fixed and associated with other pelvic disease—are very few indeed.

(1) If the retroversion is mobile, the uterus should be replaced bimanually, if necessary under anaesthesia, and a Hodge pessary should be introduced to retain the uterus in its anteverted position. This pessary should be retained in position for two months and then removed. If the patient is rendered free of symptoms operative treatment is unnecessary.

Sometimes pessary correction may be followed by a return to the retroverted position as soon as the pessary is removed with the reappearance of dyspareunia. It may, therefore, be stated that one possible indication for the surgical treatment of retroversion is dyspareunia unrelieved by pessary correction or recurring after the removal of the pessary. No enlightened young woman can reasonably be asked to wear a pessary for an indefinite period: it is aesthetically unpalatable, inconvenient and may from its very presence interfere with the physical aspects of matrimony.

(2) A fixed retroversion associated with other pelvic disease is an indisputable indication for operation. The other pelvic disease is the primary indication not the retroversion.

(3) In a very few patients who have had repeated abortions at about the tenth week, in whom no other cause can be found and who are extremely keen to do everything to achieve a baby, operation is occasionally justified.

It is very doubtful if operative treatment for mobile retroversion is justifiable unless it can be conclusively established that the patient has symptoms definitely attributable to the retroversion. By adopting the methods recommended above, the practitioner should first convince himself that this is the case before advising operation, and for this the pessary test described on p. 552 is most useful. Unfortunately many women are operated upon and the displacement of the uterus is corrected, and not only do they continue to have the symptoms which they originally possessed, which were in no way connected with the retroversion, but they acquire further symptoms, particularly low abdominal pain, which can definitely be attributed to the operation itself. Unjustifiable surgical intervention and bad clinical judgment is probably better illustrated in the various operations performed for retroversion than in any other sphere of surgery. This shortcoming of clinical judgment is now fortunately less common than in past decades of gynaecological practice where the operation of shortening the round ligaments was a frequent ornament of every operating list.

Operations for Retroversion

Ventrosuspension. In the operation of ventrosuspension, the two round ligaments are sutured together in front of the rectus muscle so that the round ligaments are not only shortened, but attach the uterus directly to the anterior abdominal wall. The peritoneal cavity is first opened by a midline or Pfannenstiel incision and any adhesions or abnormality of the appendages first dealt with. In Gilliam's operation the round ligament is first plicated by a suture—usually non-absorbable, such as thread—and bunched together close to the uterine cornu. The ends of this suture are left long. A long curved forceps is now passed between the anterior rectus sheath and its muscle proper as far as the lateral borders of the muscle. The forceps is now forcibly directed through the internal inguinal ring into the space between the two layers of the broad ligament towards the uterine cornu. The forceps point is now pushed through the peritoneum of the broad ligament and the ends of the ligature in the bunched-up round ligament withdrawn along the track of the forceps. These ends are now anchored in the anterior rectus sheath, and when tied the round ligament is drawn up against the anterior abdominal wall. If this technique is followed there will be no lateral space through which the small bowel can be strangulated.

Intestinal obstruction is a real risk of any operation for retroversion, and great care must be expended on the reperitonisation of any raw area to which small bowel may become adherent. The formation of bands by such an adhesion is always a danger to the patient, especially if she becomes pregnant.

Before closing the peritoneum, the operator should draw down the omentum behind the uterus, otherwise there is a risk of adhesions forming between the small intestine and the wound in the parietal peritoneum. The wound is closed in the usual manner.

Much ingenuity can be expended in devising different techniques for the operation of ventrosuspension, and almost every gynaecologist has his own particular method. The great advantage of promoting anteflexion by shortening the round ligaments is that enlargement of the uterus in a subsequent pregnancy is not interfered with, and obstetrical complications are relatively few. On the other hand, however carefully the operation is performed, the recurrence rate is high, and as a permanent cure for retroversion it is a poor procedure. Notwithstanding this depressing observation on the ultimate prognosis of the operation regarding permanent correction of the displacement, it is a somewhat cynical observation that although the retrodisplacement recurs the patient is quite often illogically cured of her symptoms. There must, therefore, be a considerable functional element in the symptomatology of retroversion.

For retroversion causing symptoms in patients nearing the menopause and who have finished child-bearing, total hysterectomy is a better procedure if the severity of the symptoms warrants surgery. But the real indication for the operation is not so much the retroversion as the myohyperplasia of the uterus and the diseased state of the cervix.

Retroversion of the Gravid Uterus

Retroversion of the uterus is no bar to conception, though fertility is perhaps slightly lowered. The coincidence of abortion in the retroverted gravid uterus is probably no greater than that for the anteverted, i.e. one in five of all conceptions. As the retroverted gravid uterus enlarges it rights itself spontaneously, and, apart from minor complaints of backache and frequency of micturition, no abnormal symptoms may arise. Very rarely, the uterus becomes impacted in the pelvis, and then pressure symptoms occur which lead to the patient developing retention of urine. An experienced gynaecologist can only be expected to see a retroverted gravid uterus causing retention once every two to three years.

Retention of urine is the most important and characteristic symptom of an incarcerated retroverted gravid uterus. The retroverted gravid uterus tends to sink, so that the fundus of the uterus is at a very low level in Douglas's pouch. As a result, the anterior vaginal wall and the urethra are stretched and the muscles at the base of the bladder pass into spasm. The apparent elongation of the urethra is considerable and the normal $1\frac{1}{2}$ in. may be extended to 4 in. or more. This point must be remembered when passing a catheter. The retention is not caused by direct pressure on the urethra, since a rubber catheter can always be passed without difficulty. The bladder fills with urine and forms a large abdominal tumour which is tense and tender, and projects anteriorly more than the normal gravid uterus. This tumour is fixed by the peritoneum and has no lateral or up and down movement, unlike an ovarian cyst. Patients may develop retention overflow, and have dribbling and frequent micturition. Unless treatment is adopted, cystitis is inevitable and may be serious. The rare condition of exfoliative gangrenous cystitis is now of academic interest and should never be seen in clinical practice unless the patient has refused to consult a doctor because, for instance, she wished to conceal the fact of her pregnancy.

The main symptom is retention of urine, and the possibility of a retroverted gravid uterus should always be borne in mind if this symptom is complained of at the end of the third month of pregnancy. Care must be taken in arriving at the diagnosis. A ruptured ectopic gestation with a pelvic haematocele sometimes causes retention of urine, and in any case may cause difficulty in diagnosis, because the physical signs are in many ways similar. In pelvic haematocele the cervix is pushed forwards, but the external os looks downwards, whereas with a retroverted gravid uterus the external os looks forwards, and, very characteristically, the anterior vaginal wall is stretched. Moreover, a pelvic haematocele has an indefinite outline, and is often extremely tender. If an accurate bimanual examination is possible the body of the uterus can be palpated separate from the swelling in Douglas's pouch. In both these conditions a history of slight vaginal haemorrhage may be obtained and in both the patient suffers from abdominal pain. If any doubt exists after clinical examination the patient should be examined under an anaesthetic.

Retention of urine may be caused during pregnancy by a myoma or an ovarian tumour impacted in the pelvis. Difficulty may be experienced in distinguishing such a condition from retroversion of the gravid uterus, complicated by a full bladder. The retroverted gravid uterus is soft and smooth, whereas a myoma is hard and an ovarian cyst is tense and cystic. Moreover, if the abdominal swelling is the pregnant uterus, the cervix, although pushed forwards, is directed downwards instead of forwards, as in the case of the retroverted gravid uterus. The full bladder is tense, tender and fixed, and lies more anteriorly than the gravid uterus. It is important to establish the diagnosis as, if attempts are made to replace the swelling in the pouch of Douglas and the swelling happens to be a pelvic haematocele, the patient may collapse and be gravely endangered from intra-abdominal bleeding. The diagnosis can be made with absolute precision by emptying the bladder with a catheter.

The Treatment of Retroverted Gravid Uterus with Retention of Urine. The patient should be placed in the left lateral position and a self-retaining catheter introduced with all aseptic precautions into the bladder. Sometimes the urethral meatus is drawn up into the vagina and may be found only with difficulty, but this is unusual. After the self-retaining catheter has been introduced the patient is placed in an exaggerated left lateral or Sims' position and the catheter connected by means of a long piece of plastic tubing which is passed to a uribag. The essential part of the treatment is to empty the bladder slowly. This should be done by attaching a screw-clip to the plastic tube, and allowing the urine to run away slowly, so that at least twenty-four hours is taken to empty the bladder. If this method is adopted, at the end of twenty-four hours the uterus will be found to be lying in an anteflexed position, having righted itself spontaneously. This method of treatment should be invariably successful, unless the uterus is held down by adhesions in which case an abdominal operation is necessary. If the bladder is rapidly emptied by catheterisation there is a possible danger of haemorrhage into the bladder, but the uterus remains retroverted and retention will recur.

While strongly recommending slow evacuation of the bladder, it is now felt that the dangers of rapid evacuation have been exaggerated in the past.

Acute Anteflexion of the Uterus

The uterus is sometimes congenitally acutely anteflexed, so that the body is bent forwards at an acute angle on the cervix. This condition has been described in Chapter 18 in the section dealing with Dysmenorrhoea. The acutely anteflexed uterus, or cochleate uterus, is often a maldeveloped organ associated with scanty or infrequent menstruation and infertility.

Lateral Displacements of the Uterus

In gross maldevelopment, e.g. uterus bicornis bicollis with hypoplasia, the whole upper genital tract may be congenitally displaced towards either side of the pelvis. At other times the uterus is pulled to one side by peritoneal adhesions resulting from salpingo-oöphoritis and by scars resulting from past parametritis. Alternatively the uterus may be pushed over to one side by swellings of the Fallopian tube such as pyosalpinx, hydrosalpinx, and haematosalpinx: by tumours of the ovary and by broad ligament swellings such as myomata and parovarian cysts. Intraperitoneal swellings such as appendix abscess, carcinoma of the sigmoid, and diverticulitis abscess may also push the uterus over to the opposite side. Lastly, a large acute parametric effusion may displace the uterus.

Other Displacements

Sometimes the cervix is found to be higher up than normal when a vaginal examination is made. The best examples are found when large swellings in Douglas's pouch, such as myomata and ovarian cysts, push the uterus upwards and forwards. The cervix is also higher up than normal when a myomatous polypus is being extruded and in inversion of the uterus. Similarly, if the uterus is retroverted, and particularly if the uterus is also pregnant, the cervix is higher than normal and displaced forwards.

If, on the other hand, the cervix is found to be lower than normal when a vaginal examination is made, either prolapse or the presence of congenital elongation of the cervix should be suspected.

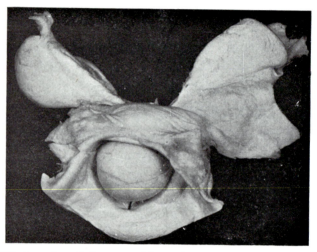

FIG. 275. Inversion of the uterus. The vagina has been cut through below and the rounded projection into the vagina is the inverted fundus of the uterus. The two ovaries lie above.

Forward displacement of the uterus is usually caused by swellings of Douglas's pouch such as myomata, ovarian tumours, pelvic abscess, and pelvic haematocele. It is very rare for the uterus to be pulled forwards by intraperitoneal adhesions except after the operation of anterior hysterotomy or Caesarean section. In such cases the uterine wound may become adherent to the abdominal scar.

The uterus is sometimes displaced posteriorly by swellings in front of it such as ovarian tumours, particularly dermoids, by parovarian cysts, or by large myomata in the anterior wall of the uterus.

Inversion of the Uterus

In inversion of the uterus the uterus becomes turned inside out. At first, the fundus is pushed down into the cavity of the uterus leaving a cup-shaped depression on the peritoneal surface. As the result of contractions of the uterus, the invagination becomes pushed further and further down until finally the whole uterus is turned inside out and hangs into the vagina. If the peritoneal surface of the uterus is inspected the Fallopian tubes, the ovarian and the round ligaments can be seen to pass down into a deep hollow in the position where the body of the uterus should be. Inversion of the uterus is described as complete or partial according to the degree to which the uterus is turned inside out (see Figs. 275 and 276).

Acute Inversion

Most inversions of the uterus are puerperal. Some are due to traction being applied to the umbilical cord when the placenta is morbidly adherent, while others are produced by squeezing a relaxed uterus immediately after delivery. Nevertheless, most puerperal inversions are probably spontaneous, although the exact aetiology is unknown. It has been suggested that the uterine muscle is defective in the region of the lower segment, and that the

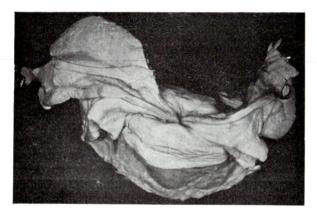

FIG. 276. The same specimen as Fig. 275, seen from above. The Fallopian tubes, broad ligaments and ovarian ligaments pass into a cup-shaped depression at the fundus of the uterus.

puerperal contractions of the body tend to invaginate the fundus into the uterine cavity. The presence of muscle defects or "crowns" in the region of the uterine fundus may also allow a dimple to occur in that region and progressive invagination to follow. Puerperal inversion of the uterus may be complete, so that the whole uterus lies outside the vagina. The condition is associated with a severe degree of shock and the inverted uterus bleeds vigorously. The treatment of acute puerperal inversion depends in the main upon the circumstances. The ideal treatment is immediate replacement. If the uterus is seen by doctor or midwife to be in the process of inverting or to have just done so then it may be easily replaced by using pressure on the inverted uterine fundus, providing only seconds have elapsed. If the placenta is attached to the uterus it must not be removed until after the replacement has been effected. In all instances the shock should first be treated by transfusion with blood or plasma substitute. In domiciliary midwifery, this must be continued until facilities for replacement of the uterus become available. The best method of performing this has been described by O'Sullivan. Once shock has been arrested, and with the least possible delay, the patient is anaesthetised. One gallon of warm sterile water is prepared ready for irrigation into the vagina, using a pressure of 3-4 ft. After gently pushing the inverted uterine fundus back into the vagina, the nozzle of the irrigator is inserted also and the vaginal orifice closed by the hands of the operator and an assistant. As much as 6 pints of fluid may be needed, the inversion being slowly corrected by the hydrostatic pressure. If this method fails, manual reposition may be attempted under deep anaesthesia. As a last resort, the abdomen should be opened and, if the inverted fundus cannot easily and without damage be pulled back into position with simultaneous pressure from the vagina, the tight cervical ring may be divided in order to restore the uterus and then repaired. In some cases abdominal total hysterectomy will be preferable if the patient is in the older age group and has had all the family that she and her husband desire. Following any of these procedures, antibiotic cover is indicated.

Chronic Inversion of the Uterus

Chronic inversion of the uterus consists of the late puerperal cases in whom the initial stages of the inversion, occurring in the immediate post-partum period, have been overlooked and those associated with the extrusion of a submucous myoma of the fundus. In the latter group the myoma must arise from the fundus, as if it arises elsewhere it becomes extruded as a polypus. The proportion of sarcomatous myomata is higher in chronic inversion than in all cases of myoma, and thus malignant change, with the tendency of the sarcoma to infiltrate the myometrium, may possibly explain why the uterus tends to become inverted. Clinically, chronic inversion associated with a fundal myoma may be suspected if the patient gives a history of severe intermittent lower abdominal pain combined with irregular vaginal bleeding. In time the myoma becomes infected and leads to profuse offensive vaginal discharge.

The diagnosis of chronic inversion is often difficult. Certain puerperal inversions escape diagnosis because the shock and bleeding are ascribed to a severe post-partum haemorrhage which is treated by transfusion and the usual resuscitative methods. The improvement in the patient masks the true diagnosis which can only be made by digital vaginal and uterine exploration. For the diagnosis to be established a cup-shaped depression must be identified in the situation of the fundus. If the inversion is complete, the cervix will be drawn up and the vaginal portion of the cervix will not be palpable. In partial inversion, if a uterine sound is introduced into the uterus, it will be passed only a short distance along the uterine cavity, and this will help to distinguish the partial inversion from a myomatous polypus of the body of the uterus. Even if the possibility of chronic inversion of the uterus is suspected, the diagnosis may not be made without anaesthetising the patient. When the tumour which protrudes through the cervix is pulled down with volsellum forceps, if the cervix moves upwards, then it is most suggestive that an inverted uterus is present. If the tumour is a polypus, traction brings down the cervix or the tumour may be pulled further through the external os without the cervix being drawn up. In chronic inversion, the inverted fundus is likely to be ulcerated and infected and thus resemble an infected fibroid polypus.

It is important to be quite certain of the diagnosis, as it is customary for myomatous polypi to be shelled out from below. If this procedure is adopted with an inverted uterus the peritoneal cavity will be opened with the risk of peritoneal infection.

Surgical Treatment. (1) Before attempting any conservative reposition or surgical correction of a chronic inversion, the patient should be treated by antibiotics with complete bed rest and local antiseptic packing with gauze soaked in flavine emulsion. These methods should effectively control the local sepsis and lessen the discomfort of reposition and the risks of peritonitis if operation is performed.

(2) *Operative:* (*a*) If it is desired to conserve the uterus in young patients, the inversion can be corrected by either a vaginal or an abdominal approach. In either instance the important step in the operation is the section of the constricting ring of the cervix after which it is easy to restore the fundus to its correct position. The transected cervix is then repaired by suture.

(*b*) If it is not desired to conserve the uterus because the patient is in her later child-bearing age or has all the children she desires, a vaginal or total abdominal hysterectomy is performed.

(*c*) For inversion caused by the extrusion of a fundal myoma, the treatment largely depends on the same arguments, e.g. vaginal myomectomy and reposition assisted by the operation of vaginal hysterotomy (cutting the cervix in the anterior midline to gain access to the tumour base) for the younger patient and vaginal or abdominal hysterectomy for the older. The significantly higher incidence of sarcoma will incline the surgeon towards the more radical abdominal operation of total abdominal hysterectomy and if, on removing the uterus, the tumour is not encapsulated, if the myometrium appears to be infiltrated or if the cut surface of the tumour is suspicious, the question of bilateral salpingo-oöphorectomy arises. This radical operation should only be performed in the first instance if sarcomatous change is reasonably certain.

Non-operative Treatment. Conservative treatment of chronic neglected puerperal inversion may be attempted with an Aveling repositor, consisting of a vulcanite cup placed in contact with the inverted fundus and pushed upwards by a metal rod supported by tapes from a waistband and shoulder straps. The treatment causes some shock and pain and should only be employed when no surgical facilities are available.

23 New Growths of the Uterus:

CONNECTIVE TISSUE TUMOURS

Myomata

Myomata are innocent new growths which arise in the myometrium. They are extremely common and occur in 10% of all gynaecological patients. It has been computed that about 20% of all women after the age of 35 have myomata.

The tumours were known to Hippocrates, who called them scleromata. They were described as fibrous tumours of the uterus during the early part of the last century. Rokitansky called the tumours fibroids, but it was Virchow who demonstrated that they were essentially leio-myomata. Although the terms fibroid and myoma are in common use, the correct terminology is leio-myoma.

The tumours are spheroidal in shape, and encapsulated so that they can be shelled out fairly easily. They are usually multiple and may attain an enormous size. John Hunter described a myoma which weighed 140 lb.

Incidence. The tumours are most common between the ages of 35 and 45, half the cases being found in patients in this decade of life. Thirty per cent.

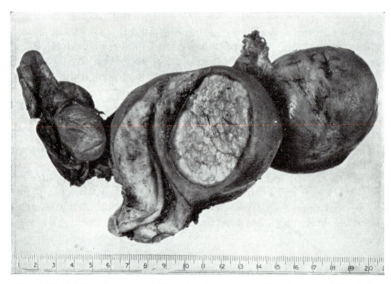

FIG. 277. Calcified intramural fibroid and subserous fibroid on the right of the picture.

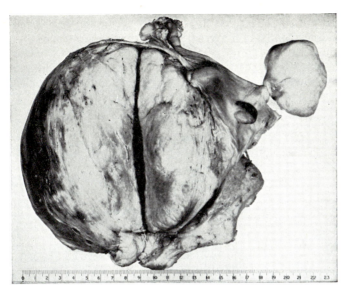

FIG. 278. Large broad ligament and smaller pedunculated subserous myomata.

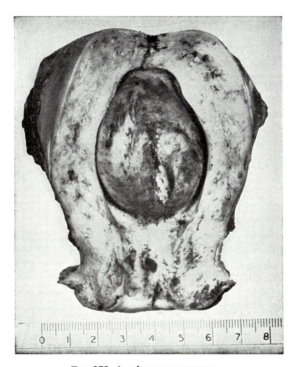

FIG. 279. A submucous myoma.

are found in patients between the ages of 30 and 40. The tumours are very rare indeed before the age of 20, but they are found not infrequently in women of post-menopausal age. In patients between the ages of 40 and 50 the distribution is as follows: Virgins 10%, nulliparae 30%, uniparae 20%, and multiparae 40%. These statistics do not account for the relative preponderance of married women over the age of 40 and are in some ways misleading. A woman who has borne a large family is far less likely to develop

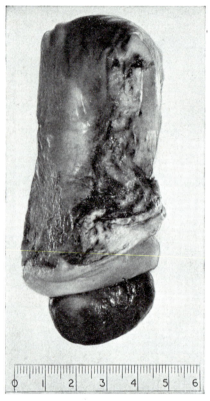

FIG. 280. Fibroid polypus being extruded through the cervix. Note the expanded rim of external os around the tumour.

myomata than a woman who has never been pregnant at all. The statistics show that 60% of myomata arise in women who have either never been pregnant or have had only one child.

Anatomy. A typical myoma has a whorled appearance when transected. The tumours are firmer in consistence than the myometrium. The capsule consists of connective tissue which fixes the tumour to the myometrium. Although not easily visible to the naked eye the capsule is clearly defined if the myoma is shelled out. The vessels which supply the tumour lie in the capsule and send radial branches into the periphery of the tumour. The blood supply of the middle part of the tumour is far less than that of the periphery, so that degeneration is most noticeable in the middle. On the other hand, in calcareous tumours, lime salts which are deposited from the blood stream are most plentifully deposited near the periphery, and quite often the radial direction of the vessels can be distinguished when a calcified myoma is examined. If the myoma has attained any great size, large vessels are found in the capsule. These vessels are best distinguished in subserous tumours,

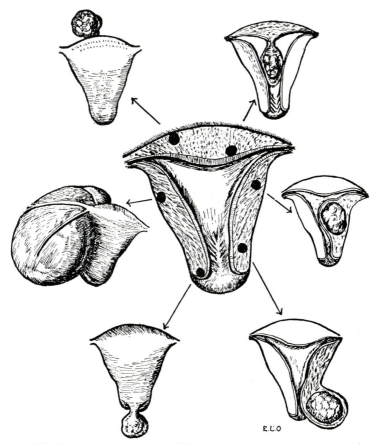

Fig. 281. The development of the different types of uterine myomata. (After Halban-Seitz).

while with large intramural myomata they can be seen beneath the peritoneal covering of the uterus and serve to distinguish the enlargement of the uterus from a normal intrauterine pregnancy.

All uterine myomata arise in the myometrium. The tumour may grow symmetrically, remaining in the myometrium, when it is termed intramural. At other times, the tumour is extruded towards the surface of the uterus so that it may project into the peritoneal cavity and, in extreme cases, be attached only by a small pedicle to the uterus. This type of myoma is referred to as subserous, or subperitoneal. In other cases the myoma is extruded into the broad ligament, forming a broad ligament myoma. The contractions of the uterus may, however, force the myoma towards the cavity, when if it projects into the uterus and is covered only by endometrium, it is referred to as submucous. The uterine contractions may force the tumours still further into the cavity, so that finally the tumour is attached only by a pedicle when it forms a myomatous polypus. Very rarely a fundal myoma projecting into the cavity of the uterus may cause chronic inversion. In other cases the myoma arises primarily in the cervix, but this situation is uncommon,

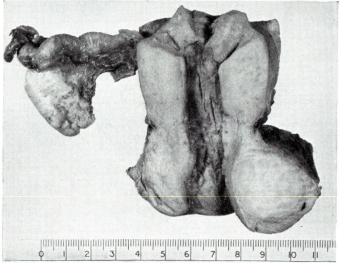

FIG. 282. Myoma growing from the cervix into the broad ligament. Compare with the last figure on the right of the preceding diagram.

cervical myomata comprising only 4% of all cases. Intramural myomata are the most common of the tumours found in the body of the uterus, the distribution being as follows:—

Intramural	73%
Submucous	16.6%
Subserous	10.4%

The majority of myomata arise primarily in the uterus, but they also arise from the round ligament, even in the inguinal canal, from the ovarian ligaments, in the uterosacral ligaments, in the vagina, and at the vulva. The tumours can therefore be classified as uterine or extrauterine, the uterine being subdivided into those which arise from the body and those which arise from the cervix (see Figs. 277–284).

The presence of the tumours in the wall of the uterus leads to hyperplasia of the myometrium. The cavity of the uterus is often distorted and enlarged, and, characteristically, the ovaries are enlarged and hyperaemic. The endometrium tends to be much thicker than normal except with submucous myomata, when it is thinned out over the surface of the tumour.

The cervix is frequently enlarged and hypertrophic in the presence of fibroids but, despite an increase in endocervical secretion, cervical erosions are not a common finding.

Microscopically the tumour consists of bundles of plain muscle cells separated from each other by connective tissue. In small tumours the muscle cells are more embryonic than those of the myometrium, the nuclei stain

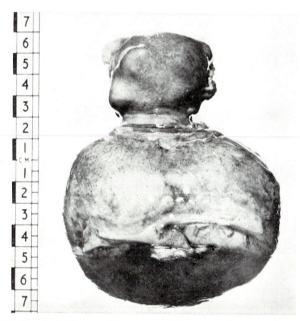

Fig. 283. Cervical Myoma : The body of the uterus lies entirely above the tumour.

deeply, and there is less cytoplasm than in a normal plain muscle cell. The histological appearances are therefore simple. Myomata, however, show a well-marked tendency to degeneration, and some degree of degeneration is present in all tumours more than about 1½ in. in diameter and in many not so large. The degenerative changes will be described later in the chapter.

Large tumours disturb the normal anatomical relations in the pelvis. Broad ligament myomata displace the uterus to the opposite side. They may burrow extraperitoneally and displace the uterine vessels and the ureter from their normal situations. Large cervical myomata displace the body of the uterus upwards, and cause pressure upon the bladder and bowel. Such tumours are extremely difficult to remove and the ureters and bladder are a natural hazard of the operation (Fig. 283).

Aetiology. There is little exact knowledge of why myomata develop. They are most common in women who are either sterile or have borne only one child, and they develop only very rarely immediately after childbirth. Large tumours mostly arise in nulliparous patients. Moreover, in 15% of cases the uterine adnexa show evidence of previous inflammation so that the Fallopian tubes are occluded and the woman is sterile. On the other hand, a uterine myoma may be a contributory factor in infertility, perhaps through distorting

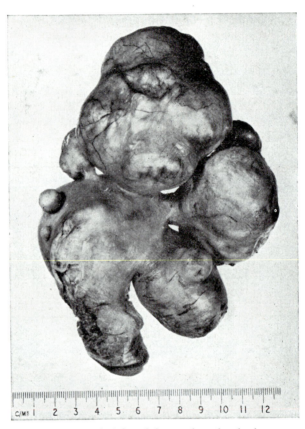

Fig. 284. The uterus is on the left and three pedunculated subserous myomata on the right.

the cavity of the uterus, and after removal of the tumour the woman may conceive. This is particularly so with the submucous myoma which acts as a natural intrauterine contraceptive device. There is little evidence that myomata arise in women of post-menopausal age, although they may persist until after the menopause without causing symptoms. Similarly they hardly ever, if ever, arise before puberty. The tumours should therefore be regarded as being related to the child-bearing period of life. They are associated with enlarged hyperaemic ovaries, a true hypertrophy of the endometrium and, mostly, with excessive menstrual loss. It has therefore been suggested that the tumours arise in association with ovarian dysfunction and that they are to some extent oestrogen-dependent. The tumours are in many ways different from innocent neoplasms, for their incidence is restricted to the child-bearing period of life and they become smaller after the menopause. Very few innocent neoplasms found elsewhere in the body undergo spontaneous retrogression. These facts have suggested that the presence and growth of myomata is an oestrogen-dependent phenomenon. This hypothesis is somewhat supported by the fairly frequent coincidence of endometriosis and endometrial hyperplasia and, sometimes, even carcinoma of the endometrium. These three conditions are also suggested to be oestrogen-dependent. Moreover, the tumours are usually multiple, as many as thirty to fifty tumours being commonly found in a single uterus. This curious multiplicity in a single organ is almost unknown elsewhere in the body.

No clue is obtained from histogenetic studies. It is well known that minute areas of embryonic muscle cells are often found in the normal myometrium which have been thought responsible for the development of myomata, and it has also been suggested that the tumours arise from the plain muscle cells of small arterioles in the uterine wall. Neither view is established and both are hypothetical. It can be shown with minute seedling myomata that there is a normal transition between myoma cells and myometrium, and that the capsule development is a relatively late phenomenon. Tumours similar to myomata have been produced in the guinea-pig's uterus as the result of prolonged administration of oestrogens. The tumour's development can be prevented if progesterone, testosterone, or desoxycorticosterone are injected. These experimental results are of the greatest importance, for they suggest a hormonal interrelation of myoma-producing and myoma-inhibiting hormones. Reports of shrinkage of myomata after the administration of androgens can be found in the literature.

General Characters

Number. In most cases the tumours are multiple, and more than a hundred myomata have been found in one uterus, when the whole uterus and perhaps the ovarian and round ligaments as well are studded with small tumours and the myometrium is soft, thickened and vascular. Single tumours are interesting as they tend to be forced into the cavity of the uterus, when they become submucous or polypoidal, and rarely give rise to chronic inversion. Similarly, large cervical myomata are usually single. There is a well-recognised form of subserous fundal myoma attached in the midline to the top of the uterus which forms a large swelling in comparison with the uterus itself, but in such cases smaller myomata are usually found in the wall of the uterus.

Size. All gradations in size are known between mammoth tumours and minute seedling myomata which can be detected only by microscopical examination.

Shape. Small tumours are spheroidal, because the development is centrifugal, with the resistance to growth uniformly distributed around the tumour. Large tumours are distorted because they project either into the cavity of the

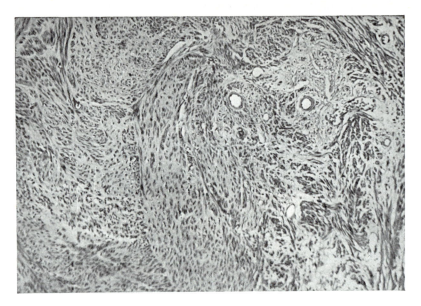

FIG. 285. Early hyaline degeneration. Note the diffuse intercellular hyaline material. ($\times$ 100.)

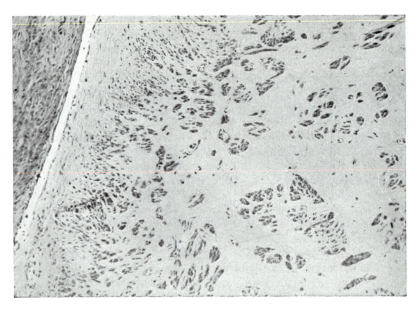

FIG. 286. Late hyaline degeneration. ($\times$ 115.)

uterus or into the peritoneal cavity, so that the resistance to their growth is distributed irregularly. Large pelvic tumours may be distorted by the pressure of the bony pelvis in which they lie.

Secondary Changes: Degenerations

Atrophy. As a result of diminished vascularity due to the natural or artificial menopause there is a shrinkage in the size of the tumour, which becomes firmer and more fibrotic. A similar change occurs in myomata after delivery, when a tumour easily palpable during pregnancy may be difficult to define six months after the puerperium.

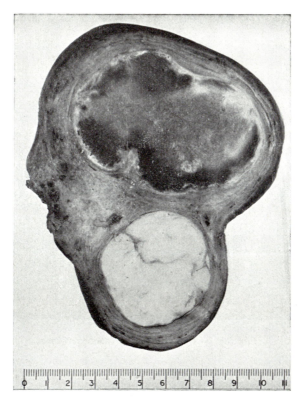

FIG. 287. Myomata, the upper one showing peripheral calcification and haemorrhage into the tumour.

Hyaline Degeneration. Some degree of hyaline degeneration is present in all tumours more than $1\frac{1}{2}$ in. in diameter. A hyaline myoma is hard and firm, and the striated appearance of the cut surface is inconspicuous. An extreme degree of hyaline degeneration causes the whorled appearance to be lost, so that the tumour has a uniform waxy appearance, but such cases are unusual. Hyaline degeneration is best identified microscopically. The outlines of the muscle cells become indefinite and the cell cytoplasm merges with a structureless intercellular matrix. The nuclei remain for a time, but eventually break up to become disorganised into the structureless hyaline material which stains uniformly pink with eosin. Hyaline degeneration is best marked in large subserous tumours. It causes no specific clinical symptoms and is only of pathological interest (see Figs. 285 and 286).

Cystic Degeneration. Cystic degeneration represents a late stage of hyaline degeneration when the hyaline material undergoes liquefaction. The tumour becomes soft, and irregular spaces filled with clear fluid are found in the middle of the tumour. Cystic degeneration is met with most frequently in large

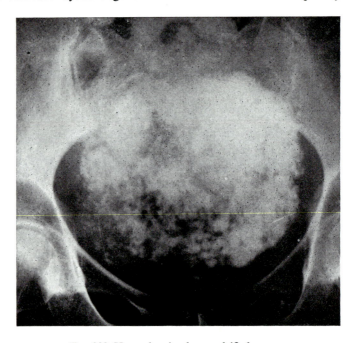

Fig. 288. X-ray showing large calcified myoma.

intramural tumours, and is best marked in the middle, probably because the blood supply is less plentiful here than at the periphery.

Cystic degeneration must be distinguished from lymphangiectasis, in which large fluid spaces filled with lymph and lined by endothelium are found in the substance of the tumour and in the broad ligaments in the region of the uterine vessels. Such dilated lymph channels may attain an appreciable size and measure a centimetre in diameter and are a frequent finding with large tumours.

Fatty Changes. Fatty degeneration of the muscle cells of myomata is relatively uncommon and most cases result from previous red degeneration. In rare instances true fat cells are found amongst the muscle cells of myomata.

Calcareous Degeneration. In calcareous degeneration, phosphates and carbonates of lime are deposited in the periphery along the course of the vessels. The best examples of calcareous myomata are those in old patients with long-standing myomata. They are found as "womb-stones" in old graveyards. Fatty degeneration may occur first, subsequently the fatty acids are changed first into soaps, and finally, by the interaction of the carbonates and phosphates of the blood, into calcium phosphate and carbonate. Very rarely true ossification ensues upon calcification. Calcareous tumours are easily identifiable by radiography (see Figs. 287 and 288).

Red Degeneration. This complication of uterine myomata develops most frequently during pregnancy, although it is not rare in cases of painful myomata in woman over the age of 40. The myoma becomes tense and tender

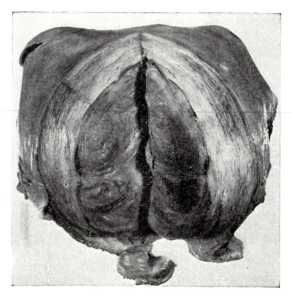

FIG. 289. Red degeneration of a myoma. Note that the encapsulated tumour shows uniform dark discoloration.

and causes severe abdominal pain with constitutional upset and fever. The tumour itself assumes a peculiar purple-red colour and develops a fishy odour. If the tumour is carefully examined, some of the large veins of the capsule and the small vessels in the substance of the tumour will be found to be thrombosed. The discoloration is possibly caused by diffusion of blood pigments from the thrombosed vessels. Histologically, apart from thrombosis, no specific appearances have been identified, although it must be remembered that previous hyaline degeneration may be present. Little is known of the exact aetiology and particularly of why only the myoma should be involved and not the myometrium. It should be noted that, although the patient is febrile with a moderate leucocytosis and raised E.S.R., the condition is an aseptic one (see Fig. 289).

Sarcomatous Degeneration. The development of a sarcoma in the tissues of a pre-existing myoma is rare. A sarcoma of the uterus may arise primarily in the myometrium or endometrium and infiltrate a myoma. Care must therefore be taken to establish that sarcomatous changes found in a myoma are not caused by the myoma being infiltrated by a sarcoma arising in some other part of the uterus. The statistics of the incidence of sarcomatous changes in myomata differ widely because the recognition of malignancy by histological means in a connective tissue tumour such as a myoma requires great experience. Moreover, small areas of embryonic tissue are frequently found in most myomata, and this tissue may very easily be mistaken for sarcoma. Probably in 0.5% of all myomata malignant change can be demonstrated. In Novak's investigation of 6,981 myomata he found thirty-nine sarcomata,

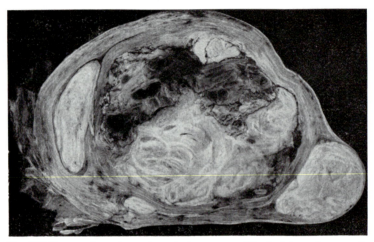

FIG. 290. Sarcomatous change in a uterine myoma. The dark irregular areas in the substance of the myoma which lie in the middle of the specimen represent areas of sarcomatous change.

an incidence of 0.56%. This is lower than the figures of previous observers and is based upon accurate histological examination. Intramural tumours are most frequently involved, after them cervical myomata, and, least frequently, subserous tumours. It is rare for malignant change to develop in a myoma under the age of 40, and 50% of cases arise between the ages of 40 and 50. The tumour is usually a leio-sarcoma, but spindle-celled, round-celled and mixed-celled tumours may be found. The tumour may erode through the capsule of the primary myoma and produce polypoidal projections into the cavity of the uterus. In most cases the diagnosis is made only after the removal of the uterus, but rapid enlargement of the myoma associated with profuse haemorrhage and pain should cause the possibility to be suspected. Similarly, in post-menopausal women, rapid enlargement of the myoma with a sudden onset of pain and local tenderness is almost pathognomonic of sarcomatous change. To the naked eye a sarcomatous myoma is yellowish-grey in colour and often infiltrated with blood. The consistence is friable and soft, quite different from the typical firm consistence of a simple myoma (see Fig. 290). One very important sign is the non-encapsulation of the tumour. All benign myomata are always encapsulated.

Other Complications of Myomata

Torsion. A subserous myoma may undergo rotation at the site of its attachment to the uterus. As a result, the veins are occluded and the tumour

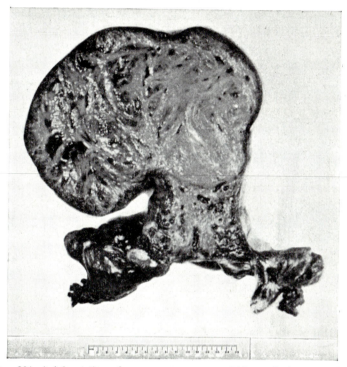

FIG. 291. Axial rotation of a myomatous uterus. This particular uterus had rotated through three half-turns (540°) carrying with it both tubes and ovaries which were also gangrenous and are seen in the lower part of the illustration. (Reproduced by kind permission of Mr. Alan Hunt.)

becomes engorged with blood. Very severe abdominal pain is experienced, and most patients are operated upon immediately. Very rarely the rotated tumour may adhere to adjacent viscera, obtain a fresh blood supply from these adhesions, and finally be detached completely from the uterus, the so-called "wandering fibroid". Axial torsion of a subserous myoma is a rare phenomenon.

Axial rotation of the whole myomatous uterus itself is seen as a very rare occurrence. In such cases a large subserous myoma is attached near the fundus, the uterus itself being only slightly enlarged, and the site of rotation is in the neighbourhood of the internal os at about the level of Mackenrodt's

19*

ligament. The symptoms are comparable with those developing with axial rotation of a subserous myoma (Fig. 291).

Inversion. Inversion of the uterus caused by a submucous fundal myoma has been described already in the previous chapter.

Capsule Rupture. Very rarely a myoma may burst through its capsule and be extruded almost completely either into the peritoneal cavity or into the broad ligament. A similar situation arises when one of the large veins on the surface of a subserous myoma ruptures and causes diffuse intra-peritoneal bleeding with the symptoms and signs of internal haemorrhage. Fortunately, this complication of myomata is rare.

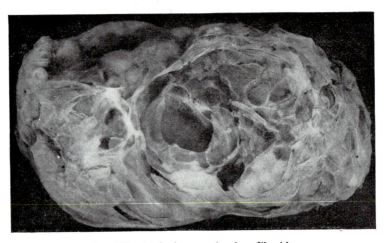

FIG. 292. Cystic degeneration in a fibroid.

Inflammatory Changes in Myomata

Infections arise most frequently in submucous myomata and myomatous polypi, because the blood supply to the lower pole of such tumours is impoverished, and this part of the tumour, by projecting into the cervical canal, or even into the vagina, is exposed to the organisms which form the vaginal flora. It is not uncommon with large polypi for there to be circulatory disturbances at the pedicle, so that the lower pole of the tumour is congested and readily infected. The surface becomes inflamed and ulcerates, and discharges a bloodstained purulent fluid into the vagina. The infection may spread upwards and involve the endometrium of the uterus itself, and it is not uncommon after the removal of such polypi for a moderately severe degree of uterine sepsis to occur. The worst infections are seen after confinement, when a submucous myoma becomes extruded into the cavity of the uterus. The severity of the infection is to be attributed to the diminished resistance of the tissues in the immediate puerperium. The tumour is rarely extruded spontaneously, when the symptoms clear up. If the diagnosis is made early in the puerperium and if the tumour is causing severe delayed post-partum haemorrhage the tumour should be removed by the vaginal route as soon as possible.

Sometimes a myoma becomes infected from an adjacent focus of sepsis such as appendicitis or diverticulitis, but it is extremely rare for it to become secondarily infected from acute adnexal inflammatory conditions such as pyosalpinx.

Adnexal Disease

As myomata are such a common occurrence it is not surprising that old pelvic inflammatory disease is sometimes found in the appendages when operating on a patient with myomata. There is no evidence to consider the two conditions in any way complementary and the adnexal disease is best regarded as a chance finding. When myomata are present the ovaries are sometimes found to be enlarged, cystic and hyperaemic. This is reasonably accounted for by the increased blood supply to the genitalia though it is naturally tempting to invoke a state of hyperoestrogenism to account for both conditions.

Lymphangiectasis and Telangiectasis

Dilatation of lymphatic channels in the substance of a myoma is not un-common. The tumour becomes soft and almost cystic to palpation, and when cut exudes large quantities of clear yellow fluid (Fig. 292). The walls of the dilated spaces are smooth and glistening, and are found on microscopical examination to be lined by endothelium. Little is known of the causation of lymphangiectasis. Dilated lymphatics are, however, found very frequently along the main uterine vessels in association with large myomata

A somewhat similar condition of the blood vessels is sometimes found in the substance of myomata, and the cases are of considerable pathological interest, for the tumours are of the nature of angiomyomata, rather than simple myomata.

Association with Carcinoma of the Uterus

Myomata of the uterus are associated not infrequently with uterine carcinomata and statistics show that carcinoma of the body was present in 20 out of 700 cases of myoma, whereas carcinoma of the cervix was present in only six, a proportion of roughly $3\frac{1}{2}$ to 1 (Novak). The higher frequency of carcinoma of the body is attributable to the tendency of both myomata and this form of carcinoma to arise in women who are either sterile, or who have had only one or perhaps two children many years before. Carcinoma of the cervix should be detected fairly easily, but carcinoma of the body is not always recognised until after the removed uterus has been examined. If a myomatous uterus causes persistent bleeding in a woman of menopausal age the possibility of a coexisting carcinoma of the body should always be borne in mind (see Fig. 293).

Myomata and Pregnancy

Although myomata may of themselves lead to infertility, pregnancy complicated by the presence of uterine myomata is extremely common.

Infertility is sometimes caused by a submucous myoma distorting the cavity of the uterus. A myoma may lead to abortion, particularly if it is of the submucous type, because the endometrium is thinned out over the tumour, and if the ovum is implanted in this situation it may not obtain the requisite nutrition because of a faulty blood supply to the choriodecidual space. The presence of a myoma may provide a purely mechanical reason for abortion by virtue of its position, e.g. impaction in the true pelvis.

During pregnancy the myoma may undergo red degeneration causing severe abdominal pain and tenderness over the tumour, together with vomiting,

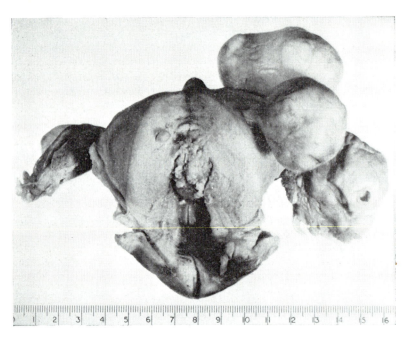

Fig. 293. Myomata with concomittant carcinoma of the endometrium.

fever and leucocytosis. Operative treatment is contraindicated, as the symptoms subside with rest in bed, and further complications such as infection are almost unknown. Myomata may appear to increase in size during pregnancy, and tumours which were previously not palpable become easily recognisable as pregnancy advances. Later in pregnancy the size remains stationary, and the tumour may even seem to become smaller. After delivery, the myoma seems to shrink as the uterus involutes. Large myomata may remain in the pelvis in the early months of pregnancy and cause severe pressure symptoms, but in most cases the tumour is drawn out of the pelvis as the pregnancy proceeds. Cervical myomata, and occasionally subserous tumours may become wedged in the pelvis and offer an insuperable obstacle to delivery, so that Caesarean section has to be performed at term. Tumours in this situation may cause retention of urine about the third month of pregnancy, similar to that seen in patients with a retroverted gravid uterus. If, when performing a Caesarean section, the tumour appears easy to enucleate, it is always a temptation to the surgeon to do so. This temptation should be firmly resisted owing to the danger of very heavy and often uncontrollable bleeding. Myomectomy and Caesarean section are also associated with a greatly increased post-operative morbidity. It is always wiser to postpone myomectomy for six months when the operation is easier and safer to perform.

The obstetrical difficulties caused by myomata during labour, such as malpresentations, inertia and post-partum haemorrhage are described in midwifery textbooks. The tendency for submucous tumours to become infected during the puerperium has already been described.

Symptoms

Although large myomata are encountered with no symptoms whatsoever, except abdominal swelling, the majority lead to characteristic symptoms.

MENSTRUAL DISTURBANCES. The most constant symptom is **menorrhagia.** The menstrual cycle remains unaltered but the duration of the bleeding is prolonged to as much as ten days, and the amount lost on each day is increased. The menorrhagia may be extreme and a severe degree of anaemia be induced. It is probable that several factors determine the severity of the menorrhagia. In the first place the endometrium is usually thickened, except over the surface of submucous and polypoidal tumours and the thick endometrium of itself causes excessive menstrual loss. Secondly, the cavity of the uterus is often greatly increased in size, so that a much larger surface than normal menstruates. Thirdly, the myometrium is soft and vascular, which tends again to cause excessive haemorrhage during menstruation. Lastly, hormonal influences probably increase the bleeding, as the ovaries are usually hyperplastic. As a rule subserous tumours have little effect upon menstruation.

Polymenorrhoea. Polymenorrhoea is another but much rarer symptom with myomata, the menstrual cycle being reduced and the duration of the haemorrhage increased. It is doubtful whether the tumours themselves cause polymenorrhoea, and it is more likely that this is the result of excessive hormone activity.

Metrorrhagia. Intermenstrual bleeding arises typically when the tumour is polypoidal or submucous. With large polypi profuse and almost continuous bleeding may occur, and if the tumour becomes infected the discharge is purulent and offensive as well. It is not uncommon for adenomatous polypi to develop in the endometrium in cases of myomata and such polypi sometimes cause slight haemorrhage during the intermenstrual part of the cycle. When irregular bleeding is encountered in a woman of menopausal or post-menopausal age the possibility of coincident uterine cancer must never be forgotten.

PRESSURE SYMPTOMS. Pressure symptoms are mostly complained of by patients with cervical myomata. Such tumours may almost fill the true pelvis. Pressure upon the bowel leads to constipation, while pressure upon the bladder causes first frequency, and, in extreme cases, retention of urine. Subserous tumours may become incarcerated in the pouch of Douglas and cause retention of urine. Small tumours growing from the anterior surface of the cervix or the lower part of the body of the uterus may press upon the bladder and cause frequency of micturition and dysuria. Urinary symptoms are usually most severe immediately before the onset of menstruation. Ureteric obstruction is probably commoner than is generally realised and would be more frequently diagnosed if intravenous pyelography were employed before operation. It is especially seen in the presence of cervical myoma and large tumours. Dilatation of the ureter and the renal pelvis can be expected to disappear within six months of operation in the absence of urinary infection. In a few cases, however, a permanent hydronephrosis may remain and require the attention of an expert urologist. Very rarely large tumours may cause a mild subacute intestinal obstruction by pressing the intestine against the promontory of the sacrum. Considering the bulk of some tumours it is surprising that the bowel is so rarely embarrassed.

Pressure on the great vessels of the pelvis causing oedema of the legs is extremely rare and unilateral oedema is almost always due to a malignant infiltration of an ovarian cancer and not the pressure of an innocent tumour of the uterus. The same remark applies to pressure symptoms on the lumbosacral plexus and obturator nerve.

Pain. Most patients with large myomata complain of a feeling of weight in the pelvis, or lower abdomen, which they sometimes describe as a heavy feeling or a boring pain. The symptom is probably caused by the weight of the tumour pressing upon the pelvic cellular tissues. Severe abdominal pain develops with red degeneration and with torsion. Adhesions are apt to form to calcareous myomata, when colicky pains may be experienced.

Severe spasmodic dysmenorrhoea arises when myomatous polypi are being extruded through the cervix. On occasion the colicky pain may be severe enough to compel the patient to rest in bed. Dysmenorrhoea of the congestive type arising a few days before the onset of menstruation is complained of by patients with large vascular myomata. The sudden onset of pain in a rapidly-forming myoma at or after the menopause strongly suggests a malignant degeneration.

Finally, it must be remembered that most fibroids are relatively painless and, if pain is a notable symptom, the fibroid has undergone infection, red degeneration, torsion, sarcomatous change or there is usually some complicating condition such as endometriosis.

Discharge. A minor degree of leucorrhoea is often complained of if the myomata are large and the cavity of the uterus increased in size, partly because of an increased secretion from the glands of the endometrium, but mainly from the endocervical glands of the hypertrophic cervix. With myomatous polypi the discharge may be bloodstained, and if the myoma becomes infected and its surface ulcerates, the discharge becomes purulent and offensive.

Infertility and Pregnancy Complications. It has already been mentioned that myomata may lead to infertility, during the investigation of which a submucous myoma may be found on clinical examination. The effect of complications of pregnancy and myomata on pregnancy have already been mentioned (p. 579).

Other Symptoms. Patients with myomata often complain of tachycardia and palpitations. The symptom is quite common and is probably attributable to the resultant anaemia. Similarly, it is common for patients with myomata to complain of indigestion.

Anaemic patients with myomata are apt to develop thromboses both before and after operation.

Abdominal Swelling. In a fairly large proportion of cases of myomata the patient's attention is first directed to an abdominal swelling which is remarkably painless. It should be remembered that subserous tumours may be accompanied by no menstrual disturbances or pressure symptoms, so that the first indication to the patient that something is wrong is the development of an abdominal tumour or increasing tightness of her clothes.

Physical Signs and Diagnosis

The patient is aged about 40, either nulliparous or having had only one or two children some years before. The patients often have attractive personalities, and are free of the depressions and introspections which mark the majority of gynaecological patients. Quite often they have a good colour, but if there has been much menorrhagia the mucous membranes are pale and the complexion sallow, although some degree of malar flush persists until a severe level of anaemia has been reached.

The typical history may be one of increasing menorrhagia associated with pressure symptoms and the development of an abdominal tumour. The abdomen is found distended below the umbilicus and an abdominal swelling may be visible. On palpation a tumour is found arising from the pelvis. It is hard and firm, with a smooth surface, although several smooth oval swellings may be palpated attached to each other. The swelling is movable from side to side, from before backwards, but with little mobility from above downwards. The swelling is harder and firmer than the pregnant uterus, not so painful as the full bladder, and not fluctuant like an ovarian cyst. The swelling is dull on percussion and is not accompanied by ascites. Quite frequently a souffle can be auscultated over the swelling. On vaginal examination the physical signs differ according to the position of the tumour. With intramural and subserous tumours the cervix is found to be continuous with the abdominal swelling, and movements transmitted to the cervix are communicated to the abdominal tumour, and, conversely, movement of the abdominal tumour leads to movement of the cervix. If the diagnosis is to be made with precision the position of the body of the uterus must be established. If the body of the uterus can be identified separate from the abdominal swelling, the latter is more likely to be an ovarian tumour or a subserous pedunctuated myoma. Both the uterus and the cervix may be displaced from their normal positions by myomata. For example, a myoma attached to the back of the uterus may push the uterus and cervix forwards, and in extreme instances the cervix may be displaced upwards and forwards, above the level of the symphysis pubis, and be out of reach of the examining finger. With large cervical myomata the cervix is usually displaced upwards while the body of the uterus, not appreciably increased in size, rests on the top of the swelling. Broad ligament tumours displace the uterus to the opposite side and myomata of the uterosacral ligaments displace the uterus upwards and forwards.

The lower pole of a myomatous polypus can be palpated by a finger placed through the external os, while if the polypus projects into the vagina the pedicle can be palpated passing upwards through the cervical canal. The possibility of the existence of chronic inversion caused by the tumour must be borne in mind, and the diagnosis established by the methods described on p. 562. A small submucous myoma can be suspected but not diagnosed by clinical examination and, if curettage fails to reveal it, only hysterography will do so by demonstrating a filling defect in the contrast medium.

Small tumours lying in the pelvis do not cause abdominal swelling, but these rarely cause difficulty in diagnosis because on bimanual examination the uterus is found to be enlarged and hard, with a bossed irregular surface. Some submucous tumours and some myomatous polypi may measure as much as 4 in. in diameter, and although lying mainly in the pelvis may be palpated on abdominal examination.

Although the diagnosis of uterine myomata is usually easily made it can present very great difficulty.

Differential Diagnosis of Abdominal Swellings

(1) **Ovarian Cyst.** A large single intramural myoma with cystic degeneration may be mistaken for an ovarian cyst. A large ovarian cyst is, however, either manifestly cystic or tense, and bimanual examination should ensure the separate identification of the uterus from the tumour. Moreover, a large ovarian cyst rarely causes menstrual disturbances and may arise at any age. A tense tender tumour projecting anteriorly in the midline should always be suspected of being the full bladder, and if necessary the patient should be catheterised to exclude this possibility.

(2) **Pregnancy.** The possibility of the abdominal swelling being the pregnant uterus should always be borne in mind. It is extremely rare for a pregnant woman to have uterine haemorrhage at regular intervals after the third month, and consequently if a patient is found to have a large abdominal swelling and gives a history of menorrhagia or regular menstruation without any period of amenorrhoea, it is unlikely that she is pregnant. Breast activity is absent and the veins on the surface of the breasts are not dilated and the development of a secondary areola is unknown. If the tumour extends high in the abdomen and *is* the pregnant uterus, either foetal movements or a foetal heart will be auscultated, and the tumour may be felt to contract under the hand. Moreover, in pregnancy, the vagina and cervix are softened and a mauve discoloration may be detected in the vagina. A hydatidiform mole may cause rapid enlargement of the uterus and be associated with irregular vaginal bleeding, and the abdominal swelling may be firm and hard, like a uterine myoma. But the other symptoms and signs of pregnancy will then be present. If any doubt remains about excluding pregnancy, a pregnancy test of the urine should be carried out. It may sometimes be clear that the uterus

contains myomata but the question has to be answered whether it is pregnant as well. Often great difficulty may be experienced in arriving at the correct diagnosis. It is better, however, to take pains to carry out every investigation, including a pregnancy test and a simple plain X-ray of the abdomen, than to open the abdomen unnecessarily.

(3) **Adenomyosis and Endometriosis Externa.** Adenomyosis interna of the uterus may cause a uniform enlargement of the uterus which simulates the presence of a myoma. The association of severe congestive dysmenorrhoea arising in a woman after the age of 35 years should suggest the possibility of adenomyosis, though some cases of myoma present this symptom. Endometriosis of the ovary may be mistaken for a myoma, though the fixity and tenderness of the tumour together with the congestive dysmenorrhoea should suggest the correct diagnosis. Both conditions can give rise to infertility and menorrhagia, which further confuses the issue.

(4) **Malignant Ovarian Tumour.** One of the classical mistakes in gynaecological diagnosis is to fail to distinguish between bilateral malignant solid ovarian tumours adherent to the uterus and myomata. The diagnosis may be impossible in spite of every care taken over the history and examination, so that the exact diagnosis is made only at abdominal operation. Most malignant ovarian tumours are, however, associated with ascites, and the presence of metastases in Douglas's pouch can be detected through the posterior fornix as hard, fixed nodules.

(5) **Pelvic Inflammatory Disease.** In other cases adnexal inflammatory tumours, like pyosalpinx, may cause difficulty in diagnosis if the swelling is adherent to the uterus.

(6) **Extrauterine Gestation.** Occasional mistakes are made with ectopic gestations so that peritubal haematoceles are regarded as subserous myomata. In both these conditions care taken over the elucidation of the menstrual history will be of the utmost service in establishing the diagnosis.

(7) **Abnormalities.** Such as bicornuate uterus may cause difficulty in diagnosis.

(8) **Carcinoma of the Cervix and Body of the Uterus.** Small submucous myomata and myomatous polypi present symptoms and signs similar to those of cervical or endometrial cancer. Persistent bleeding from a bulky uterus in a nullipara of 50 would lead to suspicion of carcinoma of the body of the uterus, and the cavity of the uterus should be explored to establish the diagnosis.

Differential Diagnosis of Myomatous Polypus

A myomatous polyp lying in the cervical canal must be distinguished from retained products of conception, from chronic inversion, and from a malignant growth. If the tumour which lies within the cervical canal is friable and bleeds easily, it is unlikely to be a myoma. With carcinoma of the cervix a cauliflower-like growth may sometimes be mistaken for a myomatous polypus. If there is any doubt about the diagnosis a biopsy should be performed.

Treatment of Myomata

In almost all myomata, treatment is necessary, either because of excessive haemorrhage or because of pressure symptoms. Occasionally, however, patients are seen where no treatment is necessary. In patients of post-menopausal age myomata may be discovered during routine examination, and if the patient is symptomless, immediate treatment is not necessary. Nevertheless, the patient should be watched, and if there is any suspicion of further growth of the tumour, operation is clearly indicated, for such growth would be suggestive of the development of sarcoma. Needless to say, the diagnosis must be made with absolute confidence. If, for example, the tumour happens to be an ovarian swelling, and not a myoma, an unpardonable mistake will be made. Similarly, symptomless myomata found during the child-bearing period of life in women who are bad subjects for operation do not require treatment, but there must be no doubt about the diagnosis before this course can be followed. Symptomless myomata are usually of the subserous type. The majority of other forms require treatment.

In general, treatment may be conservative, radiotherapeutic, or operative.

Conservative Treatment. Sometimes patients are seen who have small myomata in the uterus which produce few, if any, symptoms. If such patients are likely to marry and have children, or if they are newly married and anxious to have a family, it is better to avoid operation until the woman has had a chance to conceive. In the meantime, menorrhagia should be treated by rest and iron. Such patients are by no means infrequent, and should be examined periodically so that any rapid enlargement of the tumour may be detected. In practice, the question often arises as to whether a woman should be informed if she has small myomata in the uterus. If a woman is likely to conceive fairly soon after the diagnosis is made, it is as well to inform her of the presence of the myomata, but it should be pointed out that the tumours, though frequently becoming painful during pregnancy, have a well-marked tendency to retrogress during the puerperium.

The profound anaemia which may be caused by myomata should be corrected before the actual tumour is treated. It is an unwarrantable risk to operate upon a patient with a haemoglobin value of under 70%. Blood transfusion is the most useful method of treating this anaemia since its results are immediate so that operation can be performed before the next period begins. A prolonged course of systemic or oral iron therapy will benefit a lot of patients and though theoretically commendable, has the disadvantage that an excessive menstrual period may start during the treatment. It is much better to treat by blood transfusion followed by operation within a week. If, however, blood transfusion is not available or is considered inadvisable the general condition of the majority of patients can be considerably improved by the administration of iron to correct their anaemia and the judicious use of progestogen to control temporarily the menorrhagia.

Treatment by Radiotherapy

The mortality of hysterectomy with expert, modern anaesthesia is now so small (0.2%) that it largely removes the old argument in favour of a radiation menopause with its negligible death rate. In fact, the mortality of hysterectomy is that of anaesthesia and pulmonary embolism, and diagnostic curettage with either the insertion of radium or followed by Deep X-ray is no more immune from these particular hazards. Occasionally, however, gravely ill patients suffering from some severe medical disease will be presented to the gynaecologist and in whom a major operation should be avoided. For these patients the alternative of a radiation menopause must, therefore, be considered. If an irradiation menopause is employed, it is essential that carcinoma of the endometrium be first excluded by diagnostic curettage and to side-step this obligation is submitting the patient to an unjustifiable risk, especially as this age-group of patients is particularly liable to suffer from uterine cancer.

The presence of a submucous fibroid or an infected fibroid polypus in process of extrusion is a contraindication to irradiation since these tumours continue to bleed after the irradiation menopause has been effected.

Large tumours, owing to their liability to degeneration after irradiation treatment, may cause symptoms as severe as the original condition as a result of this degeneration.

Concomitant pelvic pathology, such as tubo-ovarian inflammatory disease or an ovarian neoplasm, is again a contraindication to radio-therapy.

The age of the patient is of importance. To induce an artificial menopause under the age of 45 may produce a severe and acute onset of menopausal symptoms such as flushes. Moreover, it has a considerable psychological effect on the patient. Modern practice, therefore, provides only the rarest indication for the employment of irradiation in the treatment of myomata.

Operative Treatment

The operative treatment of uterine myomata represents one of the most satisfactory applications of surgery. The mortality is low, the patients are cured of their symptoms and the part removed is a useless structure.

The methods available are **myomectomy,** in which the tumours are removed and the uterus conserved, and **total hysterectomy,** when the uterus and its myomata are removed *en bloc*.

Myomectomy. The removal of a myomatous polypus by the vaginal route represents one form of myomectomy and will be considered later in the chapter.

Abdominal myomectomy is performed through the peritoneal cavity with the patient lying in the Trendelenburg position. The treatment is ideal for women who are anxious to have children or who are infertile and in whom the infertility is perhaps attributable to the myoma. The most suitable patient for myomectomy is therefore a woman in the early 30s, recently married, anxious to have children, who has one or only a few myomata. On the other hand, a woman over 40 with living children, whose uterus is studded with multiple myomata, is best treated by hysterectomy. In the operation of myomectomy the myometrium over the tumour is incised and the tumour shelled out from its capsule. With a little ingenuity other intramural tumours can usually be removed either through this incision or through a second incision made through the opposite pole of the uterus. Subserous tumours are easily removed. Although a conservative measure, myomectomy has certain disadvantages as compared with hysterectomy. In the first place, haemorrhage may be experienced during the operation in spite of temporary clamps being applied to the main uterine vessels. With proper technique this objection is largely groundless. Secondly, although extreme care may

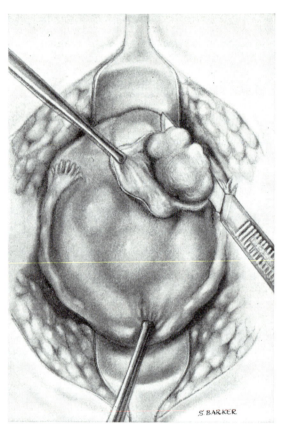

Fig. 294. Abdominal myomectomy. With small myomata the position of the capsule is found by incising into the tumour.

be taken to obtain exact apposition of the edges of the wound in the wall of the uterus, reactionary haemorrhage may occur into the peritoneal cavity or cause a haematoma in the uterus, which, even if it does not become infected, may lead to the production of adhesions with their attendant risk of acute intestinal obstruction. This is a rare but real criticism of the operation. Lastly, small seedling tumours unobserved at operation may subsequently grow, so that hysterectomy finally becomes necessary, and this occurs in about 5% of all patients treated by myomectomy. For these reasons it is probably better to restrict the use of the operation to those cases when the patient insists upon retaining the uterus so that she may have a chance of carrying a child to term, or where the youth of the patient is a strong contra-indication to hysterectomy.

Hysterectomy. Hysterectomy is the operation most frequently performed in the surgical treatment of uterine myomata. The ovaries should be retained

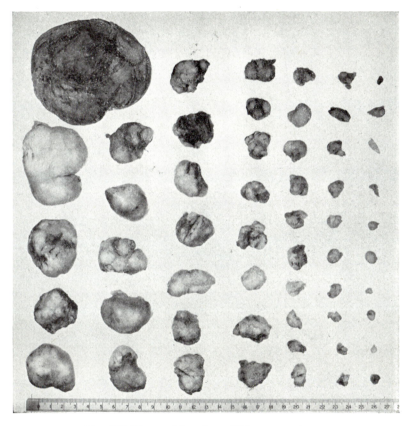

FIG. 295. The trophies of a multiple myomectomy.

unless grossly diseased; if both are removed the patient will develop meno-pausal symptoms. It is true that adnexal complications such as salpingo-oöphoritis and chocolate cysts are sometimes encountered, which necessitate the removal of both ovaries, but wherever possible one ovary should be left behind. There has been much dispute as to whether the cervix should always be removed. If the cervix is conserved it may subsequently become carcino-matous in about 1 % of cases, and this incidence has been used as an argument for total hysterectomy as a routine. If a hysterectomy is to be undertaken and the cervix is lacerated, eroded, or chronically inflamed, the whole uterus should be removed, as the diseased cervical stump will continue to give rise to some of the symptoms of bleeding and discharge for which the operation was originally indicated. Total hysterectomy is technically more difficult, with a greater risk of injury to bladder and ureters than subtotal hysterectomy. This is, however, a poor defence for the adoption of subtotal hysterectomy, since if

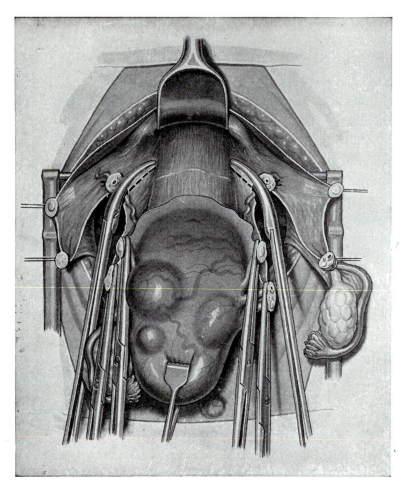

FIG. 296. Total hysterectomy. The diagram shows how clamps are placed over the parametrium. To apply the clamps the uterus is drawn over to the opposite side and the assistant carefully retracts the bladder. (From Shaw's "Operative Gynaecology," E. & S. Livingstone Ltd.)

a surgeon is incapable of performing a safe total hysterectomy he had better not perform the operation at all.

Another argument adduced in favour of preserving the cervix is that the fascial supports of the vaginal vault are left intact and subsequent vault prolapse is less likely to occur. This is, however, a purely technical problem and if a total hysterectomy is properly performed there is no greater risk of vault prolapse than if the cervix is conserved. In fact it may very well be less.

Dyspareunia does not occur as a result of total hysterectomy if the technique of the operation is correct, and coitus is in no way functionally impaired. At the present day the mortality rate of total hysterectomy is at least as low as or even lower than that of subtotal hysterectomy, in the region of 0.2%; and because of the possibility of a carcinoma subsequently developing in the cervix, the operation of total hysterectomy is favoured by modern enlightened gynaecological opinion.

In the majority of patients the operation of hysterectomy can be carried out simply and quickly, but great difficulty is experienced in the operation if the myoma is cervical or if it has burrowed into the broad ligament or backwards along the uterosacral ligament. In such cases the tumour fixes the uterus, so that the uterus cannot be drawn out of the pelvis. The tumour may dislodge the bladder and ureters from their normal situations so that the bladder is almost entirely an abdominal organ and may be injured when the abdominal incision is being made. With cervical myomata the ureters are usually pushed upwards far above their normal level as they pass forwards to enter the bladder, and quite often the ureters lie in close connection with the capsule of the tumour. Successful removal of extraperitoneal and cervical myomata depends upon finding the correct layer from which to enucleate the tumour. This layer lies a little external to the capsule, and when opened up the tumour can be shelled out of the pelvis quite easily, with little risk of damage to the ureter or bladder. If there is any coincident pelvic endometriosis the pelvic cellular tissue is fibrotic, so that difficulty may be experienced in separating the bladder from the uterus and in opening up the broad ligament to clamp the uterine vessels.

The Operative Technique of Hysterectomy

Pre-operative Treatment. The patient is given an aperient at midday on the day before operation, and bathed and shaved the same evening. On the morning of operation an enema may be given according to the particular routine of the surgeon. It is best for all patients to be catheterised in the theatre by the surgeon immediately before operation. A metal catheter is the surest instrument for emptying the bladder, and care must be taken that air is not aspirated into the bladder when the suprapubic pressure is released as the catheter is being withdrawn. The presence of air in the bladder is just as embarrassing to the surgeon as water.

Operation. The patient is placed in a moderate Trendelenburg position and the abdomen opened by a paramedian or midline incision. The uterus is drawn out of the wound, a large abdominal retractor introduced, and the intestines packed away from the operation area with packs soaked in warm saline if they tend to intrude into the area of operation.

If the ovaries and Fallopian tubes are found to be healthy and the uterus alone is to be removed, the following technique is employed. The uterus is pulled over to one side so that the tube and ovary of the opposite side are stretched and well exposed. The ovarian ligament, the Fallopian tube and the round ligament thus exposed are then divided between clamps which are placed near the cornu of the uterus. If the uterus contains large myomata, very large veins may be found in the vicinity of the cornu, so that three or four pairs of clamps may have to be applied to obtain complete haemostasis. The same procedure is now carried out on the opposite side.

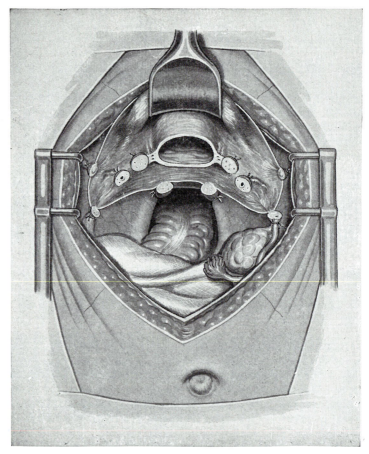

Fig. 297. Total hysterectomy. All pedicles ligatured. The right appendages are conserved. (From Shaw's "Operative Gynaecology", E. & S. Livingstone Ltd.)

The uterus is then pulled upwards and backwards and the uterovesical pouch of peritoneum exposed. This line of peritoneum is now divided transversely with scissors, from the round ligament of one side to the round ligament of the opposite side. As a result of this, the broad ligaments of the two sides can be opened up and the bladder can be separated from the front of the cervix. The bladder can then be pushed down with a gauze strip provided the correct layer is found.

The uterine vessels must now be exposed. The uterus is therefore drawn over to one side, when the uterine vessels of the opposite side will be exposed as they run upwards along the lateral border of the uterus. The uterine vessels are now divided between heavy clamps, and the uterus is firmly pulled upwards by an assistant. The bladder is now stripped away from the cervix and the upper part of the vagina. Some degree of oozing from venous plexuses is fairly common particularly near the sides of the cervix. Especial care must be taken to push the bladder well away from the sides of the cervix otherwise the ureter may be included in the clamp used for the parametrium. It is most important to make quite sure that the bladder and the ureters are stripped clear before clamps are applied to the parametrium. A clamp should be applied to the parametrium on one side of the cervix, the uterus being forcibly drawn to the opposite side and the cervix separated from the parametrium with scissors. A similar procedure is employed for the opposite side. The vagina is now opened by cutting with curved scissors from the lateral border of the vagina. The anterior lip of the vaginal portion of the cervix now comes into view. It is grasped with volsellum forceps and drawn upwards. The cervix is now completely separated from the vagina by cutting with scissors. It is sometimes convenient to apply clamps to the vaginal walls and to cut above the clamps with scissors. In this way, haemorrhage can be controlled. The uterus is now removed and a gauze pack soaked in an antiseptic such as flavine is introduced into the vagina from above. At this stage it is best to put separate clamps on the lateral vaginal plexuses of veins, otherwise there may be troublesome haemorrhage. The pedicles are now transfixed and ligatured. Some surgeons close the vagina with interrupted sutures of catgut, while others prefer to leave the upper end of the vagina open. The raw surface is covered with peritoneum and the uterosacral and Mackenrodt's ligaments together with the round ligament are fixed by transfixation sutures to the lateral angles of the vaginal vault. These three ligaments form a strong sling which prevents subsequent vault prolapse, and if this part of the operation is properly performed the chances of vaginal prolapse are minimal after total hysterectomy. The abdomen is closed in the usual way (see Figs. 296 and 297).

Although the main steps in the operation have been indicated above, variations are necessary according to the size, number, and situation of the tumours.

After-treatment. The patient is returned to bed, lying on one side until she has recovered from the anaesthetic. The patient is then placed in a more upright position and given an injection of 20 mg of omnopon or 100 mg. of pethidine which can be repeated as required to relieve the abdominal pain. Providing that no complications were encountered at operation the patient may have sips of water as soon as she is conscious. She will require adequate sedatives for the first night but will probably sleep for short periods only. The morning after operation she should sit up and may start to take fluids freely followed by light diet if no nausea is present. She gets up for bed-making in the afternoon. On the second day she has a light diet, gets up several times for short periods and has a mild aperient at night. On the third day she will probably suffer from "wind pain" which will be relieved by passing flatus; this is encouraged by giving glycerine suppositories. A post-operative enema should seldom be required. After the third day, if convalescence is normal, few symptoms are complained of. If a total hysterectomy has been performed some degree of vaginal discharge may develop at the end of the first week if the wound in the upper part of the vagina becomes infected. If the vaginal discharge is purulent and the patient has fever, the appropriate antibiotic should be given.

The great value of chemotherapy and antibiotics both for prophylaxis and treatment must be remembered. In any hysterectomy where sepsis is met with at operation prophylactic treatment should be employed immediately.

Complications

Prophylaxis. Prophylactic measures to correct or eliminate possible sources of post-operative complication should be undertaken while the patient is awaiting admission to hospital. A little time and trouble expended before operation will shorten convalescence, save bed wastage and unnecessary expense to hospital and patient.

A thorough general examination of the gynaecological patient will be undertaken at the first consultation. This may reveal:

(1) Obvious cardiovascular abnormality, in which case the fitness of the patient for operation should be assessed by a cardiologist. Well-compensated valvular disease is not a contraindication to surgery, but hypertension, so often associated with obesity, calls for rest, strict diet, sedatives and possibly a hypotensive drug. In this way many bad-risk patients can be temporarily converted into the category of "safe for operation". The commonest finding in candidates for hysterectomy is anaemia, and no patient with a haemoglobin level below 70% should be submitted to an elective operation. A course of iron will normally suffice, but in severe cases pre-operative transfusion may be necessary. In all hysterectomy patients the blood grouping and Rhesus typing should be done with the haemoglobin estimation before operation. Many patients with unsuspected anaemia will be discovered and the deficiency corrected in good time.

(2) No elective hysterectomy should be performed on a patient with acute untreated respiratory disease. Simple measures such as the interdiction of smoking and the use of pre-operative breathing exercises will do much to improve a bed chest. Chest radiography and the opinion of a physician will be required for the patient with chronic pulmonary disease, especially the known or unsuspected tuberculous infection. Such patients may need admission to a medical ward for a few weeks before they can be pronounced fit for anaesthesia and operation.

(3) Obvious local sepsis in mouth, throat, skin or vagina should be eliminated before operation, and the co-operation of the various specialists concerned should be sought if necessary.

(4) Any abnormality of the urinary tract should be investigated and, if possible, corrected before operation. It is easier to sterilise an infected urine before operation than after, and less distressing to the patient.

(5) A proper diet adequate in first-class protein and vitamin content is essential for proper wound healing.

(6) The psychological attitude of the patient to her forthcoming ordeal should be fortified by reassurance. A good morale on the part of the patient is essential and is particularly important in the menopausal woman.

(7) Other non-gynaecological symptoms should be investigated. A common example is backache, which is quite likely to be unrelated to the gynaecological lesion. An X-ray of the spine should be taken to exclude an orthopaedic lesion such as osteoarthritis or a prolapsed intervertebral disc. It is important to assess such conditions before operation so that the patient can be made aware of their significance. In this way the results of her gynaecological operation will not be misinterpreted.

Shock. The removal of a large myomatous uterus may rarely be followed by shock, particularly if haemorrhage has been free during the operation or if much traction has been necessary to pull the tumour out of the pelvis. A simple hysterectomy performed expeditiously and with small haemorrhage should never give rise to shock. Treatment consists in drip transfusion either with blood or plasma substitute. Oxygen should be administered by BLB mask until the colour of the skin improves. Morphia should not be administered until the patient has recovered from the anaesthetic, and excessive heating of the patient with electric blankets should be avoided as this only results in peripheral vasodilatation and loss of circulating blood to the vital centres.

Haemorrhage may be *primary, reactionary* or *secondary*.

Primary haemorrhage is to be expected during the actual removal of large or multiple myomata, where usually one of the uterine veins is torn. The bigger the tumour the more vascular the parametrium, hence the importance of progressive clamping and ligation as the dissection proceeds. If all pedicles are secured as they are divided there is no excuse for operating in a morass of blood.

Reactionary haemorrage occurs as the blood pressure rises on recovery from the anaesthetic. It is therefore particularly to be expected if hypotensive agents have been used. The most likely cause of reactionary haemorrhage is failure to ligate a moderate-sized vessel simply because owing to the hypotension it was not bleeding at the time of inspection. The vessels in the cut vaginal vault are likely offenders, especially the descending vaginal branch of the uterine vessels. With good fortune if these vessels are at the vault firm vaginal packing may control the bleeding—if not laparotomy is indicated. A meticulous surgical technique very largely eliminates primary and reactionary bleeding.

Secondary haemorrhage due to sepsis is a possible complication of an infected total hysterectomy. Vaginal bleeding may suddenly develop during the second week when it is necessary to anaesthetise the patient, to remove the clot from the vagina, and then to plug the vagina tightly with dry sterile gauze, the gauze being removed forty-eight hours later. As the source of the bleeding is most likely to be an infection or abscess in the region of the vaginal vault it usually represents an ill-defined generalised ooze from a friable indurated area. Any suture ligatures will immediately cut out and cause more bleeding than they control.

After severe haemorrhage of any type transfusion will be needed.

Sepsis. Sepsis may be local or it may lead to general peritonitis.

(*a*) **Local.** Infection of the abdominal wound may involve all layers and usually follows ineffective haemostasis resulting in a haematoma. It is therefore commoner in fat patients, previous scars and with post-operative chest infections. If superficial to the rectus sheath infection causes an ugly scar; if deep to the sheath it endangers the security of the abdominal wall and may result in a scar hernia. There should be no hesitation in draining all layers of a wound where oozing is either uncontrollable or likely to become so. It is almost never necessary to drain the peritoneal cavity.

(*b*) **Pelvic sepsis.** Local sepsis in the peritoneal cavity is particularly apt to occur in haematomata, which develop between the upper end of the vagina below and the peritoneum above, after total hysterectomy. These haematomata subsequently suppurate and usually discharge themselves into the vagina. A haematoma may collect in the true pelvis or in the broad ligament and when this becomes infected a pelvic abscess develops. It should be drained by the simple manoeuvre of passing a finger through the vaginal vault.

(*c*) **General peritonitis** is a rare complication of hysterectomy for myomata. If pelvic sepsis develops it tends to be restricted to the pelvis and the pelvic peritoneum is usually able to deal with the infection itself, so that spreading peritonitis is exceptional. Spreading general peritonitis is particularly apt to ensue if the bowel has been injured during operation, if a swab has been left behind or if the bladder or ureters have been injured during the operation.

Burst abdomen is a rare but unpleasant complication which may arise as a result of local haematoma formation and sepsis in the wound. There is a growing feeling among surgeons that the peritoneal suture line gives way first and that the burst occurs from within outwards. If therefore there has been difficulty in closing the peritoneum owing to its friability, or suture of it under tension, this complication is particularly to be feared, and fat patients are obvious candidates for the reason that the abdominal contents exert a disrupting force on the wound. Post-operative retching or coughing is also a significant factor. The clinical condition is an obvious one and is usually foreshadowed by pain in the wound, which gives way with a discharge of serous or serosanguinous fluid. Inspection reveals the presence of omentum or a coil of gut. In the more dramatic case several coils of bowel are found to be extra-abdominal. Immediate resuture under anaesthesia gives good results and the patients surprisingly do not develop peritonitis, though it is a wise precaution to give prophylactic antibiotics. Resuture of the wound should be undertaken in layers, using interrupted sutures, and stainless steel wire or nylon is useful when suturing the rectus sheath.

If the wound is weakened by haematoma formation or sepsis a partial disruption takes place and the patient subsequently develops an incisional hernia. This should be repaired six months after the original operation. The whole wound should be laid open from top to bottom and the peritoneal sac of the hernia excised and the edges carefully sutured. The rectus sheath is then dissected free from the rectus muscle and sutured with 36-gauge stainless steel, using interrupted sutures. The secret of secure suture is to take a wide bite well lateral to the edge of the wound, not timid nibbles which are liable to cut through. It is always wise to drain the wound for twenty-four hours as far as the peritoneum.

Urinary Complications. Abdominal hysterectomy is almost never complicated by retention of urine, the incidence being no more than 1%. This rare event will be treated by a cholinergic drug and, if this is not rapidly effective, catheterisation.

Incontinence of urine suggests the development of a urinary fistula, either vesicovaginal or ureterovaginal. In such cases catheterisation demonstrates the presence of bloodstained urine in the bladder. An occasional complication of gynaecological operations is for the ureter to be included wholly or in part in a ligature. This complication should be suspected if the patient develops a high temperature immediately after the operation without abdominal, pelvic or pulmonary signs. Careful palpation of the costo-vertebral angle will, however, usually elicit some local tenderness in the affected kidney. The usual sequel is for a ureterovaginal fistula to develop on about the tenth day after operation.

Injury to the bladder occurs either on opening the abdomen or during the dissection of the bladder from the anterior aspect of the cervix and vaginal vault. In both instances, it should be immediately recognised and repaired at once, after which an indwelling catheter is left in situ for fourteen days. These wounds heal without complications. If unrecognised, a fistula develops almost at once and is obvious within twenty-four hours of the operation. Fortunately, these fistulae discharge usually through the vaginal vault or rarely through the abdominal incision. Intraperitoneal extravasation of urine, if it occurs, gives rise to the signs of severe peritoneal irritation with a high and rapidly climbing blood urea, vomiting, distension and severe pain. The treatment is immediate exploratory laparotomy with intravenous fluid and chemotherapy. The wound should be found and the bladder closed in layers with catheter drainage or cystotomy.

Suppression of urine is a rare complication of abdominal hysterectomy, and when it occurs it is usually due to ureteric obstruction or damage at the time of operation. Bilateral obstruction is uncommon but anuria can result from the occlusion of one ureter resulting in the sympathetic failure of function on the part of the unobstructed kidney. In very rare cases the sole functioning kidney may have been obstructed where the patient only had one good kidney before operation. In severely shocked patients with a low post-operative blood pressure a temporary anuria occurs, but this should always respond to resuscitation by blood transfusion.

If no urine has been passed in twenty-four hours and the passage of a catheter shows the bladder to be empty the abdomen must be reopened and the ureters explored on both sides from the pelvic brim to the operation site. Once the obstruction has been found the offending ligature should be cut out if this is possible, or the ureter divided and reimplanted into the bladder.

Sometimes oedema or a haematoma makes these procedures impracticable, and in these desperate cases bilateral nephrostomy is essential and life-saving. Fortunately this heroic measure is seldom necessary.

Urinary infections arise fairly commonly after hysterectomy, particularly if it has been found necessary to dissect either the bladder or the ureters away from the uterus or appendages. Minor injuries to any part of the urinary system are apt to be followed by urinary infections. Similarly, catheterisation is very prone to be followed by the development of cystitis.

Phlebothrombosis is one of the most dangerous complications of gynae-cological surgery and accounts for the major proportion of operative fatalities of hysterectomy. According to the modern concept the usual site of the clot is the deep muscular veins of the calf, and the process is primarily an aseptic one and the clot is not anchored to the vessel wall by an inflammatory reaction. In 10% of cases, however, the deep pelvic veins may be affected either alone or in addition to the veins of the calf. If the pelvic veins are in-volved there is usually some pelvic sepsis and the condition is probably one of true infective thrombophlebitis and therefore less dangerous in its liability to pulmonary embolism.

Several factors contribute to the development of phlebothrombosis.

(1) The general condition of the patient. Anaemia, sepsis, obesity and prolonged illness in the recumbent position are contributory factors.

(2) Venous stasis is the most significant single factor; hence the importance of early ambulation and breathing exercises and the absolute interdiction of Fowler's position.

(3) Trauma to the leg veins by prolonged pressure on the operating table. For this reason suspension of the patient by the bent legs and the use of leg straps is to be heartily condemned. All modern operating tables should now have the corrugated non-slip mattress of Langton Hewer.

(4) An increased coagulability of the blood following operation. The fibrinogen content of the blood, prothrombin activity and platelet cohesion and number are all increased.

The diagnosis of phlebothrombosis should be made before the signs are obvious. Every patient who has undergone hysterectomy should be questioned night and morning about pain in the calf or thigh, and the legs should be examined for tenderness as a routine twice daily.

Any tenderness in the leg, especially if associated with slight oedema, should be regarded as significant. Pain on dorsiflexion of the foot (Homans' sign) is unreliable. Usually the chart will show a small rise of pulse and temperature and the patient will not feel quite so well as she should.

As soon as the diagnosis is made anticoagulant treatment should be started. It is usual to start by giving 10,000 to 15,000 units of heparin intra-venously six-hourly and 150–300 mg. of phenindione by mouth the first day. On the second day the phenindione is reduced to 100–200 mg., and the heparin may be discontinued if the patient's condition has improved. This will be shown by relief of pain in the leg and fall of temperature and pulse to normal. The aim of treatment is to hold the prothrombin level at about 20% to 25% of normal, and the dose of phenindione must be varied to achieve this. A course of treatment usually lasts five to seven days but may be continued longer or repeated. Prothrombin estimations should be done daily, and if these are not available it is safer to use heparin. Protamine sulphate to counteract the heparin should always be available.

If bleeding occurs from the wound or the vagina it may be necessary to stop treatment, and sometimes transfusion and vitamin K will be necessary. We have recently seen a very large retroperitoneal haematoma 20 cm. in diameter develop in a clean, technically faultless hysterectomy on the 13th day after anticoagulation.

The great advantage of anticoagulant treatment is that the patient is not immobilised for a long period, and in fact she can resume full ambulation after a week of bed rest with modified limb exercises.

Pulmonary Embolism. Any sudden post-operative pain in the chest, however slight, should be suspected as being due to an embolism until the surgeon is satisfied of his diagnosis. Certain clinical types are recognised:

(1) The patient has obvious phlebothrombosis in the leg and the lung infarct is merely a severe complication of this. The chest symptoms and signs are fairly obvious, such as acute pain, dyspnoea, cyanosis, tachycardia and moderate fever. A pleural rub will be found if listened for before it is masked by the small resultant effusion, and an X-ray taken twelve hours after the onset of symptoms will show the characteristic wedge-shaped area of opacity in the lung.

(2) The chest symptoms are so slight as barely to worry the patient and signs are minimal or absent. In this case a small infarct has occurred and will be absorbed without trouble though another infarct may occur later.

(3) The sudden massive fatal embolism associated with great pain, shock, rapid feeble pulse and death in a few minutes. The pulmonary vessels are in acute spasm and at autopsy a large clot is found lying across the bifurcation of the pulmonary artery.

The diagnosis of pulmonary embolism calls for an increase of anticoagulant therapy if it is already being given, or for its prompt administration in large doses until the condition is under control. It is better to give anticoagulants for a misdiagnosed chest condition than to delay treatment until the diagnosis is all too obvious.

Other Methods of Treatment. In certain rare instances anticoagulant treatment is contraindicated or ineffective. In these vein interruption should be considered. If the leg is affected the femoral vein can be tied below Poupart's ligament on one or both sides. If the pelvic veins are thought to be involved the inferior vena cava should be ligated by a transabdominal approach. This operation, though sounding formidable, is really a simple one and has been performed on two occasions by one of the authors without any untoward effects on the patient apart from temporary oedema of the legs controlled by rest and bandaging.

Lumbar sympathetic block is particularly useful for cases of femoral thrombosis associated with a painful and persistent oedema of the leg. For the best results it should be done early and may be repeated if necessary. An epidural block works equally well.

Gastrointestinal Complications

Vomiting. Post-operative vomiting is a comparatively rare complication of modern anaesthesia and should be treated by the usual nursing regime. The antihistamine drugs such as Avomine, Dramamine and Marzine are useful additions if vomiting is troublesome. Intramuscular Fentazin, 5 mg., repeated, if necessary, in four hours, is most useful where the already-mentioned drugs are ineffective. On rare occasions it may be necessary to pass a small stomach tube and wash out the stomach with a dilute solution of sodium bicarbonate. It should always be remembered that persistent vomiting is a symptom of four more serious conditions: acute dilatation of the stomach, paralytic ileus, peritonitis and intestinal obstruction.

Post-operative Gaseous Distension. This is probably the commonest complication of total hysterectomy and some degree of flatulent distension of the large bowel is almost invariable. The aetiology of the condition is obscure, but two main causes are obvious—firstly, that intestinal stasis predisposes to gas formation and, secondly, that most of the air in the gut is the result of air swallowing by the patient either during the induction of the anaesthesia or in the post-operative period, especially during retching. If post-operative distension is unrelieved, a state of paralytic ileus may result, which is a serious condition. Flatulent distension is undoubtedly less in patients who are ambulatory and in whom post-operative physiotherapy is employed.

Prevention is the best treatment of the condition. Avoidance of pre-operative enema, good anaesthesia, gentle handling of the intestine at operation and immaculate technique are all important, but the treatment of the intestine during the phase of inhibited peristalsis in the first twenty-four hours after operation is rest for the patient and the gastro-intestinal tract. 20 mgm. of morphia four- to six-hourly is therefore given, and only small quantities of fluid by mouth until peristalsis is re-established. Sometimes a glycerine suppository on the third morning after operation is helpful in promoting the passage of flatus. It is wrong to overstimulate the bowel by giving drugs such as prostigmin, acetyl choline and pituitary extract. Once the bowels have been opened no further trouble should be encountered.

Paralytic Ileus. This condition is one in which all peristaltic movement has ceased in the bowel. Both large and small gut may be affected and even the stomach. The patient usually starts with a simple post-operative distension which does not respond to treatment. The abdomen becomes progressively more distended and is tense and tender to palpation. Gut sounds are absent and the passage of a flatus tube or the giving of an enema produces little result. The pulse soon rises and the patient becomes dehydrated both from the vomiting and from loss of fluid into the paralysed bowel. The water and electrolyte imbalance soon reaches dangerous figures, and an essential part of the treatment is to keep the patient in fluid and electrolyte balance by intravenous therapy, controlled by frequent biochemical estimations. The correction of hypokalaemia alone is often sufficient to cure the condition since a low serum potassium level causes hypotonia of all types of muscle, striated, unstriated and cardiac. The distension of the bowel is best relieved by a continuous suction with a Miller-Abbott or similar tube. It is important to avoid any so-called intestinal stimulant, and this should never be given until peristaltic movement is restored to the bowel. This may take many days —as much as ten or fourteen—but need cause no anxiety if the patient is properly controlled as far as her water and electrolytes are concerned and if the distension is relieved by continuous intestinal suction.

Acute Dilatation of the Stomach. This is a very rare complication of hysterectomy although it may be seen in association with paralytic ileus. The patient is extremely ill, in a shocked condition with a rapid pulse and exhausted from the large quantities of copious vomit—several pints of dark-brown fluid may well effortlessly out of the stomach with obvious adverse effects on the electrolyte and water balance of the patient. Treatment consists in continuous aspiration of the stomach by an indwelling Ryle's tube and the replacement of the lost fluid and electrolyte by intravenous infusion.

Peritonitis. The classical symptoms and signs of this condition are pain and vomiting, localised or generalised distension of the abdomen and loss of peristalsis from the affected segments of the bowel. The secondary effects of fluid and electrolyte losses soon become apparent and the condition is sometimes difficult to distinguish from that of paralytic ileus, and in fact the two conditions often coincide. In fact, if paralytic ileus lasts long enough it must result in peritonitis, whereas with peritonitis there is always some degree of ileus from the first. In gynaecological practice the peritonitis is usually localised mainly to the pelvis, so that the signs of a general peritonitis must be somewhat modified. Treatment consists in fluid and electrolyte replacement as required, continuous intestinal suction and the administration of a broad spectrum antibiotic.

Laparotomy is only indicated in the early stages of peritonitis where damage to the gut is suspected, e.g. criminal abortion, and in the later stages to drain a localised pelvic abscess which is not amenable to simple vaginal drainage.

Intestinal Obstruction. The possibility of intestinal obstruction should always be borne in mind after gynaecological operations, and it is especially likely in pelvic inflammatory disease, in endometriosis, following myomectomy, anterior hysterotomy and, in obstetric practice, Caesarean section. The symptoms consist of pain, distension and severe vomiting. On examination the abdomen shows an acute local tenderness near the site of the obstruction, and the gut above the obstruction shows hypertonic peristalsis, while that below is atonic. A straight X-ray of the abdomen in the sitting position will show multiple fluid levels above the site of obstruction. No fluid or flatus is passed after the part of the bowel below the obstruction has been emptied, and toxaemia from dehydration and electrolyte imbalance is soon profound. The treatment consists in the restoration of fluid and electrolyte loss, treatment of shock, continuous suction aspiration of the gut followed by immediate laparotomy as soon as the patient is fit for operation.

Pulmonary Complications

Pulmonary complications are less common in operations in the lower abdomen than those in the upper abdomen, where there is interference with the diaphragm and its movement. Patients who have chronic bronchitis are liable to develop post-operative chest infections, but the worst criminal is the cigarette addict. The logical prophylactic is interdiction. The inhalation of Isoprenaline, to dilate the bronchioles, and physiotherapy to the chest are useful in preventing pulmonary infection. Post-operative physiotherapy encourages the patient to breathe and to expand the base of the lungs. If there is no physiotherapist to assist, inhalations of 10% carbon dioxide in oxygen or even the blowing of carbon dioxide itself from a tube placed close to the mouth will make the patient breathe deeply.

Atelectasis may arise as a result of a bronchus becoming plugged by inspissated mucus. This is usually heralded by a slight rise of temperature, absent breath sounds in the area affected and, if the atelectasis is fairly large, the diaphragm will be raised on the same side and there will be mediastinal shift and the apex of the heart may be displaced from its normal position. Sometimes it is possible to move the plug by stimulating the respiratory centre by the injection of nikethamide, 3 ml. intravenously. This makes the patient cough, and while the patient is coughing the abdomen should be held with one hand while gentle tapping of the chest over the affected area is performed with the cupped hand. In the case of massive atelectasis where cyanosis occurs, inhalations of oxygen should be given or bronchoscopy considered to clear the blocked bronchus.

Pulmonary embolism has already been fully discussed.

Neurological Complications

There is a certain danger in the use of Trendelenburg's position if the patient is secured by the legs, which are bent at a right-angle after the ankles have been strapped to the lower leaf of the table. The external popliteal nerve may be damaged by pressure in this position and a foot-drop result. If, however, the patient is secured by shoulder pieces, and if, for the purposes of intravenous infusion, the arm is abducted to a right-angle or more there is grave risk of brachial palsy. For this reason the authors have abandoned the use of shoulder supports and employ the non-slip mattress of Langton Hewer. This mattress allows extreme degrees of tilting without securing the patient in any way whatever. Even with this mattress, however, the arm should never be abducted to a right-angle, and if the arm has to be exposed for some manoeuvre, precautions must be taken against any excessive abduction.

TREATMENT OF MYOMATOUS POLYPI

Most myomatous polypi should be removed by the vaginal route, the only exceptions being when multiple myomata are present in the uterus in addition to the polypus. Such cases, however, are exceptional, and it has been pointed out already that a large myomatous polypus is often the sole myoma in the uterus. The removal of the uterus in cases of this kind is unnecessary, except when the tumour has caused inversion. Moreover, if the uterus is removed by the abdominal route there is some risk of peritonitis as the lower end of the polypus is usually infected. The results of vaginal myomectomy are satis-factory and the operation simple. The patient is placed in the lithotomy position and vaginal retractors are introduced. If the polypus hangs down into the vagina so that a pedicle passes through the external os, the pedicle can be ligated and the polypus excised. If, on the other hand, the pedicle cannot be reached, or if part of the polypus lies within the cervical canal, the polypus can usually be removed without difficulty by torsion. Volsellum forceps are applied to the tumour and the tumour is rotated until the tissues of the pedicle tear through. Bleeding from the pedicle is minimal or moderate and can be controlled quite easily by plugging the uterine cavity with dry sterile gauze.

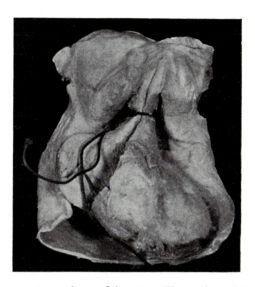

Fig. 298. A myomatous polypus of the uterus. The specimen dates from 1831. A ligature was placed around the pedicle of the polypus in the hope that the tumour would slough away. A fatal peritonitis ensued.

If the maximum circumference of the polypus has not passed through the external os and only the lower pole presents, removal is more difficult. Small tumours can usually be removed by torsion, but it may be necessary to split the cervix by the operation of **anterior vaginal hysterotomy.** A transverse incision is made through the vagina at the upper level of the anterior fornix, the bladder separated from the cervix by dissection with scissors and retracted upwards. The cervix is now divided in the midline whereby the cavity of the uterus is exposed and the myoma can then be either shelled out or removed by torsion. Haemorrhage from the tumour bed should be controlled by plugging the uterus with dry sterile gauze. The incision in the uterus is closed by interrupted sutures of catgut, after which the vaginal incision is similarly treated.

Removal of myomatous polypi is sometimes complicated by local sepsis in the uterus with pyrexia and purulent discharge. The appropriate chemo-therapy will control the infection and any anaemia must be corrected by transfusion.

SARCOMA OF THE UTERUS

Uterine sarcomata are rare tumours, comprising 4.5% of all malignant growths of the uterus. The relation to myomata is that in about 0.56% of all myomata sarcomatous change can be demonstrated (see p. 576). The tumours arise most frequently between the ages of 40 and 50, and are rare before 30, but they are not uncommon between the ages of 50 and 60. The incidence of pre-menopausal and post-menopausal sarcoma is almost equally divided. In 25% the patients are nulliparous, but parity is un-related in the aetiology.

Four types of uterine sarcomata are described. In the first, or intramural, the tumour arises in the myometrium. In the mucosal, the tumours develop from the endometrium of the uterus. In the third type the tumour arises in a pre-existing myoma, while the fourth type is a rare but interesting tumour known as the grape-like sarcoma of the cervix. The commonest form of sarcoma of the uterus is the intramural type. Histologically the tumour may be round-celled, spindle-celled, mixed-celled, or giant-celled. The com-monest form is the spindle-celled tumour which is termed a leiomyosarcoma. To the naked eye the cut surface of the tumour is haemorrhagic and irregular, without the whorled appearance of a myoma. The consistence is friable and soft. The outline is irregular with well-marked invasion of the surrounding structures and there is no capsule demonstrable. The mucosal form sometimes tends to project in the form of a polypus into the cavity of the uterus, while in other cases it spreads uniformly around the cavity of the uterus to produce a uniform enlargement.

Metastases form relatively early, the spread occurring by the blood stream, by lymphatics, by direct spread, and by implantation. As a result of blood-stream dissemination, metastases form in the lungs and kidneys. Direct spread into the peritoneal cavity leads to multiple metastases being formed over the peritoneum with accompanying ascites and large deposits in the omentum. By implantation metastases form at the vulva. It has been computed that the average duration of life from the commencement of symptoms is about two years.

Sarcoma of the uterus is diagnosed before the removal of the uterus only very exceptionally. With mucosal tumours which produce continuous bleeding, a histological examination of curettings may enable a diagnosis to be made. Again, rapid enlargement of a quiescent myoma in a woman of post-menopausal age is almost pathognomonic of sarcomatous change. Sarcoma of the uterus usually causes rapid enlargement of the uterus with profuse and irregular vaginal bleeding. Pain is present in 60% of cases and fever due to degeneration or infection may also occur in about one-third of the patients. If the tumour has encroached upon the cavity of the uterus and caused post-menopausal bleeding, diagnosis may be made by curettage. The interpretation of the histology is, however, rendered very difficult by the presence of degenerative and infective changes. After metastases have formed, the diagnosis may be made if the uterus is found to be enlarged.

Apart from the grape-like sarcoma of the cervix the diagnosis of sarcoma of the uterus is made usually after the uterus has been removed for a suspected myoma.

Treatment. The treatment of sarcoma of the uterus should consist of an extensive total hysterectomy with bilateral salpingo-oöphorectomy, followed by a full course of X-radiation therapy. If the growth is in the region of the isthmus or cervix a radical hysterectomy of the Wertheim type with bilateral lymph node excision probably offers the best chance of cure, since in many cases the glands may be involved. This can be followed by X-radiation therapy. The five-year cure rate is a little under 30% and largely depends on the type of the growth, being worst in the round-cell variety and where the growth originates in the endometrium. The presence of distant metastases is a contraindication to surgery unless of a palliative nature, e.g. to stop uterine haemorrhage.

Mesodermal Mixed Tumours (Including Botryoid and Grapelike Sarcoma)

Uterine sarcomata arise typically in the body of the uterus, while sarcomata of the cervix are very rare, and in this way sarcoma of the uterus differs essentially from carcinoma of the uterus. The grape-like sarcoma of the cervix is a very rare tumour, of great pathological interest, which is well known because of its arborescent structure and its grape-like vesicles. Pathologically the tumours should be regarded as **mixed mesodermal tumours** as they often contain cartilage, striated muscle fibres, glands, and fat. The stroma is embryonic in type, similar to the embryonal mesenchyme. Grape-like sarcoma of the cervix arises typically in adult women, metastases develop rapidly, and local recurrence follows their removal.

Somewhat similar tumours are known to develop in the vagina in children at a very early age, and such tumours contain striated muscle fibres and an embryonic stroma. Rather similar tumours sometimes develop in the body of the uterus in old women, and in this way three types of mixed tumours, namely, the vaginal tumours of children, the grape-like sarcoma of the cervix, and the mixed tumours of the body of the uterus of old women can be distinguished. Clinically the tumours are of little importance because of their rarity. In all cases the prognosis is bad, rapid recurrence following their removal.

24 New Growths of the Uterus:

EPITHELIAL TUMOURS OF THE CERVIX

Carcinoma of the uterus is regionally divided into:

(A) Carcinoma of the endometrium of the body of the uterus;

(B) Carcinoma of the cervix; this is again subdivided into:

    (*a*) Carcinoma of the portio vaginalis, comprising 80% of all cervical cancers.

    (*b*) Endocervical carcinoma which accounts for the remaining 20%.

Carcinoma of the cervix is the most frequent of all the genital tract cancers and, of all cancers occurring in women, it takes second place after cancer of the breast. The relative incidence of cancer of the cervix to that of the endometrium is 1·5 to 1·0 and the most recent figures suggest a trend towards 1·0 to 1·0. Though these two main cancers of the uterus are so closly related in their regional origin, in clinical and pathological behaviour they are in many ways totally dissimilar. Cancer of the cervix is certainly more difficult to treat and more lethal to the patient.

The relative figures of the two diseases vary from different localities and with different authorities. It should be realised that the primary origin is often obscure in an advanced cancer of the uterus in which it is impossible to differentiate a low corporeal from a high endocervical adenocarcinoma.

Aetiology

Carcinoma of the cervix occurs most frequently in multiparous women, only between 5% and 8% of patients being nulliparous. Carcinoma of the cervix occurs very rarely indeed in virgins; women who have borne large families are more apt to develop it than women who have had only one child. The age-incidence of the growth depends upon the parity of the women. In nulliparae the average age-incidence is about 57, whereas in women with six children the age-incidence falls to an average of about 39. It follows that child-bearing has some influence upon the development of the growth. A married woman of 35 is twice as likely to develop carcinoma of the cervix as a virgin of the same age; if the married woman has borne children the risk is increased tenfold. All investigators are agreed that coitus is an important factor and to some extent quantitative. The earlier a woman has coitus, the more frequently she has it, and the more diverse the number of her sexual partners, the greater the risk of carcinoma. Amongst life-long celibate nuns it is an almost unknown disease whereas carcinoma of the endometrium occurs in these patients as frequently as in the married woman. It should be remembered that coitus is no longer the privilege or preserve of the married and that, when closely questioned, an unmarried patient with carcinoma of the cervix will often admit to frequent and sometimes promiscuous coitus.

Carcinoma of the cervix very rarely occurs in Jewesses, and its incidence is more common in working-class patients than in woman of the professional class. It is, therefore, suggested that early circumcision in the male and penile hygiene are important in aetiology. The obvious extension of this hypothesis is that smegma is carcinogenic and in lower animals this has been experimentally demonstrated. Wynder found that of women exposed to circumcised males, the incidence of carcinoma of the cervix was only a little less than in those exposed to the uncircumcised, 40% as against 60%. These figures can hardly be considered as significantly supporting the carcinogenic role of smegma. Scarring of the cervix as a result of childbirth, chronic cervicitis, particularly with ectropion, and chronic discharge are generally regarded as contributory factors, although they should not be considered precancerous conditions. The age-incidence is shown in the following graph:

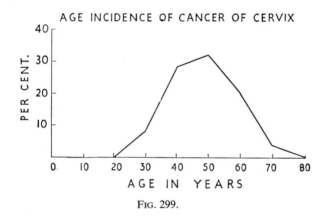

FIG. 299.

The incidence of carcinoma developing after subtotal hysterectomy varies from 0·1 to 1% according to different authorities. These figures, however, take no account of parity and represent the total incidence in all cases.

Pathology

It is customary to identify two groups of carcinoma of the cervix. In the first, the carcinoma arises from the squamous epithelium covering the vaginal portion of the cervix (Figs. 303 and 304). In the second the carcinoma develops from the mucous membrane of the cervical canal, and is referred to as endocervical carcinoma (Fig. 302). Endocervical carcinoma is less common than carcinoma of the vaginal portion in a ratio of 1 to 5. Histologically, endocervical cancers are more often squamous celled than adenocarcinomata in spite of their site of origin and this fact is often puzzling to the student. Only one cervical cancer in twenty is an adenocarcinoma; only one endocervical cancer out of four is an adenocarcinoma. Growths which arise from the squamous epithelium covering the portio vaginalis are squamous epitheliomata. It should be remembered, however, that the normal squamous epithelium covering the portio vaginalis develops by metaplasia from transitional epithelium during intrauterine life. Perhaps because of this, the squamous-celled growths of the cervix are often densely cellular. Pure adenocarcinoma of the cervix arises from the mucous membrane of the

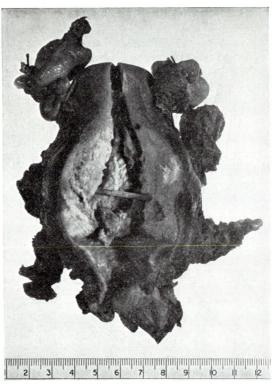

FIG. 300. Advanced carcinoma of the cervix removed by extended Wertheim's operation. The cervix has been completely replaced by growth that is infiltrating the vaginal vault and extending into the corpus above. The patient is alive and well 15 years later.

cervical canal, but this histological picture is rare and most cervical cancers are squamous in type; of all cervical cancers 94·5% as against 5·5% are squamous according to Martzloff. This preponderance of squamous cancers is in part explained by the tendency of the endocervical epithelium to undergo squamous metaplasia and this tendency increases with age. Some degree of squamous metaplasia can be found in nearly 50% of all cervices if these are submitted to careful histological examination. A similar squamous metaplasia is frequently seen in mucous polypi of the cervix.

Carcinoma of the vaginal portion of the cervix assumes one of three

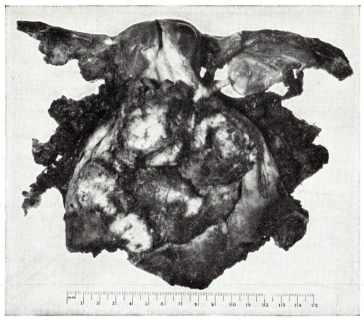

FIG. 301. Proliferative carcinoma of cervix. Note the large mass of growth replacing the cervix and distending the upper vagina.

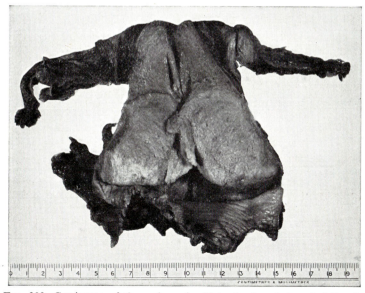

FIG. 302. Carcinoma of the endocervix. Note the barrel-shaped deformity of the cervical canal.

20*

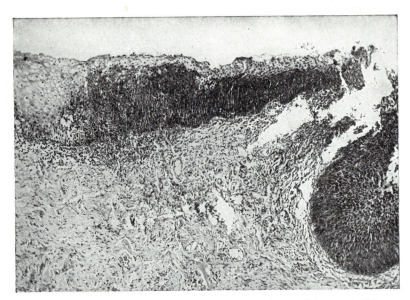

FIG. 303. The margin of an early squamous carcinoma of the cervix. Note normal epithelium on left and infiltrating carcinoma on right.

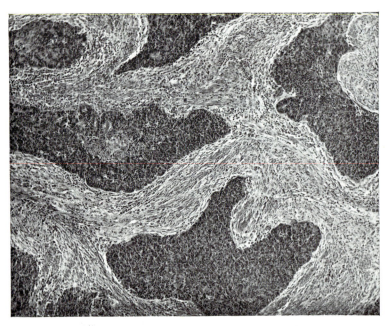

FIG. 304. Invasive squamous carcinoma of the cervix.

clinical types. It takes the form of a proliferating cauliflower-like growth which projects into the vagina (Fig. 301), it may develop as an excavating ulcer, or it assumes the form of a raised flat induration. The cauliflower or exophytic growths are very vascular and produce profuse vaginal bleeding, and, because of infection and necrosis, lead to an offensive vaginal discharge. The excavating or endophytic form does not lead to such profuse haemorrhage, the main symptom being bloodstained discharge. The tumours can be graded histologically by the appearance of the cancer cells, the cells being undifferentiated in the most malignant growths, while in the mature forms there is a tendency to develop epithelial pearls (Fig. 305). Martzloff has introduced a classification which must be mentioned since it is in common

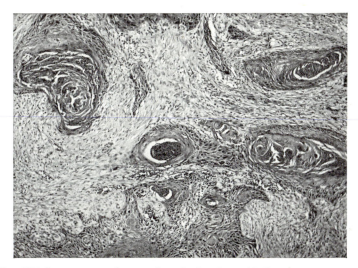

FIG. 305. Squamous carcinoma of cervix showing epithelial pearls. ($\times$ 52.)

pathological usage. This classification is based upon the cell type seen in different zones of the squamous epithelium:

(a) **The spinal cell cancer** resembles in its histological appearance the cells of the superficial layers of the epithelium. The cells possess large nuclei and the cytoplasm is abundant. Keratinisation and epithelial pearl formation may be seen. This type of cancer is, therefore, relatively mature, well differentiated and of lower malignancy than the following. The frequency of this type is 15% (Fig. 306).

(b) **The transitional cell cancer** resembles the cellular pattern of the intermediate layers of the squamous epithelium. The nuclei are more deeply basophilic, and pyknotic and the cytoplasm is scanty. The shape of the cell is rounded and there are no epithelial pearls or keratinisation. This is the commonest variety (66·8%). Its malignancy is intermediate between the spinal and the spindle cell cancers (Fig. 307).

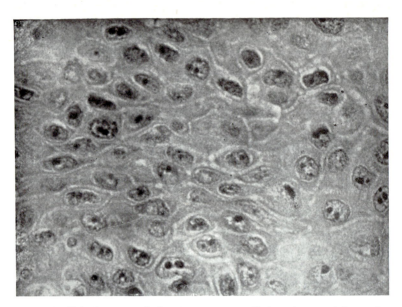

Fig. 306. Spinal cancer cells from a squamous-celled carcinoma of the cervix uteri. (Maliphant, from Macleod and Read's "Gynaecology".)

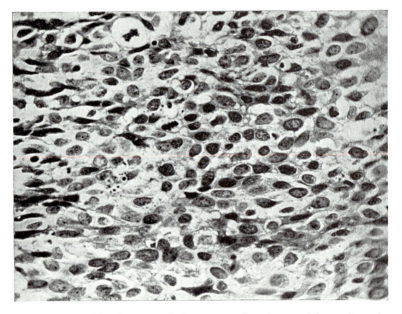

Fig. 307. Transitional cancer cells from a case of carcinoma of the cervix uteri. (Maliphant, from Macleod and Read's "Gynaecology".)

(c) **The spindle cell cancer** is the rarest (12%) and most malignant. The name aptly describes the cell shape which somewhat resembles a sarcoma. The cells have dark-staining nuclei and little cytoplasm. It has been suggested that they are derived from the basal layer of the epithelium (Fig. 308).

The remaining 6% are adenocarcinomata.

Difficulty is often experienced in distinguishing early carcinoma from erosions of the cervix. With carcinoma of the cervix, instead of the squamous epithelium of the portio being represented by a basal layer of cubical cells, a middle-celled layer of prickle cells and a superficial layer of horny cells, there is no orderly arrangement and prickle cells may not be demonstrated.

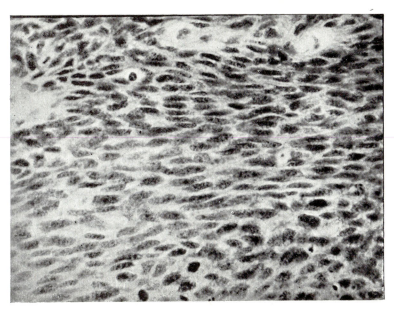

Fig. 308. Spindle cancer cells. From a case of carcinoma cervicis uteri. (Maliphant, from Macleod and Read's "Gynaecology".)

The cancer cells differ amongst themselves in size, shape and staining properties, and show active mitosis. Lastly, there is no orderly arrangement with respect to the subjacent tissues, so that the cancer cells penetrate irregularly into the subjacent stroma (see Figs. 306–308).

Mode of Spread

The primary site of origin of a cervical cancer is almost invariably at the squamo-columnar junction where the squamous epithelium of the portio vaginalis merges into the columnar epithelium of the endocervical canal. The growth may extend by direct spread, by lymphatic permeation, by the blood stream, and lastly by implantation.

Direct Spread. Direct spread is best represented by involvement of the vagina. In autopsy material the vagina is found to be infiltrated in about 86%

of cases, and with advanced growths the carcinoma may spread far down the vaginal walls. When the growth involves the upper part of the anterior vaginal wall, it can easily reach the bladder so that a vesicovaginal fistula is a frequent complication in late cases. On the other hand, involvement of the rectum is much rarer, for the growth must track down the posterior vaginal wall beyond the lower level of Douglas's pouch before the rectum can be infiltrated (see Fig. 309).

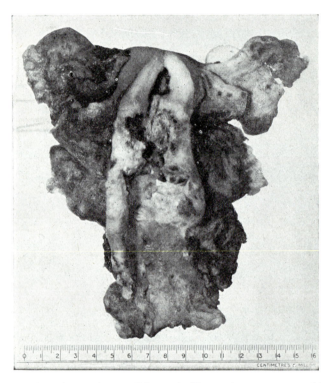

FIG. 309. Ulcerative carcinoma of the cervix. The specimen was removed by the operation of synchronous combined hysterocolpectomy. Note that the cervix has been almost entirely eroded by the growth. Note also the extent of the parametrium and paracolpos removed by this method.

Quite often the growth spreads upwards and involves first the upper part of the cervix and may then reach the body of the uterus infiltrating either the endometrium or myometrium. Involvement of the body of the uterus is necessarily more frequent with endocervical carcinoma.

Involvement of the Fallopian tubes and ovaries is very rare, in fact, ovarian metastasis in cervical cancer is said to occur only once in a hundred patients.

The parametrium is usually infiltrated quite early. Probably in the early stages the cancer cells permeate along the lymphatics which lie in Macken-rodt's and the uterosacral ligaments, and by eroding through the lymphatic channels involve the parametrium. In late stages the growth spreads directly into the parametrium and causes fixation of the uterus. The involvement of the parametrium is detected clinically by fixity of the uterus and by palpating the parametrium by rectal examination. When the involvement of the uterosacral ligaments is extensive the bowel may be partially or completely obstructed.

The bladder is involved in the majority of late stages, the growth extending either directly from the supravaginal portion of the cervix or after it has involved the upper part of the anterior vaginal wall. First the patient complains of frequency and pain on micturition, then cystitis and haematuria

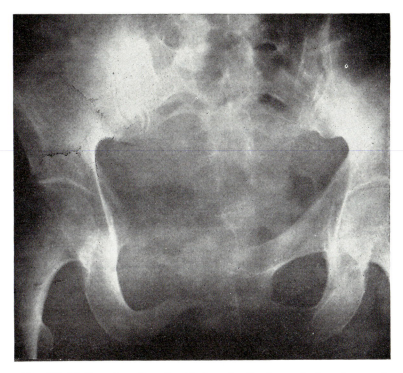

Fig. 310. Malignant erosion of pubic bone by direct spread of carcinoma of cervix.

occur, and lastly a vesicovaginal fistula develops, with incontinence of urine. The ureters become involved when the growth invades the parametrium, and occlusion of the ureters leads to the development of hydronephrosis and ascending infections of the urinary tract. 60% of those who die with carcinoma of the cervix die from uraemia as the result of invasion of the urinary tract with subsequent urinary infection.

The clinical extent of a cervical cancer is interpreted by placing the growth into one of five stages:—

Stage O   Carcinoma in situ.
Stage I   Confined to cervix.

Stage II   Spread to uterosacral and Mackenrodt's ligament and/or upper
              third of vagina.
Stage III   Fixation to pelvic wall and/or lower two-thirds of vagina with
              no cancer-free area between the cervix and the pelvic wall.
Stage IV   Involvement of bladder or rectum or distant extrapelvic
              metastases.

It will be found to be helpful and instructive if the clinical limits of the
growth are mapped out on the chart illustrated (see Fig. 311). If the patient is
subsequently treated by operation a second chart should be filled in. This
includes the pelvic glands. A comparison of the clinical and pathological
charts will often show considerable variation between the true (pathological)
extent and the presumed (clinical) findings.

Lymphatic Permeation. The lymphatic drainage of the cervix is to the small
glands in the parametrium, and thence to the obturator, external iliac and
hypogastric glands. The hypogastric glands which are particularly involved

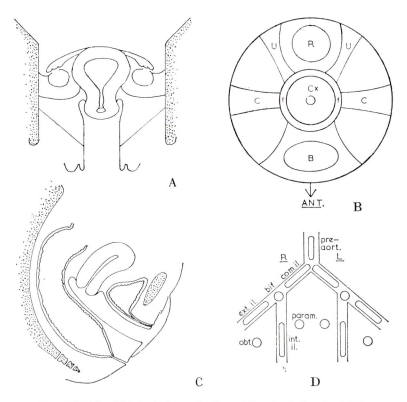

FIG. 311. After histological examination of the glands the chart D is

                    marked as follows: present–clear   :
                                          present–involved:

are those which lie below the level of the bifurcation of the common iliac artery. In carcinoma of the cervix the glands may be involved early in the course of the disease, and as they cannot be palpated by bimanual examination it may be difficult to determine how extensive the growth may be, except

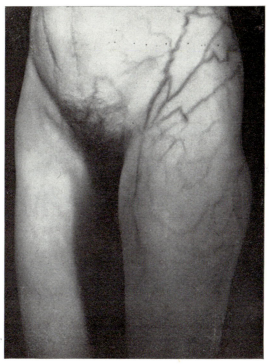

FIG. 312. Left-sided venous obstruction due to a mass of malignant glands occluding the left common iliac vein.

by abdominal operation. It is rare for the aortic and lumbar glands to be infiltrated with growth, most patients dying before the growth extends beyond the pelvis (see Tables V and VI and Fig. 312).

In some advanced cancers of the cervix the malignant cells spread down the anterior vaginal wall deep to the epithelium and finally ulcerate through

TABLE V. *Node Involvement*

Total operations	138
Iliac adenectomies	38
Wertheim's hysterectomies, laparotomies, etc. . .	100
Node-involved cases	74 (53·5%)
Node-free cases	64

TABLE VI.   *Groups of Nodes Involved*

	Right	Left	Total
Parametrial	5	1	6
Obturator	31	41	72
External iliac	39	44	83
Hypogastric	11	11	22
Iliac biurcation	18	17	35
Common iliac	22	17	39
Aortic	11	13	24
Inguinal*	1	2	3

* Inguinal nodes not removed as a routine.

the skin in the region of the vestibule. These distant vaginal metastases are attributed to retrograde lymphatic or venous spread.

Blood Stream. As the venous drainage of the cervix belongs to the systemic and not to the portal system, metastases in the liver in carcinoma of the cervix are relatively uncommon. It is exceptional for carcinoma of the

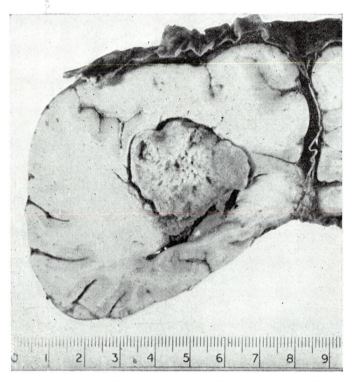

FIG. 313. Metastasis of carcinoma of cervix in lateral ventricle of brain.

cervix to spread by way of the blood stream except with anaplastic growths when metastases are found in lungs, liver, bone and kidneys (see Fig. 313).

Metastases in distant organs are found in about 50% of patients at autopsy. At operation, as opposed to autopsy material, it is rare, however, unless the growth is advanced, to find dissemination of the carcinoma outside the pelvis (see Fig. 314).

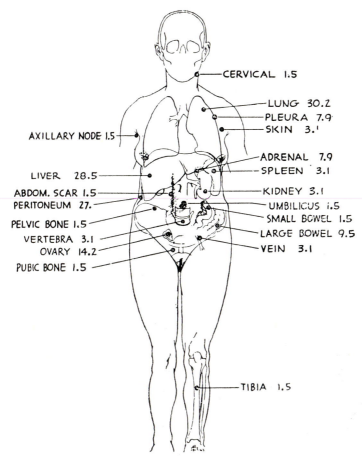

CERVICAL 1.5
LUNG 30.2
PLEURA 7.9
SKIN 3.1
AXILLARY NODE 1.5
ADRENAL 7.9
SPLEEN 3.1
LIVER 28.5
ABDOM. SCAR 1.5
KIDNEY 3.1
PERITONEUM 27.
UMBILICUS 1.5
SMALL BOWEL 1.5
PELVIC BONE 1.5
LARGE BOWEL 9.5
VERTEBRA 3.1
OVARY 14.2
VEIN 3.1
PUBIC BONE 1.5
TIBIA 1.5

FIG. 314. Sites and incidence of metastases from carcinoma of cervix. (Henriksen, *Amer. J. Obst. & Gyn.*)

Symptoms

There are four main symptoms of carcinoma of the cervix, namely: haemorrhage, discharge, cachexia and pain. By far the most important of these is haemorrhage. Other symptoms develop in late stages, but are not so important in diagnosis, for by then the recognition of carcinoma of the cervix offers no difficulty.

Haemorrhage. The typical haemorrhage in carcinoma of the cervix is superimposed upon normal menstrual bleeding, so that in the early stages the woman can distinguish that in addition to her normal menstruation she has irregular haemorrhage. In most instances the haemorrhage follows coitus and takes the form of a trickle of blood which may persist for several days. Strains and other exertions may initiate the haemorrhage which tends to persist for a longer time the more advanced the growth becomes. Vaginal bleeding in women of post-menopausal age should always be suspected as being caused by carcinoma of the cervix, and all parous women with inter-menstrual bleeding of any type or with any form of vaginal bleeding super-imposed upon normal menstruation should always be examined vaginally to exclude the presence of carcinoma of the cervix. This examination should, without exception, include cytological screening as described in Chapter 4, p. 133. Women expect some irregularity of the menses when they reach meno-pausal age and are apt to regard any irregular bleeding as being due to the menopause. In consequence they are reluctant to be examined vaginally, but medical practitioners should insist upon a careful vaginal examination, both digital and visual, to exclude the presence of carcinoma of the cervix. The normal menopause consists of a gradual diminution of flow, duration and frequency of the periods and all patients showing deviation from this standard should be examined to eliminate a genital tract cancer. As with most forms of carcinoma early cases respond well to treatment, whereas with late cases the possibility of obtaining permanent cure or even some measure of relief is small. The cauliflower type of growth is usually very vascular and is apt to bleed vigorously on touch, or even with speculum examination. If *severe* vaginal bleeding follows upon simple digital examination of the cervix it is almost certain that the patient has a carcinoma. With endophytic growths and those which are scirrhous in type, bleeding is not a well-marked symptom, and some patients may complain only of an offensive discharge, but these patients are few. Sometimes the vaginal bleeding is considerable and a severe degree of anaemia results, but it is very rare for the haemorrhage to be fatal. The source of the haemorrhage is the dilated capillaries of the vascular growth. Finally it should be emphasised that any woman in the cancerous era, who has irregular or post-menopausal bleeding and whose clinical examination is unsatisfactory should be submitted to a thorough examination under an anaesthetic including biopsy of the endocervical canal and endo-metrium—so-called fractional or differential curettage.

Discharge. The vaginal discharge in carcinoma of the cervix is blood-stained and has a characteristic offensive odour. The discharge originates from necrotic areas on the surface of the growth, and the degree to which it is bloodstained depends partly on the vascularity of the carcinoma and partly upon trauma. With endophytic growths offensive vaginal discharge is often a more dominant feature than irregular haemorrhage. In women of post-menopausal age a watery vaginal discharge may be complained of as an early symptom.

Cachexia. Cachexia is well marked in advanced growths. The woman is anaemic and shows symptoms and signs of incipient uraemia, with loss of appetite, headaches, and sickness. Weight loss is obvious and sometimes extreme.

Pain. Pain is nearly always a late symptom. If the growth infiltrates the parametrium, some degree of parametritis is usual. If the glands below the bifurcation of the common iliac artery are extensively infiltrated with carcinoma, the obturator nerve becomes involved and the woman develops referred pain in the knee and along the inner side of the thigh. If the bladder is infiltrated with growth, urinary symptoms and pelvic pain develop, while in advanced cases if the carcinoma spreads laterally and backwards to the pelvic wall, the sacral plexus may be infiltrated with growth, with resultant pain along the back of the thighs. It should be emphasised that the presence of pain has no value whatsoever in the diagnosis of operable cancer of the cervix. There is one notable exception to this dictum. A pyometra may result from stenosis and blockage of the cervical canal whereby the uterine cavity becomes infected. A pyometra produces fever and constitutional signs, raised white count and a painful tender, slightly enlarged uterine body. Pyometra should always be suspected with this clinical picture and the diagnosis is obvious on dilatation of the cervix when pus, usually blood-stained, readily escapes.

Other symptoms arise in late cases, such as painful and frequent micturition, incontinence of urine due to vesicovaginal fistula, painful defaecation because of proctitis and obstruction and pruritus because of vaginal discharge.

Physical Signs

Just as there are four main symptoms of carcinoma of the cervix, so there are four main physical signs. In the first place the cervix bleeds on touch, secondly, it is friable, thirdly, the cervix is fixed and has lost its mobility either due to malignant infiltration of the parametrium or because of the invariable parametritis due to the infection, and fourthly, there is induration either of the cervix itself or, in advanced cases, of the surrounding structures.

In most cases digital examination of the cervix is followed by **profuse vaginal bleeding.** The bleeding is particularly well marked when the growth is of the cauliflower type, but with endophytic tumours the bleeding is not so severe although it always arises if the examining finger is pressed firmly into the growth. The bleeding is caused by trauma, small capillaries being opened when the growth is damaged by the examining finger. Scirrhous tumours are less friable and not so vascular as exophytic growths. Bleeding on examination is a physical sign not restricted to carcinoma of the cervix. It is present with vascular erosions, mucous polypi, myomatous polypi, and retained products of conception, but only with the last is it comparably profuse.

The carcinomatous area is **friable,** but again the degree of friability depends upon the type of growth, the exfoliating or exophytic forms being easily broken up by the examining finger while hard scirrhous endophytic tumours are less friable. If the cervix is examined with a speculum it will be found that a blunt probe can be pushed into the tissues of the growth while the healthy non-malignant tissues of the cervix are resistant. The more friable the growth the more bleeding follows the examination. Friability is one of the most important signs of carcinoma of the cervix. Myomatous polypi are not friable, mucous polypi and vascular erosions are not broken up by the examining finger, but retained products of conception projecting through the cervical canal are as friable as vascular cauliflower growths of the cervix.

The third sign, **loss of mobility** due to infection or malignant parametrial permeation, is always appreciable to the examining finger. The normally mobile cervix has lost its mobility and on passing a speculum a vascular ulcerating growth of the cervix is apparent. In advanced cases the superficial parts of the growth become necrotic so that minute grey sloughs are scattered over the surface of the tumour. Obvious infection of a cervical growth is not of itself diagnostic of a carcinoma, though in combination with bleeding, fixity and induration it is most suggestive. It should be remembered, however, that the lower pole of a myomatous polypus is usually infected and necrotic, and the rare growth, grape-like sarcoma of the cervix, has a similar appearance. Retained products of conception are nearly always infected if they project through the cervical canal. Apart from grape-like sarcoma an infected myomatous polypus or retained products of gestation are not associated with fixity of the cervix.

The fourth sign is **induration.** In advanced carcinoma of the cervix there is well-marked induration of the cervix and surrounding tissues, so that the cervix is fixed. In early cases the induration may be difficult to detect, particularly if the growth is of the exophytic type. The induration may be detected in the parametrium, particularly along the uterosacral ligaments when a rectal examination is made.

In advanced cases other physical signs may develop. The growth may extend along the vaginal walls or it may extend forwards towards the base of the bladder, when a firm induration may be detected above the level of the anterior fornix. Cystoscopic examination of the bladder is an essential part of the investigation of any case of cancer of the cervix, and this becomes imperative if there are any urinary complications such as pyuria or haematuria. If a vesico-vaginal fistula has developed there is incontinence of urine, and urine may be seen trickling down the vagina. It is rare for affected lymphatic glands to be palpable either by abdominal or bimanual examination. If the growth has extended far along the uterosacral ligaments a rectal examination will demonstrate this induration, and in very advanced cases there may be some degree of stenosis of this part of the bowel. It has already been pointed out that it is rare for metastases to be found above the level of the pelvic brim. The metastases which form at the vulva by retrograde spread along the lymphatics which lie deep to the anterior vaginal wall are only seen in advanced cases.

With endocervical carcinoma the cervix is expanded and firm and the characteristic feature is its barrel shape. Often the external os is dilated so that the finger placed in the cervical canal palpates the friable growth. At other times, although the external os is closed, the growth may advance downwards and be visibly infiltrating the tissues around the external os. Haemorrhage always follows bimanual examination in endocervical cancer.

The general signs of anaemia and cachexia are found only with advanced growths.

Diagnosis

The history given by the patient should lead to the suspicion of the presence of a carcinoma of the cervix, and it is important always to examine the patient carefully and not to dismiss her as merely suffering from irregular menstruation. As in all branches of medicine, mistakes in diagnosis are usually due to incomplete investigations and to this day, although succeeding generations of medical students have had impressed upon them the importance of examining suspected patients vaginally, a fair percentage of those with carcinoma of the cervix who are sent up to hospital have received previous conservative treatment from their medical practitioners for several weeks before it is decided that a vaginal examination is necessary. Unless a practitioner has considerable skill in gynaecological practice he should always suspect carcinoma of the cervix in any woman with irregular vaginal bleeding. As a general rule, the diagnosis is made without difficulty if the cervix is examined both digitally and visually. Cytological examination is now almost obligatory and while providing additional evidence of malignancy it is never to be regarded as a substitute for a thorough clinical examination. A negative smear may be reassuring but it is never infallible. Many women who present the symptoms of cervical cancer avoid consulting their doctor for various reasons, such as fear, modesty, ignorance, prejudice and a conviction that irregular menopausal bleeding, or even post-menopausal bleeding is an inevitable accompaniment of the change of life. At least half the patients with cervical cancer behave in this way.

If a carcinoma of the cervix is suspected, a vaginal examination should be made and the cervix examined for the signs of bleeding on examination, friability, infection and induration. Next, the cervix should be examined with a speculum and tested for friability with a blunt-pointed probe, if there is any doubt about the diagnosis. If the diagnosis of carcinoma of the cervix is made, the next step is to make a rectal examination and to palpate the uterosacral ligaments to determine the degree of involvement, either by carcinoma or by inflammation. The mobility of the uterus, detected by bimanual examination, will indicate the degree to which the surrounding structures, particularly the bladder and parametrium, are infiltrated by the growth. The body of the uterus should be identified if possible. If it is found to be enlarged, the possibility of the presence of a pyometra should always be borne in mind. In some cases of carcinoma of the cervix the growth produces stenosis of the cervical canal and the cavity of the uterus collects secretions which become infected and lead to the formation of a pyometra. If a pyometra is suspected its presence should be excluded before resorting to radium treatment, because the radium emanations are apt to lead to an ascending extension of the intrauterine sepsis with resultant and often quite severe pelvic peritonitis. In some clinics the bacteriology of the cervical discharge is investigated before radium treatment, and systemic chemotherapy may be used.

It is very important to determine whether there is involvement of the urinary tract in a case of carcinoma of the cervix, for the prognosis depends to a great degree upon the extent to which the bladder and ureters are involved in the growth. If the bladder is infiltrated a history of frequent, painful micturition with pyuria or haematuria may be obtained. All patients should be investigated by cystoscopic examination before operative treatment is decided upon. If the bladder is infiltrated with growth the earliest sign of involvement is the development of a bullous oedema at the base of the bladder. In more advanced cases a depression forms, due to contraction of the growth in this situation, while in late cases the growth can be seen by cystoscopy to ulcerate directly into the bladder. In every carcinoma of the cervix an intravenous pyelogram must be performed before any operative or radiation treatment is considered. The presence of ureteric obstruction affecting one or both kidneys profoundly alters the prognosis and may well be the determining factor in the line of treatment adopted (see Table VII).

TABLE VII.   *Extent of Tumour and Renal Lesions.*

	Total cases	Abnormal pyelograms
Stage I	37	3 (8·3%)
Stage II	75	15 (20%)
Stage III	17	12 (70%)
Stage IV	17	12 (70%)

It is also important to know the exact state of the urinary tract before treatment so that any operative or radiation damage involving the ureter or bladder can be fairly assessed. Pre-operative pyelography also provides a control for subsequent urological studies after treatment.

Diagnosis of Carcinoma of the Cervix in its Earliest Stages

One half of all patients suffering from cancer of the cervix present themselves for examination when the growth has already reached stage III or stage IV. This means that in half of the cases seen, the growth is already so advanced that the prognosis for complete cure is poor. Moreover, half of the patients who present themselves for treatment have already had irregular vaginal bleeding for as long as three months, while in a quarter of the patients seen, irregular haemorrhage has been present for at least six months. Apart from instruction to the general public, two methods of investigation have been introduced. The first is the method of vaginal smears introduced by Papanicolaou, Traut and Meigs. They have shown that after appropriate staining methods, simple vaginal smears taken with a pipette enable malignant cells to be identified in both carcinoma of the cervix and carcinoma of the body, though the diagnosis rate of the former is very much higher and more accurate than the latter, 98% to some 55%–60%. The staining of smears requires a special stain similar to Shorr's and the interpretation of the films requires considerable cytological knowledge and experience. An extension of this method is the surface biopsy using the special spatula described by Ayre and already referred to in a previous chapter. By this method of surface biopsy and by the use of vaginal smears a small number of clinically unsuspected cancers have been diagnosed and treated with excellent prognosis. The chief value of the method is that a positive smear demands a full cervical biopsy from which a definite histological diagnosis should be made. The method is also of great value as a follow-up check after irradiation by which radio-resistant cases can be diagnosed and treated surgically if active cancer cells are demonstrated.

The second method of attack is with the help of the colposcope by which the cervix is examined under high magnification with binocular vision (see p. 137). It is suggested that all women attending gynaecological out-patients should be examined in this way, and that suspected cases should be carefully followed up week by week if necessary. The original work was carried out by Hinselmann, who described three types of epithelium covering the vaginal portion of the cervix. In the first type the epithelium is squamous and stains brown with iodine. The second type is described as ectopic, when the epithelium is high columnar and is derived from the mucous membrane of the cervical canal. This ectopic epithelium is illustrated by the red areas of congenital and glandular erosions. The red epithelium becomes white after painting with acetic acid or 5% silver nitrate. With the help of the colposcope the mouths of the glands can be seen opening on to the red epithelium. In the third type the epithelium is unstable; squamous epithelium is replacing and growing over the columnar epithelium, and in this way small Nabothian follicles are being produced.

Atypical forms of epithelium can be recognised. Hyperkeratosis and lichenification are common and are seen well in cases of prolapse of the cervix. After a time the superficial horny cells of the leucoplakia areas are shed, leaving the basal area behind, which can be identified with the colposcope. The Schiller test can be performed with great exactness with the colposcope. Early or established carcinomatous areas are iodine-negative and this absence of staining is highly suggestive of malignancy, as are the irregular vascular patterns diagnostic of this condition, which are readily interpretable by the colposcope.

Carcinoma in Situ

Intra-epithelial Carcinoma, Pre-invasive Carcinoma, Cancer of the Cervix Stage O.

This is a lesion in which the whole thickness of the squamous epithelium is replaced by cells histologically resembling those of invasive cancer. Stratification of the cells is absent but there is no penetration beyond the basement membrane—hence the term intra-epithelial carcinoma. Careful observation of a number of patients, whose cervix has shown such a lesion, has demonstrated that in a few, about 30%, actual invasive cancer does eventually develop though it may be ten or more years before such a malignant change is frankly obvious. In other patients who have been carefully observed for several years the condition has been seen to regress.

There is no macroscopical lesion by which carcinoma *in situ* can be recognised on clinical examination and most cases will be discovered on routine section of a cervix removed for some other reason. Most of the patients have no symptoms. Bleeding after vaginal examination or coitus has been the reason for further examination in a small number. The average age for carcinoma *in situ* is 38 years as against 48 for true invasive cancer of the cervix, so that post-menopausal bleeding is unlikely to be a helpful symptom. Routine cytological screening of gynaecological outpatients and those attending Family Planning Clinics provide the most likely material for the diagnosis

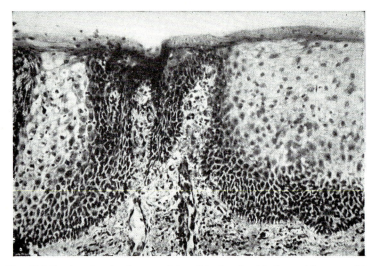

FIG. 315. Section showing hyperactivity of the basal epithelium with reasonably normal differentiation into the superficial layers. Ayre; "Cancer Cytology of the Uterus." Grune & Stratton Inc. (× 105).

of this otherwise symptomless condition. Absence of staining is of great value in indicating the most likely area for further histological investigation.

The histology of carcinoma *in situ* presents a difficult and debatable problem and in order to understand it a little the reader should be fully conversant with three histological pictures encountered in the cervix.

The first of these is epidermidisation of the columnar epithelium of the endocervix and its glands. This squamous metaplasia is found at all levels in the cervical canal and is particularly well marked in some cervical polypi. Nulliparous cervices are affected and there is no evidence that the lesion is in any way precancerous. The condition is found at almost any age and it is uncertain what part inflammation plays in its production. It is important to recognise this innocent lesion since the inexperienced histologist might regard it as precancerous or actually malignant.

The second condition has been termed basal-celled hyperactivity and is frequently seen at the edges of an erosion. The basal cells of the squamous epithelium are notably hyperplastic and may be many layers deep, occupying far more than their normal share of the epithelial thickness. Although the nuclei are hyperchromatic, mitotic figures are absent and the cells, all lying with their axes in one direction, retain their polarity (see Fig. 315).

The third condition is carcinoma *in situ*. In this the cells are anaplastic, mitotic figures are present, and the axial arrangement of the cells is haphazard; in other words polarity is lost. The cells are of varying sizes with hyperchromatic nuclei. Within the epithelium the picture is really indistinguishable from invasive cancer. There is no differentiation of the epithelium into its

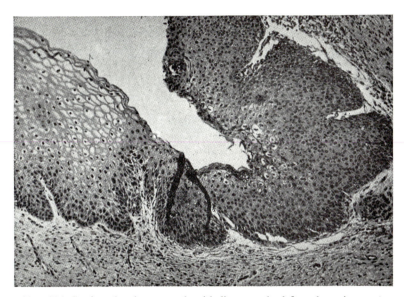

FIG. 316. Section showing normal epithelium on the left and carcinoma *in situ* on the right side of the picture. Ayre; "Cancer Cytology of the Uterus." Grune & Stratton Inc. (×110).

various layers and there is complete absence of the normal stratification. The basement membrane, however, is intact (see Fig. 316).

If these histological concepts are accepted the question next arises as to whether carcinoma *in situ* does develop into true invasive cancer. Novak, Te Linde and Galvin and several other American writers are convinced that it does in about 30% though an average of ten years may elapse in the process.

The treatment of carcinoma *in situ* is still somewhat controversial. As the disease is slow in its progress no hasty decision in favour of radical surgery is called for and this is certainly so in the case of younger patients who may desire children. In such patients the cervix should be treated by a thorough cone biopsy and the patient examined at three- to six-monthly intervals. A deterioration in the picture would call for total hysterectomy and the appearance of active invasion would indicate the same treatment as for a stage I carcinoma of the cervix.

In older women who have borne as many children as they desire a total hysterectomy with a reasonable cuff of the vaginal vault is the logical treatment.

Operability

As soon as a carcinoma of the cervix is suspected on clinical grounds, the diagnosis will be confirmed by surface biopsy and cytological examination which, again, must be confirmed by cold cone or knife biopsy. It is best to admit the patient for this examination so that the biopsy can be taken in optimum conditions. The surgeon then makes a thorough and planned examination of the pelvis and exactly maps out the extent of the growth as it appears to him at this time. His findings are recorded on the chart illustrated (Fig. 311). He is thus able to reach a reasonable conclusion as to what stage the cancer should be allocated and whether it is operable, suitable for radiation or, at worst, neither. Signs of inoperability are complete fixity of the cervix and parametrium to the lateral pelvic wall which is invaded by growth, extensive infiltration of the vagina, and the presence of extra-pelvic metastases. Moreover, the condition of the patient should be borne in mind. Fat women, old women, and patients with cardiovascular and chronic respiratory diseases are not ideal subjects for extensive abdominal operations.

Prognosis

The degree of spread of the growth will indicate the prognosis. The average duration of life with carcinoma of the cervix after the development of symptoms is about eighteen months. If the vagina is extensively involved, if a vesicovaginal fistula is present, or if there is evidence of ureteric obstruction and pyelonephritis, the prognosis is gloomy, whatever treatment is employed. On the other hand, in early cases, whether operative or radiotherapeutic treatment is chosen, the end-results are fairly good. Some cases, however, which seem favourable for radiotherapy do not necessarily respond well, and conversely, surprisingly good results may be obtained in advanced cases. Failure to respond to a full course of radiation treatment can be diagnosed by the surface biopsy method of Ayre or by actual biopsy of the tumour. The presence of active cancer cells, e.g. the persistence of mitotic activity, a high percentage of resting or potentially malignant cells, an unchanged percentage of degenerate or differentiating cells as compared with the original histological picture are all signs of insensitivity to radiation. These findings constitute a strong indication for surgical treatment. Efforts have been made to grade carcinoma of the cervix histologically and to compare the response of the different grades of tumours to radiological treatment. Broders was able to group together four grades of carcinoma of the cervix, Grade I being represented by tumours with cell nests and highly differentiated cells. In the fourth grade the cells are anaplastic in type. Little reliance is now placed upon the histological method of grading tumours with respect to their radio-sensitivity, and this method has been largely relegated to a purely academic importance.

Differential Diagnosis

It has already been stated that the diagnosis is established without difficulty as a rule if the patient is carefully examined. Moreover, the greater the experience of the practitioner the less likely is he to have difficulty in making a diagnosis. Nevertheless, certain conditions may produce rather similar pictures. In the first place, a chronically inflamed cervix with laceration and ectropion may cause discharge and bleeding and give an appearance rather similar to that of carcinoma of the cervix. An area of ectropion is, however, smooth and glistening and not friable. The ectropion may be associated with scarring of the vaginal wall as a result of laceration during childbirth, and the scarred area of the vaginal wall may be mistaken for the induration of carcinoma. If there is any doubt in making the diagnosis the practitioner should refer the case to an experienced surgeon for biopsy. The surface biopsy of Ayre and examination by the colposcope are of great value in assessing such a lesion. The most helpful feature of colposcopy is that the observer is enabled to designate the exact site on the cervix at which the biopsy must be taken. This localisation of the suspect area greatly enhances the accuracy of cancer diagnosis.

Schiller introduced a clinical test in which the cervix is painted with Lugol's solution. The healthy squamous epithelium covering the portio stains a deep brown, due to the glycogen content of its cells, while the high columnar epithelium of an eroded area does not alter its colour. If the area of carcinoma is infected or necrotic the cells do not stain with iodine, but before ulceration and infection the squamous carcinoma cells appear as grey areas, for they do not contain the glycogen-like substance possessed by normal vaginal epithelium. The test is suitable for suspect cases of early carcinoma of the cervix, but its main service is to exclude the presence of carcinoma in a suspicious erosion.

Sometimes difficulty is experienced in distinguishing between a cauli-flower-growth of the cervix and various forms of polypi. Mucous polypi do not often give rise to difficulty, because their surface is smooth and glistening. Old-standing mucous polypi, however, become covered with squamous epithelium by metaplasia of the original columnar epithelium and may project as firm vascular tumours from the cervix into the vagina.

It is rare, however, for such polypi to be ulcerated and they are seldom friable nor is the cervix fixed or indurated. Myomatous polypi are often ulcerated and may bleed on examination, but their consistence is firm and they have a characteristic spherical shape. A pedicle may be felt passing upwards through the cervical canal towards the cavity of the uterus.

Retained products of conception may project through the cervical canal and give rise to difficulty in diagnosis, as they bleed on examination, produce an offensive discharge, and are friable. A careful investigation of the history should help in establishing the diagnosis and a histological examination of a portion removed for section will confirm the clinical findings.

The rare tumour, grape-like sarcoma of the cervix, is diagnosed with precision only by histological examination. Sometimes carcinoma of the body of the uterus spreads downwards to involve the cervix, and may project through the external os. The distinction between an endocervical carcinoma and this form of growth is sometimes possible by a histological examination but this is largely an academic exercise since the treatment for both these types of cancer is the same.

Very great difficulty may be experienced in distinguishing between carcinoma of the cervix and a primary sore of the cervix, as a primary sore may resemble very closely an early carcinoma. A chancre, however, can occur anywhere on the portio and may not be necessarily related to the squamo-columnar junction. A chancre produces a rounded ulcer with a firm base and only slightly elevated edges. Smears should demonstrate the spirochaete. The diagnosis can be confirmed by histological examination of the portion removed. Later in the course of the disease secondary manifestations of syphilis will develop and the serological test will be positive.

Tuberculosis of the cervix is a very rare disease but it produces an appearance rather similar to that of carcinoma of the cervix. There is considerable tissue destruction and the typical tuberculous granulation tissue may be seen in the base of the ulcer, which is tough but not friable, unlike a malignant ulcer. Microscopical examination of the portion removed will establish the diagnosis.

Treatment of Carcinoma of the Cervix

The treatment of carcinoma of the cervix is either operative or by radiation. Advanced growths are unsuitable for operative treatment and the signs of operability have already been discussed. Extensive infiltration of the bladder, the presence of vesico-vaginal fistula, extensive infiltration of the vagina or parametrium, are usually contraindications to operative treatment, unless some form of exenteration is performed. The operations of radical hysterectomy and lymphadenectomy are difficult and extensive, so that unless the general condition of the patient is good, the primary mortality is of the order of 1–3%. At the present day it is customary to allocate carcinoma of the cervix into one of five stages, depending upon the degree of development of the growth.

Stage O. Intraepithelial, non-invasive carcinoma *in situ*.

Stage I. The growth is restricted to the cervix and the uterus is movable (see Figs. 317–320).

Stage II. The uterus retains some degree of mobility. The growth involves the parametrium but not as far as the pelvic wall and there is a definite cancer-free space between the parametrium and the pelvic wall. It may also spread downward to involve the upper one-third of vagina in the region of the fornices (see Figs. 321 and 322). This stage is sometimes divided into Stage II (parametrium) meaning that the parametrium is involved but the upper vaginal third is clear, or Stage II (vagina) in which the parametrium is clear but the upper third of the vagina is involved. Frequently the two subdivisions co-exist.

Stage III. The mobility of the uterus is restricted and the parametrium is infiltrated with growth. There is no cancer-free space between the parametrium and the pelvic wall which is actually infiltrated by the malignant

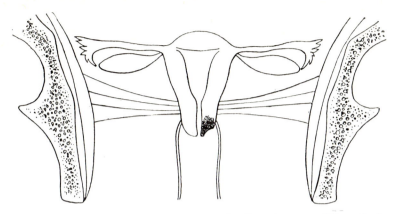

FIG. 317. Carcinoma of the cervix, Stage I. Ulcerating type. (Neuweiler.)

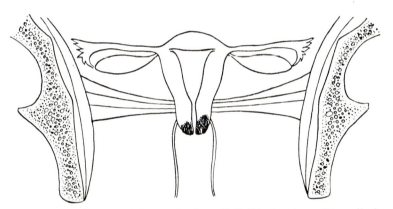

FIG. 318. Carcinoma of the cervix, Stage I. Infiltrating type. (Neuweiler.)

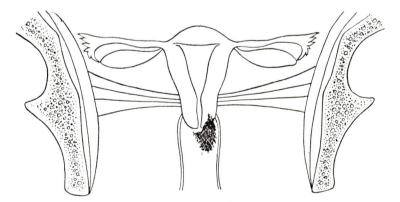

FIG. 319. Stage I. Cauliflower type.

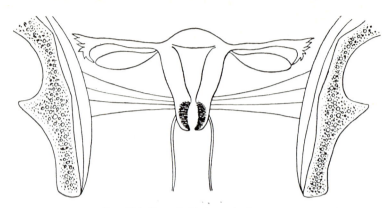

FIG. 320. Stage I. Endocervical type.

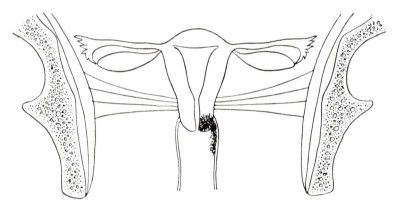

FIG. 321. Stage II. Infiltration of the vagina.

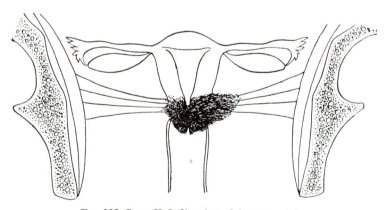

FIG. 322. Stage II. Infiltration of the parametrium.

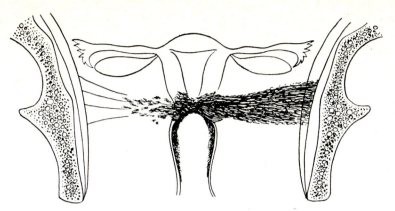

FIG. 323. Stage III. Infiltration of the parametrium together with the whole of the vagina. Fixity of the parametrium by malignant invasion into the pelvic wall.

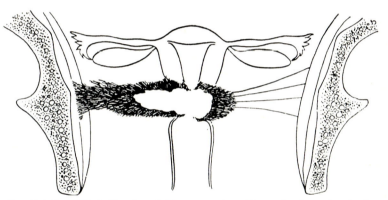

FIG. 324. Stage III. Infiltration of the parametrium. The vagina is not involved.

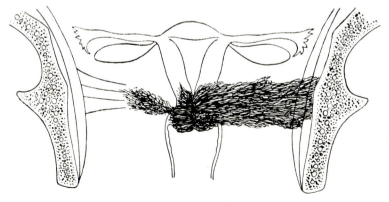

FIG. 325. Carcinoma of the cervix, Stage III. Infiltration of the parametrium as far as the periosteum, but not through it. (Neuweiler.)

process. The vagina is extensively infiltrated and metastases may be present
in the lower two-thirds of the vagina, but not beyond the introitus (see Figs.
323, 324 and 325).

Stage IV. The uterus is fixed, both parametria are infiltrated to the pelvic
walls and the growth involves the bladder and/or the rectum, and the whole
of the vagina. The presence of extra pelvic metastases also places the carcinoma in Stage IV, even if the primary growth is not advanced beyond, say,
Stage II (see Fig. 326).

The classification is imperfect as all such classifications must be, but so far
as the practitioner is concerned, it indicates to him how cases can be graded

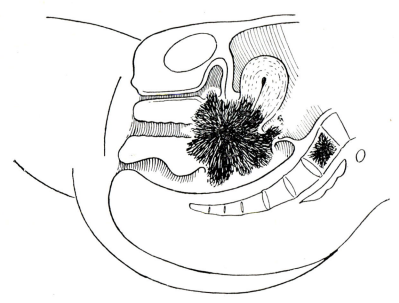

Fig. 326. Carcinoma of the cervix, Stage IV. Infiltration into the rectum
and bladder, together with bone metastases. (Neuweiler.)

according to the extent of the growth. It is obvious that Stage I and Stage II
cases may be operable; while Stage III or Stage IV cases are unlikely to be
cured by any ordinary operation, though some form of exenteration may be
considered if radiation treatment is contraindicated, e.g. by vesicovaginal
fistula.

The operability rate depends upon other factors than the degree of development of the growth. The patient may be a bad subject for surgery. She may
be fat or have chronic cardiovascular or respiratory disease. Also, the majority
of gynaecological surgeons would refrain from operating upon a woman
advanced in years however early the growth might be unless her general
condition was otherwise excellent. Modern anaesthesia, chemotherapy and
pre- and post-operative treatment have greatly extended the scope of surgery.

With surgery the extended abdominal hysterectomy perfected by Wertheim is the operation of choice in this country, although complicated vaginal hysterectomies are still employed on the Continent. Statistics show that whatever method of treatment is employed, whether radiotherapy, Wertheim's operation, or extended vaginal hysterectomy, the percentage of five-year cures is similar, so that so far as end-results are concerned with a consecutive series of patients there is little to choose between the individual methods. With early operable cases good results are obtained both by surgery and by radiotherapy, but radiotherapy has a smaller mortality compared with surgery. It should be remembered that radiotherapeutic techniques are constantly improving whereas the scope of surgical development has reached its acme. For these reasons the modern tendency it to employ radiotherapy which combines local applications of radium with deep X-ray therapy to the pelvis rather than surgery, except in certain cases to be discussed later, e.g. those in which lymphatic glandular involvement is likely.

The best radiotherapeutic figures are those published by Kottmeier of Stockholm for 1949 and 1950:

Stage I . . . . . 89·9% 5-year cure rate
Stage II . . . . . 52·8% 5-year cure rate

For adenocarcinoma of the cervix the figures are slightly inferior for Stage I, 73·2%. These figures represent the highest achievement so far obtained by radiotherapy.

The best comparable surgical figures are those published by J. V. Meigs from Boston, Massachusetts:

Stage I . . . . . 81·8% 5-year cure rate
Stage II . . . . . 61·8% 5-year cure rate

His series is small, only 100 cases, but it represents the best that surgery can achieve. Similar figures have been presented in this country by Currie of Leeds.

A comparison of these two sets of figures shows that the best radiation and the best surgical results in Stage I and Stage II are similar. In a large series of cases the primary operative mortality would slightly favour radiation and the morbidity, e.g., from urinary complications such as ureteric fistulae (7% in Meigs' cases) would further favour radiation.

One great argument in favour of surgery is the question of an involved lymphatic field. According to Meigs, radiation cannot sterilise an involved lymphatic gland though Kottmeier doubts this contention. According to Dobbie of Birmingham 15% of Stage I cases have involved glands and 47% of Stage II. This may account for Meigs' results from surgery in Stage II being slightly better than Kottmeier's, and Dobbie's figure of 47% involved glands in Stage II cases almost exactly corresponds with the salvage rate from radiation of 52·8% in Kottmeier's figures. Surgery on the other hand can and does cure cases with involved glands though the 5-year cure rate is halved when the glands are malignant—22% as against 53% of gland-free cases in Bonney's series, and 32·9% as against 65·2% gland-free cases from the Royal Prince Alfred Hospital, Sydney. As it is impossible to know whether the glands are involved or not by any known clinical test, this fact provides ammunition for the surgical argument. In fact some gynaecologists now employ a bilateral lymphadenectomy as a routine after a full course of radiotherapy, in order to eradicate any actual or potential gland metastases. This operation represents a logical step forward in the attack on the gland-involved case. The introduction of new and improved methods of super-voltage therapy offers a promising method of attack on the cancer-involved glands. Blaikley and in America Morton do believe that radiation can deliver

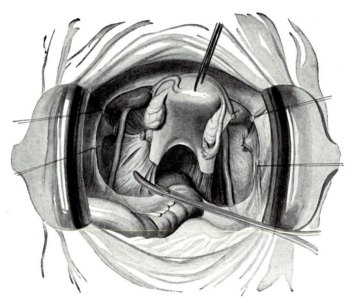

FIG. 327. Wertheim's operation. After division of the uterine vessels and the dissection of the ureters, the peritoneum of Douglas's pouch is divided, the uterus pulled forwards, and the uterosacral ligaments clamped and divided. (Peham-Amreich.)

a cancericidal dose to malignant glands in the pelvic wall and this is supported by Kottmeier. If their contentions are supported, the five-year salvage rate of cancer of the cervix will have advanced a further notable step.

Wertheim's Operation. The operation should be restricted to early cases and the signs of operability have already been described. One of the great advantages of the method is that an opportunity is afforded of inspecting and palpating the lymphatic glands in the pelvis. The vaginal operation for carcinoma of the cervix does not allow the lymphatic glands to be palpated or removed, for which reason it has never found favour with British surgeons.

Preoperative treatment consists in improving the general health, by blood transfusion if the patient is anaemic, by local antiseptic douching or applications, and systemic chemotherapy in an endeavour to limit or control the sepsis. Extradural anaesthesia gives a better exposure, because of complete relaxation, than inhalation anaesthesia, and some form of hypotensive anaesthesia is also a great help in ensuring a bloodless field of operation.

The patient is placed in the Trendelenberg position and the abdomen opened by a long subumbilical median incision and the pelvis examined for metastases and the mobility of the uterus determined. A search is made for extra-pelvic metastases, e.g. involved aortic glands. If the case is inoperable the abdomen is closed. If operation is undertaken the uterovesical fold of peritoneum is first incised and the bladder separated from the cervix. If the

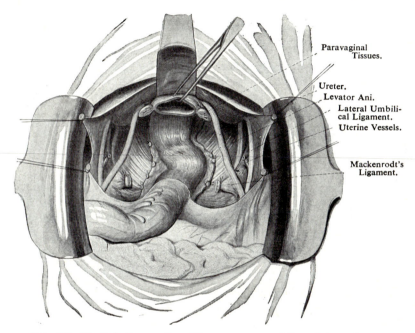

Paravaginal Tissues.

Ureter.
Levator Ani.
Lateral Umbilical Ligament.
Uterine Vessels.

Mackenrodt's Ligament.

Fig. 328. Wertheim's operation. The appearance of the pelvis at the completion of the operation before covering the raw area with peritoneum. The ureters, rectum and bladder have been cleared of the pelvic cellular tissue, and the ligaments have been divided. (Peham-Amreich.)

bladder is extensively involved it is best to stop the operation and close the abdomen, unless an anterior exenteration is to be performed. This consists of bilateral uretero-intestinal implantation and removal of the bladder as well as the uterus and upper vagina. After the separation of the bladder the infundibulo-pelvic folds and the round ligaments are divided between clamps as in pan-hysterectomy, and then the uterus is pulled forcibly to one side. The next step consists in dissecting out the ureters from the parametrium as far as the point at which they enter the bladder. The uterine arteries are now clamped and divided close to their origin, the ureters retracted out of the way and the parametrium and uterosacral ligaments divided as far from the uterus as is possible. The bladder is separated from the vagina as far down as possible and the vagina cut through below the level of a special clamp placed on the mobilised vagina. The amount of vagina removed should always be the upper half at least and, if the vagina is infiltrated as in Stage II, a greater length of vagina must be removed—two-thirds. The purpose of using this clamp is to prevent septic material from being disseminated over the raw area in the pelvis and also to reduce the possibility of the development of implantation deposits from the cervical growth. All lymphatic glands along the internal iliac vessels and below the bifurcation of the common iliac artery are now removed, as well as the external iliac glands. It is best to drain the raw area into the vagina by packing with gauze. The raw area

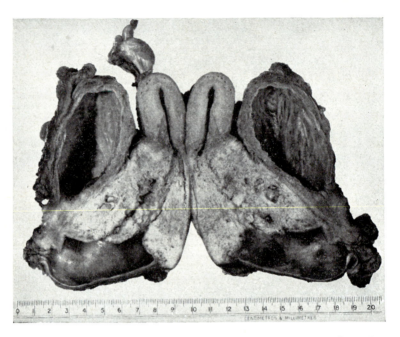

FIG. 329. Anterior exenteration. The specimen has been bisected from the front. Note the large growth invading the anterior vaginal wall and bladder.

in the pelvis is now covered with the peritoneal flaps and the abdomen closed (see Figs. 327 and 328).

Complications which are apt to develop are those mentioned in the previous chapter, where the operation of total hysterectomy was described. After Wertheim's operation the patient is very likely to be shocked and has to be treated accordingly. Sepsis, taking the form either of local sepsis in the raw area in the pelvis or peritonitis, is a possible complication, but it should respond to antibiotics. The urinary complications are very important. Many patients suffer from retention and urinary infections are very common. Most surgeons advise the use of a self-retaining catheter for ten days after the operation. Injuries to the ureters and bladder may lead to the development of fistula, and if both ureters have been ligatured the patient will develop suppression of urine. Interference with the blood supply of the ureter may lead to a urinary fistula. It will be remembered that the ureter receives branches from the aorta, the internal iliac artery, the uterine artery and the superior vesical artery. If the internal iliac branch is cut, the wall of the ureter is likely to undergo avascular necrosis so that a urinary fistula develops, usually about the tenth post-operative day. Further details of the operation are beyond the scope of this book.

Taussig's Operation (*Extra-peritoneal lymphadenectomy*). This operation consists in the block dissection of all lymphatic glands below the bifurcation

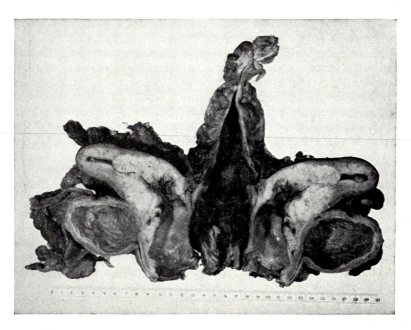

Fig. 330. Total exenteration. The specimen has been bisected from the front into the rectum and shows involvement of bladder, urethra, anterior vaginal wall and rectum by growth.

of the aorta after the carcinoma of the cervix has been treated by a full course of radiation. An incision is made parallel to Poupart's ligament and an extra-peritoneal approach is used. By this method all the external iliac, common iliac and internal iliac glands can be removed on both sides.

Pelvic Exenteration. This method has been employed by Brunschwig in the treatment of advanced carcinoma of the cervix, vagina, vulva and corpus. The bladder, uterus, vagina, and sometimes the rectum, are removed, and the ureters transplanted into the large intestine, which is brought out of the abdomen to leave a wet colostomy. The operation has a primary mortality rate of about 25%. Technically, it presents no great difficulty. In his first 100 cases Brunschwig has produced eleven five-year survivals. Whether the operation is justified on humanitarian grounds is a matter for the individual practitioner and surgeon to decide. This decision depends largely on the fortitude of the patient and her psychological constitution (see Figs. 329 and 330).

Radiotherapy. Details of radiotherapy in carcinoma of the cervix are described in a later chapter.

CARCINOMA OF THE CERVICAL STUMP

The incidence of cancer occurring in the residual cervical stump after subtotal hysterectomy is difficult to assess. Way has recorded thirty-four cases out of a total of 2,468 cervical cancers, an incidence of 1·3% of all cervical cancers seen. Of these stump cancers twelve appeared within two years of the subtotal operation and were probably present at the time of operation but unrecognised as such by the surgeon. The age incidence of these cancers is less than that of cervical cancer in general, twenty-six of the thirty-four cases occurring in the 30–50 age group, largely because in this younger age group the surgeon held the mistaken idea that the preservation of the cervix was essential to coital function. Way assesses the incidence of cancer occurring in the cervical stump after subtotal hysterectomy as 1·9% though most authors would place it at something under 1%.

The clinical findings and diagnosis of this condition are similar to those already described for carcinoma of the cervix. The prognosis and treatment, however, are very different. The removal of the body of the uterus allows the growth a ready access to the bladder, uterovesical peritoneum and rectum and most cases when seen are incurable by operation. Adequate radiation is also seriously prejudiced by the inability of the operator to place an intrauterine tube in position, so that he has to rely solely on vaginal radium applicators and deep X-ray therapy. The proximity of the unguarded bladder limits his total dosage and the five-year salvage rate is 12·9%.

As the operation of total hysterectomy becomes universally performed, the incidence of stump carcinoma will diminish and, it is hoped, ultimately disappear. The incidence of stump carcinoma is sufficient to justify total hysterectomy in all cases and an experienced gynaecological surgeon should have no excuse for performing the subtotal operation.

Summary of the Treatment of Cancer of the Cervix

(1) Radiation is the treatment of choice in all cases of Stage 1.

(2) Radiation is probably the treatment of choice in cases of Stage II though it is logical to employ a subsequent bilateral lymphadenectomy to attempt to eliminate the high percentage of involved lymphatic glands (47%).

(3) An extended Wertheim's operation with bilateral lymphadenectomy is a justifiable procedure for Stage II cancers and should give a slightly better cure rate than radiation—62% as compared with 53% for radiation in the best hands.

(4) The 5-year cure rate for the best surgery in Stage I is slightly inferior to that of the best radiation—82% as compared with 90%.

(5) The immediate mortality and morbidity rates of the best surgery are slightly greater than those of radiation.

(6) When a cancer of the cervix has failed to respond to radiation it should, if possible, be treated surgically.

(7) Adenocarcinoma no longer provides an absolute indication for surgery as used to be stated. Kottmeier claims a 73% cure rate in Stage I cases of adenocarcinoma. Some surgeons, however, can justifiably claim to get better results with surgery in this histological type.

(8) Stage III cases are best treated by radiation in the first instance unless there is some contraindication, e.g. pyometra or adnexal inflammatory masses, which should be dealt with before radiation treatment is started. In Stage III radiation gives better results than surgery.

(9) In late cases Stage III and IV in which radiation is either contraindicated or has failed owing to radio-insensitivity of the growth some form of pelvic exenteration may be considered if the general condition of the patient is favourable and if the growth is confined to the pelvis. Extra-pelvic metastases are an absolute contraindication to any surgical treatment.

(10) Certain cases are unsuitable for radiation and should be treated surgically. If the uterus contains fibroids or if a pyosalpinx is present, surgery is the preferable choice. Some authorities, Kottmeier for instance, remove the fibroids and the pyosalpinx and follow the operation by a course of radiation, but most surgeons would agree that if the abdomen is opened for these reasons and the cancer is operable, surgery should be employed with bilateral lymphadenectomy.

(11) Finally the best results in cancer of the cervix will be obtained in a large centre where an experienced surgeon and an experienced radiotherapist see all cases in joint consultation and plan the treatment in close co-operation and harmony, so that each case is assessed as an individual problem.

25 New Growths of the Uterus:

EPITHELIAL TUMOURS OF THE BODY
CARCINOMA OF THE ENDOMETRIUM

This is the second most common cancer in the female genital organs, the cervix being the first. Its malignancy is much lower than that of carcinoma of the cervix. The proportion of carcinoma of the body to that of the cervix is in the region of 1 to 1·5 and the peak age incidence is about 55 years (see Fig. 331). As the years pass the incidence of cervical to corporeal cancer

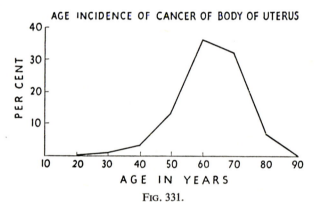

AGE INCIDENCE OF CANCER OF BODY OF UTERUS

Fig. 331.

diminishes. In the 1930 era it was seven or eight to one, whereas now in some districts it is nearly equal. It is usually a disease of post menopausal women. In about 30% the patients are nulliparous. Way has drawn attention to the interesting fact that carcinoma of the body of the uterus is associated with a late menopause, obesity, hypertension, the presence of fibroids and a high incidence of diabetes in many patients and he wonders if some primary pituitary factor may not account for this syndrome. The clinical significance of this syndrome is that the type of patient who has endometrial cancer is a poor surgical risk. Obesity and hypertension are perhaps the two most implacable enemies of surgeon and anaesthetist and, apart from the technical hazards of operating on such patients, their post-operative morbidity from chest complications, phlebo-thrombosis and infection places them in a special category of bad surgical risks.

The patient who has endometrial cancer is, therefore, likely to be:

Obese: She is, in fact, significantly heavier than the patient who has a cervical cancer.

Associated with this obesity, she tends to have *hypertension.* Bastiaanse found 64% of his patients with carcinoma of the corpus to have a systolic blood pressure of over 150 mm. of mercury.

The coincidence of *diabetes* is significant. Way found that 29% of patients with carcinoma of the endometrium had clinical diabetes or diabetes diagnosed on laboratory investigations. A further 43% of his patients had an abnormal glucose tolerance test, suggesting that they were incipient diabetics. The high incidence of diabetes with cancer of the endometrium has been confirmed by American workers. The clinical importance of this finding is that all patients with carcinoma of the endometrium must have a sugar tolerance test performed before operation.

The actual age at which the *menopause* occurs is *deferred*. In Way's series, 54% of patients with cancer of the endometrium menstruated after the age of fifty years with an average age for the menopause of 51·5 as compared to 46·5 for those patients who did not develop cancer of the endometrium.

Apart from these well defined clinical associations, there are two additional features which merit attention.

An interesting observation has been made by Novak regarding the coincidence of hyperplasia of the endometrium and carcinoma of the corpus in post-menopausal women. He found twenty-five cases out of a total of 104 cases of carcinoma of the endometrium to show clear evidence of endometrial hyperplasia. He suggests that an excess of oestrogen production may be responsible for both conditions. In some instances where the urinary oestrogen has been estimated it has been found to be high. The association of endometrial polypi with carcinoma of the endometrium in 5–7% of cases may be explained in the same way, namely that the polypus is produced as a result of endometrial hyperplasia due to an excess of oestrogen.

The high incidence of carcinoma of the endometrium with the feminising tumours of the ovary, granulosa cell and theca cell tumours has been noted; 15 endometrial cancers in 87 feminising tumours of the ovary (Dockerty), 6 out of 16 (Haines) and 4 out of 66 (Ingram and Novak). This coincidence strongly suggests that carcinoma of the endometrium may be an oestrogen-dependent disease.

A number of patients have been reported in whom there is a strong familial tendency towards the disease. The mother and sisters of a patient have been operated upon for carcinoma of the endometrium or may have died from it. Corscaden quotes a family background of cancer in 12–28% of patients suffering from endometrial cancer.

Pathology

The growth is an adenocarcinoma which starts as a small papillary excrescence from the endometrium of the body of the uterus. Microscopically it has a typical structure of an adenocarcinoma, the malignant cells being cubical or columnar in shape, larger than the epithelial cells of the healthy endometrium, with large nuclei which show mitotic division. The carcinoma cells infiltrate the myometrium by direct spread and permeate along the lymphatics, but not with the same rapidity as in the case of carcinoma of the cervix.

To the naked eye, in early cases the growth takes the form of a disc-like excrescence on the endometrium, the surface being irregular and vascular, bleeding easily and discharging blood and infected secretions into the cavity of the uterus. This has been described as the circumscribed type of growth. With more advanced growths the cancer infiltrates the myometrium and spreads over the endometrium as well, so that the uterus becomes symmetrically enlarged and finally the whole cavity of the uterus is lined by friable ulcerated growth, the so-called diffuse type (see Figs. 332 and 333).

Histological Classification of the Biopsy Material. Most authors agree that endometrial carcinoma should be divided into three grades of increasing malignancy and increasing powers of permeation and metastasis. The ultimate prognosis can be very considerably based on this grading.

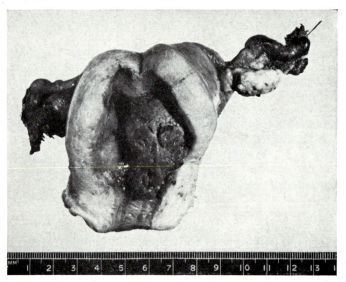

Fig. 332. Adenocarcinoma of the endometrium presenting as a polypoid mass in the cavity of the uterus.

1. Grade I. The most differentiated, which has been called adenoma malignum, and which is frequently confined to the endometrium. The histological picture is one of adenomatous hyperplasia and is at first limited to the glands of the endometrium. The single epithelial layer, however, becomes multiple and heaped up and, sooner or later, the confines of the basement membrane are broken through and the stroma is invaded. Once this has occurred, the histological label is one of invasive carcinoma but, before this invasion is obvious, the pathological diagnosis presents one of the biggest problems in exact diagnosis. This perplexing state of affairs gave rise to the famous dictum of Halban, "Nicht Karzinom, aber besser heraus," and any thoughtful gynaecologist would be inclined to agree with his verdict. Some writers have called this carcinoma *in situ*, largely on the appearance of the

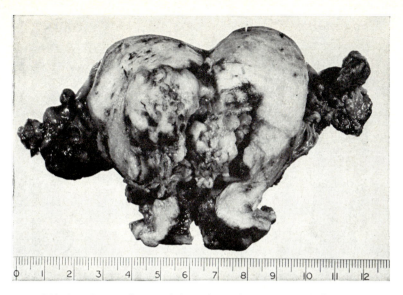

FIG. 333. An adenocarcinoma of the endometrium. The growth forms a large tumour projecting into the cavity of the body of the uterus.

cells which are large with abundant eosinophil cytoplasm and pale nuclei. Their general appearance is quite distinct from that of the normal glandular epithelium which may coexist in other areas of the section. The basement

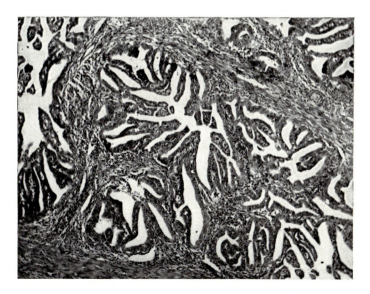

FIG. 334. Low power section of well differentiated adenocarcinoma of the endometrium. The adenoid pattern is preserved. (×52.)

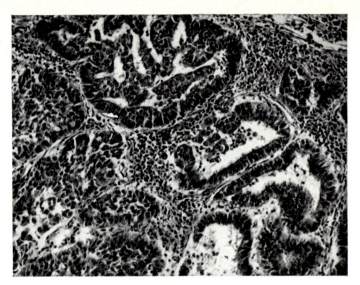

Fig. 335. High power of Fig. 334. (×116.)

membrane is intact and the stroma is not invaded. It is in Grade I that extra
uterine metastasis is rarest and that the prognosis is best, five-year surviva
rates of 85% and over being reported (Figs. 334 and 335).

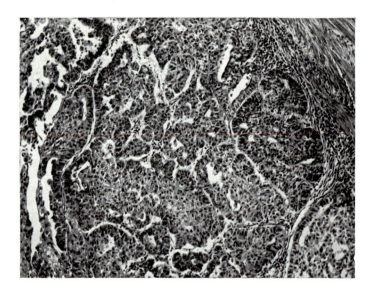

Fig. 336. A less well differentiated adenocarcinoma but one in which the
adenomatous pattern is still preserved. (×76.)

2. In Grade II the glandular differentiation is still present, clearly recognisable but less distinct. Interspersed with an adenomatous pattern are cell masses in which no gland formation can be seen. The general appearance is one of obvious malignancy, and this type of growth is far more invasive than Grade I. Extra-uterine spread and metastasis are more frequent and the prognosis from surgery or radiation is less favourable than in Grade I (Fig. 336).

3. In Grade III the picture is one of complete histological anaplasia. There is no glandular architecture, and it is often difficult to say whether this is a sarcoma or a carcinoma on superficial microscopic inspection. Invasion

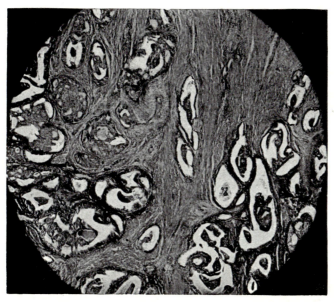

FIG. 337. Carcinoma of the body of the uterus. The growth is an adenocarcinoma. It is infiltrating the myometrium, which lies above and to the right.

of the stroma is widespread, and only an occasional adenomatous-like structure will suggest the diagnosis. Many of these sections have been labelled as sarcomata. The prognosis is naturally the worst in this of the three grades and invasion and metastasis are most extensive. The significance of this grading is seen in the end-result of treatment, 90% survival in Grade I as against 10% in Grade III.

Gross Pathological Classification. It is time that some international classification of carcinoma of the endometrium was accepted as it is in carcinoma of the cervix, so that an intelligent comparison of the end results of surgery and radiation could be compiled. Attempts have been made by many writers to stage the disease (Crossen, 1937; Corscaden and Covell, 1954) and the following tentative division into stages is suggested.

Stage I.   Carcinoma limited to endometrium and myometrium intact.

Stage II.   Myometrium invaded but serosa intact and no obvious extra-uterine involvement (Figs. 336 and 337).

Stage III.   Serosa involved, lymph node metastasis, ovarian invasion, bladder and/or rectum involved. Any one of these structures involved separately places the growth in Stage III, but it is still operable. No extra-pelvic metastases obvious.

Stage IV. Extrapelvic metastases present—therefore inoperable and largely untreatable by any means (Fig. 341).

From a treatment and prognostic point of view, Stages I and II are favourable and should give a five-year cure rate of 85% for Stage I and, depending

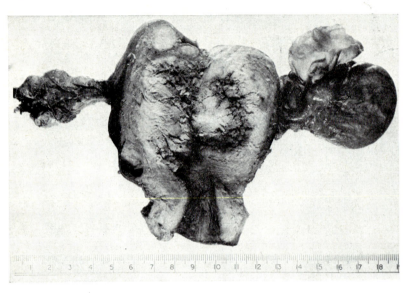

Fig. 338. A specimen to show a Stage II carcinoma of the endometrium. The muscle is deeply and extensively infiltrated but has not yet reached the serosa.

on the depth of myometrial involvement, if superficial 74%, if deep 41% in Stage II (Corscaden). Stage III will naturally carry a poor prognosis and a reduced operability rate and, in this stage, most anaplastic growths will be found as in Stage IV. By a similar reasoning, a Stage III growth with an anaplastic histology should demand a complete pelvic lymphadenectomy as the chance of glandular involvement is greater than in the more differentiated type of carcinoma.

It will be seen from the above considerations that a pre-operative study of the histology obtained by curettage and an examination of the degree of invasion of the myometrium in the removed uterus will give the surgeon a fairly accurate idea of the scope of his operation and place the treatment on a more scientific basis. A strong plea is therefore made to all surgeons to consider this problem along these suggested lines.

Lymph Node Invasion. The attitude of surgeons towards lymph node metastasis in carcinoma of the endometrium has, in the past, varied from complacency to defeatism. It was either considered that the growth was a relatively slow-growing one with late lymph node metastasis or that, when the lymph nodes were invaded, dissemination was too wide to warrant any form of treatment. It was with some justification agreed that lymphatic spread should travel by the ovarian lymphatics to the aortic glands and that, once these were involved, the case was hopeless. It has been found in practice that, with the lower corporeal situation of the growth, many of these cancers behave like a carcinoma of the cervix and spread initially to the hypogastric group of nodes and that a complete pelvic lymphadenectomy in such will give a small but reasonable chance of survival. The actual incidence of lymph node metastasis is not yet settled and will not be until more cases are treated by radical operation with complete pelvic lymphadenectomy. Javert (1952) reports a very high incidence of 28·6%. Rickford (1954) gives 23·6%, while Winterton (1954), who has been a protagonist of the extended operation, reports only 7%. These figures must vary with the extent, situation and histological pattern of the growth and, until all these facts are reported together, it is impossible to be conclusive. A tentative figure is probably between 10 and 20%, sufficiently large to justify a pelvic lymphadenectomy in every case of low corporeal growth, of growth invading the myometrium deeply and of growth which is histologically Grades II and III, i.e. poorly differentiated or anaplastic.

Vaginal Recurrences. All surgeons are too well aware that one of the common sites of recurrence after total hysterectomy and bilateral salpingo-oöphorectomy for carcinoma of the endometrium is the vaginal vault (13·3% —Rickford (*vide supra*)). Whether this is due to the spill and implantation of viable cancer cells at operation or to the pre-existence of vaginal spread not clinically demonstrable is debatable, but its frequency demands a more realistic treatment of the vagina as a potential source of recurrence. Either the vagina should be radically and generously removed as in a Wertheim's operation, as a primary operative procedure, or radium should be applied post-operatively to the vagina as advocated by Read (1955), 50 mg. for thirty-six hours on the fourteenth post-operative day. It is a possibility that the combination of radium and surgery will lower the incidence of vaginal metastasis.

In order to reduce the potential danger from the spill of cancer cells when performing hysterectomy for carcinoma of the endometrium, Percival (1952) has devised an occlusive clamp which he claims is superior to packing or suturing the cervix. In the accompanying fig. 339 the clamp unit A consists of sharp-toothed upper and lower jaws, supported by strong arms converging at a hinge 1½ in. distant; the opening and closing of the jaws is controlled by a rachet mechanism B neatly located in the hinge. The control lever C of the rachet lies parallel to the arm of the lower jaw, where it may be disengaged readily by a simple device D on the carrier forceps E when the clamp is approaching the cervix in the vagina. This allows the clamp to be introduced in the closed position through the narrow introitus of the nulliparous patient, and then to be opened when the roomier vagina is reached so that it can grip

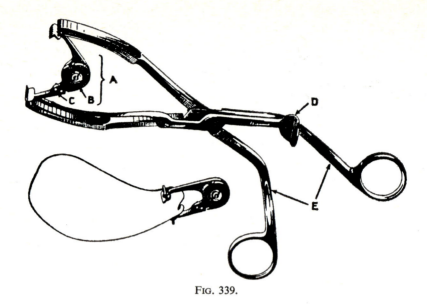

FIG. 339.

and compress the cervix. Immediately before the final compression of the cervix, the rachet on the clamp is allowed to come into action merely by operating the disengaging lever D on the carrier forceps. Full compression is thus securely maintained. The carrier forceps are then easily slipped off the clamp by a slight opening movement of the handles. The clamp, which is made in two sizes (standard and large), takes up very little room in the vault and in no way interferes with the hysterectomy.

If a surgeon believes in the spill theory, he should, when operating on a carcinoma of the endometrium, occlude not only the cervix but tie both tubes at the fimbriated ends as there is a genuine risk of peritoneal contamination from the tubal ostia.

Ovarian Metastases. These metastases are of importance from the surgical point of view. There is no doubt that in a certain number the metastases form by implantation upon the surface of the ovary while in others the ovaries are involved by lymphatic spread, the carcinoma cells reaching the ovary by way of the medulla. In a third group there is a coincident tumour of the ovary, with a carcinoma of the body of the uterus. These tumours have been investigated by Werner (1939) and by Wilfred Shaw, amongst others, and it seems that the ovarian carcinoma is sometimes coincident in development with the carcinoma of the body of the uterus. It is also well known that malignant ovarian and Brenner tumours are sometimes associated with a carcinoma of the body of the uterus. These observations demonstrate that in the surgical treatment of carcinoma of the body it is essential to remove both Fallopian tubes and both ovaries.

Symptoms

The most characteristic symptom of carcinoma of the body of the uterus is post-menopausal haemorrhage or irregular intermenstrual bleeding in the pre-menopausal or menopausal patient. It must never be forgotten that carcinoma of the endometrium can occur in quite young women. The bleeding is continuous without rhythm or definite frequency. In most cases the bleeding is only moderate and severe haemorrhage is rare. It is usually associated with

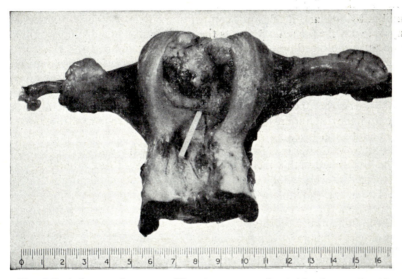

FIG. 340. A danger of curettage. The uterus was perforated by the curette at the margin of the carcinoma. The site of injury is indicated by the white rod. Perforation is always a hazard when the growth has infiltrated the myometrium deeply.

some degree of offensive discharge caused by the ulcerated growth, but this is not so characteristic a symptom as with carcinoma of the cervix.

Pain is sometimes complained of, when it is described as colicky and is attributed to contractions of the uterus. Pyometra is quite a common feature of cancer of the endometrium. This complication gives rise to pain, fever, leucocytosis and general constitutional disturbance. The pain is of a dull, aching nature and localised to the hypogastrium and the enlarged, tender uterus. Other symptoms arise only in late cases when, for example, the growth infiltrates the surrounding structures or when cachexia results from the presence of an old-standing infected growth.

Physical Signs

In women of post-menopausal age the most certain sign of carcinoma of the body of the uterus is to see blood emerging from the external os. The uterus is enlarged, though not appreciably, except when the disease is advanced. A small normal uterus, however, does not by any means exclude the presence of an endometrial cancer. It should be remembered that carcinoma of the body of the uterus tends to develop in patients who may have uterine myomata, and the possible coincidence of these two tumours should always be borne in mind.

Diagnosis. As in carcinoma of the cervix, the essential symptom is irregular and usually post-menopausal bleeding. The source of the bleeding, however, is not available for inspection and palpation and its importance is not so readily obvious, and it does not compel immediate diagnosis. Valuable time may be lost while the patient awaits the confirmation of a diagnostic curettage or because the bleeding, initially slight, does not impress the gynaecologist sufficiently. Quite a number of the patients may have had oestrogen for menopausal symptoms and it is, not unnaturally, thought that the bleeding is due to this treatment. While the authors admit readily that in many instances this may be the correct diagnosis, the penalty of such a dangerous conclusion is too great and they maintain that, oestrogen or no oestrogen, all patients with post-menopausal bleeding should be screened by examination and curettage under an anaesthetic. It is freely admitted that many unnecessary curettages will be performed if this dictum is rigorously obeyed but, equally so, many unsuspected cancers will be discovered at an early stage favourable to operation. The actual catchment rate is roughly 1:10, i.e. one carcinoma of the endometrium for every ten diagnostic curettages performed for this type of post-menopausal bleeding.

Cytological diagnosis is not as accurate in endometrial as cervical cancer and the ordinary vaginal and cervical smears will probably miss half the true positives. Hecht (1956) has elaborated an aspiration smear technique whereby a suction specimen is taken direct from the endometrium with a special cannula and syringe. By this method he now claims an accuracy of 85%. Though an appreciable advance, this is not yet good enough and, at the time of writing, diagnostic curettage must remain our most reliable method of diagnosis. The great value of cytology is in diagnosing the rare and clinically unsuspected cancer.

Diagnostic Localisation of the Carcinoma. In carcinoma of the endometrium the exact situation of the growth must be known. It is reprehensible and dangerous to treat a carcinoma of the endocervix as if it were an endometrial adenocarcinoma arising in the fundus, and yet this unhappy mistake is all too often made. The authors would like to draw a critical line at a purely arbitrary level well above the isthmus and, for purposes of treatment, any growth, no matter what its site of primary origin or what its histology, should be treated either by radiation or surgery as a carcinoma of the cervix if it was found to encroach below that arbitrary level. It is hoped that all surgeons will carefully examine this suggestion and that when they are considering treatment of an endometrial cancer which has extended into the isthmus and upper endocervix will either perform an extended Wertheim's operation with complete pelvic lymphadenectomy or treat it with radium and radiotherapy as adequately as if it were a carcinoma of the endocervix. It is this type of endometrial cancer that most frequently invades the lymphatic glands in the

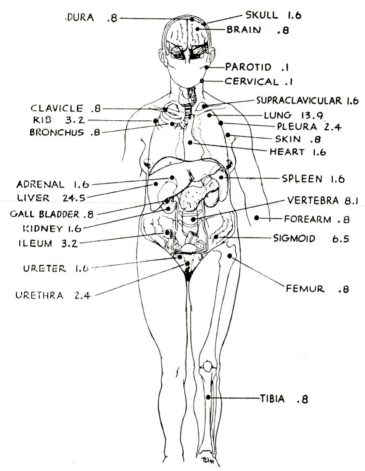

FIG. 341. Sites and incidence of metastases from carcinoma of the uterine body. (Henriksen, *Amer. J. Obst. & Gyn.*)

pelvis and which gives poor results from total hysterectomy and bilateral salpingo-oöphorectomy (Fig. 342).

Fractional Curettage. In order to establish the true situation of an endometrial cancer the diagnostic operation of fractional curettage is recommended. This is considered of such importance that it is here described in some detail.

It is assumed that the portio vaginalis of the cervix has been excluded by inspection, palpation, colposcopy (if indicated) and scrape or surface

biopsy after the method of Ayre. (1) The first specimen is obtained by curetting the endocervix with a small sharp curette before the canal is dilated. If
the endocervix is normal little or nothing will be obtained in the way of a
histological specimen, in which case a cytological smear should be made.
This specimen is labelled No. 1, endocervix. (2) The cervical canal is now
dilated and a small sharp curette is introduced as far but no further than the
isthmus—that is, 1 cm. above the internal os, which can usually be felt via
the curette as a small circular constriction at the top of the endocervix. This is
specimen No. 2. If specimen No. 1 or No. 2 is positive for a carcinoma, then
the patient should be treated as if she had a carcinoma of the cervix. (3) The
fundus is next explored at each cornu, and these specimens are labelled No.
3A right, and No. 3B left.(4) The anterior and posterior surface of the uterus
is finally explored and these specimens are individually labelled.

The ideal procedure is to obtain six separate curettings, though, in practice,
only endocervical, isthmic, fundal and corporeal may be secured. A study
of this material should enable the surgeon to localise the situation of the
growth.

Differential Diagnosis

Although the symptoms and physical signs of carcinoma of the body are
relatively simple, there is often difficulty in establishing the diagnosis. In the
first place, a fair proportion of women with carcinoma of the body are either
virgins or nulliparae, so that a vaginal examination with the use of a speculum
may be difficult. In every post-menopausal haemorrhage some form of
carcinoma of the genital organs should first be thought of, particularly
carcinoma of the cervix or of the body of the uterus or of the ovaries. Other
growths, such as carcinoma of the vagina and vulva, can usually be demonstrated without difficulty.

Post-menopausal uterine bleeding is a not uncommon symptom with
carcinoma of the ovaries, particularly with the rare granulosa cell tumours
of the ovaries. If bimanual examination demonstrates the existence of an
adnexal tumour in a woman of post-menopausal age suffering from uterine
bleeding, it is reasonable to assume that the adnexal tumour is an ovarian
growth producing bleeding from the endometrium. The bleeding in such cases
is usually due to an oestrogenic proliferation of the endometrium and the
correct treatment is to remove the uterus as well as both appendages.

Senile vaginitis causing bleeding and offensive discharge in women of
post-menopausal age often gives rise to difficulty in diagnosis. The bleeding
in this condition is never more than slight whereas in carcinoma of the body it is
usually heavier. The vaginitis can be recognised by speculum examination
of the vaginal wall, but the two conditions may be coincident. Even so, it is
an essential precaution that the uterus should be curetted and the curettings
examined microscopically.

Sometimes small adenomatous polypi develop in the endometrium of the
body of the uterus in women of post-menopausal age and give rise to symptoms similar to those of carcinoma of the body. Another difficulty is that the
polypi may escape the curette as their pedicles are often small. Curettage will

usually exclude the presence of carcinoma, although it does not necessarily establish the diagnosis of adenomatous polypus.

Very exceptionally myomata become extruded into the cavity of the uterus and cause post-menopausal bleeding, and tuberculosis of the endometrium sometimes causes uterine bleeding when it arises in patients after the menopause.

The abuse of oestrogen as a panacea for all menopausal symptoms is an all too common cause of post-menopausal oestrogen withdrawal bleeding. As it is impossible to reach a certain diagnosis without curettage this drug is responsible for a large number of unnecessary operations and the wastage of valuable beds, money, patients' and hospital time is serious. Oestrogen must now rank as one of the commonest causes of post-menopausal bleeding.

Treatment and Prognosis

The time-honoured treatment of endometrial carcinoma has been a total hysterectomy with bilateral salpingo-oöphorectomy, irrespective of the situation and the invasion of the growth and its histological characteristics. It is apparent that the better operative risk has been selected and the operability percentage of all patients seen has averaged around 75 per cent. Corscaden and Covell (1954) report a five-year survival rate of 64%, and Rickford (1954), 74% of all patients operated upon by them. It is hoped that these figures can be improved by a more rational approach to the problem and that to submit a patient to a blind total hysterectomy and bilateral salpingo-oöphorectomy is not good enough. The following suggestions for treatment are therefore submitted:

1. Fractional curettage of all patients in whom carcinoma of the endometrium is suspected will, in most instances, give an accurate idea of the situation of the growth.

2. Histological grading of the curettings will establish the degree of malignancy.

3. A careful examination under anaesthetic at the same time will give a good idea of the operability.

4. An assessment of the general condition of the patient will help to decide her fitness or not for radical surgery if this should be otherwise indicated.

When all this data is available, the surgeon can make a reasonable decision about the best treatment.

1. If the growth is situated in the fundus and is well differentiated (Grade I), a total hysterectomy and bilateral salpingo-oöphorectomy with removal of the upper half of the vagina should be adequate. When removed, the uterus should be bisected and the extent of the myometrial invasion determined on the spot. If the myometrium is deeply invaded, a bilateral pelvic lymphadenectomy should be performed on the assumption that lymph node involvement is more likely than in the less or not involved myometrium. It is assumed that the patient is fit enough for this more extensive operation.

2. If fractional curettage suggests that the growth has invaded below the

critical line situated above the isthmus, it is to be treated as a carcinoma of the cervix and either a radical Wertheim's operation with bilateral lymphadenectomy performed or a full course of radiotherapy given with or without subsequent operation as above. The former is obviously reserved for the fit patient. (Fig. 342.)

3. If the growth is anaplastic (Grade III and some cases of Grade II) histologically, it is suggested that the uterus should be packed with multiple radium sources after the technique described by Kottmeier (1954), since this method ensures that every part of the uterus receives adequate radiation. In good-risk patients this intracavitary radium application can be followed in two weeks' time by an extended hysterectomy and bilateral salpingo-oöphorectomy and pelvic lymphadenectomy. This latter refinement will ensure the removal of potentially invaded nodes and will provide in the future valuable information about the incidence of lymph node involvement. Marshall (1951) has reported 91·5% cure-rate from radium and surgery in a small series and Corscaden (1956) 82·8%. Corscaden strongly advocates pre-operative radium followed by surgery. Payne (1952) has compared a

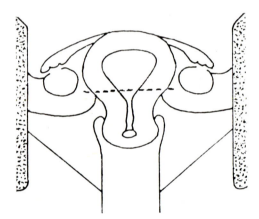

FIG. 342. Illustration of uterus to show the critical line. Any endometrial cancer which has extended below this line must be treated as though it were a carcinoma of the cervix. (After Shaw's "Operative Gynaecology," E. & S. Livingstone Ltd.)

92·9% cure-rate with radium and surgery to a 80·4% cure-rate from surgery alone. Some of these results are undoubtedly due to selection, but they do show what can be achieved. There is therefore little doubt that radium pre-operatively and surgery will be more frequently used in the treatment of endometrial carcinoma in the future.

4. For the obese, hypertensive and poor-risk patient, radium alone will cure about 55% of patients. Kottmeier (1953) reported a five-year absolute cure-rate of 60·2%, but 12·9% of his patients were operated on after radiation and these should naturally be deducted from the figure of 60·2%.

Summary of Treatment of Cancer of the Body of the Uterus

(1) The treatment of this condition should be operation—total hysterectomy and bilateral salpingo-oöphorectomy with removal of the upper half of the vagina to prevent vault recurrences. This operation is satisfactory only if the growth is above the ctitical line (see Fig. 342) and if it has not infiltrated deeply into the myometrium.

(2) If the growth has been found on fractional curettage to arise in the region of the isthmus or to encroach by spread into the endocervix the case should be considered to be an endocervical cancer and treated as such, and either a full scale Wertheim's operation performed or a full course of radiation given. Pelvic lymphadenectomy should be performed as for cancer of the cervix.

(3) Some surgeons will treat true carcinoma of the body by some combined form of pre-operative irradiation followed by surgery. The results of this method may well show an improvement over surgery alone but it is still under trial in this country. The anaplastic type of growth is the one most logically treated by this combination of radiation and surgery.

(4) If an ordinary total hysterectomy and bilateral salpingo-oöphorectomy is performed it is wise to employ post-operative radium to the vaginal vault as advocated by Read.

(5) In patients unsuitable for surgery the intrauterine packing with multiple radium sources after the method of Heyman gives results a little inferior to operation. If radium is used for this growth this is the best method.

(6) If, during a diagnostic curettage for suspected endometrial cancer, the surgeon suspects that he has perforated the uterus there is a real danger of localised pelvic peritonitis and dissemination of the growth. He must therefore proceed to perform a laparotomy and deal with the growth, if present, under the above headings 1 or 2 (see fig. 340).

26 Radiotherapy in Gynaecology

by

DAVID B. L. SKEGGS, M.A., B.M., F.F.R., D.M.R.T.

Consultant Radiotherapist to the Royal Free Hospital, London.
Honorary Consultant Radiotherapist to the Royal Northern Hospital, London.

Radiotherapy has gradually assumed a more important part in the treatment of gynaecological cancer over the past forty-five years since intracavitary radium was shown to be a highly effective form of treatment, particularly for the early squamous cell carcinoma of the cervix. The treatment of more advanced disease by external irradiation was by no means certain and, in fact, sometimes even proved hazardous. The earlier X-ray machines lacked the penetrating power of modern equipment and in order to deliver an adequate dose to a deep seated pelvic tumour were liable to cause severe skin reactions and later pathological fractures of the femur.

The introduction of cobalt teletherapy units and other forms of mega-voltage equipment has revolutionised the treatment of pelvic neoplasia because of specific advantages which are characteristic of mega-voltage irradiation (1 million volts and above). These include:

(1) The maximum dose absorbed by the tissue occurs deep to the skin; the skin reaction, therefore, is no longer the limiting factor in the course of treatment.

(2) All tissues, regardless of their chemical constituents, will absorb the same amount of irradiation. The risk of causing bone damage is thus greatly reduced. Deep X-rays (250 kV) by contrast are differentially absorbed by tissues of high atomic weight and therefore are liable to cause bone damage.

(3) The beam, having a highly penetrating quality, can deliver an adequate dose to the tumour by means of a simple field arrangement whereas, with deep X-ray therapy, complicated multi-field arrangements are necessary.

The advent of super voltage irradiation has completely altered the whole concept of radiotherapy for pelvic disease, so that it is now possible to administer a radical dose to the lymph nodes on the lateral pelvic wall, even in the larger patients, by means of external irradiation. As a result, cure rates have improved and radiotherapy is playing an even more important role.

The radiotherapist requires an intimate knowledge of the behaviour and spread of tumours, tempered with an understanding of the basic physical principles that apply to ionising radiation. Ionising radiation encompasses all forms of radiation that transfers its energy as a result of causing secondary ionisation. This will include alpha, beta and gamma emission from radio-active isotopes, and X-rays and high energy electrons generated by machines. To understand how these agents are employed to obtain the best effect, the following basic physical principles must be understood:

(1) Ionising radiation obeys the Inverse Square Law. The intensity of radiation from a given source falls off inversely with the square of the distance from that source. The implication of this is relevant to the use of radio-active sources in the form of implants or applicators. These will achieve a high dose to the tissues in direct relationship to the source but due to the rapid fall off of radiation intensity away from the source, adjacent organs will be spared from high dose irradiation. At the same time, it must be remembered that lymph nodes, even at a relatively short distance from the source, will also be spared.

(2) The penetrating power of X- and gamma-radiation is proportional to its energy. In clinical practice, the radiotherapist has available machines which will generate X-rays at any energy between 10,000 volts and 30 million volts. The particular energy he will select will be governed mainly by the depth of the lesion to be treated. Also, the characteristic of mega-voltage irradiation in sparing the skin and bones is of the utmost impor-tance when treating the pelvis.

(3) X- and gamma-irradiation are absorbed exponentially in tissue and have an infinite range. This necessitates most careful treatment planning to limit as much as possible the irradiation of tissue outside the designated tumour volume.

(4) Electrons, for practical purposes, have a limited range which is pro-portional to their energy. The range is approximately 1 cm. for every 3 million electron volts. This form of irradiation has a special application for treatment of superficial conditions, such as carcinoma of the vulva. By selecting the appropriate energy of an electron beam for a particular tumour which has to be treated, the whole tumour volume can be irradiated to high dosage with relatively complete sparing of the underlying tissues.

Tumour Sensitivity. The susceptibility of tumours to irradiation damage is very variable, but in general, the more cellular a tumour is and the more primitive its constituent cells are, the more likely it is to be radio-sensitive. Tumour sensitivity is divided into three grades:

High Sensitivity:	Some anaplastic tumours.
	Dysgerminoma.
Medium sensitivity:	Squamous cell carcinoma.
Low sensitivity:	Some adenocarcinomata.
	Fibrosarcoma.

This histological guide to radio-sensitivity is invaluable to the radiotherapist. Coupled with his knowledge of the extent and likely spread of a given tumour, he will have the necessary information to determine the exact volume that will be required to be irradiated and the appropriate dosage that should ensure successful treatment.

Cell Survival

Successful treatment is dependent upon the normal, healthy tissue surrounding a tumour being able to survive the maximum dose of irradiation required to ensure complete destruction of all the malignant cells in that tumour. Healthy tissue can usually survive a cancericidal dose of irradiation and subsequently undergo normal cellular division. However, this margin of tissue tolerance is indeed narrow when it is considered in terms of the dosage that is known to be necessary to sterilise any but the more radio-sensitive tumours. Any factor that may jeopardise this marginal advantage of normal tissue over tumour, can prove critical to the success of the treatment. The radiation dose required to sterilise tumours is variable, but for a given tumour increases in proportion to the size of that tumour. The explanation for this is that all malignant cells must be destroyed for the treatment to achieve a cure, and the larger a tumour becomes, the smaller will be the mathematical chance of every malignant cell present being destroyed. For this reason, smaller doses can prove curative when dealing with a small residuum or microscopic invasion of disease.

Oxygen Effect

Fully oxygenated cells have been shown to be approximately 2·5 times more susceptible to a given dose of irradiation than are anoxic cells. The significance of this fact becomes apparent when it is realised that in most tumours, 1% of the cells are poorly oxygenated and are therefore protected to some extent from irradiation. Furthermore, in larger tumours the percentage of anoxic cells is liable to increase as the mass outgrows its blood supply. This protective effect of anoxia on tumour cells may be increased by the patient being anaemic and by other factors such as chronic infection, or scarring which result in some diminution of the blood supply to the tumour.

Dosage

When prescribing treatment, the radiotherapist is constantly considering the limits of tolerance of the normal surrounding tissues before selecting a dose to be given to the tumour. Certain organs, such as the kidneys and small bowel, tolerate irradiation poorly and will require to be given special thought if they are likely to come within the zone of irradiation. In pelvic irradiation, the limiting factors to tolerance are the rectum and any loop of small bowel which may be incarcerated in the pelvis as a result of post-operative adhesions.

Tissue tolerance and the ability to recover from irradiation are progressively reduced as the total volume irradiated is increased. Thus, if the region being treated is of a limited volume it is possible to prescribe a high dose with safety. For example, when radium is used to treat carcinoma of the cervix it is customary to give a dose between 7,000–8,000 rads at point A (2 cm. above and 2 cm. lateral to the cervix). This is possible because only a limited volume receives this high dose, the intensity of which diminishes rapidly in the surrounding tissues. In contrast, if it is necessary to irradiate the whole pelvis, it is dangerous to prescribe much in excess of 5,000 rads in five to six weeks for such a large volume. Furthermore, on the few occasions when it is essential to treat the whole abdomen, a dose of 2,500–3,000 rads should not be exceeded.

Treatment Planning

To achieve the ideal of irradiating the smallest volume possible, precise knowledge of the tumour location is essential for the radiotherapist. This is only possible as a result of close co-operation with the surgeon. Meticulous operation notes are essential and the use of silver clips as markers at special

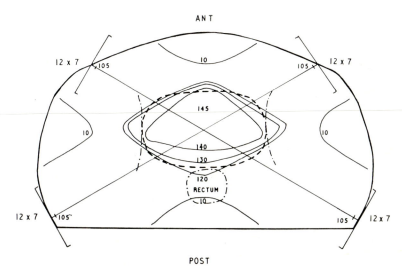

FIG. 343. Plan of a standard four field arrangement used to give external irradiation to the pelvic cavity. The figures denote intensities of irradiation relative to a 100% applied dose given to each of the four fields.

sites can prove invaluable. This information, together with knowledge of likely direct and lymphatic spread of a tumour, enables the therapist to describe the exact volume in the patient that should be treated. This volume is then drawn in on a cross-section contour taken of the patient. It then remains for the physicist, with the guidance of the radiotherapist, to devise the most appropriate and efficient field arrangement for that particular situation.

At a glance, one can see from this plan not only what dosage the tumour volume itself is receiving, but also the doses being received by other sites of interest such as the bladder and the rectum. Much time is devoted to devising these plans and the accuracy of the treatment may be confirmed by means of a simulator which takes radiographs of the exact volume that will be treated by the therapy machine (Fig. 343).

Joint Consultations

Joint consultations between the gynaecologist and radiotherapist are essential to ensure the fullest possible evaluation of each new case in turn. Also, with a better understanding of what either specialty can achieve, the patient will receive the treatment which is best suited to her particular disease

Carcinoma of the Cervix

Since the earliest days when radium was introduced as an effective form of treatment for this disease, the techniques used have been repeatedly modified and improved. The two principal systems, originally devised in Paris and Stockholm, have retained these names and are similar in the

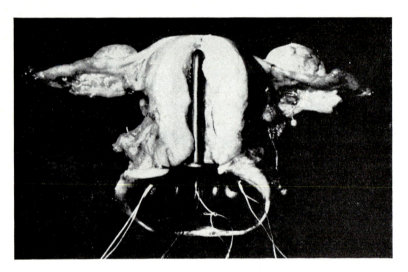

Fig. 344. Cross section of an operative specimen demonstrating the correct positioning of the radium in a "Manchester" insertion. (From Shaw's "Operative Gynaecology", 3rd Ed. E. & S. Livingstone).

method of distribution of the radium. In both instances, a long central source is employed for the uterine canal in conjunction with two or possibly three sources, according to the size of the vagina, in the vaginal vault, The reasoning behind this particular positioning of the radium is to achieve a pear-shaped distribution of irradiation which will include not only the primary growth, but also as much as possible of the parametrium which is the primary region of spread.

The difference between the two systems is the concept of dosage. In the Paris method, a smaller amount of radium (which is removed daily for cleaning) is applied continuously for five days. For the Stockholm technique, a heavier loading of radium is used which is inserted on three separate occasions, with intervals of seven days between the first two insertions and a further fourteen days before the last insertion. The actual content of the

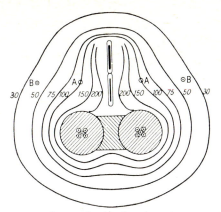

FIG. 345. Isodose curves of a standard radium insertion using the Manchester technique for carcinoma of the cervix uteri. The dose at point A is taken as 100%. From Paterson R. " The Treatment of Malignant Disease by Radium and X-Rays ", Edward Arnold.)

radium used may be adjusted to suit the particular requirements of the patient being treated and in fact, varies from one treatment centre to another. The central tube usually contains 50 mg. of radium and the boxes are loaded with 25 mg. of radium.

The Manchester Method

The Manchester method is a variation of the Stockholm technique and uses rubber ovoids loaded with radium in place of the platinum boxes for the vaginal vault. Three different sizes of ovoid are available which, together with varying sizes of spacers, allows full flexibility to ensure optimum irradiation of the vault (see Figs. 344, 345 and 346).

Standard Loading of Manchester Sources:

Intrauterine tubes:	Long	..	35 mg (15+10+10)
	Medium	..	25 mg (15+10)
	Short	..	15 mg.
Vaginal ovoids:	Large	..	25 mg. (5+10+10)
	Medium	..	20 mg.
	Small	..	15 mg. (10+5)

A conventional Manchester treatment will consist of two insertions, each lasting 72 hours, with a seven-day interval between the two operations.

Choice of Treatment

Each patient should be examined under an anaesthetic and assessed jointly by the gynaecologist and radiotherapist before any plan of treatment is formulated. At this time, a cystoscopy will be performed and also a biopsy will be taken from the tumour. The cure rate for carcinoma of the cervix is closely linked to the staging of the disease (see p. 635). If the results of surgery and radiotherapy in the treatment of carcinoma of the cervix are compared,

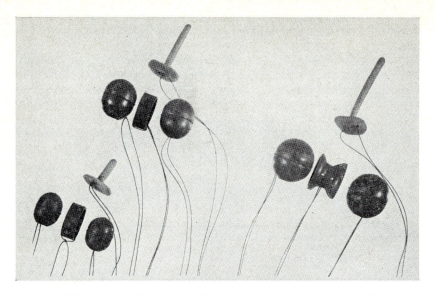

FIG. 346. Large, medium and small radium sources as used in the "Manchester" method. Note in each instance, the spacer in place between the two ovoids. (From Shaw's "Operative Gynaecology", 3rd Ed. E. & S. Livingstone.)

the cure rates achieved in Stage I and Stage II cases are comparable by either method. Therefore, the choice of treatment can be a personal matter, especially if the surgery and radiotherapy at a centre are of an equally high standard. But, when it comes to the selection of treatment for Stage III and Stage IV tumours, radiotherapy is the treatment of choice. Endocervical tumours are frequently adenocarcinomata and have a sinister reputation as they are often stony hard and respond poorly to irradiation. For this type of tumour, radical surgery is the treatment of choice.

Preparation of Patients for Radium:

The patient should be admitted three days before the operation to allow time for routine pre-operative treatment. A low residue diet is given and, if necessary, an enema or suppositories should be given so that the large bowel is empty at the time of the radium insertion.

Each patient will require an intravenous pyelogram and chest X-ray. As there is always a possibility of a urinary infection, a mid-stream specimen of urine should be cultured and if necessary appropriate treatment implemented. A full blood count is performed and if the haemoglobin level is less than 10 gm. (70%) it will be necessary to correct this by means of transfusion, because anaemia may cause some degree of cellular anoxia, which can protect tumour cells from the irradiation. If there is any evidence of pelvic infection, this must be treated before starting the radium treatment as irradiation is liable to cause an exacerbation of infection. A vaginal swab should be taken for culture and antibiotic treatment commenced immediately.

The Insertion of Radium

In this country, it is customary to insert radium under a general anaesthetic. The patient is placed in the lithotomy position and after a self-retaining catheter has been inserted into the bladder, the cervix is dilated to a sufficient extent to allow the uterine source to be inserted with ease. The longest source that can be accommodated by the canal is selected and then, with the maximum speed to minimise the amount of radiation exposure to the staff, the radium is inserted. According to the system being used, ovoids or boxes are then positioned in the fornices to give the radiation distribution which has been calculated to be best suited to the particular patient. Special care is then taken to stabilise this arrangement by packing paraffin gauze against the radium in such a way that the rectum and bladder are displaced away from the radium to avoid the risks of an excessive radiation reaction. Ideally at this stage a radiation probe should be inserted both into the bladder and into the rectum in order to establish the level of radiation dosage being received by these organs. Serious damage may be caused by excessive irradiation and if the probe readings should prove to be unacceptably high, it will be necessary to take out the pack and reposition the radium. Antero-posterior and lateral X-rays of the pelvis are taken to check the position of the radium; it is then possible to deduce the exact position of the radium in the body and to calculate the dosage of irradiation at different sites.

Radium Dosage:

The radium dosage is calculated with respect to the amount of irradiation received at two theoretical points, A and B. Point A lies 2 cm. above and 2 cm. lateral to the base of the radium tube in the cervical canal. This point approximates to the position in the pelvis where the uterine artery and ureter cross. Point B lies 3 cm. lateral to point A and roughly corresponds to the position of the obturator nodes. A standard Stockholm course of radium gives the following dosage distribution:

Point A   —   8,000 rads.
Point B   —   1,500 rads.
Side wall of pelvis   —   1,000 rads.

This type of dosage distribution is potentially curative for Stage I tumours and also for Stage 2A tumours. Any disease extending to the side wall of the pelvis, however, will be inadequately treated and can only be effectively irradiated by supplementing the dosage to the gland fields by means of external irradiation. Before the advent of super-voltage equipment, this proved technically to be very difficult, especially in fat patients. With modern machines, it is no problem to irradiate the pelvic glands and this in itself has led to alteration of the radium techniques being used. Today, radium is seldom used entirely alone, even in clinical Stage I disease, because lymphangiography has revealed that approximately 15%–20% of patients who have clinical Stage I disease do, in fact, have lymph node involvement.

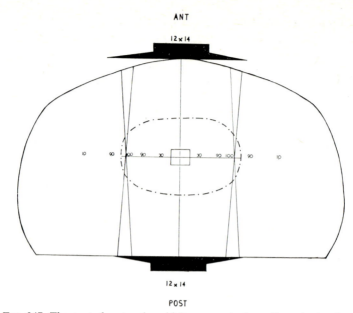

FIG. 347. The central rectangle, which represents the radium, is the site of
most intense irradiation. The figures denote the percentage contribution
from the supplementary external irradiation. The specially shaped lead
filters in the beam are designed so that the centre receives minimal dosage
and the maximum dosage occurs at the side wall of the pelvis.

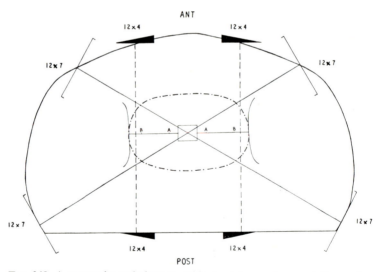

FIG. 348. A composite technique to achieve maximum dosage at the cervix
with homogeneous irradiation at a lower dose level to the rest of the pelvis.

Combined Radium and External Irradiation

The pear-shaped dosage distribution which results from the classical methods of radium insertion is by no means ideal when it comes to giving supplementary treatment to the gland fields by means of external irradiation. Although in principle, especially with the earlier cases, the aim is to give a rather higher dose to the primary tumour, it is essential to give the tissues in the parametrium and the side wall of the pelvis, homogeneous irradiation. To "key-on" external irradiation to an irregularly shaped isodose from the radium inevitably must result in zones of over-dosage or under-dosage. As a result, there has been a move away from the classical radium insertions to the use of mid-line radium alone, with no sources in the lateral fornices. This enables the external irradiation to the pelvis to be supplemented to that of the radium with a far higher degree of accuracy and consequent improvement in results.

Figures 347 and 348 display how this supplementary treatment is given. In the first instance, the pelvic irradiation is given by parallel opposed fields. This beam is directed through a lead filter which is shaped so that the thickest part of the filter, nearest to the centre, will absorb the greatest amount of irradiation and this absorption decreases progressively away from the centre of the field. As a result, the central portion of the pelvis which has received high dosage from the radium, receives a smaller contribution from the external irradiation. This situation is reversed the further you progress from the centre where there has been a much smaller contribution from the radium.

In the second method (Fig. 348) the whole pelvis is treated to a dose of 3,000 rads by the use of four oblique fields, and then the underdosed glands on the side wall of the pelvis are given supplementary irradiation by means of two pairs of small parallel opposed fields, using wedged filters. The ultimate aim of these combined techniques is to give 7,000 rads to point A, a considerably higher dose to the cervix itself and 5,000 rads to the gland fields in the rest of the pelvis. In Stage III tumours, where the disease is already involving the side wall of the pelvis, more emphasis is placed on the external irradiation of the pelvis which is given a dose of 5,000 rads throughout. This may then be supplemented by a single radium insertion to contribute a further 2,000 rads to point A.

Timing of Treatment

It is debatable whether the radium insertion should be performed before or after the external irradiation. When more than one insertion of radium is planned, I prefer the radium insertions to be given as the initial treatment for the following reasons:

(1) If at the time of the proposed second insertion there is a clinical impression, subsequently confirmed by histological examination, that the tumour is not responding to the irradiation, the treatment policy can be altered immediately in favour of surgery.

(2) If the positioning of the radium proves unsatisfactory or if it is impossible to locate the canal for the main central source, the treatment policy with regard to subsequent irradiation can be adjusted at this stage.

There are occasions when it is prudent to initiate the treatment with the external irradiation. If there is extensive associated local infection, an initial 3,000 rads to the whole pelvis will help greatly to improve this. Likewise, if the tumour has caused sufficient distortion of the normal anatomy of the cervix to make it difficult to locate the canal, it is wise to start with external treatment. After about 3,000 rads, the tumour usually will have regressed sufficiently to allow easy insertion of the radium.

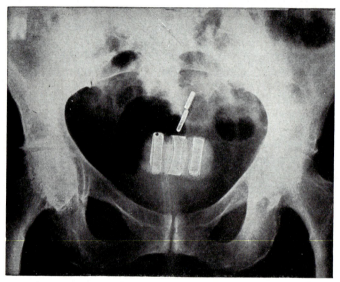

FIG. 349. X-ray of pelvis, showing positioning of radium in a "Manchester" insertion. Note that the central opacity between the two ovoids is, in fact, a spacer and *not* a third radium-containing ovoid. (Macleod & Read, "Gynaecology".)

Pre-operative Irradiation

Some gynaecologists prefer their patients to have a radium insertion prior to surgery. There is no doubt that this can be helpful in reducing the tumour mass and thereby helping to eliminate any infection before the operation. Whether it improves results by diminishing the risk of malignant cells disseminated at the time of operation causing metastases, is another matter. If pre-operative radium is given, no more than two insertions should be attempted because the resultant reaction may greatly complicate the dissection. Also, the impaired circulation that results from irradiation may cause delay in healing.

Post-operative Radiotherapy

Pelvic irradiation following surgery for carcinoma of the cervix is only indicated when the surgery has been incomplete or when histological examination of the lymph nodes shows that there has been infiltration by the tumour.

Recent Advances in Therapy

1. New Isotopes

Radium is a potentially dangerous source of irradiation because its active principle, radon, is a gas. If a radium tube should be damaged, there is a risk that the radon could escape and be inhaled. Therefore, radium is gradually being withdrawn from centres and is being replaced by sources loaded with caesium or some other suitable isotope.

2. "After-Loading" Techniques

A further improvement is the introduction of "after-loading" techniques, which are designed to overcome the irradiation hazard to nursing and medical staff, as well as to other patients sharing the same ward. In similar fashion to the conventional radium insertion, a catheter of special design is inserted into the uterine canal. After its position has been checked by means of radiographs, the patient is transferred to the treatment room where the catheter is connected to the special unit which contains the radio-active sources held in readiness for use. The therapist then leaves the room and the radio-active source is transferred by remote control into the patient. After the calculated time of exposure has elapsed, the radio-active source will automatically be withdrawn back into the protective container. The patient can then be disconnected from the unit and returned to the ward.

3. Hyperbaric Oxygen

The results of treating Stage III tumours are poor and it seems likely that one reason for these bad results is that these tumours outgrow their blood supply and the resultant anoxia partially protects the malignant cells from the irradiation. To overcome this factor, some centres have been irradiating the more advanced cases in special chambers under conditions of hyperbaric oxygenation and the results so far appear to be encouraging.

Carcinoma of the Cervical Stump

The prognosis for this type of tumour is not quite so good as that for a straightforward carcinoma of the cervix, as the natural barriers to tumour spread are no longer present. However, if the remaining cervical canal is sufficiently long to accommodate a radium source the tumour may be treated by means of radiotherapy in the same manner as described for carcinoma of the cervix.

Carcinoma of the Corpus Uteri

Carcinoma of the corpus uteri is nearly always an adenocarcinoma of the endometrium which in general responds poorly to irradiation, and surgery should be relied upon as the primary form of treatment. The place of radiotherapy is usually confined to a supplementary role, being recommended for post-operative pelvic irradiation when the tumour is poorly differentiated, or has either invaded locally or metastasised more widely. The degree of sensitivity of corporeal carcinoma to radiotherapy is variable.

Figures 350 and 351 are lymphangiograms of a patient with carcinoma of the corpus uteri with widespread lymphatic involvement, especially of the para-aortic lymph nodes. The nodes were treated widely by means of cobalt teletherapy using an inverted Y-shaped field. Although it was possible to give such a large treatment volume only 4,000 rads in five weeks, it can be seen that there has been an excellent response. It is always worth while attempting treatment in circumstances such as these in the hope that the tumour may prove to be radio-sensitive.

Carcinoma of the corpus uteri has a tendency to involve the vaginal vault post-operatively. The importance of removing a generous cuff of the

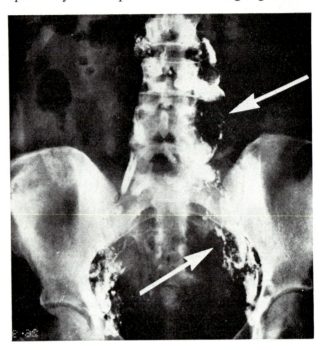

Fig. 350. Lymphangiogram of a patient with carcinoma of the corpus uteri showing massive lymph node involvement confirmed by biopsy.

vagina at operation cannot be over-emphasised, but many surgeons prefer to endorse this measure by giving radium therapy to the vaginal vault either before or after the operation. Pre-operative treatment consists of a single radium insertion and the hysterectomy is then performed two to four weeks later, by which time the radiation reaction will have subsided. If post-operative vault irradiation is preferred, this will be undertaken a few weeks after operation, as soon as the vault has healed satisfactorily. A specially designed vaginal applicator with a central source of radium is inserted under general anaesthesia. The upper half of the vagina will be treated and a radium source of appropriate length will be selected to cover this area. A dose not exceeding 4,000 rads at 0·5 cm. tissue depth should be given.

There are some centres that rely upon radiotherapy as the preferred method of primary treatment for carcinoma of the corpus uteri. The Stockholm method of packing the uterine cavity with multiple small sources of radium is used and this is subsequently supplemented by external irradiation to the gland fields.

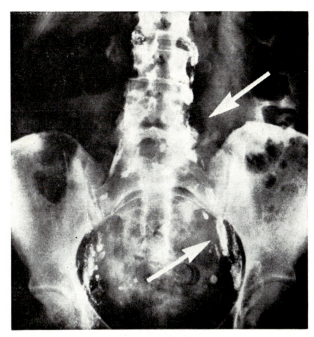

FIG. 351. Lymphangiogram of the same patient following irradiation of the involved nodes. Note the decrease in size of the nodes, as indicated by the arrows.

Chorion Epithelioma

This is a rare condition that deserves special mention. It is a highly radiosensitive tumour but in spite of this the results, even when combined with radical surgery, have been poor. The introduction of cytotoxic drugs has completely altered the management of these tumours and a 70% five-year survival rate can now be expected. The drugs that have proved most effective are Methotrexate and Velbe, but Actinomycin D is at times used when the tumour does not respond to the first two agents.

Tumours of the Ovary

The prognosis with these tumours, except for granulosa cell tumours and dysgerminomas, is very poor. The treatment of choice is total hysterectomy and bilateral salpingo-oöphorectomy. Formerly, the uterus was frequently conserved at the time of operation so that it might act as a carrier for radium at a later date, but there is no virtue in doing this. From the radiotherapeutic aspect, subsequent treatment to the pelvis can be given more efficiently by external irradiation. Furthermore, the uterus is a possible site for spread of the tumour and on this account alone should be removed. If by chance the tumour should be ruptured during the course of its removal, it is advisable to instil Thiotepa mgm. 45 into the peritoneal cavity before closure, in the hope that this cytotoxic agent will destroy any viable malignant cells that have been released. Even if after opening the abdomen it becomes apparent that a radical operation is not possible, it is still advisable to remove as much as possible of the tumour mass together with the omentum as this procedure alone, followed by pelvic irradiation, can give good palliation.

Post-Operative Radiotherapy

Most radiotherapists agree that the following circumstances necessitate post-operative pelvic irradiation:

(a) Local spread of the tumour beyond the ovary.
(b) Involvement of the other ovary by tumour.
(c) Lymph node metastases.
(d) Peritoneal seedlings in the pelvis.
(e) Rupture of the tumour at the time of removal.

This treatment will take the form of external irradiation to the lymph node drainage of the pelvis in much the same way as for other forms of pelvic neoplasia. An exception is made with a dysgerminoma as this tumour behaves in a similar manner to a seminoma, spreading up from the iliac nodes to involve the para-aortic lymph chain. With these tumours, it is essential to have a lymphangiogram which acts as a guide in planning the treatment, which will cover the whole lymph chain from the level of the xiphisternum down to the external iliac lymph nodes. Even if there is no clinical evidence of involvement, the survival rate is greatly improved by this treatment. These tumours are very radio-sensitive and a dose to the glands of 3,500 rads in four to five weeks will prove fully adequate.

Cytotoxic Drugs

These are of special importance in the management of ovarian tumours. Chlorambucil, Thiotepa and Cyclophosphamide are the three drugs which are most consistently effective. Thiotepa is especially renowned for its depressant effect on the bone marrow but no cytotoxin should be given without adequate facilities for repeated blood counts and experience in the management of cytotoxic therapy. Up to 40% of tumours may respond in some degree to these drugs, and in instances of widely disseminated disease, cytotoxic therapy should always be attempted after the planned course of radiotherapy has been completed.

Carcinoma of the Fallopian Tube

This is the rarest site for a gynaecological cancer. With few exceptions, these tumours are adenocarcinomas. They should be managed by means of radical surgery, followed by post-operative telecobalt therapy such as would be given for a carcinoma of the corpus uteri.

Tumours of the Vagina

These are almost entirely squamous cell carcinomas which are only moderately sensitive to irradiation. The tumour usually arises from the upper part of the posterior vaginal wall. If radical surgery is to be successful, it may be necessary to exenterate the pelvis, to divert the urine and form a colostomy. If the tumour is one of the less common variety which involves the lower two-thirds of the vagina, surgery will entail not only removal of the vagina, but also a total vulvectomy. It is not surprising that radiotherapy is normally selected as the primary treatment.

If the tumour is at the vault, the treatment will be similar to that prescribed for carcinoma of the cervix, using a combination of local radium plus external irradiation for the gland fields. In the lower half of the vagina, the tumour may be suitable for interstitial irradiation, using radium needles. A single plane implant is usually all that is necessary but great care must be taken to be certain that none of the needles penetrates either the urethra, bladder or rectum. If this form of treatment is not suitable, a radium applicator may be made for the patient with the radium so arranged to give a surface dose of 10,000 R. to the lesion.

Metastatic deposits in the vagina are by no means unknown and may arise from a carcinoma of the corpus uteri or very rarely from a left-sided hypernephroma. The treatment is the same as for a primary tumour and the usual practice is to use radium needles to implant the deposit. Sometimes, with a small lesion it may be more satisfactory to use gold seeds for the implant.

Carcinoma of the Urethra

This is a rare tumour and more usually involves the external part of the urethra, in which case it may be successfully treated by means of a cylindrical radium needle implant. This will surround the urethra in which is positioned a self-retaining catheter that remains in place for the duration of the implant. According to the size of the tumour, a dose of 6,000–7,000 R. in six to eight days will be prescribed. Tumours involving the posterior part of the urethra tend only to give rise to symptoms when they are far advanced and therefore their prognosis is poor.

Carcinoma of the Vulva

This disease is usually associated with leucoplakia or other pre-malignant hypertrophic changes. 96% of the tumours are squamous cell carcinomas but other epithelial tumours, such as Bowen's disease, malignant melanoma and basal cell carcinoma may rarely occur. The vulva tolerates irradiation poorly, partly due to the persistent presence of secretions and partly as a result of the inevitable trauma from the anatomical position of the tumour. Radical vulvectomy is the treatment to be preferred and radiotherapy is only prescribed when surgery is contraindicated. In this situation, the treatment can be given either by means of an electron beam, which has the virtue of treating only to a limited depth, or an extensive radium implant may be performed. The dose for this implant will be limited to 5,000–6,000 R. in eight days on account of the unusually large area that has to be treated.

Carcinoma of the vulva (and sometimes carcinoma of the urethra) frequently metastasises to the inguinal lymph nodes. Here again, the treatment of choice is surgery, performing a full block dissection. The groins tolerate irradiation poorly as a result of the perspiration which is liable to accumulate in the groin creases, especially of fat people. Also, the constant movement of the lower limbs plays its part in aggravating what would otherwise be a mild reaction. However, with high energy irradiation it is sometimes possible to give these glands 5,000 rads in 4–5 weeks and this should be attempted if there are contraindications to surgery.

Malignant Ascites

This is a most distressing condition and frequently occurs in the latter stages of carcinoma of the ovary. It is essential to have the fluid examined to confirm the presence of malignant cells. There is a 50% chance that the condition may be improved by the administration of either cytotoxic drugs or radio-active gold into the peritoneal cavity. There is little to choose in the response rate between the radio-active gold and the cytotoxic drugs and therefore a drug such as Thiotepa should be selected in preference to the radio-active gold, which is not without its hazards. Apart from the danger emanating from the radio-active gold in the patient to all her attendants, there is also some risk of the gold causing adhesions, intestinal obstruction and, very occasionally, fistula formation in the patient. Therefore, gold should only be used in those cases when cytotoxic drugs have failed to be effective; if the blood count is satisfactory, between 100 and 150 mC. of radio-active gold may be instilled into the peritoneal cavity. The gold must flow in freely and if there should be any suspicion that the ascitic collection is loculated, the gold must not be injected. After administration, the patient is "postured" every 15 minutes for about $1\frac{1}{2}$ hours in order to ensure that the colloidal gold is evenly distributed over the peritoneal lining to help it achieve its best effect.

Hormone Therapy

In recent years, more interest has been taken in the use of various hormones to control tumours which are known sometimes to be restrained by these drugs. With gynaecological tumours, the most successful hormone has proved to be Progesterone. Large doses are necessary (Provera 100 mg. t.i.d.) and about 20% of metastatic disease from carcinoma of the corpus uteri may be expected to respond, if only temporarily.

NON-MALIGNANT CONDITIONS

Pruritus Vulvae

The treatment of this condition with superficial irradiation should, with very few exceptions, be resisted. There is usually a straightforward underlying pathological cause and if it should be associated with leucoplakia, this in itself is a direct contraindication to treatment with radiotherapy, being a pre-malignant condition. If no underlying cause can be detected, small doses of superficial irradiation (75 R. × 4, at weekly intervals) no doubt will be effective temporarily, but before long the patient will be requesting a further course of treatment.

Artificial Menopause

The main indications for an artificial menopause are as follows:
1. Endometriosis.
2. Metropathia haemorrhagica.
3. Dysfunctional uterine haemorrhage.
4. Carcinoma of the breast, as an ablative form of hormonal therapy.

In all these situations, this treatment is symptomatic and where possible in the first three instances, appropriate surgical treatment is preferable. In the last instance, for carcinoma of the breast, surgical removal of the ovaries is also to be preferred as the effect on the hormonal environment is immediate.

The decision to establish a radiation menopause is usually prompted by some underlying medical condition which makes surgery undesirable. The usual method of creating this artificial menopause is by means of external irradiation to the ovaries. In the past, it was commonplace to induce it by means of local irradiation with radium, inserting a standard source into the uterine canal and leaving it in place for 24 hours. This technique is now seldom used and external irradiation is the method preferred. Before embarking on this treatment, it is essential that the patient should be examined under an anaesthetic and a curettage be performed to ensure that no underlying malignant pathology is causing the symptoms.

The technique of the treatment is simple and causes the patient the minimum of disturbance. The pelvis is irradiated by means of a pair of parallel opposed fields, large enough to be certain of covering the ovaries wherever they may be lying, and the treatment is given in four or five fractions in as many days by means of cobalt teletherapy. The actual dosage to be prescribed varies according to the age of the patient. In a younger woman, a dose of 800 rads to the ovaries will be effective but with a patient nearer the age of the natural menopause, a dose in the region of 500–600 rads will be adequate. Very occasionally, the treatment may cause a little nausea, in which event a suitable anti-emetic drug may be prescribed. The patient should be warned that she may well have one further normal menstrual loss, but after this occasion any form of bleeding must be regarded as being abnormal and must be investigated. A rule should be made that the patient is seen two months after the induction of this menopause in order to confirm that there has been no further bleeding.

REACTIONS TO RADIOTHERAPY

These will occur at the time of treatment, or at a later date, possibly even years later.

Early Reactions

Radiation Sickness: This syndrome includes not only symptoms of anorexia, nausea and sometimes vomiting, but also there may be headaches, lassitude and a loss of general sense of well being. The cause of these symptoms is uncertain, but they occur most frequently when extensive volumes are being irradiated with large doses. It seldom occurs when radium is being used but by contrast, when the whole abdominal cavity is being treated by radio-active gold, this may be a feature. In common with other forms of sickness, suggestion can play an important part and positive reassurance at the start of treatment is important. If symptoms develop in spite of this, anti-emetic drugs such as Fentazin or Maxolon are usually effective and it is seldom necessary to have to reduce the amount of daily treatment.

Blood Changes: At the start of treatment, it is essential to have a full blood count and this should be repeated at weekly intervals during the course. The first cells to be affected by irradiation are the lymphocytes and in time there may be some reduction in the number of polymorphs and later, in the platelet count. Any drop in blood count that occurs is generally only slight unless a large volume of bone marrow is being irradiated.

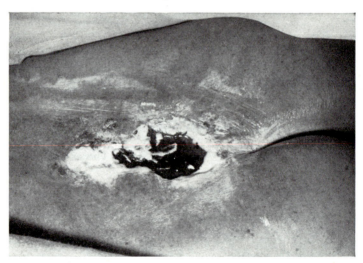

FIG. 352. Deep radiation burn with necrosis of skin and extensive loss of tissue down to the sacrum from which large sequestra of dead bone periodically were discharged. This patient was treated elsewhere for carcinoma of the cervix before the introduction of the modern techniques, and such a severe accident should never be seen.

Skin Reactions: High energy radiation as a general rule does not cause severe skin reactions. As previously mentioned, the groins and vulva are most susceptible to irradiation but reactions at these sites can be reduced by the patient having regular warm baths (without using soap) and, after carefully drying the skin, talcum powder should be freely applied (Fig. 352).

Mucosal Reactions: The mucosa responds to irradiation in similar fashion to the skin, by developing an erythema, which may progress to exudation and later desquamation. These changes are best seen in the vagina, following

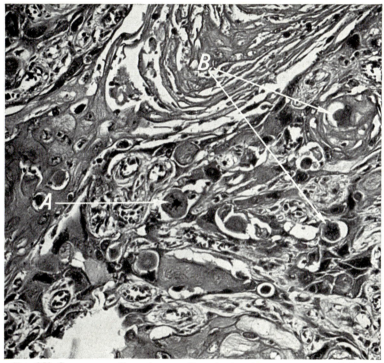

FIG. 353. Squamous cell carcinoma of cervix showing response to radiation. Note nuclear disintegration (karyorrhexis) at A, and widespread vacuolation of the malignant cells at B. (× 210.)

local use of radium, and will gradually regress over the next two weeks or so, especially if there is no associated infection. When the bladder is affected, symptoms of cystitis develop but the most troublesome symptoms occur with bowel reactions. If the small bowel is being affected, the patient will have frequent bowel actions associated with colic. These are danger signs, as small bowel tolerates irradiation poorly and the treatment each day must either be reduced or suspended for a while. Large bowel reactions take the form of the patient having to defaecate frequently and at times she may pass nothing more than mucus; tenesmus may also occur. These symptoms usually improve with some reduction in the daily dose of irradiation but, at times, it may be necessary to prescribe hydrocortisone suppositories.

Late Reactions

SKIN CHANGES are not often seen following mega-voltage irradiation but after treatment with radium it is usual to see some atrophic changes. The vaginal mucosa becomes pale and less moist and there is a tendency for the canal to contract. Adhesions may form at the vault which sometimes occlude the cervix from view.

Radiation Fibrosis: Radical treatment will give rise to a certain amount of fibrosis, and this is most apparent in patients who have had extensive disease. When tumour is destroyed by irradiation, it is replaced by scar tissue and at times this may feel indistinguishable from recurrent growth. The slow progression of these signs, coupled with absence of symptoms of active disease usually confirm the diagnosis.

Pathological Fractures: These still do occur occasionally, even with mega-voltage therapy. They should be treated in the normal way and usually heal without difficulty.

Bowel: These late reactions can take various forms, according to the part of the intestine involved. If it is the small intestine, a malabsorption syndrome with a macrocytic anaemia may develop, due to a deficiency of folic acid uptake. In less severe cases, there may be only an increased liability to diarrhoea with any dietary indiscretion.

In the case of large bowel reactions, these are usually associated with excessive dosage from faulty positioning of radium. Fibrosis may occur at the recto-sigmoid junction which at times is so severe that a complete stricture results and a colostomy becomes necessary. In the milder cases, the patient may pass small amounts of blood in her stools. Proctoscopic examination usually reveals an area of telangiectasia which is the cause, and conservative treatment, recommending a low residue diet and the use of hydrocortisone suppositories, is the best policy.

From time to time, patients may develop intestinal obstruction following radical pelvic irradiation. It usually occurs within 18 months of treatment as a result of adhesions which develop if an exudative reaction of the bowel occurs at the time of treatment. These adhesions can be extensive and their division is not an easy task.

Bladder: High dose changes in the bladder can usually be explained by faulty positioning of radium. The presenting symptom of haematuria results from mucosal telangiectasia which, if persistent, may require local cauterisation to halt the bleeding.

Fistula Formation between the vagina and either bladder or rectum is frequently attributed to the radiotherapy, but careful assessment usually confirms that the presence of active disease is responsible.

27 Endometriosis

By definition endometriosis is the presence of ectopic endometrium in any situation outside its normal location, namely, the lining of the cavity of the uterine body. It is advisable to demand certain histological criteria before labelling ectopic glandular elements as endometriosis even if these glandular islets have the appearance of endometrium on superficial examination. These criteria are:—

(1) An appearance in which the lining epithelium resembles that of endometrium.

(2) The presence of typical endometrial stroma surrounding the glandular spaces.

(3) The ectopic endometrium should be responsive to the endocrine stimulus of oestrogen and, to a lesser degree, of progesterone so that it is capable of a miniature menstruation. This response is seen in the characteristic appearance of cystic glandular hyperplasia in some lesions and the much less frequent saw-tooth, crenated appearance typical of the progestational phase of the cycle. Moreover if the patient with endometriosis becomes pregnant the heterotropic endometrium may show a decidual reaction in its stromal cells.

(4) The content of these ectopic endometrial glands is dark, altered, tarry menstrual blood.

(5) The presence of pigment-laden scavenger macrophages in a deep layer surrounding the endometrial cyst lining. These pseudo-xanthoma cells are large and polyhedral and contain haemosiderin. They somewhat resemble the granulosa lutein cells of a corpus luteum.

By no means all areas of clinical endometriosis fulfil all these diagnostic demands. For instance, the intracystic pressure in a large tarry cyst will destroy the lining epithelium which is no longer recognisable as endometrial in origin and it is then by inference and circumstantial evidence that the diagnosis is made. Response to progesterone is relatively rare so that secretory changes in the epithelial lining of endometriosis is particularly diagnostic. Nor should undue reliance be placed on the presence of pseudo-xanthoma cells as these scavengers also surround a corpus luteum or follicular haematoma, the contents of which are also tarry and the pathology of which has nothing to do with endometriosis. From these remarks it will be realised that the histological corroboration of a clinically suspected endometriosis is far from easy or certain.

General Observations. Having defined the histological criteria by which an endometriosis can be accepted as such, certain further observations can be added. The condition is pathologically peculiar since endometriosis is essentially benign and yet it possesses the powers of invading healthy, adjacent structures. In this propensity it is unique. The suffix -oma should, therefore, be replaced by that of osis-, since -oma suggests a neoplastic process. Adenomyoma and endometrioma are consequently better termed adenomyosis and endometriosis. It is true that endometriosis results in a tumour in the strict sense of the word which means a swelling but not in the sense that tumour has tended to acquire, namely a neoplastic process. Ferreira and Clayton in 1958 could find only twenty-three authentic instances in the literature of carcinoma developing in an area of endometriosis.

The disease is one of adult sexual life, as is to be expected from its definition in paragraph one of this chapter and it is rare indeed to find it active in post-menopausal women. It may also be regarded as an oestrogen-dependent disease. The peak incidence is the decade 30–40 and the patient is either nulliparous in over 50% or has had only one or at most two children several years previously. The association of endometriosis and infertility may explain the greater incidence amongst the affluent classes where family limitation is more effectively employed than in the lower social grades who have more children and less endometriosis.

It is far commoner than is clinically or pathologically conceded and, if carefully looked for at every laparotomy, will probably be found in 20 to 25% of all patients. This figure might well be increased if the surgeon were to request his pathologist to examine histologically all grossly suspicious areas. The activity of endometriosis does not necessarily last during the whole of the reproductive era and spontaneous regression may occur. There is often evidence of this when a hysterectomy is performed in the 40 to 50 age-group in the dense adhesions and the finding of a few old collections of dark encysted blood. The incidence of pregnancy in a patient known to have endometriosis, proved by previous laparotomy, has a genuine, if largely inexplicable inhibitory effect on the activity of endometriosis. This antagonism between fertility and endometriosis is well recognised clinically and is certainly used therapeutically in the encouragement to become pregnant given to patients who have had conservative operations for endometriosis. The production of a state of pseudo-pregnancy by long term heavy dosage of gestogens has an inhibitory effect on endometriosis (see later under treatment).

Situations of Endometriosis. Endometriosis should be divided into: *internal endometriosis or adenomyosis*, a condition in which islets of endometriosis penetrate from the basal layer of the endometrium into the myometrium. The clinical behaviour and pathological features of adenomyosis interna are rather different from those of endometriosis externa and will be considered in detail later. It is sufficient now to separate it from *endometriosis externa* which comprises all those situations of endometriosis anywhere outside the myometrium. Scott, whose experience in this condition is unparalleled, lists the following situations of endometriosis externa according to their frequency of incidence. Out of a total of 516 patients with histologically proved endometriosis externa:—

(i)   One or both ovaries were in-
      volved in   .   .   .   .   412 (or 79.8%)
      In many instances the ovarian
      situation was one of multiple
      involvement of other organs.

(ii) Pelvic peritoneum including sur-
      face of uterus and tubes   .   .   79
      Pouch of Douglas and utero-
      vesical pouch 264

(iii) Uterosacral ligaments alone   .   19
      (but many of (ii) included the
      uterosacral folds so that the
      actual involvement of uterosacral
      ligaments is greater than 19)

(iv) Rectovaginal septum   .   .   37 ⎫ In all these the recto-
(v)   Anterior rectal wall .   .   . 24⎫| sigmoid would be in-
      and sigmoid colon   .   .   .   4⎭ ⎬volved and in many of
                                          | section (ii)—pelvic peri-
                                          ⎭ toneum.

(vi) Small bowel   1
      Appendix   7
      Omentum   3

(vii) Abdominal scars   .   .   . 4
      Perineal scars 4

(viii) Umbilicus   4
      Processus vaginalis   .   .   . 4

(ix) Bladder 5

This total of situations exceeds the 516 patients as many of the endometrioses were multiple, affecting more than one organ or area.—

From a perusal of the above table and that on the next page, four main situations for endometriosis are readily recognisable:—

(1) Endometriosis or adenomyosis interna in the uterus.

(2) Endometriosis externa in the ovary.

(3) Endometriosis of the pelvic peritoneum involving the ovary and the recto-sigmoid.

(4) Distant extra-pelvic endometriosis in scars, peritoneal hernial sacs, umbilicus, appendix and more distant, apparently extracoelomic situations—perineum, arm, leg and pleura.

The clinical picture and the treatment of each is a little different so that it is advisable to consider each separately later.

Distribution of Endometriosis (after Masson)

Uterus	1,852
Ovary	904
Pelvic peritoneum and pouch of Douglas	511
Large bowel	360
Fallopian tube	200
Ligaments of uterus	192
Bladder or peritoneum of bladder	62
Rectovaginal septum	67
Vaginal wall	44
Cervix	45
Abdominal wall	37
Small bowel	35
Caecum	18
Umbilicus	11
Appendix	15
Ureter	8
Femoral hernia	2
Labia	1
Vesicovaginal septum	1
	4,365

Other rare distant situations in which endometriosis has been described are the arm (Navratil), the thigh (Schlicke) and the pleura and diaphragm (Brews).

Aetiology

The Implantation Theory. Sampson was the first to maintain that implantation of regurgitated endometrium explains the majority of chocolate cysts of the ovary and of pelvic endometriosis. He presented a formidable mass of evidence in support of this theory, showing that substances injected into the cavity of the uterus permeate along the Fallopian tubes and can be demonstrated at a later date over the pelvic peritoneum. It is also well known that menstrual blood is often found in the pelvis at laparotomy during normal menstruation and Halban has found endometrial tissue in this fluid. Similarly, grafting experiments have shown that the endometrium can be implanted on to the peritoneum, and during pregnancy a decidual reaction comparable to that found in the endometrium has been demonstrated in the stroma of these heterotopic endometrial proliferations. Secretory hypertrophy can sometimes be demonstrated in the affected areas during the menstrual cycle, and it is probable that some degree of menstrual bleeding occurs from them during menstruation itself. In other words, the heterotopic proliferations may be influenced by the normal hormonal control of the menstrual functions. It is definitely established that menstrual regurgitation is a fairly frequent pheno-menon, so that there is much evidence in support of Sampson's theory. The so-called adenomyomata in laparotomy scars after pelvic operations, such as Caesarean section, can most satisfactorily be explained by assuming that pieces of endometrium become implanted in the wound during the operation. Convincing support to Sampson's theory of retrograde menstruation, im-plantation and spread has been provided by the experimental work of Scott, Te Linde and Wharton. They chose the female rhesus monkey since this primate is a cyclically menstruating animal and is known to be capable of developing spontaneous endometriosis.

(1) Ten monkeys were surgically modified so that the uterus menstruated into the abdominal cavity. Six developed endometriosis.

(2) Six monkeys were surgically modified so that their uterus menstruated into the musculature of the abdominal parietes. All these animals developed endometriosis outside the peritoneal cavity and unconnected with the peri- oneum so that the peritoneum cannot be claimed to have had any part in its production. (Contrast with the serosal metaplasia theory later.) The con-clusion from this experimental work is that menstrual fluid can produce endometriosis and that it can do so independently of the peritoneum. Inci-dentally, endometriosis has been produced in the abdominal wall of a human patient by injection of menstrual fluid.

The recent investigations of Hughesdon provide strong additional evidence to fortify the implantation theory. He studied the case histories of twenty-three patients with the addition of two of his own in whom some uterine abnormality had caused gross retrograde menstruation. Some of the causes were developmental atresias, others acquired stenosis or obstruction of the cervix. Fifteen of these twenty-three patients had developed obvious external endometriosis and, in most of the others, there was some presumptive evidence of it, such as adhesions and the presence of blood cysts.

Hughesdon next noted that the critical time interval during which retro-grade menstruation must occur before the development of external endo-metriosis was one to three years, which was similar to that of the experimental rhesus monkeys. The longer the retrograde menstruation occurs, the more likely the development of endometriosis. One possible explanation of this long latent interval is that endometriosis develops not so much by implanta-tion as by induction, that is that the implant itself dies but exerts an inductive effect by its short-lived presence on the host tissue—serosa or sub-serosal mesenchyme, causing a metaplasia into endometrium. A similar inductive effect has been seen in the ovary where the presence of an ovum is capable of modifying the stromal cells of the ovary into theca cells which are highly specialised.

Whatever the method of initial production of the endometriosis, whether by implantation or by induction, the resulting lesion is always at first on the surface of the ovary and not in its substance. The primary position is anti-hilar, i.e. on the opposite side to the hilum and adjacent to the ovarian fimbria where it would be expected to find its first lodgement after tubal regurgitation. The reaction of the ovary to the presence of endometrial tissue

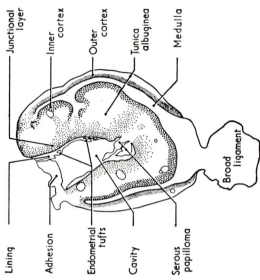

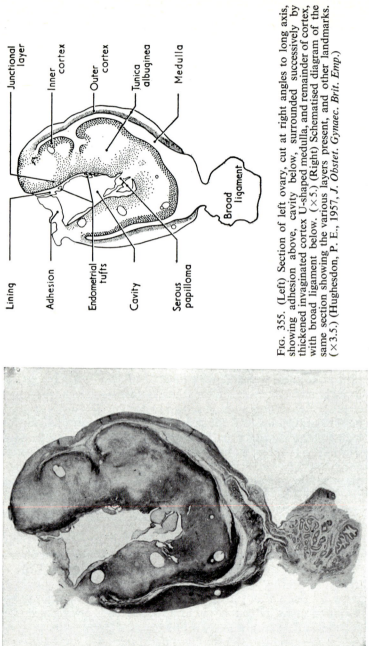

Fig. 355. (Left) Section of left ovary, cut at right angles to long axis, showing adhesion above, cavity below, surrounded successively by thickened invaginated cortex U-shaped medulla, and remainder of cortex, with broad ligament below. (×5.) (Right) Schematised diagram of the same section showing the various layers present, and other landmarks. (×3.5.) (Hughesdon, P. E., 1957, J. Obstet. Gynaec. Brit. Emp.)

is one of buckling and scarring whereby the endometriosis is drawn into a pit, the walls of which are gradually formed by an incurling of ovarian cortex. The shape of this pit resembles a large brandy glass or balloon, the lip of which becomes increasingly contracted until it is sealed by granulation and scar tissue—thereby producing a typical chocolate cyst. The proof of this theory lies in the histological demonstration of two layers of cortex in the cyst wall of the endometriosis—one inner adjacent to the endometriosis and one outer separated by an intervening zone of medulla (Fig. 355).

The Serosal Theory. The serosal theory, which is also called the Iwanoff-Meyer coelomic metaplasia theory, explains almost all forms of chocolate cysts of the ovaries and pelvic endometriosis as due to metaplasia of the peritoneal mesothelium. It is well known that the peritoneal mesothelium frequently undergoes metaplasia and becomes converted into high columnar epithelium, particularly in inflammatory lesions in the pelvis and especially with ectopic gestations. The epithelium of the Müllerian system is primarily derived from the primitive mesothelium of the coelom. The serosal theory therefore postulates that endometriosis externa is due to proliferation of this epithelium and that chocolate cysts of the ovaries and pelvic endometriosis are caused by a similar conversion of the surface epithelium of the ovaries and peritoneal mesothelium. The serosal theory in this way accounts for all forms of endometriosis except adenomyosis interna and it explains even the rare tumours of the umbilicus, endometriosis in hernial sacs, and of laparotomy scars when it is assumed that the peritoneal mesothelium grows into the scar tissue. The supporters of the coelomic metaplasia theory argue that the great objection to Sampson's theory is that the endometrium shed at the time of menstruation is necrotic and non-viable and represents the end-result of a progressive avascular necrosis. Even if some part of the endometrium were shed in a relatively viable state it would be unlikely to survive the interval occupied in its passage from the uterus to its site of alleged implantation and would arrive in a non-viable condition. The experimental work of Scott, Te Linde and Wharton on Rhesus monkeys and the recent publications of Hughesdon can be said to have silenced this reasonable but theoretical objection. The suggestion that the presence of menstrual regurgitation acts as an inductor and evokes a metaplastic change in the coelomic mesothelium or submesothelial mesenchyme provides a neat and happy marriage of this hitherto incompatible couple. The present authors are at the moment, content to leave the matter here.

Hormonal Influence. Whatever the initial genesis of endometriosis, it can be fairly stated that its development depends on the presence of active circulatory ovarian hormone. It is a disease of those decades of a woman's life in which ovarian activity is at its height; it is unknown before puberty and extremely unusual after the menopause. It is a frequent associate of one well-known hyperoestrogenic condition—metropathia haemorrhagica—though, strangely, pregnancy, a state in which there are very high levels of oestrogen in the blood, inhibits it. One explanation of the immunity of the pregnant is that the high level of oestrogen is here constant whereas in other hyperoestrogenic states, it is fluctuant. Extragenital endometriosis can be caused to

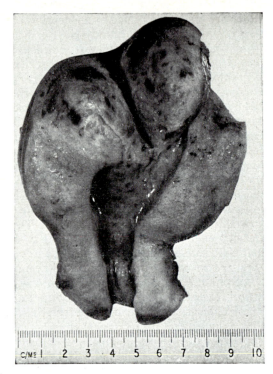

Fig. 356. Adenomyosis of the uterus. The uterus is enlarged asymmetrically, and the rounded dark areas consist of spaces full of blood. The enlargement is caused by hyperplasia of muscle cells surrounding areas of endometrium which have bled during menstruation.

regress by bilateral ovarian removal or destruction by irradiation. The hormone likely to be most responsible is oestrogen and this explains the association of endometriosis and metropathia haemorrhagica. The inhibition of endometriosis by pregnancy has been explained by the high circulating progesterone at this time. Kistner of Boston claims control of endometriosis by inducing a state of pseudo-pregnancy by a long course of orally active progestational steroid—nor-ethynodrel. Meigs maintained that endometriosis is caused by prolonged hyperoestrinism, and that the higher social classes are affected most because they restrict pregnancy.

Morbid Anatomy and Histology

I. Endometriosis Interna or Adenomyosis is quite a common finding, 21·5% of all hysterectomy specimens removed for whatever reason. In this condition the origin of the myometrial endometriosis is a downgrowth of the basal layer of the endometrium which invades deeply into the muscle. Superficial invasion is extremely common and presents no gross macroscopical evidence of its presence, only being detected on histological examination. It is especially seen with cystic glandular hyperplasia in metropathia. The diffuse type of adenomyosis affects a large part of the uterus though one wall may be more involved than the other. Sometimes a localised area of adenomyosis is seen confined to a small region of the uterus where it forms an asymmetrical enlargement clinically indistinguishable from a myoma. This condition has been

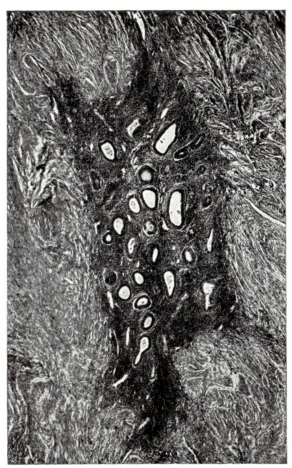

FIG. 357. Adenomyosis uteri. Note the island of endometrial glands with associated stroma deep in the myometrium. (× 33.)

called an adenomyoma but a preferable term is localised adenomyosis. Occasionally, a small localised adenomyosis projects into the cavity of the uterus to form the so-called adenomyomatous polyp. In well-marked generalised adenomyosis interna the uterus is symmetrically enlarged. The affected area is softer in consistence than an intramural myoma, and when incised has a peculiar striated appearance with tiny grey soft areas interspersed amongst the striations. Adenomyosis is never encapsulated as is a myoma and the affected area merges into normal myometrium. Occasionally small collections of blood can be distinguished which are found on microscopical examination to consist of glands filled with blood. Microscopical examination of uterine adenomyosis shows the presence of gland spaces similar to those of the glands of the endometrium surrounded by cellular stroma, again similar to the stroma of the endometrium, while around this cellular stroma lies normal myometrium. The gland spaces do not usually show secretory hypertrophy during the menstrual cycle although this alteration can sometimes be detected.

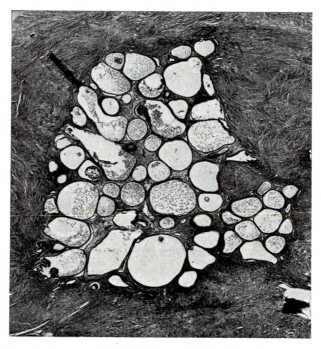

FIG. 358. Adenomyosis uteri. Note the marked glandular dilatation. ($\times$ 16.)

The reason suggested for this glandular inactivity is that the adenomyosis is derived from the basal or inactive layer of the endometrium. This explanation is somewhat hypothetical since it is from this layer that the proliferative endometrium is regenerated after menstruation and this endometrium is far from inactive. The stroma cells, moreover, undergo marked decidual reaction during pregnancy (Figs. 356–358).

Adenomyosis is not often associated with endometriosis externa. There is, however, an exception, when the adenomyosis is derived from an extension of external endometriosis into the myometrium from without, that is from the serosal surface. In this condition the uterus behaves no differently from any other affected structure except that the myometrium modifies the extent of the invasive process more effectively than the ovary and controls the expansion of the endometrial cysts. In fact, the histological appearances of this external adenomyosis as it is sometimes called, are no different from those of internal endometriosis. The origin is, however, different and the coincident pelvic endometriosis obviously causative. Careful section of the specimen will

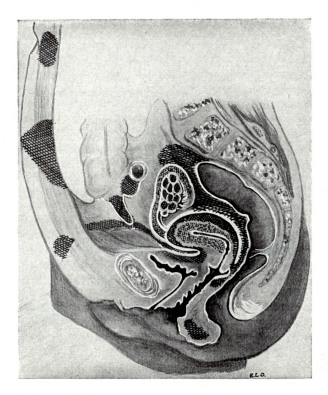

FIG. 359. The distribution of pelvic endometriosis. The types illustrated are those of the umbilicus, laparotomy scars, round ligament, appendix and small intestine. Adenomyosis interna of the Fallopian tube and uterus are shown with a different shading. Adenomyosis externa of the uterus and Douglas's pouch, the sigmoid, the rectovaginal septum and the ovary are also shown. Lastly, the rare form of the perineal endometrioma is illustrated. (After Halban-Seitz.)

demonstrate the pathway of entry and the surface of the uterus itself shows pigmented, puckered and indrawn areas of endometriosis. This type of adenomyosis, being associated with endometriosis externa and pelvic endometriosis will be considered under that heading since it is really only an extension into the uterus of the generalised pelvic condition.

Clinical Features of Adenomyosis Interna. In nearly all instances the main presenting symptoms is menorrhagia of fairly severe degree. Half the patients will complain of a feeling of weight in the pelvis which is worse in the premenstrual phase and about a third will have congestive dysmenorrhoea. Infertility is a frequent symptom.

The physical signs are either (*a*) a symmetrical enlargement of the uterus if the adenomyosis is diffuse. The enlargement rarely exceeds that of a three months pregnancy and is usually diagnosed as a fibroid. If, however, a woman of 35 to 40 gives a history of menorrhagia with accompanying dysmenorrhoea, whose periods have before been painless, a shrewd observer will always consider the possibility of adenomyosis. (*b*) If the adenomyosis is localised and circumscribed usually in the region of one cornu, the enlargement is asymmetrical and the resemblance to a myoma is more close. A myoma of this size is rarely painful unless degenerate which, again, is unusual for so small a tumour. Therefore a painful, asymmetrical enlargement of the uterus should suggest the correct diagnosis.

Treatment. As most of these patients are about forty years of age and the likelihood of conception is small and since it is technically often impossible to excise the tumour and conserve a healthy uterus capable of child-bearing, the correct treatment is total hysterectomy. If the condition is strictly limited to the uterus and the ovaries are not involved, there is no need to remove them. In true adenomyosis interna, the ovaries are usually not affected. In younger women, in whom a localised adenomyosis is found confined to one cornu of the uterus, a localised excision is sometimes feasible and this conservative resection is reasonable if the patient is particularly anxious to have a child. She should be warned that the price of conservatism, though laudable, may be another operation at a later date.

II. Endometriosis Externa. Endometriosis externa by strict definition includes all those varieties of endometriosis not resulting from a downgrowth of the basal layer of the endometrium into the uterine muscle—the adenomyosis or endometriosis interna already described. It also includes those examples of adenomyosis of the uterus in which the ectopic endometrial islets have entered the uterus from outside its cavity—that is, by invasion from an external endometriosis on the serosal surface. As the lesions are so often multiple involving, for example, ovary, pelvic peritoneum and rectosigmoid, topographical divisions are largely artificial.

(1) *The most frequent site of external endometriosis is the ovary*, 80% of all lesions being situated here.

(2) *The second most frequent site is the pelvic peritoneum* of the pouch of Douglas, especially that of the uterosacral folds and the anterior surface of the pouch in relation to the upper one-third of the vagina, the back of the cervix and uterus. From here the process may spread to:

(3) *The anterior wall of the recto-sigmoid*, forming a densely adherent mass of uterus, bowel and ovary and invariably obliterating the pouch of Douglas so that the recto-sigmoid is firmly fixed to the back of the uterus. The obliteration of the pouch of Douglas is one of the most constant and characteristic signs of pelvic endometriosis. The adhesions are of a dense cartilaginous nature and can only be unravelled by a cutting instrument, blunt dissection being usually impossible and frequently dangerous.

(4) From here the endometriosis naturally spreads to the *recto-vaginal septum* and may even present as small dark blue or purple discrete spots in the posterior vaginal fornix.

It is convenient from the clinical, pathological and surgical viewpoint to consider all these varieties of endometriosis as one unit since they frequently co-exist though one organ may be the most obviously involved.

(1) **Chocolate Cysts of the Ovaries.** Chocolate cysts of the ovaries represent the most important clinical manifestation of the proliferations. The affected ovary is enlarged and its outer surface is white and thickened. The ovary and Fallopian tube are prolapsed and fixed to the back of the uterus, to the back of the broad ligament and perhaps to the sigmoid colon as well by dense

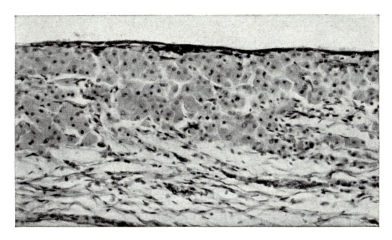

Fig. 360. Chocolate cyst of the ovary. Above lies the cavity of the cyst which is lined by endothelial cells. Beneath the endothelial lining are large poly-hedral deeply staining pseudo-xanthoma cells.

relatively avascular adhesions of pelvic endometriosis. Separation of the ovary from these attachments is difficult, and during the separation it is customary for the cyst in the ovary to rupture and discharge dark brown altered blood into the peritoneal cavity. Usually the cyst measures about two inches in diameter, but small chocolate cysts are not uncommon, while rarely large tumours as much as nine inches in diameter may be encountered. The disease is obviously bilateral in about a third of all cases (see Fig. 361). If, however, the good ovary is examined carefully, it will often be found to show on its surface a small thickened area, a shaggy roughness or a dark pinpoint blood spot. This otherwise unaffected ovary, when carefully sectioned, will often show early microscopic evidence of invasion.

To the naked eye the affected ovary after removal shows obvious thickening of the tunica albuginea, and vascular red adhesions are particularly well marked on the under surface of the ovary. The cyst fluid is thick and similar to that contained in a haematocolpos. The inner surface of the cyst wall is vascular and contains areas of dark brown tissue.

The histology of chocolate cysts of the ovaries is extremely difficult. In some cases the cysts are lined by an epithelium which is usually columnar with a tendency to the formation of papillae. Beneath the epithelium a zone of tissue containing large cells with brown protoplasm, polyhedral in shape and closely resembling lutein cells, is nearly always found. These pseudo-lutein cells are probably large macrophages or scavenger cells, and their brown or yellow coloration is due to the ingested blood pigments such as

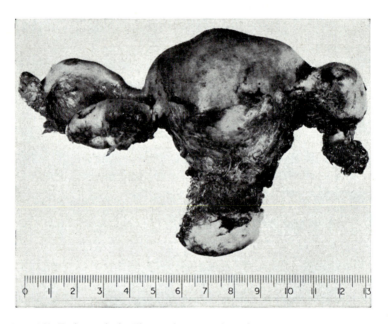

FIG. 361. Endometriosis. The specimen consists of the uterus, both Fallopian tubes and ovaries. The back of the specimen has been photographed. The ovaries are covered with areas of endometriosis and the lower part of the back of the uterus is extensively involved.

haemosiderin (see Fig. 360). In the commonest forms of chocolate cysts the epithelial lining is either incomplete or is represented only by flattened endo-thelial cells, although these cells tend to become columnar in the region of crypts and pockets in the wall. With old-standing cysts, when hyaline tissue has been deposited beneath the surface epithelium, the epithelium may occa-sionally become high columnar with a well-marked tendency to the formation of papillae and a subjacent cellular stroma may be developed. It is exceptional for tissue closely resembling the endometrium to be found forming part of the lining wall, although such tissue is sometimes seen, and when present is absolutely diagnostic.

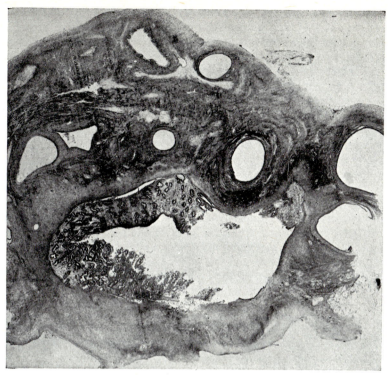

FIG. 362. Ovarian endometriosis. Note the large cyst with an incomplete lining of active endometrium. (× 8.)

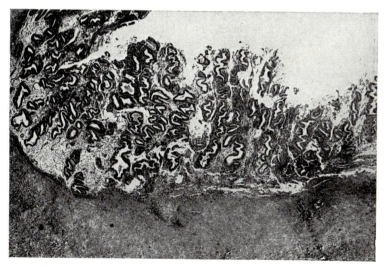

FIG. 363. A higher magnification of Fig. 362 showing a secretory pattern. This is an unusual feature of endometriosis. (× 20.)

(2) **Pelvic Endometriosis.** A minor degree of pelvic endometriosis is extremely common. If, during hysterectomy for myomata, the uterus is drawn forcibly upwards and forwards, it is quite common to see minute black cysts beneath the peritoneum in the region of the uterosacral folds. These indurated dark spots have been given a number of descriptive, if picturesque, terms such as powder-shot burns or *les yeux de perdrix*. These areas are often surrounded by dense scar tissue which restricts the mobility of the uterus. In more severe cases the affected area is not only fibrotic but covered with red vascular adhesions which fix the bowel and adjacent structures firmly to Douglas's pouch and to the back of the uterus. The areas of fibrosis are important because they can be detected easily on vaginal examination. Well-marked pelvic endometriosis is usually associated with the presence of chocolate cysts in the ovaries, when the ovaries and Fallopian tubes become fixed to the back of the uterus and to the sigmoid colon. Small areas of endometriosis are often found in the uterovesical pouch. It is very exceptional, however, for endometriosis to be found above the level of the pelvic brim. Occasionally small areas form on the mesentery and may even cause intestinal obstruction. On histological examination areas of pelvic endometriosis show the presence of glands similar to those of the endometrium, but the similarity is not always very striking and it is unusual for the glands to be surrounded by a stroma comparable to that of the endometrium. The glands sometimes undergo secretory hypertrophy. Similarly, the stroma undergoes decidual reaction during pregnancy (Figs. 362 and 363).

Symptoms of Ovarian and Pelvic Endometriosis

Not by any means all patients with endometriosis have symptoms referable to this particular disease. It is quite frequently found when performing a hysterectomy for myomata that well established endometriosis co-exists. Moreover, if the back of the uterus and the uterosacral ligaments are carefully inspected during all hysterectomies for conditions other than endometriosis, evidence of its presence can often be found in thickening of the uterosacral ligaments, roughening of the peritoneum, adhesions of the ovaries to the back of broad ligament, and multiple small dark-brown or black pinpoint puckerings or nodules. The practised gynaecologist can identify this evidence at a glance and accurately state that endometriosis is or has been present.

Pain. This is usually a deep-seated dull ache appreciated in the region of the mid-pelvis and referred to the sacrum, lumbar region, rectum and lower abdomen. When a chocolate cyst of an endometriosis leaks or ruptures, it gives rise to an acute pain simulating appendicitis. Rupture and leakage is far commoner than generally acknowledged, largely because these patients are operated on by general surgeons, suspecting an acute appendicitis. Others are diagnosed as an extra-uterine gestation. Both these mistakes are reasonable and only avoidable if a most careful history is taken from the patient and a competent bimanual pelvic examination performed.

Dysmenorrhoea. Any woman over 30 who suddenly develops congestive dysmenorrhoea, not primarily having suffered from it, should suggest a diagnosis of endometriosis somewhere. In actual fact, only half the patients suffer from dysmenorrhoea. The pain occurs before, during or even after menstruation and is due to a congestion of the functional ectopic endometrium and an increase in intracystic tension due to menstruation. It is at this time that a cyst is likely to undergo spontaneous rupture when, as stated, the pain becomes acute and resembles that of any acute intra-abdominal emergency.

Disturbances of Menstruation are as common as congestive dysmenorrhoea. Menorrhagia, often with a shortened cycle, is usual but irregular bleeding is not caused by endometriosis.

Dyspareunia is especially notable if the endometriosis involves the utero-sacral ligaments, recto-vaginal septum or results in a fixed, tender retroversion of the uterus.

Infertility is, perhaps, one of the most constant symptoms of endometriosis. The cause of it, however, is obscure. It is certainly not due to blockage of the Fallopian tubes as it is a characteristic of endometriosis that these are almost always patent and, if occluded, the occlusion is due to some pathological process other than the endometriosis.

Bowel Symptoms. It is not surprising, since the rectosigmoid is so often involved in the endometriosis, that increasing constipation or discomfort during defaecation should occur. A rarer feature is attacks of diarrhoea and tenesmus due to irritation of the bowel wall. As constipation is so common this symptom tends to be overlooked. It is important, however, as extensive involvement of the bowel wall can lead to a subacute intestinal obstruction. Of greater importance is the differential diagnosis of carcinoma of the colon because the two conditions so closely resemble each other in their physical signs. As endometriosis of the bowel is essentially a serosal involvement it is unusual for the process to invade further than the muscular coat, but it can ulcerate into the lumen on rare occasions and cause cyclical bleeding from the bowel. As proctoscopy will then reveal the ulcerating area it is a natural error to suspect it to be malignant.

Bladder Symptoms. Involvement of the bladder is extremely rare and rarer still is ulceration in the mucosa. When this occurs cyclical haematuria results or unexplained attacks of periodic urinary infection.

(3) **Endometriosis of the Rectovaginal Septum.** The proliferation may spread downwards along the rectovaginal septum or backwards to infiltrate the wall of the rectum and cause rectal symptoms and even stenosis. Various types are described. In the usual form there is a diffuse induration arising in the neighbourhood of the peritoneum of Douglas's pouch which spreads downwards. At other times the endometriosis may produce a papillary excrescence in the upper part of the posterior vaginal wall. There are usually several small blue-domed cysts protruding into the posterior fornix which may later ulcerate and cause cyclical or irregular bleeding. At first sight the symptoms and signs strongly suggest a carcinoma but biopsy should be diagnostic. These patients usually present with painful defaecation as their main symptom. Such examples can be explained best as metaplasia of the obliterated peritoneal mesothelium below the floor of the pouch of Douglas; others probably arise from the peritoneum of the pouch itself and penetrate through the posterior vaginal wall.

Physical Signs. If one or several of the preceding symptoms are present and bimanual examination reveals a fixed and often bilateral appendage swelling with, possibly, a fixed tender retroversion of the uterus and if the examination produces pain similar to that of which the patient complains, the diagnosis should be easy and usually accurate. Large cystic swellings are usually tense and mistaken readily for myomata. Their fixity is, however, a characteristic of endometriosis and is rare with myomata, nor, unless they are degenerate, are myomata tender on examination. If, apart from the swelling in the appendages, the uterosacral ligaments and the pouch of Douglas feel thickened and shotty with multiple small nodules palpable through the posterior fornix, the diagnosis becomes reasonably certain. A fixed retroversion, tender on bimanual examination, in a young woman aged about 30 who gives no history suggestive of pelvic inflammatory disease, should at least suggest a possible diagnosis of endometriosis. With practice, the diagnosis will be made more frequently and accurately, provided its possibility is not forgotten.

Differential Diagnosis

(1) *Chronic salpingitis and salpingo-oöphoritis.* Pelvic inflammatory disease, apart from the history, so closely mimics endometriosis in the symptoms and signs that errors in diagnosis are frequently exchanged between the two. Both produce pelvic pain, congestive dysmenorrhoea, menorrhagia or alteration in menstruation, sterility and dyspareunia. Endometriosis may, if there is a leakage of blood contents, even produce leucocytosis, a raised E.S.R. and moderate fever. The physical signs of both are fixity and tenderness of the uterus and appendages with, possibly, appendage swellings. The only difference is that in endometriosis the tubes are patent, and if gestogen is given for a month in high dosage it provides a reasonably accurate therapeutic test, since endometriosis should respond whereas pelvic inflammatory disease will not.

(2) *Multiple small myomata*, unless degenerate, are painless and can usually be manipulated to demonstrate their mobility. Inadequate examination is usually the cause of error here.

(3) *Ovarian cancer* with metastatic deposits in the pouch of Douglas is sometimes mistaken for endometriosis. The history, the pain, the age of the patient and other symptoms suggestive of endometriosis are against the diagnosis of cancer but the physical signs, apart from tenderness, are very similar to those of an ovarian neoplasm.

(4) If the rectosigmoid is involved sufficiently to cause an alteration in bowel habit or, in the rare event of bleeding occurring into the bowel lumen from an invasive endometriosis, carcinoma of the bowel is, perhaps, a commendable error. In fact, this is a mistake that should be made so that sigmoidoscopy and biopsy can exclude the more lethal disease.

(5) If a chocolate cyst ruptures, all possibilities in an acute abdominal catastrophe must be visualised, including a ruptured tubal gestation though the most frequent error is to operate for acute appendicitis.

Treatment

The treatment of this condition depends somewhat upon the age of the patient and the severity of the symptoms.

Obviously in a young woman, it is important, if possible, to conserve reproductive capacity and if, at laparotomy, some reasonably healthy ovarian tissue can be salvaged in one or both ovaries, an ovarian cystectomy should be performed. Table VIII shows that the pregnancy rate after a conservative operation is by no means to be despised and Te Linde supports this dictum. Should such a conservative operation result in pregnancy, the condition may well become stationary and the present authors know of one patient who, after such an operation for proved bilateral endometriosis, had four successful pregnancies and two miscarriages over a period of thirteen years. Jeffcoate reports similar results.

TABLE VIII. *Pregnancy Rate in External Endometriosis of the Ovaries following Conservative Surgery* (Whitehouse and Bates, 1955)

Authors	Year	No. of cases	Relief of symptoms (expressed as percentages)			Pregnancy rate (per cent.)
			Cured	Improved	Failed	
Read and Roques	1929	14	71·5	19·2	19·3	—
Keene and Kimbrough	1930	21	95·3	4·7	—	28·0
Pemberton	1937	107	71·0	—	29·0	15·0
Counsellor	1938	98	56·2	19·8	24·0	6·0
Holmes	1942	24	29·1	54·1	16·6	12·6
Bacon	1949	138	49·3	21·0	29·7	26·8
Beacham	1949	43	95·5	—	4·5	37·0
Counseller and Crenshaw	1951	48	60·0	28·0	12·0	20·8
Whitehouse and Bates	1954	46	70·0	15·0	15·0	45·7

It is not always possible, however, even in young women, to find sufficient healthy ovary to render a conservative operation worth while and, in fact, both ovaries may be hopelessly disorganised by chocolate cysts in which the ovary itself is represented merely by a capsule adherent to adjacent viscera. When operating on such patients, the surgeon has no choice but to perform a difficult and sometimes hazardous bilateral salpingo-oöphorectomy and total hysterectomy. It is important to remove the uterus since it may be or may become involved in the ovarian endometriosis. After the performance of this operation, other areas of endometriosis will be found in the pelvis and these may be treated by fulguration. Too much attention need not be paid to the meticulous ablation of these secondary situations of the disease since ovarian removal will immediately result in their regression. When operating on external endometriosis, the surgeon must proceed with great caution, using meticulous technique, since the dense adhesions which involve the large and small bowel may well lead to damage of these structures. The endocrine therapy of endometriosis is discussed later.

III. Intestinal Endometriosis. In a survey of this subject, Macafee and Hardy Greer (1960) have published some interesting facts.

(*a*) The true incidence of intestinal endometriosis in 7,177 patients in the world literature was 880—12%.

(*b*) The situation in the involved bowel was as follows:—

Sigmoid, rectum or rectosigmoid . . .	72·4%
Recto-vaginal septum	13·5%
Small bowel	7·0%
Caecum	3·6%
Appendix	3·0%
Elsewhere	0·5%
	100·0%

(*c*) In their own Belfast series, Macafee and Hardy Greer found twenty-nine instances of intestinal endometriosis distributed as follows:—

Bowel involvement without obstruction .	11
Bowel involvement with obstruction . .	8
Involvement of recto-vaginal septum . .	5
Involvement of appendix	5

Of the 8 patients with bowel obstruction, the situation of the obstruction was ileal in 7 and sigmoid in 1. The cause of the obstruction was usually involvement of the terminal ileum in a right-sided ovarian endometriosis.

(*d*) The world literature for bowel obstruction in 371 intestinal endometrioses was 100 or 27% obstructed.

(*e*) The site of the obstruction is more usually sigmoid than ileal—13 sigmoid to 3 ileal in McGuff's 16 patients. The large bowel is, in the authors' opinion, far the commoner site of obstruction. This is in disagreement with the Belfast figures.

The importance of these observations is that obstruction of the bowel by endometriosis is not unusual, and owing to a clinical and radiological resemblance to carcinoma, a mistaken diagnosis may lead to an unnecessarily mutilating operation. Endometriosis of the sigmoid and rectosigmoid is most likely to be confused with carcinoma and the following table (modified) from Macafee and Greer should help to differentiate the two.

	Endometriosis of Colon	*Carcinoma of Colon*
Incidence:	Very rare.	Extremely common.
Age:	25–45.	40–60.
Weight loss:	Little or none.	Marked.
Constipation:	Intermittent, associated with menses.	Progressive and of short duration.
Bleeding on defaecation:	Rare and, if present, only at menses.	Frequent.
Fertility:	Low.	Normal.
Dysmenorrhoea:	Frequent and progressive.	No relationship.
Sigmoidoscopy:	Intact mucosa. No bleeding.	Gross ulceration and bleeding.
Barium enema:	Long filling defect — intact mucosa.	Short filling defect — irregular mucosa.
Biopsy:	Conclusive.	Conclusive.

	Endometriosis of Colon	*Carcinoma of Colon*
Palpation:	(1) Stricture does not encircle bowel.	Stricture encircles bowel.
	(2) Tumour is relatively mobile in bowel.	Tumour fixed to bowel and immobile apart from it.
	(3) No enlarged glands in mesentery.	Glands present in mesentery.
	(4) Serosa and muscularis primarily involved.	Mucosa primarily involved and serosa less so.
Other evidence of pelvic endometriosis:	Present and obvious.	Absent.

Since carcinoma of the colon and diverticulitis have several features in common, diverticulitis and endometriosis may be confused.

The Treatment of Intestinal Endometriosis

(1) If the patient is young and obstruction is present, there is little question that the obstruction must be relieved by resection of the affected segment and anastomosis. Conservative surgery of the ovarian endometriosis may be justifiable.

(2) If the patient is 40 or over and there is intestinal obstruction, resection of the affected segment and total hysterectomy and bilateral salpingo-oöphorectomy or at least bilateral salpingo-oöphorectomy should be performed.

(3) If there is an obvious but non-obstructive bowel lesion and the patient is young, conservative resection of the ovarian endometriosis, if feasible, should be performed and every encouragement given to the patient to become pregnant. Treatment by oral progestogens is very useful in this class.

(4) If the patient is over 40 or has all the family she wants, total hysterectomy and bilateral salpingo-oöphorectomy should be carried out in the hope that the surgical castration will limit the progress of the bowel lesion.

IV. Endometriosis in Unusual Situations. Many of these occur outside the true pelvis and even at some distance from it. Some are extensions of a pelvic endometriosis, e.g. endometriosis in the utero-vesical pouch and bladder. Others are the result of implantation in abdominal or perineal wounds. Often the endometriosis is the sole and obvious example of the disease and the pelvic organs appear to be free of it. These isolated lesions are difficult to explain unless the theory of coelomic metaplasia is accepted. It must, for example, be remembered that a tongue of coelom projects into the processus vaginalis (endometriosis of groin), into the umbilicus (endometriosis of umbilicus) and even into the perineum (perineal endometriosis). Coelomic remnants may be nipped off in the developing limb buds and thus explain endometriosis in the arm and leg.

Another possibility is that these extra-pelvic areas of endometriosis arrive by lymphatic or even vascular embolism. At all events, endometriosis has been demonstrated convincingly in pelvic lymphatic glands and there is no reason why microscopic islets should not travel as emboli in the blood stream. Novak reports a recent instance of a pulmonary tumour for which a lobectomy was performed during pregnancy, in which the tumour mass consisted of decidua.

Situations

(1) **Endometriosis of the Round Ligament and Hernial Sacs in the Groin.**
Endometriosis of the round ligament arises most frequently in the inguinal
canal though occasionally the swellings develop in the labium majus. Tumours
as large as 5 cm. in diameter have been described. These tumours consist of
glandular elements embedded in plain muscle. Areas of endometriosis are
sometimes found in hernial sacs both in the inguinal and femoral canals,
when a tender swelling is produced at the extremity of the sac which usually
swells and causes local pain during menstruation. The swelling consists
mainly of dark altered blood with vascular adhesions, and on microscopical
examination is found to contain glands similar to those of the endometrium.

(2) **Endometriosis of the Umbilicus.** Several reports of this condition have
now accumulated. The clinical feature is the appearance of small, dark-blue
nodules which enlarge at the time of menstruation and are under increased
tension causing a type of extra-uterine localised dysmenorrhoea. A few have
actually been noticed to bleed externally. Histologically, they fulfil the criteria
of endometrium. The interest in this situation lies in the explanation of it.
It is known that lymphatic and vascular channels connect the umbilicus with
the pelvis via the obliterated hypogastric vessels and Cullen's sign in extra-
uterine gestation is one example of how the blood of a pelvic haematocele
may cause a pigmentation and discoloration of the umbilical area. The
presence of a coelomic tongue in the umbilicus has already been mentioned
and this is stressed by the metaplasia exponents.

(3) **Endometriosis in Laparotomy Scars and Perineal Wounds, Episiotomy
Scars and the Scar of a removed Bartholin's Cyst or Abscess.** This is rare when
compared with endometriosis in general. Nicholson has analysed the reported
cases and shown that although the swellings usually develop after operations
upon the uterus, particularly after Caesarean section, they sometimes arise
after pelvic operations such as ventrosuspension. They have also been known
to develop after the removal of ovarian tumours. Usually a diffuse induration
develops in the scar which swells up and becomes painful during menstruation. At other times a sinus forms and menstrual blood is discharged from the
sinus coincidentally with menstruation. In 1942 Greenhill collected 300
examples of scar endometriosis with the following incidence:—

Operation

Ventrofixation	113
Caesarean section	41
Hysterotomy	49
Other openings made in the uterus, e.g.	
myomectomy	26
Adnexal operations	51
Appendicectomy	18
Vulval, vaginal and peritoneal scars	43
All others	49
	——
	390
	——

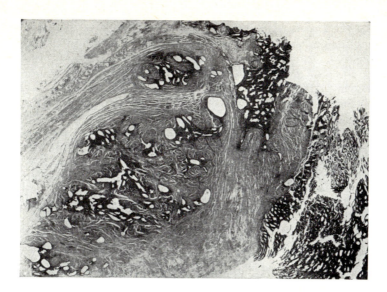

FIG. 364. Endometriosis of the bladder wall. The patient complained of cyclical haematuria. (*Courtesy Dr. A. M. Thomas.*)

The occurrence of endometriosis in appendicectomy scars is particularly interesting (see Fig. 359).

The most likely explanation is that scar endometriosis represents a direct implantation of endometrial fragments at operation and this is easily understood if the uterus is opened. The appendicectomy endometriosis is explained by suggesting that the patient was menstruating at the time of the operation and that the surgeon implanted fragments of regurgitated endometrium from the pelvis. This is comparable to some of the successful implantation experiments designed to produce endometriosis in the abdominal wall. By a similar method, perineal endometriosis is explained by either a coincident curettage or by subsequent menstruation into the granulation tissue of an operation wound which was undergoing delayed healing.

(4) **Endometriosis of the Bladder.** This is very rare and is explained by postulating an infiltration of the bladder from an area of endometriosis in the uterovesical pouch. Patients suffer from haematuria, usually cyclical, and vascular bleeding areas are found in the fundus of the bladder (see Fig. 364).

(5) **Endometriosis of the Omentum.** Although the omentum is frequently adherent to an area of pelvic endometriosis, it is rare for it to be involved in the actual process (see Fig. 365).

(6) **Endometriosis of the Cervix.** Fibrocystic disease, though considered here, has in all probability been wrongly termed endometriosis. The multiple cystic spaces do not contain altered blood but mucus and the lining is not endometrium but a low mucus-secreting columnar epithelium. Moreover,

there is no adjacent area of stroma around the glandular spaces (Fig. 366).

True endometriosis of the cervix does occur and two varieties are described: Extrinsic (the commoner) and intrinsic. In extrinsic, the endometriosis invades the cervix from a pelvic endometriosis via the uterosacral ligaments or from the posterior fornix via the recto-vaginal septum. It is, therefore, part of an extensive pelvic endometriosis, though sometimes the lesion is isolated. The symptoms are pain, dysmenorrhoea and deep dyspareunia. On inspection,

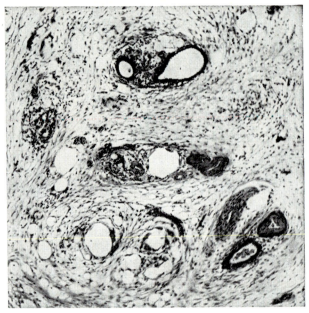

Fig. 365. Photomicrograph of omentum, showing islands of endometriosis. (Measday B., 1961, *Brit. med. J.*)

the characteristic dark blood cysts may be seen. On palpation, there is a firm, irregular tumour which may bleed on examination. It is, however, tough and never friable which helps to exclude the likely diagnosis of carcinoma.

Intrinsic endometriosis of the cervix is a true cervical adenomyosis interna and very rare.

One very plausible theory that explains some cervical endometrioses is that at menstruation endometrial fragments are implanted on the raw areas left after cauterisation and that these surface implants behave exactly as in ovarian endometriosis. In view of the frequency of cauterisation, this theory is reasonable.

The treatment of all extra-pelvic endometrioses is local excision. Provided that the condition is isolated and not part of an extensive pelvic endometriosis, nothing further is needed. Obviously, if pelvic endometriosis co-exists, it requires treatment in its own right.

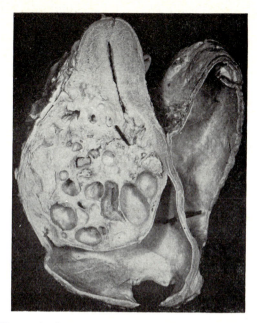

FIG. 366. Fibrocystic disease of the cervix. The bladder lies to the right, the vagina below, while a rod passes through a vesico-vaginal fistula. The tumour filled the pelvis and caused difficulty in micturition and defaecation.

Salpingitis Isthmica Nodosa. This condition, described by Chiari, is less frequent than in previous years. It takes the form of localised nodules in the isthmus of the Fallopian tube, which on microscopical examination are somewhat similar to uterine adenomyosis.

It is now questioned whether chronic pyogenic and tuberculous salpingitis are sometimes causative. The condition is produced by downgrowths from the mucous lining of the Fallopian tube into the muscle wall, which undergoes hyperplasia (see Fig. 429, page 778).

This condition has sometimes been called endosalpingiosis and is really an invasion of tubal musculature—or tubal myometrium—by the lining epithelium of the tube. The characteristic epithelial pattern of the ectopic lining may give the clue and these gland spaces have no stroma. Morevoer, they do not menstruate, so that it is probably incorrect to call the condition tubal adenomyosis or endosalpingiosis. The term, however, is so descriptive that it is retained. If it is remembered that tubal epithelium is morphologically derived from the same structure—the Müllerian duct—as the endometrium, there is no reason to regard endosalpingiosis as illogical behaviour. It is merely one further example of "heterotopic Müllerianosis". The condition is usually symptomless and the diagnosis made only after histological examination. It is therefore, of academic interest.

Stromatous Endometriosis. This is a rare tumour which can be regarded as an example of adenomyosis interna in which only the stromal elements of an endometriosis are present and there are no glandular spaces. Histologically, the cells certainly look like stroma. It is disputed whether they invade the myometrium from the endometrium or whether they already exist in the myometrium and merely undergo proliferation.

The result is a soft enlargement of the uterine wall usually mistaken for a myoma or an adenomyosis, It is, however, less firm than either of these. A feature of the condition is the presence of broad based fleshy polypoidal protrusions into the cavity of the uterus, which account for the menorrhagia or post menopausal bleeding. If fixed by broad ligament extension, this is demonstrated on bimanual examination.

The symptoms are menorrhagia or irregular uterine bleeding.

The treatment is hysterectomy and, at operation, the characteristic rubbery consistence will be appreciated. One interesting feature, which is diagnostic, is a tendency for elastic extensions of the tumour to penetrate along the uterine and broad ligament veins. These vermiform projections, when seen at operation, should suggest the diagnosis.

The tumour is locally malignant though pulmonary metastasis has been reported and tends to recur after hysterectomy often several years later. This feature and the fact that it can occur after the menopause and radiation has suggested that it is a form of low malignancy sarcoma.

Treatment of Endometriosis by Endocrines

While it has been stressed in this chapter that the treatment of endometriosis is essentially a surgical problem, there are certain patients who, owing to their youth, are undesirable as subjects for radical measures such as total hysterectomy and bilateral salpingo-oöphorectomy. There are others who may have been treated by conservative operations, such as bilateral partial oöphorectomy, in whom the condition recurs soon after operation. It has been noted that pregnancy, possibly because of its high titre of progesterone, is inhibitory to endometriosis and, arguing from this premise, a number of workers, notably Kistner of Boston (Mass.) have induced a state of pseudo-pregnancy using the potent, orally-active, synthetic progestational steroid nor-ethynodrel. A course of treatment lasts six months to two years or more in increasing dosage up to 40 mgm. daily. Kistner claims control of the endometriosis with regression of the lesion. This promising alternative to or adjuvant of surgery has now had extensive clinical trial and its value is now undisputed. The control rate of endometriosis under this treatment should be in the region of 80%, but a number of women abandon the course because of the side effects of nausea, headaches, breast discomfort and water retention actually amounting to oedema. One very valuable aspect of hormone therapy is that of confirming diagnosis by a therapeutic test.

Cyclical hormone therapy using nor-ethynodrel or nor-ethisterone has become more popular as a method of controlling endometriosis, especially after surgical removal of the majority of the disease. A dose of 5 mgm. is given daily from the 5th to the 26th day. This dose suppresses ovulation and some people prefer to give patients a high dose progestational contraceptive pill, which will often suppress the recurrence of endometriosis for many years.

In the married patient who wants or who is advised to have a family nor-ethynodrel (5 mgm.) or nor-ethisterone (5 mgm.) is given from the 15th to the 26th day of the cycle. This is frequently sufficient to control the endo-metriosis without suppressing ovulation.

It should always be remembered that in patients who have been castrated by surgery or radiation for endometriosis oestrogens should not be used in the treatment of subsequent menopausal symptoms, because the residual areas of the disease may be reactivated.

28 Diseases of the Ovaries

The majority of ovarian tumours take the form of cysts, and three types of cyst are recognised. The first is a retention cyst of the Graafian follicle, but as the cyst may arise at any stage of development of the follicle, it may take the form either of a follicular cyst or of a corpus luteum cyst. In the second type the cyst is a neoplasm. The third type is a cyst filled with altered blood due to ovarian endometriosis or haemorrhage into a corpus luteum.

It is important to distinguish between a retention cyst and a neoplasm which assumes the form of a cyst. The simplest type of the latter is a cystoma, a unilocular cystic swelling lined by active epithelium, either cubical or columnar, which shows a tendency to proliferation and the formation of intracystic growths. Quite frequently the neoplasm has the structure of a multitude of cystomata which are agglomerated. A tumour of this kind is called a serous cystadenoma or a pseudo-mucinous cystadenoma, the common multilocular ovarian cyst. On the other hand, a retention cyst is lined by flattened epithelium and its origin is from the granulosa cells of the Graafian follicle or corpus luteum.

In the present chapter the retention cysts and the neoplasms of the ovaries will be described. Inflammatory lesions of the ovary will be considered in Chapter 29, while the chocolate cysts of the ovaries, which are different from either retention cysts or new growths, have been discussed under endometriosis in the previous chapter.

Cysts of the Follicle System

Ripening and atresia of follicles, together with proliferation and retrogression of the corpus luteum are normal physiological processes. A Graafian follicle or a corpus luteum may become cystic through overactivity and it may be difficult to decide whether or not a cyst of this kind should be regarded as pathological. One of the greatest difficulties in gynaecological surgery is to decide at operation whether an enlarged and cystic ovary contains physiological or pathological cysts.

Inability on the part of the inexperienced to make this differential diagnosis has cost many an innocent ovary its life. Needless to say, the right ovary, being accessible through the muscle-splitting incision of McBurney, has been the more frequent victim of misguided surgical enthusiasm.

The distension or retention cysts of the follicular system can be classified as:—

(1) Follicular cysts.
(2) Corpus luteum cysts (menstruation, pregnancy, persistent corpus luteum and haematoma).
(3) Granulosa lutein cyst and theca lutein cysts.

The aetiology of these various retention cysts is obscure but two facts are accepted:—

Excess of chorionic gonadotropin, pituitary gonadotropin or therapeutically administered gonadotropin, human pituitary gonadotropin (H.P.G.), human menopausal gonadotropin (H.M.G.) and human chorionic gonadotropin (H.C.G.) are all associated with multiple cyst formation in the ovary. Incidentally clomiphene is also associated with cyst formation in the ovary. The best example of this is the compound granulosa lutein cysts found in the ovary in hydatidiform mole where the chorionic gonadotropin reaches a very high level.

A hyperaemic state of the ovary which results in congestion is an undoubted cause of retention cysts. Retroversion, pelvic congestion due to inflammation, increased blood supply due to the presence of myomata are all examples of ovarian congestion in which a cystic state of the ovary is found.

FOLLICULAR CYSTS

Follicular cysts arise either from ripening or atretic follicles. They should be regarded as pathological if they are more than an inch in diameter, or if the ovary is studded with a series of small cysts of this kind. Follicular cysts are at first always lined by granulosa and theca interna cells, but the granulosa cells show signs of retrogression although hypertrophied theca interna cells often persist at the periphery. The ovum degenerates and disappears early but the granulosa and theca cells may persist in a functionally active state for some time. In the case of the oestrogenic follicular cyst of metropathia haemorrhagica, this activity may last for many months. As a rule, however, mounting intracystic pressure causes atrophy of the lining cells with loss of function. For this reason the life span of a follicular cyst is a self-limited one and surgical interference is very seldom indicated or justified. Follicular cysts are thin-walled and contain translucent colourless fluid.

Different forms of follicular cysts are recognised. (1) In the first, called **Hydrops folliculi,** a single large follicular cyst is present in the ovary. This condition is very unusual, and must be distinguished from a cystoma simplex, which has a very similar appearance and is a new growth. The distinction is not always possible even by histological examination.

(2) If the ovary and tube are matted together by adhesions as the result of previous inflammation of the appendages the ovary frequently contains several medium sized cysts up to two inches in diameter. Follicular cysts are not uncommon in the large hyperplastic ovaries of patients with myomata.

(3) A rather similar type of cyst is invariably present in **metropathia haemorrhagica** (p. 463), although the cyst associated with metropathia retains some at least of its granulosa cells in a state of activity, and indeed the granulosa cells may show some degree of luteinisation.

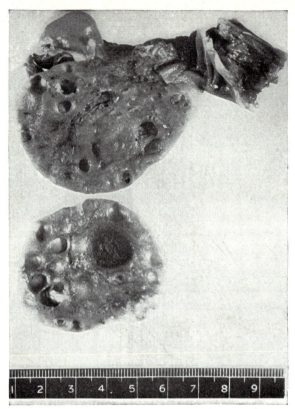

Fig. 367. Multiple follicular cysts of the ovaries.

(4) **In sclerocystic disease** (sometimes also called polycystic ovary) the ovary is symmetrically enlarged with a thickened white tunica albuginea and its cortex is riddled with small follicular cysts of about $\frac{1}{4}$ in. to $\frac{1}{2}$ in. in diameter. There is an associated state of hyperplasia in the theca cells of the stroma, so-called hyperthecosis ovarii. Well-marked sclerocystic disease is infrequent. As many as thirty small cysts may be found in the same ovary. The peritoneal surface of the ovary is free of adhesions, without evidence of previous inflammation of the appendages. Normal corpora lutea are formed, although they tend to be hyperplastic. The disease usually arises in young women and the appearances are exactly similar to that seen in the Stein-Leventhal ovary associated with virilising symptoms. It is therefore reasonable to assume that such an ovary produces androgen. Sclerocystic disease is rare apart from the Stein-Leventhal syndrome (Fig. 367).

(5) **Stein-Leventhal Syndrome.** This is a virilising syndrome seen in young women. The patient develops secondary amenorrhoea and infertility, obesity, hirsutism and acne; breast development may be subnormal. The adrenal is

not at fault since the 17-keto-steroid excretion is normal. At operation, there is a bilateral ovarian enlargement up to three times the normal size and the ovaries contain many cysts in the lining of which theca cells may be identified. It is thought that these theca cells are the source of the androgen. The condition is often amenable to surgical correction by bilateral wedge resection, a form of partial oöphorectomy (Fig. 368).

Follicular Haematomata

Small follicular haematomata are common, particularly in cases of uterine myomata. To the naked eye the ovary contains haemorrhagic cysts and occasionally the haematoma may burst into the peritoneal cavity and cause diffuse intraperitoneal bleeding of a severity equal to that met with in ruptured ectopic gestation. The haematoma is usually small and is restricted

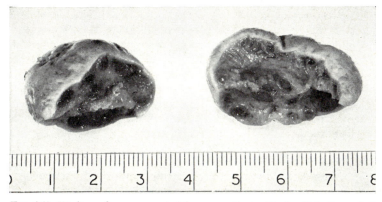

Fig. 368. Wedges of ovary resected from a patient with the Stein-Leventhal Syndrome. Even after resection, adequate ovarian tissue was preserved and the patient later became pregnant. Note the enlargement of the ovary against the scale.

to the wall of the follicle, as the granulosa cell layer is non-vascular and the membrana limitans externa separates the vascular theca interna from the cavity of the follicle. These haematomata are, therefore, almost invariably restricted to the theca interna layer. Except for the rare cases in which the haematoma bursts into the peritoneal cavity, follicular haematomata have no clinical importance.

It should be mentioned, however, that the old altered blood contents of a retention cyst, into which a haemorrhage has occurred, become tarry and give rise to one variety of chocolate cyst. When ruptured at operation with the liberation of a small quantity of tarry or chocolate contents, it is tempting for the operator to make an erroneous diagnosis of endometriosis. This common mistake is frequently the cause of quite unnecessary and unjustifiable radical surgery. In all probability, more tarry or chocolate cysts of the ovary are due to haemorrhage into retention cysts than to endometriosis.

Corpus Luteum Cysts

Corpus luteum cysts are not infrequent in early pregnancy. They may be as large as 6 cm. in diameter. They are thin-walled and contain clear yellow fluid. The wall of the cyst contains the normal convulutions of the corpus luteum. Corpus luteum cysts should not be regarded as pathological cysts of the ovary. They are more likely to represent the result of overactivity of the corpus luteum. Corpus luteum cysts rarely cause localising symptoms and are usually found on routine examination. If an ovarian cyst is found in the early weeks of pregnancy a corpus luteum cyst should be suspected and operation should be delayed, since a corpus luteum cyst subsequently becomes smaller as pregnancy advances. If an immediate operation is performed and the corpus luteum cyst removed, the patient is likely to miscarry unless the pregnancy has advanced beyond the 14th week, after which time the placenta takes over the manufacture of progesterone and oestrogen.

Very rarely a corpus luteum cyst remains functional for a variable period beyond its normal life span. The excess of circulating progesterone can cause a state of pseudo-pregnancy with amenorrhoea of short duration followed by fairly prolonged uterine bleeding. The clinical picture, therefore, resembles early pregnancy followed by abortion, metropathia haemorrhagica in which the clinical signs are exactly similar, or even an ectopic gestation. Curettage reveals a secretory pattern endometrium thus distinguishing it from metropathia haemorrhagica, and the condition is always spontaneously cured if correctly diagnosed.

Corpus Luteum Haematomata

Corpus luteum haematomata are somewhat similar to follicular haematomata. With a corpus luteum haematoma the blood is effused not only into the theca interna layer, but also amongst the granulosa lutein cells, as at this stage of development of the follicle the granulosa layer has become vascularised. In consequence the haematoma involves the granulosa lutein layer and the cavity of the corpus luteum. Occasionally diffuse intraperitoneal bleeding with collapse and shock follows the rupture of a corpus luteum haematoma.

In this case a diagnosis of extra-uterine pregnancy may be made with reasonable justification and the abdomen opened when the true nature of the condition is immediately obvious.

Granulosa Lutein Cysts, the Lutein Cysts of Hydatidiform Mole and Chorion Epithelioma

The incidence of lutein cysts in the ovaries in cases of hydatidiform mole and chorion epithelioma is well known. They may occur following attempted induction of ovulation by Follicle Stimulating Hormone and Human Chorionic Gonadotropin. The cysts are almost invariably bilateral and arise in about 60% of cases of hydatidiform mole and 10% of cases of chorion epithelioma. The ovaries are often enlarged to as much as 4 in. in diameter, and each ovary may contain as many as fifteen or twenty cysts of this kind. The surface of the ovary is free of adhesions, but a nodular appearance is produced by the cysts projecting under the surface. Large cysts as big as 3 in. in diameter have been described. The cysts are thin-walled, contain a yellow fluid and frequently a fibrinous or gelatinous substance is formed in the cavity. The inner walls of the cysts are unevenly covered with greyish-yellow material. The cysts are of the nature of granulosa lutein cysts as they are all derived from follicles and show well-marked luteinisation of both granulosa and theca interna cells. The granulosa lutein cells are as large as those found in the mature corpus luteum of the menstrual cycle but they are not arranged in folds and convolutions are absent. The cysts are almost certainly produced as the result of an increase in the chorionic gonadotropic hormone in the blood stream. Not only do they correspond in their histology to the luteinised follicles produced in the ovaries of animals after the injection of this hormone, but it is well established that this hormone is formed in large amount in cases of hydatidiform mole and chorion epithelioma. These large cystic ovaries sometimes undergo torsion during the course of the pregnancy and cause acute abdominal symptoms which demand immediate operation. Compound granulosa lutein cysts invariably atrophy after removal of the causative hydatidiform mole and though their spontaneous regression may take several months no active treatment is ever indicated apart from the complication of torsion.

Theca Lutein Cysts

Theca lutein cysts probably represent a later phase of the granulosa-lutein cyst in which the granulosa cells have atrophied and disappeared, and in which the theca interna cells persist with some evidence of luteinisation. The terms granulosa-lutein and theca lutein, therefore, represent two stages of the same disorder.

Symptoms of Retention Cysts. In most instances there are no symptoms and the discovery is a chance one made on routine bimanual pelvic examination or at operation.

Pain. It is tempting, but unwise to incriminate a cystic ovary as the cause of pain in one or other lower quadrant. The removal of the cystic ovary rarely cures the pain and even the conservative operation of ovarian cystectomy is usually unsatisfactory.

Menstrual disturbances. The follicular cyst of metropathia haemorrhagica gives rise to a state of superthreshold oestrogen, causing temporary amenorrhoea followed by prolonged threshold bleeding. A persistent functional corpus luteum can cause temporary amenorrhoea. Epimenorrhoea is caused by a congested multicystic ovary in association with intra-pelvic inflammatory disease.

Infertility is seen in metropathia and the Stein-Leventhal syndrome.

Mittelschmerz or pain at ovulation time is sometimes seen in association with a sclerocystic ovary and is presumed to be due to an excessive intra-cystic tension. This type of pain can occur with normal ovaries.

Haemorrhage into a retention cyst may cause rupture and intra-peritoneal bleeding with all the symptoms and signs of an acute abdominal emergency such as ectopic gestation. Observation over twelve hours almost always shows a dramatic improvement in the patient's condition, though many will undergo a laparotomy.

Treatment. Cysts and haematomata of the Graafian follicle require no treatment unless they have attained a considerable size or are the source of excessive intraperitoneal bleeding. When such a cystic ovary is encountered during the course of a hysterectomy for some benign lesion in a woman before the menopause, it is a common practice to remove that ovary. This is illogical since it has been shown that frequently only one ovary remains active for some years before the menopause, and in such a case this is likely to be the cystic one, so that the aim of conserving ovarian function is defeated by its removal. If anything has to be done the cyst should be punctured with a needle and collapsed or enucleated by ovarian cystectomy or excised by partial oöphorectomy and the bulk of the functional ovary thereby conserved.

OVARIAN NEOPLASMS

The neoplasms of the ovary form an extremely complicated array of tumours which is difficult to classify pathologically. The majority of the tumours take the form of cysts or cystadenomata and most of them are innocent. The tumours must be distinguished from chocolate cysts or endometriosis of the ovary; chocolate cysts are not true neoplasms as they regress after the cessation of ovarian function. Nevertheless, chocolate cysts are physically similar in many ways to a true neoplastic cyst. Broad ligament cysts found in the outer part of the broad ligament and usually called parovarian cysts also present similar physical signs.

The classification of ovarian tumours is in many ways unsatisfactory. The majority of tumours are epithelial in type and may take the form of simple cystomata, papillary cystadenomata with intra-cystic growths and pseudomucinous tumours which may reach enormous dimensions and which are filled with pseudomucin. Malignant tumours of epithelial origin may resemble in their histology the innocent tumours mentioned above, e.g. pseudomucinous cystadeno-carcinoma. The connective tissue tumours usually take the form of an innocent fibroma, while the malignant tumours comprise sarcomata and the specialised tumours which correspond in their histology with embryonic tissues found in the ovary. The teratoid tumours which consist of dermoids and solid teratomata may possibly be derived from the sex cells.

This time-honoured system of classification has been replaced by a more modern classification which takes into consideration the structures from which the ovarian tumours are derived. The cystoma simplex and the cystadenoma papillare are undoubtedly derived from the surface epithelium of the ovary, when the surface epithelium undergoes metaplasia into epithelium which is similar to that in the Fallopian tube. The process of development of the tumours can sometimes be traced with a fair degree of accuracy. The pseudomucinous tumours may be derived in a similar way, although this theory is not universally accepted. The pseudomucin in the tumours has been shown to be altered mucin, and it is believed that downgrowths from the surface epithelium undergo metaplasia into cervical epithelium. This theory explains the high columnar epithelium of such tumours, and the pseudo-mucin content is regarded as comparable to the cervical mucus. The resem-blance of the lining epithelium of a pseudomucinous cyst to that of the large gut has suggested that these cysts are in reality teratoid tumours in which the entodermic elements have outgrown and predominated over all the other elements. In support of this theory, dermoid cysts and pseudomucinous cysts are sometimes found in combination. Willis regards this hypothesis as wholly speculative and points out that the high columnar epithelium of the pseudomucinous cyst is really dissimilar from that of the gut and that the association of dermoid cysts is fortuitous.

The dermoid cysts and teratomata may possibly arise from the sex cells themselves, and such tumours clearly belong to a specialised group. The rare chorion epithelioma of the ovary should also be classified with these tumours since it is essentially a tumour of trophoblastic origin. The con-nective tissue tumours probably arise from the connective tissue cells of the ovarian cortex.

In addition to the tumours mentioned above, other ovarian tumours have been identified which consist of cells similar to the embryonic cells found either in the foetal ovary or in the foetal testis. These tumours require a separate grouping.

Before attempting a classification of ovarian tumours of which many show an epithelial structure, it is pertinent to ask how, in a structure such as the ovary which is morphologically derived from the mesenchyme of coelomic mesothelium, does an epithelial structure come to exist at all. Some explana-tion of this histological paradox must be forthcoming, however speculative it may be.

Serosal or Coelomic Mesothelial Cell Metaplasia. The Müllerian duct from which the Fallopian tube, uterine body and cervix, and upper vagina are derived originates from the intermediate cell mass of mesenchyme close to the germinal ridge which is destined to become the ovary. The mesenchyme of the Müllerian duct is ultimately differentiated into three different types of epithelium—tubal, endometrial and cervical. The squamous covering of the vagina is essentially an upgrowth from the urogenital sinus and need not be considered here. This potential for metaplasia may be the explanation of some of the epithelial tumours found in the ovary, especially if it is accepted that inclusion bodies—the so-called Walthard inclusions—are quite common in the ovarian cortex. These inclusion bodies are regarded as being derived from the surface mesothelium of the ovary and, under some unknown stimulus, are thought to have the potential of differentiation into Müllerian epithelium. This is called Müllerianosis, an ugly but descriptive word. This differentiation into epithelium resembling that of the Fallopian tube produces a papillary cystadenoma, that resembling the endometrium—endometriosis, and that resembling the cervical epithelium, a pseudomucinous cystadenoma. Malignant varieties of these give rise to primary adenocarcinomata and more primitive carcinomata. In support of the inclusion body—Walthard inclusion—theory is the fairly frequent finding of Walthard cell rests in the vicinity of pseudomucinous cystadenoma.

The Teratomatous Origin Theory. This theory originated by Meyer and supported by Novak suggests that a pseudomucinous cyst is the end result of a teratoma from the totipotential cells of which a number of well differentiated tissues have been derived. Thus cartilage, teeth, thyroid and gut structures may be obvious on histological examination. If one structure predominates at the expense of the others, eventually all evidence of its rivals disappears. The tall columnar epithelium of a pseudomucinous cystadenoma certainly bears some resemblance to the endodermic epithelium of the large bowel as does cervical epithelium and both are mucus-secreting. Moreover, small pseudomucinous cysts are sometimes found in teratomata. One further argument in favour of this theory is provided by the struma ovarii, a tumour of thyroid tissue, obvious histologically and sometimes functionally active, causing thyrotoxicosis. The struma ovarii is believed primarily to be derived from a teratoma containing thyroid tissue, which has become predominant and has eliminated the other elements originally present in the tumour. Although Willis disregards the teratoma theory, it must be conceded that it does explain the presence of epithelial structures in the ovary.

TUMOURS ARISING FROM THE SURFACE EPITHELIUM OF THE OVARY

1. **Innocent.**
   - (*a*) SIMPLE SEROUS CYSTADENOMA.
   - (*b*) PAPILLARY SEROUS CYSTADENOMA.
   - (*c*) PSEUDOMUCINOUS CYSTADENOMA.
   - (*d*) BRENNER TUMOUR.

2. **Malignant.**
   - (*a*) SEROUS CYSTADENOCARCINOMA; PSEUDOMUCINOUS CYSTADENO-CARCINOMA; SOLID CARCINOMA.
   - (*b*) MESONEPHROMA.

METASTATIC TUMOURS

(*a*) **Typical,** from primary carcinoma of the stomach, intestine, breast, uterus.

(*b*) **Atypical,** Krukenberg tumour.

TUMOURS ARISING FROM THE CONNECTIVE TISSUES OF THE OVARY

1. **Innocent,** FIBROMATA.

2. **Malignant,** SARCOMATA.

TUMOURS ARISING FROM THE OVUM

(a) DERMOID CYSTS.
(b) SOLID TERATOMATA.
(c) CHORION EPITHELIOMA.
(d) STRUMA OVARII.

TUMOURS ARISING FROM PRIMITIVE MESENCHYME

(a) **Feminising**—Granulosa cell, theca cell, luteoma.
(b) **Neuter**—Disgerminoma.* (Seminoma.)
(c) **Virilising**—Arrhenoblastoma. Suprarenal cortical tumour. Hilus cell tumour.
(d) **Mixed**—Gynandroblastoma.

The above classification is probably imperfect. For example, it is not established that dermoid cysts and some solid teratomata arise from the ovum itself.

Much work is in progress on the nature and origin of functioning ovarian tumours. In the past, classification has been made largely upon the histological appearance of the tumour and its apparent similarity to tissue of similar function in other sites. With a greater understanding of steroid chemistry this difficult problem will become clearer. Already it has been shown that certain luteomas are capable of elaborating androgen as well as the structurally similar progesterone and it is likely that such ambivalent properties will be found to be possessed by other functioning ovarian tumours. (Compare for example the virilising properties of the sclerocystic ovary of the Stein-Leventhal Syndrome).

Pathology of Ovarian Neoplasms

Cystoma Simplex or Simple Serous Cystadenoma. This ovarian tumour is a simple unilocular cyst, thin-walled, containing clear serous fluid, lined by a single layer of ciliated epithelium. The tumour is relatively rare and arises with equal frequency at any decade of life. The tumours are bilateral in 6·6% of cases. Very rarely the tumour may form a large swelling but the average size of the cyst is about 10 cms. in diameter. Although it is described as a separate entity, it is most widely accepted to be a variety of cystadenoma papillare in which the papillary processes have either not developed or have atrophied. Some cystomata of this type are confused with follicular retention cysts (Fig. 369).

---

* In deference to Robert Meyer who first named this tumour in 1930 " Disgerminoma " (Dis = two, germinoma = tumour of gonad) because of its occurrence in two separate sites—ovary and testis—this title is preserved.

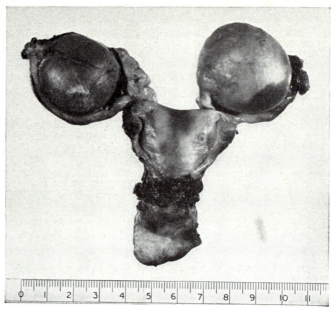

FIG. 369. Bilateral cystoma simplex. This cyst is always difficult to differentiate from a simple distension cyst of follicle.

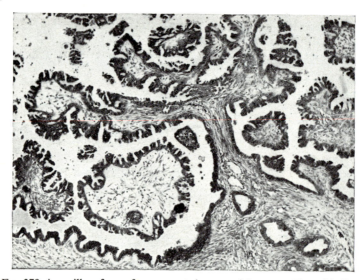

FIG. 370. A papillary form of serous cystadenoma of the ovary. The epithelium, though hyperplastic, is undoubtedly benign. (× 60.)

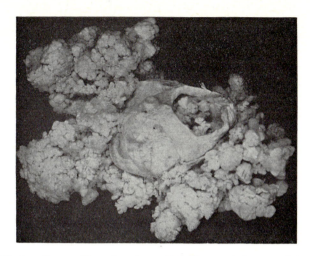

FIG. 371. A surface papillomatous form of papillary cystadenoma of the ovary.

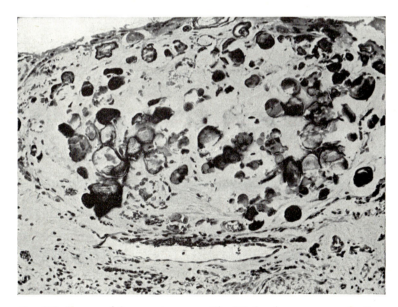

FIG. 372. An area of the same tumour as Fig. 371 showing psammoma bodies. (× 140.)

Cystadenoma Serosum Papillare (Papillary serous cystadenoma). The tumour is usually unilocular except for large cysts which are multiloculated, although it is rare for more than three or four loculi to be present. The cysts are thin-walled, contain clear serous fluid, and are lined by ciliated epithelium. The fluid contains the serum proteins albumen and globulin. The tumours are fairly frequent, the incidence being 8·67% of ovarian neoplasms, and they may produce large swellings. They are bilateral in a third of all cases. The tumours may arise at any age and there is no particular age-incidence. The cysts contain papillomata in the wall and two forms of papillomata

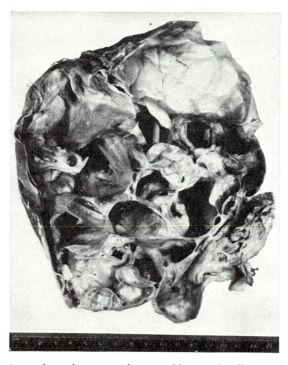

FIG. 373. A pseudomucinous cystadenoma with many loculi, several of which intercommunicate.

are recognised, namely, the stationary and the proliferating. In the stationary type, the papillae take the form of small warts on the inner surface of the tumour. In the proliferating type the papillomata are arborescent and plentiful, and may almost fill the contents of the cyst. The surface epithelium is active, but there is no invasion of the basement membrane. A frequent finding in histological sections of these tumours is the presence of calcified granules, called psammoma bodies, within the cyst wall. These psammoma bodies occur in both benign and malignant papillary tumours. In some cases the papillomata are spread over the outer surface of the cyst when they lead to ascites, and occasionally similar papillomata are scattered over the pelvic peritoneum.

Although the tumours are actively proliferating they are not necessarily malignant, even if the macroscopic appearance at laparotomy is most sinister. The histological picture, is, however, not always as clear cut as just described. A number of these cysts are encountered where the epithelial cell lining is more than one cell thick and a many layered hyperplastic appearance suggests the possibility of malignancy. The presence of mitotic figures is suggestive but not conclusive and the best guide is whether or not the basement membrane has been breached with invasion of the subjacent stroma. If this is seen, carcinoma should be diagnosed. Exact interpretation of the histology is sometimes impossible and the diagnosis can only be finally made on the subsequent clinical progress of the patient (see Figs. 370–372).

The two ovarian tumours above described, namely, the cystoma simplex and the cystadenoma papillare are now regarded as representing forms of ovarian Müllerianosis. It is established that the epithelium which lines these tumours is similar to that which lines the normal Fallopian tube. The cysts are undoubtedly neoplasms, yet the papillary cystadenoma associated with papillomata disseminated over the peritoneum is paralleled almost exactly by pelvic endometriosis which illustrates another example of ovarian Müllerianosis. In one case, the heterotopic epithelium is that of the Fallopian tube; in the other, it is endometrial in type. The great distinction between endometriosis and the papillary cystedenoma is that endometriosis is not a neoplastic condition.

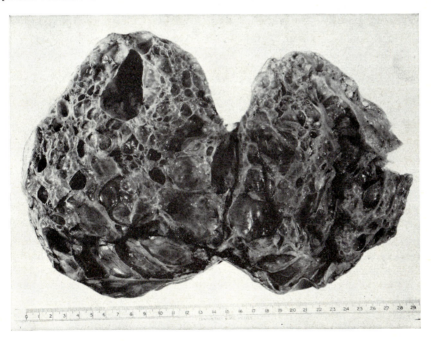

FIG. 374. Another pseudomucinous cyst, the upper pole of which is actively proliferating to produce a mass of small daughter cysts.

Pseudomucinous Cystadenoma. This form of ovarian cyst is the commonest of ovarian neoplasms, the incidence being approximately one-third. Both ovaries are affected in roughly one-tenth of all pseudomucinous cysts. The cyst is smooth, with a glistening white surface, and is multiocular. In young, actively growing tumours, the loculi are small, and produce a honeycombed appearance, but with old-standing tumours, as the result of cohesion of adjacent loculi, only a relatively small number are present, although it is

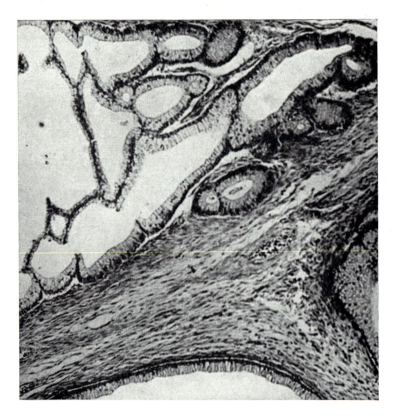

FIG. 375. A pseudomucinous cystadenoma.

quite common even with old-standing tumours for a small zone of actively growing tissue to be recognised in one pole of the swelling. The tumours contain pseudomucin which closely resembles mucin except in its chemical properties, for example, it is not precipitated by the addition of acetic acid. The average pseudomucinous cystadenoma removed at operation is at least 6 inches in diameter, and it may reach mammoth dimensions, quite a number of tumours weighing more than 200 lbs. having been described. The tumours are as mentioned 10% bilateral and they arise with equal frequency in the three decades of life, between the ages of 30 and 60. Although they arise in patients under 30 and over 60, their incidence at these ages is much less than between 30 and 60. They sometimes cause post-menopausal bleeding, but they rarely give rise to other symptoms except a dull dragging pain in the abdomen. Uterine bleeding associated with pseudomucinous tumours is not of endocrine origin and if such a uterus is examined microscopically the characteristic changes in the endometrium as seen in hyperoestrinism will not be found. In spite of the enormous size which the tumours may attain the operation of removal is usually carried out quite simply without shock or mortality. In some cases the tumours burrow extraperitoneally and may be extremely difficult to remove (see Figs. 373 and 374).

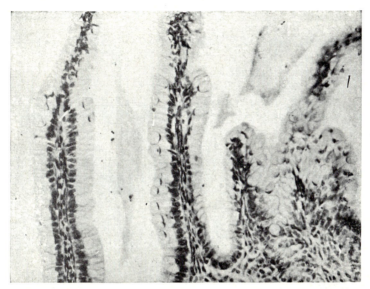

FIG. 376 Pseudomucinous cystadenoma of the ovary, showing the structure of the epithelium.

Histology. The tumour is composed of a series of loculi separated from each other by connective tissue. Each loculus is lined by high columnar epithelium, the cytoplasm of which is translucent. The nucleus is usually flattened out against the base of the cell. Large ovoid cells are usually found amongst the tall columnar cells and are displaced away from the basement membrane towards the cavity of the loculus. In proliferating tumours the epithelium is heaped up to form papillomata but large papillomata are relatively uncommon. In actively growing tumours areas of degeneration are commonly found, probably because epithelial elements of the tumour out-strip their blood supply in their growth, so that adjacent loculi communicate. Although the tumours are frequently actively proliferating it is relatively rare for them to become malignant, and probably in not more than 6% can true malignant change be demonstrated (see Figs. 375 and 376).

The Brenner Tumour. This tumour usually arises in women of post-menopausal age and can be regarded as a benign fibro-epithelial growth. It is almost always unilateral and small, although large tumours have been described up to 18 lbs. in weight. Its gross appearance resembles that of a fibroma and it is almost always macroscopically solid. It sometimes displays on section a yellow tint which a fibroma does not and this colour change should always suggest the diagnosis of a Brenner tumour. It is sometimes found in combination with a teratoma or a granulosa cell tumour or a pseudo-mucinous cystadenoma. It sometimes is associated with uterine bleeding, possibly oestrogenic. Microscopically, the tumour consists of fibromatous connective tissue which surrounds nests of epithelial cells arranged in columns

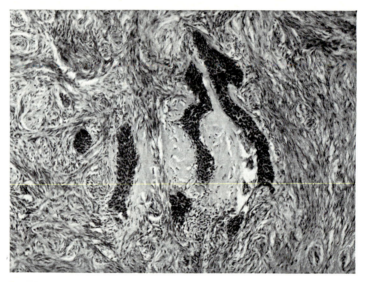

FIG. 377. Brenner tumour. (× 75.) Note nests of epithelial cells surrounded by fibromatous connective tissue.

or cords and the cells are sometimes transitional or squamous in type. The cells are strikingly uniform in type and obviously benign. Under high power examination the nuclei possess a longitudinal groove so that they have been described as resembling puffed wheat. This nuclear peculiarity is found in the cells of a Walthard inclusion, a finding that strongly supports the theory that Brenner tumours arise from Walthard cell islets. These islands were first described by Werth in 1887 and, later, by Walthard in 1903. An area of central liquefaction is commonly seen and this gave rise to the old term oöphoroma folliculare, owing to its resemblance to a Graafian follicle. The epithelial islands are surrounded by a fibromatous connective tissue and, unless this characteristic is seen, a Brenner tumour should not be diagnosed. Sometimes the central area of liquefaction in the epithelial islands compresses the cells in a peripheral direction and several small cysts may be formed in this

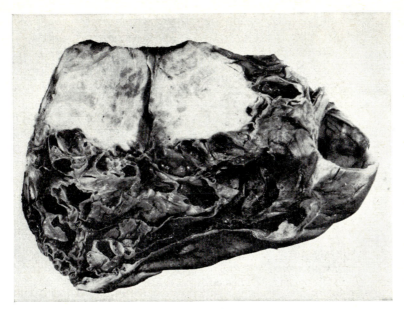

F IG. 378. A combined Brenner tumour (solid area) and multilocular pseudomucinous cystadenoma.

way. In some instances, areas of typical pseudomucinous epithelium are seen
in Brenner tumours and there is no doubt that some pseudomucinous cysts
arise in conjunction with Brenner tumours. Not only are pseudomucinous
cysts associated with Brenner tumours but some fibromata are similarly
derived. For this reason all fibromata removed at operation should be carefully sectioned for evidence of the characteristic Brenner tumour histology.

The Brenner tumour is one of the rarest ovarian tumours and until recently
was regarded as invariably benign. A few recent reports of malignancy
in a Brenner tumour must now be accepted as authentic but this feature
is exceedingly rare. The greatest age incidence is after the menopause in the
50 to 60 year period and over 60% occur in women after the age of 45 years.
These tumours produce no characteristic symptom although, in common
with fibroma of the ovary, ascites has been reported and, on rare occasions,
Meig's syndrome (*vide infra*) p. 735. The tumour has no endocrine activity
and, in those cases in which it has been described as having oestrogenic
function, the tumour has in fact been a variety of thecoma. The microscopic
appearance of the stroma of a Brenner tumour certainly bears a strong
resemblance to theca cells which are well known to be oestrogenic (Figs.
377 and 378).

Ovarian Carcinomata. Ovarian carcinomata are extremely common,
comprising at least 15–25% of all ovarian neoplasms. The malignant tumours
may be secondary deposits in the ovaries from a primary growth elsewhere in
the body and probably about 20% of all ovarian carcinomata are metastatic.

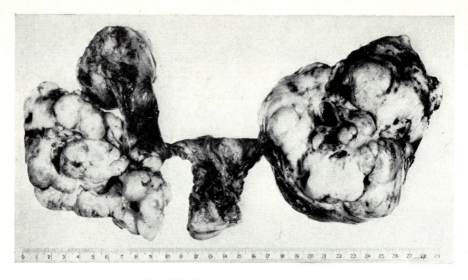

FIG. 379. Bilateral ovarian carcinoma.

The incidence of malignant change occurring in a previously benign cystadenoma is difficult to assess as many ovarian cancers which are malignant
from the start are partly cystic. It is, perhaps, fair to say that:—

    (*a*) 5% of benign pseudomucinous cystadenomata become malignant.
    (*b*) As much as 50% of the proliferating papillary cystadenomata are,
        by behaviour though not necessarily by exact histological criteria,
        malignant.
    (*c*) 1.7% of innocent dermoid cysts develop epidermoid carcinoma.

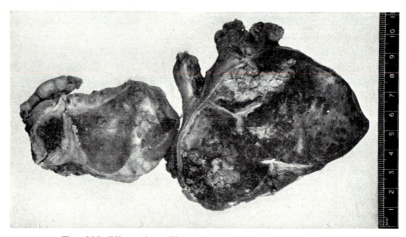

FIG. 380. Bilateral papillary cystadenocarcinoma of the ovary.

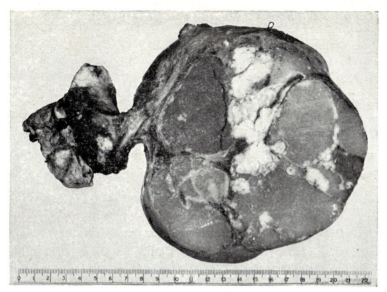

FIG. 381. Pseudomucinous cystadenocarcinoma of the ovary. Note the solid areas suggesting malignancy.

The pathology of primary ovarian carcinomata is extremely difficult and a detailed description of the different types is beyond the scope of this work. A simple method of classification is to group the primary carcinomata of the ovary into the following types:—

A. Cystic: (*a*) Papillomatous or serous (Fig. 380).
        (*b*) Pseudomucinous (Fig. 381).
B. Solid (Fig. 379).

The primary cystic carcinomata are the more common. At least half are bilateral.

C. W. Taylor's figures are instructive:—

(1) Serous papillomatous cystadenocarcinoma	.	.	105
(2) Pseudomucinous cystadenocarcinoma	.	. .	34
(3) Anaplastic solid carcinoma	. . .	.	. 23
Teratoid tumours: malignant .	.	.	. 9
			171

Criteria of Malignancy. It is often difficult to decide on histological examination whether an ovarian tumour is benign or malignant, since some benign tumours show marked epithelial activity. The following points should be helpful in reaching a diagnosis of malignancy:—

(1) Multiplication of the single epithelial layer.

(2) Invasion of the basement membrane and supporting stroma by epithelial elements.

(3) Atypical features of the epithelial cells such as altered staining capacity, irregular size, shape and situation of the nuclei, giant nuclei and mitotic figures (Fig. 382).

Grading of Malignancy. Taylor has attempted to grade the malignancy of ovarian tumours both macroscopically and histologically on the percentage of 5-year survivors after operation. The malignancy of the gross sub-divisions is as follows, expressed as a 5-year survival percentage:—

5-year Survival Rate of Various Types of Ovarian Cancer

Pseudomucinous cystadenocarcinoma	47·2%
Serous papillomatous cystadenocarcinoma . . .	10·2%
Solid carcinoma	8·0%

The histological division is into three grades:—

GRADE I: Well differentiated glands of adult structure; little infiltration of stroma and minimal nuclear changes (Fig. 382).

GRADE II: Glandular and papillary structure maintained but malignancy unquestioned.

GRADE III: Anaplastic cancer almost completely dedifferentiated with little or no recognisable glandular structure.

The five-year survival rates of these three grades were Grade I—65·5%; Grade II—8·9%; Grade III—2·4%.

It is a fair, if perhaps cynical, comment to suggest that many of the Grade I survivors were examples of borderline malignancy.

Serous Papillary Cystadenocarcinoma. These tumours are characterised by the presence of papillomata in the cyst wall. The papillomata are thick and friable and usually quite different from the delicate arborescent papillomata of innocent tumours. The papillomata infiltrate the wall of the tumour and ulcerate through to the peritoneal surface. The ensuing peritoneal irritation gives rise to ascites and secondary deposits become disseminated over the peritoneum. Various histological types can be distinguished of which the commonest is the papillary cystadenocarcinoma. It is usually unilocular, containing serous fluid, and has large friable papillomata in the cyst wall. The histology of this form of tumour is interesting because the tumour consists of a series of villous-like processes. The core of each villus contains a large vessel and the malignant cells are packed closely together being fusiform in shape and showing a tendency to squamous metaplasia (see Fig. 380).

In papillary cystadenocarcinomata, as in innocent papillary cystadenomata, psammoma bodies are quite frequently seen. Psammoma bodies are not found in pseudomucinous tumours, benign or malignant, and the significance of their presence is not understood.

Pseudomucinous Cystadenocarcinoma. Malignant changes in pseudomucinous cysts occur in only 5% of all such cysts, so that the majority of pseudomucinous cystadenocarcinoma arise as primary tumours. The tumours

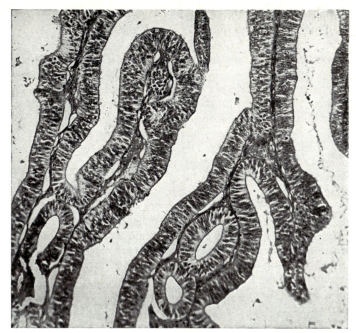

FIG. 382. Well differentiated pseudomucinous cystadenocarcinoma. Note the epithelial activity and compare with Fig. 375. (× 140.)

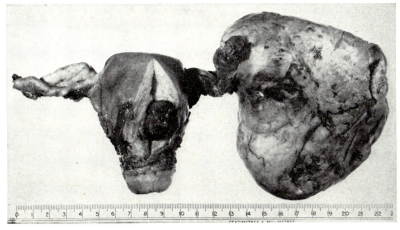

FIG. 383. Primary solid carcinoma of the ovary.

consist of a series of loculi which are irregular in shape and lined by a thick layer of malignant epithelium. Superficially, therefore, the structure resembles that of an innocent pseudomucinous cystadenoma with well-marked malignant change in the epithelium (see Figs. 381 and 382).

Solid Carcinomata of the Ovary. Here the carcinoma takes the form of a solid tumour although nearly always there is some attempt at the formation of loculi. The tumours vary in their histological characters according to their malignancy. They have been classified into various types according to their cellular pattern, e.g. adenocarcinoma, the commonest and most important variety; scirrhous, where the connective tissue between the malignant cells predominates; medullary, where the epithelial elements predominate and plexiform, which resembles the scirrhous. These histological subdivisions are largely of academic interest (see Figs. 379 and 383).

Mesonephroma. This tumour, originally described by Schiller, was believed to originate from mesonephric remains in the ovary. They may also arise anywhere in the pelvis along the pathway of the primitive mesonephric duct and have been described in the vagina and the parovarian region. This view is not accepted at the present day and the tumours are regarded as a separate form of carcinoma of the ovary. The characteristic histological feature of this rare and obscure tumour is the presence of projections which superficially resemble a glomerular tuft, the epithelium of which has a hobnailed appearance. It tends to metastasise via the blood stream to the lungs and other distant sites.

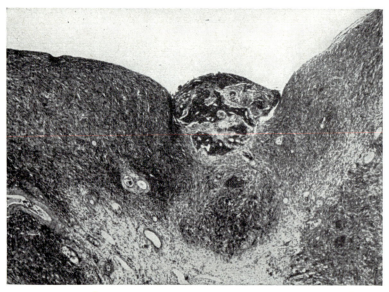

FIG. 384. A metastasis on the surface of the ovary from a primary carcinoma of the breast. (× 44.)

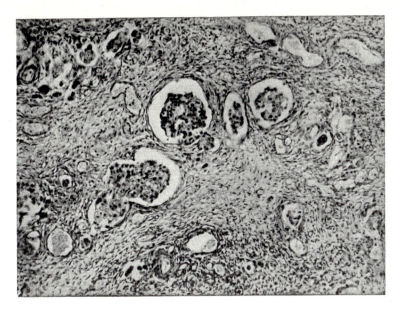

Fig. 385. Metastases of carcinoma of the stomach in the medulla of the ovary. To the naked eye the ovary appeared normal, but the lymphatics of the medulla contain a large number of malignant cells, the ovary being involved by retrograde lymphatic spread.

METASTATIC CARCINOMATA

Ovarian metastases are common from primary growths of the gastro-intestinal tract, notably the pylorus, colon and, rarely, the small bowel; they occasionally occur from the gall bladder and pancreas. They may also occur in late carcinoma of the breast, as much as 30% of all autopsy material from breast cancer (Fig. 384). Carcinoma of the corpus (10%) and cervix (1%) of the uterus also metastasises, as would be expected, to the ovary owing to the close relationship of their lymphatic drainage. Carcinoma of the corpus is ten times more likely to metastasise to the ovary than that of the cervix. The reason for this is that the ovarian lymphatics drain the corpus directly whereas the cervical metastases tend to bypass the ovarian lymphatics and to travel by way of the hypogastric and aortic glands. In autopsy material the incidence of secondary deposits in the ovary is higher than that of primary growths. With clinical material the position is different, and probably only about 20% of clinically malignant ovarian tumours are secondary deposits from primary growths elsewhere. The other 80% comprise primary ovarian carcinomata. Two forms of secondary carcinoma of the ovary are recognised. In the first the growth corresponds in its histology with the primary growth. Dissemination to the ovaries takes place either by implantation from meta-stases within the peritoneal cavity or by retrograde lymphatic spread. Both ovaries are replaced by solid carcinomata and multiple secondary deposits are usually disseminated over the peritoneum. A curious feature is that the ovarian tumours are much larger than the other secondary deposits, which is explained by supposing that the ovaries form a much better environment for the growth of malignant cells than the other intraperitoneal viscera.

These secondary ovarian cancers have the following features. They are solid, with irregular surfaces, and nearly always bilateral. Ascites is common and other obvious peritoneal metastases are present, notably in the omentum which is often replaced by an enormous solid malignant plaque. The method of ovarian infiltration is either by surface implantation or by retrograde lymphatic permeation (Fig. 385). Both methods are probably operative and histological examination is rarely able to reveal by which route the metastases occurred.

The second type of secondary ovarian carcinoma is the Krukenberg tumour.

The Krukenberg Tumour. There is an unfortunate inclination on the part of clinicians and pathologists to call any ovarian metastasis from a primary gastro-intestinal cancer a Krukenberg tumour. This type of tumour should only be diagnosed if it conforms to the following pattern: Krukenberg tumours are almost invariably bilateral. They have smooth surfaces which may, however, be slightly bossed, and they are freely movable in the pelvis.

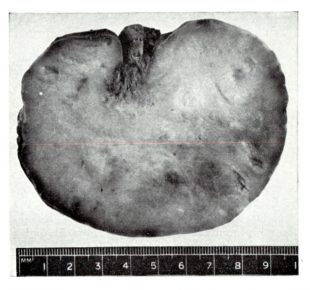

FIG. 386. Krukenberg tumour of the ovary. The tumour has a solid waxy appearance with an intact capsule free of all adhesions. The cut surface is reniform and preserves the shape of the ovary.

There is no tendency to form adhesions with neighbouring viscera and there is no infiltration through the capsule. The tumour retains the shape of the normal ovary and has a peculiar solid waxy consistence, although cystic spaces due to degeneration of the growth are common (Fig. 386). Histologically the tumour has a cellular or myxomatous stroma amongst which are scattered large signet-ring cells. These cells are ovoid in shape with a granular cytoplasm and the nucleus is compressed against one pole of the cell so that the outline of the cell resembles a signet-ring (Fig. 387). The tumours are secondary growths in the ovary and most often arise from a primary carcinoma of the stomach 70%, large bowel 15% and breast 6%. The Krukenberg tumour outstrips the primary growth in size, and unless the histology of the tumour is known the case may be regarded as one of primary malignant ovarian carcinoma, particularly as the tumours are usually freely movable without obvious intraperitoneal metastases. The tumours almost certainly

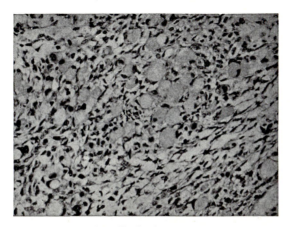

FIG. 387. Krukenberg tumour.

arise by retrograde lymphatic spread; the carcinoma cells pass from the stomach to the superior gastric lymphatic glands which receive the lymphatics from the ovary. Retrograde lymphatic spread can be demonstrated in early cases when carcinoma cells are found infiltrating the ovary by way of the lymphatics in the medulla. The older theory of direct cellular spill of cancer cells via the peritoneal cavity is challenged by the fact that the capsule of a Krukenberg tumour shows no evidence of malignant penetration from outside, whereas in certain early cases malignant cell nests have been demonstrated in the medullary lymphatics, where they presumably arrived by a retrograde permeation from the gastric primary. Interesting and rare instances have been reported where a typical Krukenberg tumour was alleged to present as a primary neoplasm, no gastro-intestinal focus being demonstrable. It is probable that a minute undetectable gastro-intestinal growth was present but unrecognisable at autopsy. It is curious that such a small primary cancer can give rise to so large and obvious a metastasis.

Coincident Carcinoma of the Ovaries and the Body of the Uterus. Cases of coincident carcinoma of the ovaries and the body of the uterus are not unknown. In some cases the growth is primary in the body of the uterus and forms secondary deposits in the ovaries. In other cases, particularly with very malignant ovarian tumours, the primary growth is in the ovaries and secondary deposits reach the cavity of the uterus either by lymphatic permeation or by implantation via the Fallopian tube. Another group of cases is well recognised in which the ovarian carcinomata are histologically different from the carcinoma of the body of the uterus. Any postmenopausal bleeding associated with an ovarian tumour should suggest the possibility of a coincident endometrial carcinoma and this possibility always demands the removal of the uterus as well as the ovarian tumours.

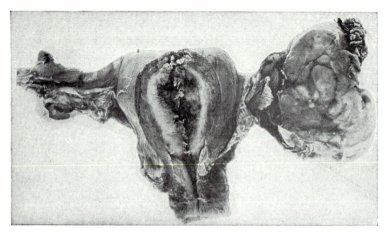

FIG. 388. A coincident carcinoma of the body of the uterus and of the ovary. On the right the ovary is replaced by carcinoma. In such a specimen it is often difficult to determine which is the primary site.

Metastases of Ovarian Carcinomata. The earliest and most important metastases from ovarian carcinomata are the multiple secondary deposits which form over the peritoneum. The malignant cells of the primary growth erode through the capsule of the tumour and become disseminated over the peritoneal cavity. The cells become implanted on the peritoneum and form friable papillomata which lead to ascites. The secondary deposits are always most numerous in Douglas's pouch and in the omentum, though in an advanced ovarian cancer it is quite common to find every single intraperitoneal organ and surface studded with growth, and hardly a single square centimetre unaffected. The secondary deposits in Douglas's pouch can be felt on vaginal examination, and this sign is of the greatest importance in the establishment of the diagnosis that an ovarian tumour is malignant. The secondary deposits in the omentum are interesting because they illustrate the phagocytic properties of this structure.

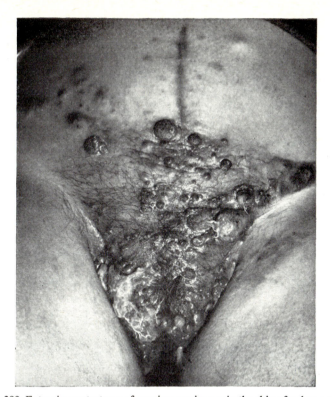

Fig. 389. Extensive metastases of ovarian carcinoma in the skin of vulva, mons and operation site.

Bilateral Character of Ovarian Tumours. Ovarian tumours show a considerable tendency to be bilateral. This tendency is particularly well marked with malignant tumours, and it has been computed that about 70% of primary ovarian carcinomata are bilateral, while in almost all cases of secondary tumours both ovaries are involved. Even when not macroscopically infiltrated serial section will reveal microscopic invasion. Innocent cystic tumours are bilateral in about 16% of cases. There is reason to believe that even with malignant ovarian tumours the two ovaries are attacked simultaneously by the disease and that the involvement of one ovary by secondary deposits from the other is very exceptional. With secondary ovarian carcinomata, if the involvement is by retrograde lymphatic spread, one would expect both ovaries to be involved simultaneously. Similar remarks apply when implantation of carcinoma cells is the cause of development of secondary deposits in the ovaries.

Metastases in the Uterus. In advanced carcinoma of the ovaries the tumour becomes adherent to surrounding structures so that the uterus is directly infiltrated by the growth. The peritoneal surface of the uterus is also infiltrated in some cases by carcinoma cells disseminated over the peritoneum. Rarely, metastases form in the endometrium of the uterus as the result of carcinoma cells passing along the Fallopian tube into the cavity of the uterus. In some cases of carcinoma of the ovaries secondary deposits are formed in the vaginal walls, and such metastases correspond to those found in cases of chorion-epithelioma and of carcinoma of the body of the uterus.

Metastases in Operation Scars. It is not uncommon after the removal of malignant ovarian tumours for metastases subsequently to form in the operation scar and to spread to the adjacent skin (Fig. 389).

Spread by Way of Blood Stream. It is rare for carcinoma of the ovaries to spread by way of the blood stream, but with very malignant tumours metastases may be disseminated in this way. It is therefore important to take a chest X-ray of all suspectedly malignant ovarian tumours.

Lymphatic Spread. It is rare to find clinical evidence of lymphatic permeation with carcinoma of the ovaries. The regional lymphatic glands of the ovaries are the para aortic and the superior gastric glands which are impalpable clinically. Sometimes, however, the malignant cells permeate to the mediastinal glands when they may ulcerate into the pleural cavity and cause pleural effusion. Sometimes secondary deposits may be found above the left clavicle in the posterior triangle of the neck, where they have arrived via the main lymphatic ducts in the mediastinum. It should be remembered that the secondary deposits disseminated over the peritoneum permeate into the sub-peritoneal lymphatics so that the pelvic glands become infiltrated.

The most important metastases of malignant ovarian tumours are those which form on the peritoneum and lead to the development of large tumours in the omentum. Most patients with advanced carcinoma of the ovaries die as the result of the ascites, exhaustion and cachexia. It must also be pointed out that secondary deposits of carcinoma of the ovaries rarely involve the liver, because the ovarian vessels belong to the systemic system and not to the portal system like those of the intestine and stomach.

Tumours Arising from the Connective Tissues of the Ovary

Of the innocent connective tissue tumours of the ovary fibromata are the most common. Pure myomata are rare tumours and very few other innocent connective tissue tumours have been described.

Ovarian Fibroma. This tumour, which is not uncommon, comprises about 3% of ovarian neoplasms and has no particular age incidence. The tumour is oval in shape with a smooth surface and large veins which are always noticeable in the capsule. The consistence is firm and harder than that of a uterine myoma. The tumour frequently undergoes degeneration so that cystic spaces are found towards the centre and calcareous degeneration is not uncommon. The tumours are usually about 15 cm. in diameter but they sometimes become much larger than this and may weigh as much as 50 lbs. Torsion may occur with the larger tumours (see Fig. 390).

Microscopical examination shows the tumour to be composed of a network of spindle-shaped cells which closely resemble the spindle cells of the ovarian cortex. The cellular pattern is strikingly uniform and there is no attempt at any nuclear activity. The association of Brenner tumours with ovarian

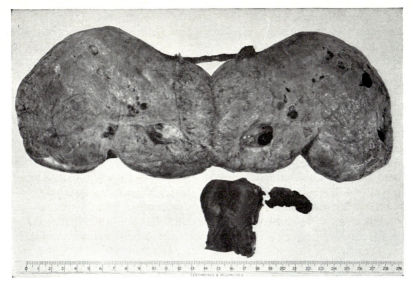

Fig. 390. Fibroma of ovary (above) and the uterus (below).

fibroma has already been mentioned. In large tumours the connective tissue cells are elongated and an intercellular matrix becomes prominent. The tumours are often accompanied by ascites. Sometimes the patient has hydrothorax and the combination of an ovarian fibroma with ascites and hydrothorax, usually right-sided, is referred to as Meigs' syndrome. There has been

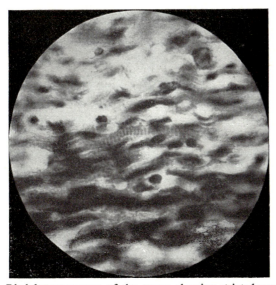

Fig. 391. Rhabdomyosarcoma of the ovary, showing striated muscle cells.

much speculation on the mechanism by which the hydrothorax occurs and it is now generally accepted that the diaphragm is porous either by reason of minute foramina or via the lymphatics. Meigs' syndrome can occur with other solid ovarian tumours such as granulosa cell tumours and Brenner tumours. It should be emphasised that the diagnosis of Meigs' syndrome may provide a trap for the unwary, i.e. the pleural effusion associated with a lung metastasis secondary to an ovarian cancer.

Three types of fibroma are recognised. In the first the tumour takes the form of a surface papilloma on the ovary. In the second type there is a small encapsulated fibroma arising in an ovary so that normal ovarian tissue can be recognised at one pole of the tumour. In the third type the fibroma replaces the ovary completely.

Sarcoma. Ovarian sarcomata are rare tumours and many tumours labelled as sarcomata have been misdiagnosed histologically and were in reality granulosa cell tumours or anaplastic carcinomata. In fact an anaplastic carcinoma so much resembles a sarcoma that it has even been dignified by the name of carcino-sarcoma. This term we deprecate. Sarcomata arise most frequently after the menopause, particularly in multiparae. They give rise to

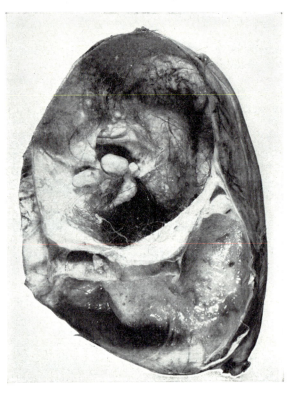

FIG. 392. Benign dermoid cyst of the ovary. Note the tooth in the embryonic node and hair arising from the wall.

multiple metastases. Rhabdomyosarcoma of the ovary has been described (see Fig. 391). This is probably more accurately to be considered one form of mixed mesodermal tumour (*vide supra* page 391).

Tumours Allegedly Arising from the Ovum

Under this heading are included dermoid cysts and solid teratomata.

Dermoid Cysts. Of all cystic tumours of the ovary 5–10% are dermoids. Dermoid cysts are usually unilocular swellings with smooth surfaces, seldom attaining more than 15 cm. in diameter. They contain sebaceous material and hair, and the wall is lined in part by squamous epithelium which contains hair follicles and sebaceous glands. Teeth, bone, cartilage, thyroid tissue and bronchial mucous membrane are often found in the wall. Sometimes the sebaceous material may be collected together in the form of small balls, and as many as 1,000 sebaceous balls of this type have been counted in a dermoid

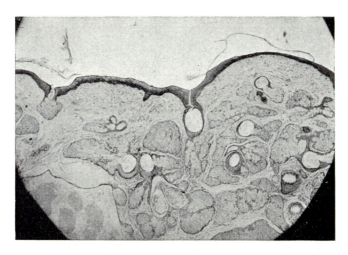

Fig. 393. Dermoid cyst of the ovary. The cyst is lined by squamous epithelium. Sebaceous glands open into the cavity of the cyst. Hair follicles are also present.

cyst. The inner surface of the dermoid cyst is always irregular and contains what is called a "focus" or "embryonic node," from which the hairs project, and in which the teeth and bone are usually found. The nomenclature "dermoid cyst" is inaccurate, for in addition to ectodermal tissues, tissues from both the mesoderm and endoderm are usually found in some part of the tumour. Moreover, though squamous epithelium usually lines the cyst, columnar and transitional types are also found. It is extremely rare for pancreas or liver tissue and intestinal mucous membrane to be found in the wall of a dermoid cyst (see Figs. 392 and 393).

Dermoid cysts frequently arise in association with pseudomucinous cystadenomata to form a combined tumour, part of which consists of a dermoid cyst while the rest has the characteristic structure of a pseudomucinous cystadenoma. Perhaps as many as 40% of dermoid cysts are combined tumours of this kind. This association suggests that the origin of the two forms of ovarian tumour is related.

Multiple dermoid cysts in the same ovary are well recognised and it is often quite usual to find three separate dermoids, and extra-ovarian dermoid cysts arise occasionally in the lumbar region, in the uterovesical septum, in the parasacral region, and in the rectovaginal septum. The combined tumours tend to arise in patients between the ages of 20 and 30, while simple dermoid cysts have a maximum age incidence between 40 and 50. The tumours may, however, arise at any age. They are not infrequently bilateral, 12%.

Dermoid cysts are innocent ovarian tumours but epidermoid carcinoma occurs in 1.7% of all dermoids and sarcomatous changes have also been described. Usually a squamous celled carcinoma develops from the ectodermal tissues but mammary carcinomata and malignant thyroid tumours have been described.

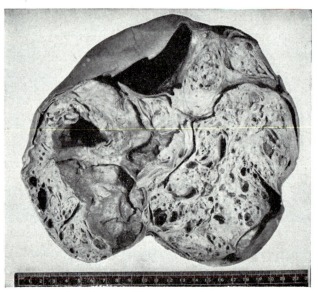

Fig. 394. A solid teratoma of the ovary.

Solid Teratoma of the Ovary. These tumours are very rare. They are mainly solid and the cut surface has a peculiar trabeculated appearance. Almost invariably large loculi are found beneath the capsule. The solid part of the tumour contains cartilage and bone, while hair and sebaceous material are found in the cystic spaces. The solid area also contains plain muscle, brain tissue, glia, pia mater, and intestinal mucous membrane. The attempted formation of a rudimentary eye has been described and even the recognisable pattern of a foetus has been simulated—the so-called embryoma. As a rule, however, the formation is conglomerate, without order or arrangement. Most solid teratomata of the ovary are malignant tumours because of sarcomatous change, but a fair proportion, probably about 20%, are innocent (see Fig. 394).

Primary Chorionepithelioma of the Ovary. This is a very rare tumour and corresponds to the chorionepithelioma of the testis which is strangely enough commoner than its ovarian counterpart. It must, of course, be distinguished from an ovarian metastasis from a primary trophoblastic tumour in the uterus.

Struma Ovarii. This tumour consists of thyroid tissue similar to that of a thyroid adenoma. The tumour is solid, consisting almost entirely of thyroid tissue and should be clearly distinguished from a dermoid cyst with thyroid tissue in its wall. To the naked eye the tumour resembles a small pseudo-mucinous cystadenoma, but the material contained in the vesicles is colloid and gives the reactions for iodine. Some cases lead to the development of

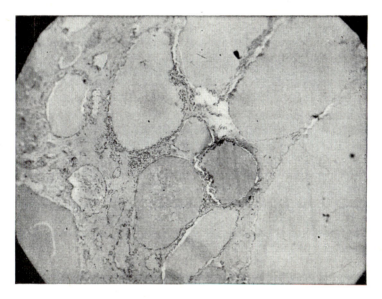

FIG. 395. Struma ovarii showing spaces filled with colloid.

thyrotoxicosis. Most of the tumours are innocent, but malignant thyroid tumours have been recorded. The histogenesis is supposedly a dermoid in which the thyroid tissue preponderates at the expense of the other elements (see Fig. 395).

Carcinoid Tumours of the Ovary. An interesting and recently described tumour of the ovary, sometimes primary and sometimes metastatic, is the argentaffinoma. It occurs as a malignant change in a benign dermoid cyst and presents as a solid yellow tumour with the characteristic histological property of reducing silver salts being derived from the specialised Kultschitzky cells of the intestine (compare the appendix). It produces 5-hydroxytryptamine with attacks of flushing and cyanosis.

TUMOURS ARISING FROM PRIMITIVE MESENCHYME (MESENCHYMOMA)

A. Feminising functioning mesenchymoma

Granulosa Cell Tumour. Granulosa cell tumours are interesting growths of the ovary, as they are composed of cells closely resembling the granulosa cells of the Graafian follicle.

Clinical Features. Granulosa cell tumours are fairly common and represent 10% of all solid malignant ovarian tumours. They can occur at any age and before and after the menopause. The main clinical features depend upon the oestrogenic activity of the tumour and only the larger ones cause pain and abdominal swelling. Feminising tumours secrete oestrogen which the tumour has metabolised from progesterone in the same manner as the normal ovary.

(*a*) When occurring before puberty, a precocious puberty results with development of secondary sexual characteristics, hypertrophy of breasts and external genitalia, pubic hair and myohyperplasia of the uterus. The endometrium shows an oestrogenic, anovulatory pattern. Removal of the tumour causes regression of all these manifestations.

(*b*) When occurring in adult life, the oestrogenic effect is less remarkable than in the prepubertal state. There is no change in the secondary sexual characteristics since these are already established. The effect on the endometrium is that of hyperoestrinism in general, i.e. an exaggerated proliferative pattern with cystic glandular hyperplasia. Thus there may be a super-threshold level of blood oestrogen, leading to amenorrhoea, followed by prolonged bleeding. In fact, the behaviour of the endometrium closely resembles that of metropathia haemorrhagica, another condition in which hyperoestrinism occurs.

(*c*) In the postmenopausal patient, the most remarkable feature is postmenopausal bleeding. The secondary sexual characteristics are less affected though hypertrophy of the breast is sometimes seen. The whole state of the patient has been likened to that of an Indian summer in which she recaptures some of the features of her lost youth. The uterus shows myohyperplasia and cystic glandular hyperplasia exactly as in metropathia. Removal of the tumour causes a regression of all these symptoms and sometimes the additional symptoms of a second menopause (Fig. 399).

Macroscopical Features. The tumours vary in size from tiny to gross, the average being 10 cm. in diameter. The shape is oval and the consistence soft. The cut surface is reticular or trabeculated with areas of interstitial haemorrhage, and it often shows yellow areas. The outer surface is smooth and often lobulated (Fig. 396).

The cells are arranged either in cords or trabeculae, and are often surrounded by structureless hyaline tissue, which resembles the glass membrane of an atretic follicle. Moreover, small Call-Exner bodies can usually be found in some part or other of the tumour; it will be remembered that these small cyst-like spaces are a characteristic feature of the granulosa cells of the Graafian follicle. Three histological types of granulosa cell tumours have been identified: (*a*) an early undifferentiated form which consists of a solid mass of

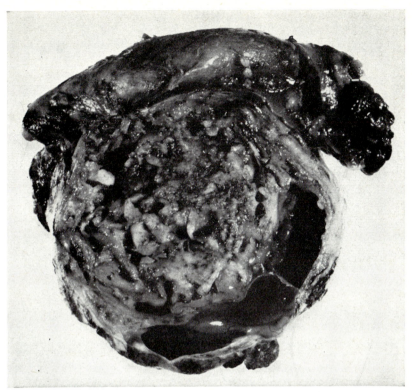

FIG. 396. Granulosa cell tumour of the ovary. The tumour shows the typical haemorrhagic areas.

granulosa cells, (b) a trabecular form, Fig. 398 (c) a folliculoid type in which the granulosa cells are grouped around spaces filled with secretion (Fig. 397). Most granulosa cell tumours are encapsulated and appear to be clinically benign. This appearance of the gross specimen and the histological picture may both be misleading as judged by the subsequent recurrence of the tumour. This recurrence may be delayed for many years, long after the arbitrary five-year period is passed. Jones and Te Linde report fatal recurrence at 18, 20 and 22 years and one of the authors has noted a fatal recurrence at 10 years. Kottmeier says that malignant recurrence occurs in 50% of granulosa cell tumours within ten years, and Haines and Jackson, reporting on the Chelsea Hospital series, are in agreement. It is, therefore, wise to regard at least 50% of granulosa cell tumours as malignant and the term granulosa cell carcinoma is thus justified.

There is a certain correlation in this, as in other malignant ovarian tumours, between the histological appearance and the malignancy. A well differentiated folliculoid pattern is 10% malignant while an anaplastic, almost sarcomatous appearance is 65% malignant.

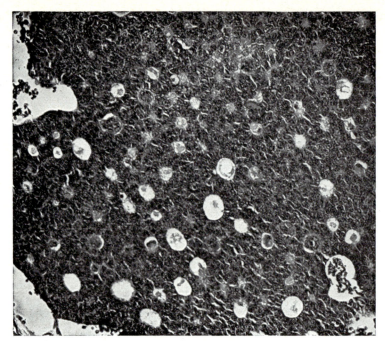

Fig. 397. Granulosa cell tumour, folliculoid pattern. Note the arrangement of the tumour cells into "rosettes" (Call-Exner bodies). (× 170.)

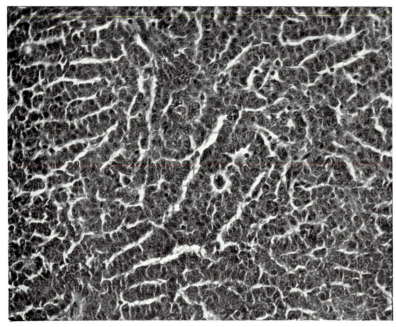

Fig. 398. Granulosa cell tumour, cylindromatous pattern. Note the branching columns of tumour cells. (× 200.)

The metastases are interesting, because the opposite ovary first becomes involved, then metastases develop in the lumbar region and, finally, secondary deposits become scattered in the mesentery, the liver and mediastinum.

Association of Carcinoma of the Endometrium with Granulosa Cell Tumours. There is strong evidence that carcinoma of the endometrium may be associated with feminising tumours of the ovary in post-menopausal women. It has been estimated that in one-fifth of oestrogenic ovarian tumours an endometrial cancer will develop. If this is established the role of excessive oestrogen production in endometrial cancer is significant. Biggart and Macafee give the

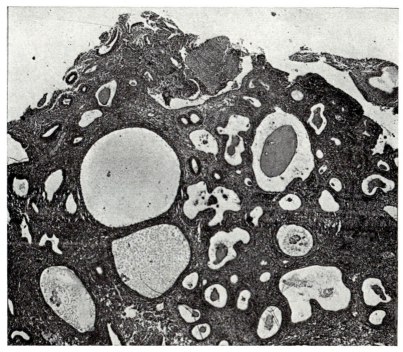

FIG. 399. Cystic glandular hyperplasia of endometrium resulting from a granulosa cell tumour. The patient, aged 79, had post-menopausal bleeding. (× 33.)

incidence of endometrial carcinoma as occurring in 16·6% of granulosa cell tumours, and Matthew 12%. A theca cell tumour is four times more commonly associated with endometrial cancer than the granulosa cell tumour.

Theca Cell Tumour. This tumour is seen only rarely and usually arises after the menopause. It is nearly always unilateral and forms a solid mass. The cut surface is often yellow in colour and, if stained selectively, lipoid material is characteristically present. The tumour consists of spindle-shaped cells reminiscent of an ovarian fibroma together with fat-laden polyhedral cells which resemble the theca lutein cells of the Graafian follicle. The tumour is intensely oestrogenic and causes post-menopausal haemorrhage. The tumour is usually innocent, but malignant forms have been described. It has been shown recently that both granulosa cell tumours and theca cell tumours may show luteinisation of their cells, with the result that progesterone is secreted and secretory hypertrophy can be demonstrated in the endometrium. There is recent evidence that certain luteinised tumours are capable of producing androgen, instead of progesterone, so that their function is virilising rather than feminising.

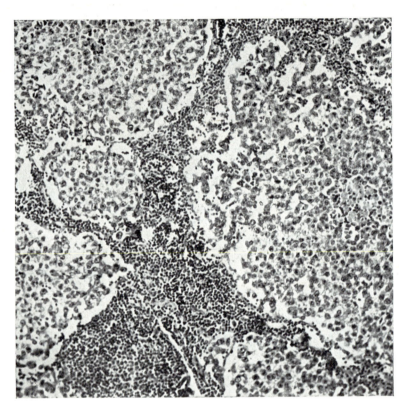

Fig. 400. Ovarian disgerminoma. Note the lymphocytic infiltration amongst the masses of large tumour cells. (× 120.)

B. Neutral Mesenchymoma

Disgerminoma. This tumour corresponds exactly to the seminoma of the testis and its incidence is one-third that of the granulosa cell tumour. It usually arises in young women or in children, with an average incidence at the age of 20. The tumour is solid with a peculiar elastic rubbery consistence with a smooth, firm capsule. The cut surface is yellow or grey with areas of degeneration and haemorrhage. The size is variable, usually moderate, though large tumours have been described. They are usually unilateral, occasionally undergo torsion and may, like all solid tumours, be associated with ascites.

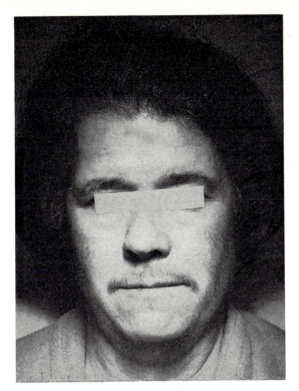

FIG. 401. A patient with ovarian arrhenoblastoma. Note the hirsutism.

The tumour consists of large cells arranged in bunches or alveoli. Lymphocytes and giant cells are always found amongst the tumour cells. This appearance of large dark-staining nuclei with clear, almost translucent cytoplasm and lymphocytic infiltration of the fibrous septa, is immediately diagnostic (see Fig. 400). The tumour is neutral and does not secrete either male or female sex hormones. A number of patients with a disgerminoma of the ovary have been reported to show genital abnormality, with hypoplasia or absence of some part of the genital tract. It has been reported in pseudohermaphrodites. Such congenital abnormalities are not caused by the disgerminoma and its removal has no beneficial effect upon them. The malignancy of disgerminoma is similar to that of the granulosa cell tumour and depends largely on the findings at laparotomy.

(1) A unilateral tumour confined to one ovary is relatively benign.

(2) The presence of active invasion of the pelvic viscera is naturally of grave import though not hopeless.

(3) The presence of extra-pelvic metastases in the general peritoneal cavity and glands, omentum or liver renders the outlook hopeless.

A fair estimate of the malignancy is 33–50%.

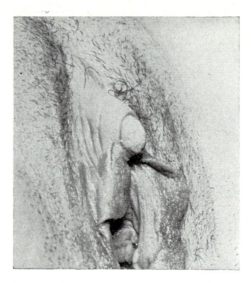

FIG. 402. Hypertrophy of the clitoris in the same patient as Fig. 401.

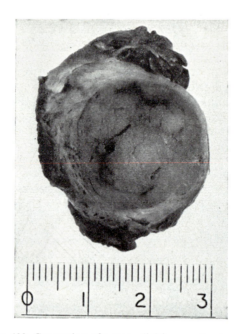

FIG. 403. Cut section of a masculinising ovarian tumour.

C. Virilising Mesenchymoma

and other virilising tumours of the ovary.

(1) **Arrhenoblastoma.** These tumours are extremely rare and usually arise in young women. The tumours are virilising and cause amenhorrhoea, hirsutism, mammary atrophy and hypertrophy of the clitoris. The incidence of malignancy is probably higher than in the oestrogenic tumours.

The clinical features are defeminisation—atrophy of the breasts and amenorrhoea—followed by masculinisation—hirsutism, acne, deepening of voice

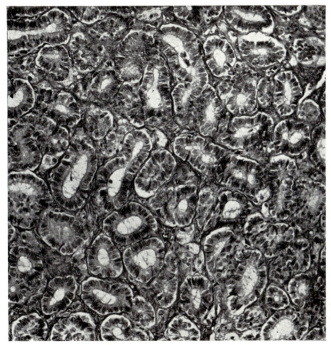

FIG. 404. High power magnification of arrhenoblastoma. Note the well-differentiated tubules simulating the seminiferous tubules of the testis. (× 170.)

and hypertrophy of the clitoris. A pelvic examination reveals a small to moderate sized ovarian swelling, usually about 2–3 in. in diameter; rarely, a tumour of 6 in. or more is found. Bilaterality is a rare feature and only one ovary is usually affected (90%). Curiously the literature contains a few associated with pregnancy. The gross appearance is that of the other mesenchymomata. On histological examination, the tumour shows all grades of differentiation from the testicular adenoma with almost perfectly reproduced seminiferous tubules to a sarcomatous anaplastic variety where, apart from lipoid-containing cells the diagnosis is usually made on the endocrine behaviour of the tumour (Figs. 401–404).

(2) Gynandroblastoma

A tumour which is referred to as a gynandroblastoma has been described which combines the characteristics of the granulosa cell tumour and an arrhenoblastoma.

(3) **Adrenal Cortical Tumours of the Ovary.** These tumours have some resemblance to adrenal cortex when examined microscopically and have been called hypernephroma, masculinovoblastoma, virilising luteoma or clear-celled tumour. These various appellations show that the constituent cells resemble the large clear cells of the adrenal cortex or lutein cells of the corpus luteum. Whatever their true origin, they are very rare tumours which are sometimes masculinising.

(4) **Hilus Cell Tumour.** A rare virilising tumour arising from cells in the ovarian hilum has been described in women past the menopause. One interesting feature of the hilus cell tumour is the presence of Reinke crystals in the cells, a distinguishing feature of the Leydig or interstitial cells of the testis.

Histogenesis of Ovarian Tumours

Fibromata. Small ovarian fibromata are fairly common tumours forming white rounded excrescences in the cortex of the ovary. The tumours arise from the stroma cells of the cortex of the ovary. Histologically a fibroma and a Brenner tumour have a close resemblance, apart from the inclusion of the epithelioid Walthard rests in the latter. With subsequent growth a capsule becomes differentiated and the tumour grows at the expense of the normal ovarian tissue, so that finally the ovary is completely replaced by the fibroma. The structure of a large ovarian fibroma is not unlike that of the stroma of the ovarian cortex, except that the constituent cells are more primitive in type.

With small fibromata it is not uncommon to see hyperplasia of the covering surface epithelium, which tends to become invaginated into the fibroma to give an appearance resembling that of a fibroadenoma. Large fibroadenomata of the ovary, however, are extremely rare.

Cystoma Simplex and Papillary Serous Cystadenoma. These tumours almost certainly originate from downgrowths of the surface epithelium of the ovary into the cortex. Small downgrowths of this sort are extremely common, even in normal ovaries, and small cysts, only recognised by microscopical examination, are fairly frequent. The cystoma simplex originates in invaginations of this kind. Papillary forms result from intracystic growths into such tumours, and it has been shown that the development of intracystic growths arises early in the life-history of the papillary cystadenoma. Papillary serous carcinomata of the ovary arise when the intracystic growths become malignant.

The origin of the tumours from downgrowths of the surface epithelium of the ovary is generally accepted and the tumours are regarded as examples of ovarian Müllerianosis. It is also recognised that the epithelial lining of the tumours is similar to that of the Fallopian tubes.

Granulosa Cell Tumours. Granulosa cell tumours consist of cells identical with the granulosa cells of Graafian follicles and theca cell tumours of cells similar to those of the theca interna cells. As both types of tumour may arise

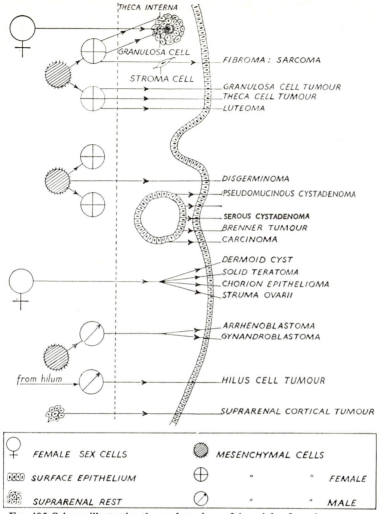

THECA INTERNA

GRANULOSA CELL

STROMA CELL

FIBROMA : SARCOMA

GRANULOSA CELL TUMOUR
THECA CELL TUMOUR
LUTEOMA

DISGERMINOMA
PSEUDOMUCINOUS CYSTADENOMA

SEROUS CYSTADENOMA
BRENNER TUMOUR
CARCINOMA

DERMOID CYST
SOLID TERATOMA
CHORION EPITHELIOMA
STRUMA OVARII

ARRHENOBLASTOMA
GYNANDROBLASTOMA

from hilum

HILUS CELL TUMOUR

SUPRARENAL CORTICAL TUMOUR

FEMALE SEX CELLS   MESENCHYMAL CELLS

SURFACE EPITHELIUM   "   "   FEMALE

SUPRARENAL REST   "   "   MALE

FIG. 405. Scheme illustrating the modern views of the origin of ovarian tumours.

after the menopause, when there are no Graafian follicles in the ovaries, the tumours cannot be regarded as being derived from mature cells of this type. They are therefore regarded as originating in mesenchymal cells which have been differentiated sexually. The arrhenoblastoma is regarded as being derived from mesenchymal cells of the male type which for some reason or other are found in the ovary. Disgerminoma can be explained on the assumption that it originates in mesenchymal cells before their sexual differentiation into male and female types (see Fig. 405). The theca cell is regarded as the master hormone producer in the ovary and its versatility is now well recognised, cf. the androgenic effects of hyperthecosis in the Stein-Leventhal syndrome where the theca cell is reasonably suspected as being androgenic.

Teratoid Tumours. The origin of these tumours is much disputed. Ideas of parthenogenesis and enclosed blastomeres are now unfashionable. Dermoid cysts never contain trophoblastic or gonadic tissue and the absence of chorionic tissue eliminates the idea that a dermoid cyst develops as a result of parthenogenesis or from an enclosed blastomere. On the other hand, malignant solid teratomata probably arise from toti-potent cells, i.e. cells

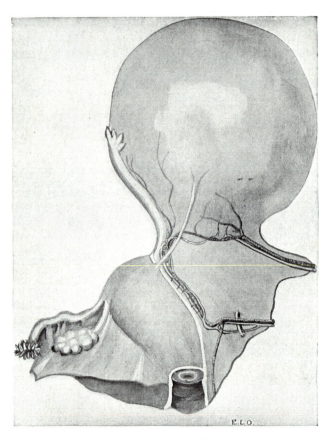

Fig. 406. The pedicle of an ovarian cyst showing the relations of the ovarian vessels, the ovarian ligament and the Fallopian tube, together with the anastomosing branch of the uterine artery. (After Stoeckel.)

which are capable of producing ectodermal, mesodermal and entodermal structures.

Pseudomucinous Cystadenomata. Although this tumour is the commonest of all ovarian tumours, its origin is unexplained. The cells of the tumour are paralleled in the body only by those of the cervix and the large intestine. The two present-day theories are (*a*) that the tumour represents an example of ovarian Müllerianosis, with metaplasia of the ovarian surface epithelium into cervical epithelium. Towers has actually demonstrated this transition from Walthard's epithelium into the high columnar epithelium of a pseudo-mucinous cyst. (*b*) That the tumour arises from large intestine elements of a dermoid cyst.

Brenner Tumour. This tumour is often associated with pseudomucinous cystadenoma, where there is probably some relation between their origins. The similarity to Walthard inclusions has already been noted and this suggests that Brenner tumours, like Walthard inclusions, are derived from the germinal epithelial layer of the ovary.

Complications of Ovarian Tumours

Axial Rotation: Torsion. Torsion of an ovarian cyst is a very common complication, and in about 12% of ovarian tumours which come to operation the tumour has undergone axial rotation. Chocolate cysts and malignant ovarian tumours are usually fixed by adhesions, so that it is very rare for these types of ovarian tumour to undergo torsion. On the other hand, parovarian cysts and the broad ligament cysts which will be described in the next chapter are the most likely pelvic tumours to undergo torsion, probably because they develop in the outer part of the broad ligament and come to lie above the infundibulo-pelvic fold, so that they have a greater degree of mobility than an ovarian tumour. In most cases the cyst is about 10 cm. or over in diameter when it undergoes torsion, and it is very exceptional for the tumour to rotate while it lies in the pelvis. After it has risen above the level of the pelvic brim it acquires a much greater degree of mobility and is therefore more prone to

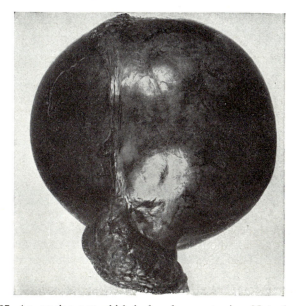

Fig. 407. An ovarian cyst which had undergone torsion. Note the intense congestion.

rotate. Occasionally very large tumours undergo rotation. Because of the high incidence of pseudomucinous cystadenomata, torsion is most frequently seen with this tumour. There is no particular age incidence. The right and left sides are involved with equal frequency. Usually the tumour rotates so that its anterior surface turns towards the patient's right side. It is not uncommon for the tumour to be rotated through three or more complete circles. As the result of rotation the veins in the pedicle become occluded, so that the tumour becomes congested, and after a time there is interstitial haemorrhage in the wall of the tumour and into the loculi. The increased tension causes severe

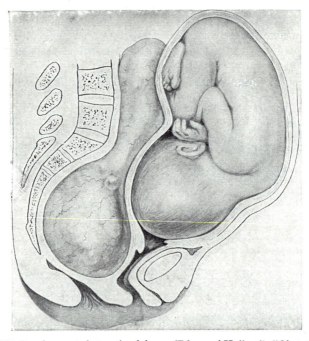

Fig. 408. Ovarian cyst obstructing labour. (Eden and Holland's "Obstetrics.")

abdominal pain, together with the signs of peritoneal irritation. Subsequently, adhesions form to surrounding structures, so that the omentum and intestines become attached to the tumour, and on rare occasions the cyst may become infected. It is, however, extremely rare for the tumour to undergo necrosis from occlusion of the arteries in the pedicle.

A variety of hypotheses has been advanced to explain why rotation develops. The contraction of adhesions, asymmetrical growth, and movements of the sigmoid colon have been suggested to explain the rotation of an ovarian cyst. These hypotheses do not explain why the tumour may be rotated through as many as three complete circles. Moreover, the pedicle of the tumour is attached to its inferior pole. It is obvious that a tumour would be more likely to undergo axial rotation if it were to hang down under the influence of gravity from an attachment high up in the abdomen. The most probable explanation of rotation of an ovarian cyst is that the cause is haemodynamic. It is suggested that some violent movement—a history of which is almost invariably obtained in cases of torsion—initiates the twist, and as a result the ovarian artery itself becomes twisted. The pulsation in the vessel will then cause a series of tiny impulses to be transmitted to the pedicle, each of which will aggravate the twist. After a time the degree of torsion will be such that the veins in the pedicle become occluded when the patient will complain of severe abdominal pain (see Figs. 406 and 407).

Rupture. Rupture of an ovarian cyst may be traumatic or spontaneous. Traumatic rupture results from direct violence to the abdomen. It may happen during labour when a cyst is impacted in Douglas's pouch in advance of the presenting part (Fig. 408). It is not uncommon for a small thin-walled retention cyst to rupture during bimanual examination. The patient then experiences sudden abdominal pain but no after-effects are to be expected apart from a transient rise in pulse rate.

Spontaneous rupture of ovarian cysts is not uncommon. With malignant ovarian tumours, particularly those of the papillomatous type, the carcinoma cells infiltrate through the connective tissue capsule to ulcerate into the peritoneal cavity. Similarly, with innocent papillomatous serous cystadenomata a similar process takes place. The most interesting cases of spontaneous rupture are, however, those arising with actively growing pseudomucinous cystadenomata. Sometimes the epithelial elements of the growth grow so rapidly that the connective tissues of the capsule are unable to keep up with them, so that a spontaneous rupture of the tumour is the result and pseudomucinous material is discharged into the peritoneal cavity. In most cases there is no serious after-effect, but very rarely the condition called pseudomyxoma of the peritoneum develops.

Pseudomyxoma of the Peritoneum. In this condition the peritoneal cavity is filled with coagulated pseudomucinous material which is adherent to the omentum and intestines. The findings at laparotomy almost exactly resemble boiled sago pudding. The material cannot be removed completely at operation because of its attachment to bowel, and the condition tends to recur after operation. Pseudomyxoma of the peritoneum in women is usually associated with a pseudomucinous cystadenoma of the ovary, but it has been reported in association with a mucocele of the appendix. The condition is recognised in men, when it is associated either with a mucocele of the appendix or with a carcinoma of the large intestine. In pseudomyxoma of the peritoneum the mesothelium of the peritoneum is converted, in part, into high columnar cells which are histologically similar to those lining a pseudomucinous cystadenoma of the ovary, and these cells secrete the mucinous material into the peritoneal cavity. The prognosis in pseudomyxoma of the peritoneum is bad, even after the ovaries and the appendix are removed.

Infection. Infection of ovarian tumours is infrequent. Most cases follow acute salpingitis, when the cyst becomes involved by direct spread. The cyst may become infected during the puerperium as part of an ascending genital tract infection. Infection may also follow torsion when, as the result of adhesions to the intestine, the tumour becomes directly infected. Infection by the blood stream is very uncommon. Infected ovarian tumours are always adherent to adjacent viscera and occasionally discharge their contents into the rectum.

Extraperitoneal Development. Some ovarian tumours burrow extraperitoneally during their development and may spread upwards into the perinephric region. The removal of these tumours is extremely difficult and there is, moreover, a danger of injuring the ureter. During dissection and removal of such a cyst large vessels may be torn in the retroperitoneal space and subsequent leakage of blood will form a retroperitoneal haematoma. Such a haematoma gives rise to considerable shock and will require drainage. Transfusion will also be necessary.

Clinical Features of Ovarian Tumours

Age Incidence. It has been stated already that serous cystomata and papillary cystadenomata have no especial age incidence. Pseudomucinous cystadenomata occur most frequently between the ages of 30 and 60, with equal proportion during the three decades between these ages.

Dermoid cysts occur most frequently between the ages of 40 and 50, and in the decade between 20 and 30, but they may be seen at any age.

Fibromata may occur at any age, but they are most common between 30 and 40. Malignant ovarian tumours are most frequent between the ages of 50 and 60, and approximately two-thirds of all cases of malignant ovarian tumours appear after the age of 50. Nevertheless, malignant ovarian tumours are sometimes found in young women, when they tend to be particularly malignant.

Secondary ovarian carcinomata are met with most frequently in patients between the ages of 35 and 50. There is no clear evidence that parity is related to the development of any type of ovarian tumour.

Innocent Ovarian Tumours

Symptoms. Although innocent ovarian cysts frequently give rise to enormous tumours they cause relatively few symptoms. Indeed, in innocent ovarian tumours the patient's attention is first directed to the abdominal swelling. The average pseudomucinous cystadenoma removed at operation is about the size of a football, and it is not until the tumour has reached this size that it causes sufficient abdominal enlargement to make the patient realise that something is wrong.

Ovarian tumours hardly ever affect the menstrual functions. It is unusual for the rhythm of menstruation to be disturbed by innocent ovarian tumours even though they are bilateral. Menorrhagia is hardly ever present in cases of ovarian tumour. Amenorrhoea is a rare symptom. It should be remembered, however, that multilocular cysts are not uncommon in women of menopausal age, so that the appearance of a large ovarian cyst coincides fortuitously with the onset of the menopause. Even with malignant ovarian tumours, when both ovaries are involved, it is unusual for the patient to develop amenorrhoea.

Pressure symptoms may be encountered in patients who have large ovarian tumours. Mammoth tumours lead to embarrassment of respiration and to palpitations as the result of pressure upon the diaphragm, while venous obstruction may cause the patient to develop bilateral oedema of the feet. Urinary symptoms sometimes develop with ovarian tumours. Frequency of micturition is a relatively common complaint, probably because of pressure upon the bladder, and very rarely retention of urine may develop, through the tumour becoming incarcerated in the pouch of Douglas. Gastro-intestinal upset and dyspepsia are surprisingly rare with innocent tumours but may be the first symptom and, possibly, the only one of an ovarian cancer. Bowel symptoms are almost unknown in cases of ovarian tumour, probably because most tumours are cystic and the soft consistence is insufficient to obliterate the lumen of the bowel. Pain is a rare symptom with innocent ovarian tumours, irrespective of their size, and if present should always suggest the possibility of malignancy. In fact, it may be stated that, apart from the accidents of torsion, rupture and infection, an innocent ovarian tumour should be painless (Figs. 409 and 410).

With large ovarian cysts it is not uncommon for the patient to develop what is referred to as ovarian cachexia, when she becomes emaciated. Such cachexia has no relation whatsoever to the development of malignant change in the tumour, and it may be of an extreme degree even though the tumour is innocent.

Axial rotation of an ovarian cyst leads to extremely severe abdominal pain. Sometimes the severity is comparable to that of a perforated gastric ulcer. The patient may become shocked and collapsed, with subnormal temperature and a weak thready pulse. Nausea and vomiting are common symptoms and later distension and constipation develop. Subsequently, the temperature rises and the pain remains constant and severe. On examination, the abdomen moves poorly and is distended. The cyst is tense and tender, and there is acute local tenderness and rigidity of the abdominal wall. The increased tension alters the consistence of the tumour, so that there may be difficulty in establishing that the abdominal tumour is cystic. Difficulty may therefore arise in diagnosis, and the tumour may be mistaken for a uterine myoma undergoing red degeneration. The abdominal physical signs may be similar to those obtained in cases of concealed accidental haemorrhage, if the torsion occurs in a pregnant patient.

Infection of ovarian cysts is a rare complication, but it should be suspected if there is abdominal tenderness, rigidity and pyrexia associated with the presence of the ovarian cyst.

Physical Signs

The typical ovarian cyst forms an abdominal swelling detected by inspection. The abdominal wall can be seen to move over the swelling when the patient takes a deep inspiration. The tumour is symmetrically situated in the abdomen and is not more prominent to one side of the midline. On palpation the upper and lateral limits of the tumour can be defined, but it is usually found impossible to identify the lower pole of the tumour except in the case of relatively small cysts with a long pedicle. The surface of the tumour is smooth, although it may be slightly bossed with multilocular cysts. Small cysts are usually movable from side to side, but large tumours filling the abdomen and tumours which have burrowed extraperitoneally are fixed. The consistence of the tumour is tense and cystic and a fluid thrill can be elicited. Sometimes a cyst is flaccid, when a well-marked fluid thrill is obtained and the tumour has not the tense consistence of a typical ovarian cyst. It is not uncommon for hard areas to be palpated, even in large ovarian cysts. These areas, in pseudomucinous cystadenomata are composed of small loculi which

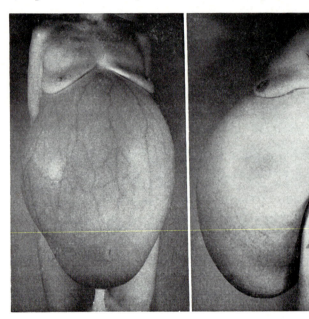

FIG. 409. A very large benign pseudomucinous ovarian cyst which weighed 108 lb. Note the prominent veins, displacement of the umbilicus, and oedema of the lower abdomen.

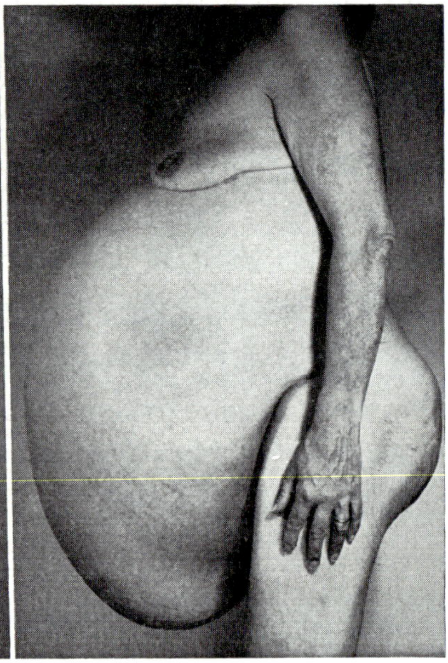

FIG. 410. A lateral view of the same patient. Note the lumbar lordosis.

give the tumour an almost solid feeling on palpation. All patients with an ovarian cyst should be examined carefully for ascites, since the presence of ascites is strong evidence that the tumour is malignant. Sometimes, however, well-marked ascites is met with in cases of ovarian fibromata. On auscultation an ovarian tumour is silent and on percussion it is dull over the centre of the abdomen but resonant in the flanks which are occupied by the dispossessed large and small bowel. This sign is reversed in ascites. The legs should be examined for oedema. Bilateral oedema is present with large innocent tumours which cause increased intra-abdominal pressure. Oedema of the feet, and particularly unilateral oedema, is also found with malignant tumours, when the fixed pelvic mass compresses the iliac veins.

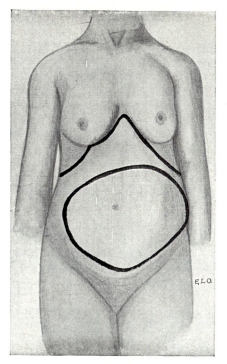

FIG. 411. Ovarian cyst. This tumour lies fairly symmetrically in the abdomen, a little more on one side than on the other. The upper border is defined below the costal margin and there is no displacement of the thoracic viscera. (Menge Opitz.)

The physical signs found on bimanual examination differ according to the size of the tumour. With small tumours the uterus can be identified without difficulty, and the ovarian cyst can be outlined bimanually, so that the whole of the surface of the cyst can be palpated. The cyst usually displaces the uterus to the opposite side if it extends into the pelvis. With large cysts it may be difficult to outline the uterus, and pressure upon the abdominal swelling may cause the cervix to descend into the vagina and the uterus is pushed down into the pelvis. Even with large cysts the lower pole of the tumour should be palpated, either through the anterior or posterior fornix. The firm rounded lower pole of the tumour has a characteristic feel, and fluctuation can usually be obtained between the fingers placed in the vagina and the external hand. It is important to identify the position of the uterus if possible, as mistakes in diagnosis with innocent ovarian cysts are almost always due to failure to identify the body of the uterus separate from the tumour. The physical signs of an ovarian cyst may be simulated very closely by a cystically degenerate myoma and the diagnosis cannot be made with accuracy unless the position of the body of the uterus is established. The cardinal sign that distinguishes a mobile ovarian from a uterine tumour is that when the ovarian tumour is raised up by the abdominal hand the cervix remains stationary to the vaginal fingers. In all cases the pouch of Douglas should be examined carefully during the pelvic examination, as the presence there of hard nodules is strong evidence that the tumour is malignant (Fig. 411).

Differential Diagnosis

The abdominal physical signs of an ovarian cyst may be simulated by a full bladder, a pregnant uterus, a myoma, ascites and other abdominal tumours such as hydronephrosis, mesenteric cyst or retroperitoneal tumour and tuberculous peritonitis especially if encysted by coils of adherent intestine. A full bladder is tense and tender, fixed in position, projecting anteriorly more than an ovarian cyst, and a catheter should be passed to establish the diagnosis.

A pregnant uterus should always be thought of whenever a tumour is found arising from the pelvis. It should be remembered that patient abdominal palpation of the gravid uterus will almost always detect painless uterine contractions. The exclusion of pregnancy offers no difficulty if a careful bimanual examination is made. Appropriate investigations such as X-rays, ultrasonic examination and a pregnancy test will confirm or refute the diagnosis. Mistakes are made because the possibility is not considered.

A myoma is usually hard and firm, without the tense cystic consistence of the typical ovarian cyst. Bimanual examination should establish that the tumour is continuous and movable with the cervix (see also p. 583).

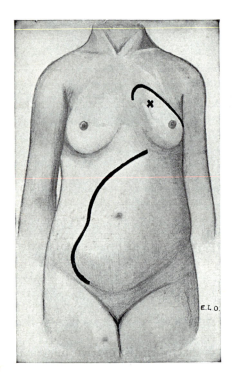

FIG. 412. Hydronephrosis. The tumour lies to one side of the midline. It passes upwards to the level of the costal margin of that side and there is bulging in the left flank. The cross indicates the position of the apex beat in the third space, while the black line over the thorax represents the upper limit of cardiac dullness. (After Menge Opitz.)

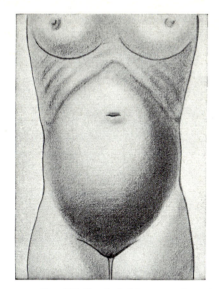
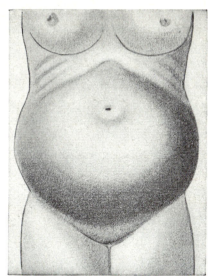

FIG. 413. On the left is a case of ovarian cyst, while on the right is the abdomen of a case of ascites. In acites the abdomen spreads much more laterally than in the case of an ovarian cyst. (After Neuweiler.)

There is sometimes great difficulty in distinguishing between a large ovarian cyst and ascites. With a large ovarian cyst the percussion note over the tumour is dull, whereas both flanks are resonant. In ascites the note is dull over the flanks, while the abdomen is tympanitic in the midline and, moreover, the physical signs of shifting dullness may be obtained. Large veins are often present in the skin of the abdomen in cases of ascites, but such veins are not uncommon with large ovarian cysts. Even with large ovarian cysts the lateral borders of the tumour may be palpable and the tumour may have some degree of mobility (see Figs. 413 and 414).

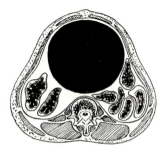
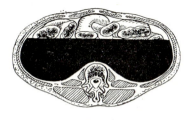

FIG. 414. On the left a cross section of the abdomen is shown from a case of an ovarian cyst, while on the right is a cross section from a case of ascites. With an ovarian cyst the intestines are displaced dorsally while with ascites the intestines lie immediately beneath the abdominal wall. (After Neuweiler.)

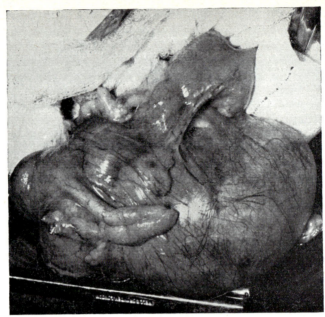

Fig. 415. A mesenteric cyst photographed at operation. The caecum and appendix lie to the left and the terminal ileum is situated above the cyst. The tumour was thought to be an ovarian cyst on clinical examination.

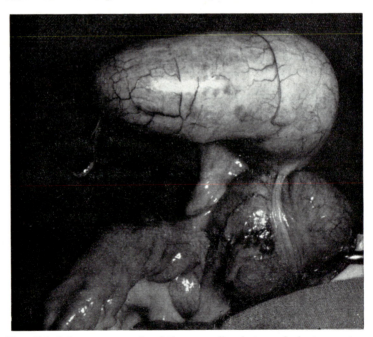

Fig. 416. A large mucocoele of the appendix photographed at operation. The caecum lies below on the right and the terminal ileum on the left. Clinically diagnosed as an ovarian cyst.

The most difficult cases are those of tuberculous peritonitis with ascites, when it may be impossible to establish the diagnosis without laparotomy. Encysted tuberculous ascites may be difficult to distinguish from an ovarian cyst, because the encysted fluid lies in the pelvis and projects into the abdomen to form an abdominal tumour. In most cases of tuberculous peritonitis the patient has lost weight, is pyrexial and suffers from night sweats and there may be other signs of tuberculosis in the body. A diagnostic curettage may reveal tuberculous involvement of the endometrium.

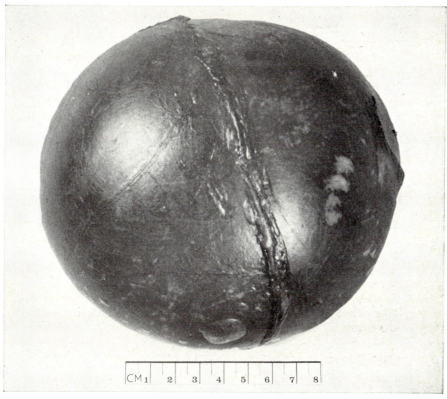

Fig. 417. Renal cyst, at first thought to be an ovarian cyst. The correct diagnosis was however confirmed by intravenous pyelogram.

Difficulty is sometimes experienced by students in distinguishing between an obese abdomen and an ovarian cyst. Some women of menopausal age put on weight very quickly and come up for medical advice complaining of what they term an abdominal tumour. Not infrequently the abdomen is prominent and held rigid. The surest method of excluding an ovarian cyst is to percuss the abdomen below the level of the umbilicus. If the note is tympanitic an ovarian cyst can be excluded, although the signs elicited by palpation may be indeterminate. Examination under an anaesthetic may be necessary.

Other tumours may cause difficulty in diagnosis; for example, a large hydro-nephrosis may project forwards into the abdomen. Such a tumour always penetrates back into the loin and is situated high up in the abdomen, well above the pelvis. Investigations by intravenous or retrograde pyelography will establish the diagnosis. Other tumours such as enlarged spleen, mucocoele of the appendix or gall-bladder, hydatid cysts, and pancreatic cysts should always be considered if the physical signs of an ovarian cyst are atypical, and if the tumour lies in the mid or upper abdomen (see Figs. 412, 415 and 416).

Small ovarian cysts which lie in the pelvis are usually palpated without much difficulty. They are movable, with a tense consistence and a smooth rounded surface. It may be difficult to establish the diagnosis with accuracy if the tumour is fixed, when such conditions as ectopic gestation, hydro-salpinx, and pyosalpinx have to be excluded. One of the most important points to bear in mind in the consideration of the differential diagnosis is the tendency for innocent ovarian tumours to be free of symptoms.

If in doubt regarding the exact clinical diagnosis, additional information may be provided by:

(1) Examination under an anaesthetic, after emptying the bowel and bladder, enables a more thorough and exact diagnosis to be made.
(2) Culdoscopy or peritoneoscopy if available.
(3) Hystero-salpingography may show distortion or displacement of the tube by a small cyst.
(4) Radiography may demonstrate a soft tissue shadow, or teeth in a dermoid. Gynaecography with carbon dioxide intraperitoneal insuffla-tion is a further diagnostic refinement.
(5) Intravenous pyelography will exclude a hydronephrosis and may show smooth indentation of the dye in the bladder in the later pictures.
(6) In all suspected ovarian cancers, a barium meal should be performed to exclude a gastro-intestinal primary carcinoma in, for example, the pylorus.

Clinical Features of Malignant Ovarian Tumours

It is important to establish whether the ovarian tumour is innocent or malignant before operation.

(1) Age. Most malignant ovarian tumours arise in women of menopausal or post-menopausal age. Malignant tumours which arise in younger women are of rapid growth and cause well-marked cachexia.

(2) Pain. Malignant ovarian tumours almost always lead to fairly severe abdominal pain, and the symptom of pain is much more pronounced than with innocent tumours.

(3) Abnormal uterine bleeding. In women of post-menopausal age, vaginal bleeding may be complained of and this symptom is typical of granulosa cell tumours. With bilateral malignant ovarian tumours in women under meno-pausal age amenorrhoea is a very rare symptom even when both ovaries are completely replaced by carcinoma.

(4) Bilateral tumours. In most cases the condition is bilateral so that two tumours are found, the incidence of bilateral tumours with malignant growths being far higher than with innocent tumours.

(5) Ascites. Perhaps the most important clinical sign of malignancy is the development of ascites, and in all cases of ovarian tumour careful examination should be made for the physical signs of ascites.

(6) Other tumour masses. In advanced cases secondary deposits in the omentum can be palpated in the upper abdomen. The pouch of Douglas should be carefully examined for nodules, and if hard fixed nodules about $\frac{1}{2}$ in. diameter are felt through the posterior vaginal fornix it is almost conclusive that the tumour is malignant.

(7) Fixity of the tumour is often though not invariably suggestive of malignancy or endometriosis.

(8) Extreme cachexia develops in the later stages and such complications as unilateral oedema in the lower limb, pleural effusion and even involvement of lymphatic glands in the left supraclavicular fossa may be found.

(9) Radiological demonstration of bone or pulmonary metastases.

Post-menopausal Bleeding with Ovarian Tumours. Post-menopausal bleeding is a characteristic symptom with granulosa cell tumours and thecomata. Uterine haemorrhage may also develop in patients with malignant ovarian tumours which are not of this type, and occasionally innocent tumours such as pseudomucinous cystadenomata and fibromata are associated with uterine bleeding. The association of carcinoma of the body of the uterus with a malignant ovarian tumour is not unusual and this possibility should be borne in mind. It is therefore essential to perform a diagnostic curettage to exclude endometrial malignancy and when removing any ovarian tumour at or after the menopause it is our invariable practice to perform a total hysterectomy and bilateral salpingo-oöphorectomy. This guiding principle should never be transgressed.

Treatment of Ovarian Tumours

Treatment of ovarian tumours is surgical except in the case of obviously inoperable malignant growths. Even in a clinically inoperable case most surgeons would prefer to perform a laparotomy to confirm the true state of affairs by intra-abdominal examination and by biopsy of the tumour. Sometimes the most hopeless case is amenable to a palliative local operation which relieves the patient of her tumour and much of her pain and discomfort. The operation for removal of an ovarian tumour is performed through the abdomen under general anaesthesia. A paramedian or median incision should be made, and, as a rule, the tumour removed entire, as it may be impossible to recognise that a tumour is malignant by naked-eye examination, and if the tumour is ruptured or tapped, malignant cells may be scattered over the peritoneum. Obviously benign tumours such as dermoid cysts and simple cystomata encountered in young women may, however, be locally excised retaining a portion of normal ovary which is then oversewn. With mammoth tumours and in the case of large tumours in aged and enfeebled women, the tumour can be tapped immediately the abdomen has been opened so that the

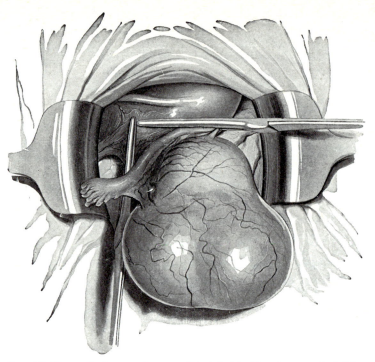

Fig. 418. Removal of an ovarian cyst of the left side. The clamp on the left has been placed on the infundibulo-pelvic ligament. The clamp on the right encloses the ovarian ligament, the Fallopian tube, and part of the broad ligament. (Peham-Amreich.)

tumour can be drawn through a reasonably small incision. Moreover, it is very rare for a mammoth tumour to be malignant. After the tumour has been drawn through the abdominal incision the pedicle is clamped. The pedicle of an ovarian cyst consists of the infundibulo-pelvic fold laterally, either the mesovarium or broad ligament in the middle, while at the uterine end are found the ovarian ligament and the isthmic portion of the Fallopian tube. Except in the case of small tumours the Fallopian tube is stretched over the surface of the tumour and has to be removed at operation. It is best to place three clamps on the pedicle, one on the infundibulo-pelvic fold, one on the broad ligament, and the third on the ovarian ligament and isthmic portion of the Fallopian tube. With large tumours huge veins traverse the pedicle, and it is best to duplicate the clamps before excising the tumour. The pedicle is put on the stretch after the tumour has been pulled out of the abdomen, and unless the veins are securely clamped they may retract through the clamp and cause retroperitoneal bleeding which may be difficult to control. The pedicle is then transfixed and ligated and covered with a peritoneal flap dissected from the lateral wall of the pelvis and the abdomen closed in the usual way (see Figs. 418 and 419).

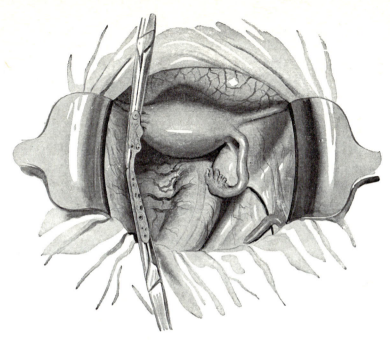

Fig. 419. The pedicle which is left after the removal of a large ovarian cyst. (Peham-Amreich.)

In most cases the operation is extremely simple to perform, but if the tumour has burrowed extraperitoneally great difficulty may be experienced in its removal. It must be shelled out by careful and patient dissection and nothing must be cut or clamped until identified with certainty otherwise there is a grave risk of damage to the ureter.

Shock is a very rare complication of the removal of large innocent tumours, patients being unaffected by the sudden release in abdominal pressure. The after-treatment is similar to that outlined in Chapter 23 in the description of the operation of hysterectomy. The particular complication is post-operative bleeding from an inadequately ligatured pedicle leading either to intraperitoneal bleeding or an extraperitoneal haematoma. Adhesions to the pedicle with subsequent intestinal obstruction should be regarded as the results of bad technique, and large pedicles should always be covered either by the sigmoid colon or by a peritoneal flap dissected from the lateral wall of the pelvis or by the round ligament.

The treatment of malignant ovarian tumours is surgical where possible and the best results are obtained after removal of both ovaries and the uterus by total hysterectomy and bilateral salpingo-oöphorectomy. The removal of malignant ovarian tumours may be extremely difficult, as the growth may become adherent to surrounding structures, so that the tumours and the uterus are firmly fixed in the pelvis.

The treatment of inoperable malignant ovarian tumours is unsatisfactory, particularly if there is well-marked ascites or if metastases are disseminated over the peritoneum and the omentum.

The question of postoperative radiation is much debated. In early operable cases with only local and removable metastases the addition of radiotherapy will probably improve the five-year salvage rate by 10%. With advanced extra-pelvic and irremovable metastases in the upper abdomen radiation has little to offer.

If faced with a malignant pelvic mass, widespread peritoneal metastases and a large mass of growth in the omentum, the surgeon should remove the primary tumour by bilateral salpingo-oöphorectomy and perform total hysterectomy; he should then excise the whole omentum and deal with any obvious and easily resectable masses. For example, the sigmoid may be involved in growth which is either actually causing or about to cause obstruction. If the patient is fit, a local palliative resection is often feasible and easy. This somewhat radical surgery will often pay a surprising dividend if only for a limited time and the patient is enabled to enjoy a further period of comparative well being and to die a more congenial death from distant metastases. In this hopeless and lethal disease, any relief from surgery is logical and justifiable and the present authors have one such hopeless patient under their care alive and clinically free from growth 15 years after operation. It is our present practice to treat all patients with advanced and technically inoperable ovarian cancer along these lines and subsequently to give a full course of a cytotoxic drug.

Ovarian cancer is an evil disease which paralyses most surgeons into an attitude of frustration and despair. Appalled and mesmerised by the inoperable mass which confronts them, they tend too readily to accept this inoperability and many an abdomen is closed after a perfunctory inspection and palpation. The patient is sent home to die without any treatment except the confirmation of a biopsy report. It is sincerely suggested that this defeatist attitude should be changed and that in every patient where it is possible, a palliative resection should be courageously carried out, not in the expectation of a cure so much as in a genuine attempt to relieve the more obvious symptoms of the disease. This should be followed by a full course of cytotoxic drugs. The reward of this treatment will be a relief of suffering, a prolongation of happier and more comfortable life and, very occasionally, a remarkable and inexplicable five-year survival.

CHEMOTHERAPY IN OVARIAN CANCER

Chemotherapeutic drugs offer a rational and reasonable method of attacking advanced gynaecological cancer, which has always been a most depressing and virtually impossible condition to treat. A number of different cytotoxic drugs are already available which may be used to modify the progress of, and occasionally even arrest the advance of ovarian cancer. Indeed in some instances it is possible to eradicate at least for a time all clinical evidence of disease.

A portion of growth removed at operation can be kept alive on tissue culture and then subjected to the effects of various drugs to ascertain the sensitivity of the tumour to the cytotoxic agents available. In this way a drug sensitivity of the tumour is obtained and the best possible cytotoxic agents can then be administered to the patient.

Varieties of Cytotoxic Drugs

The antimetabolites. These are folic acid antagonists which act by preventing rapidly dividing cells from utilising materials which are essential for the formation of nucleic acids, upon which mitosis depends. Methotrexate (amethopterin) and aminopterin are actual folic acid antagonists; 6-Mercaptopurine is a purine antagonist and 5-Fluorouracil is a pyramidine antagonist which blocks methylation. Methotrexate may be given orally in a short course (25 mg. daily for five days) or as a longer course (5–10 mg. three to six times weekly for eight weeks). It may also be given by intramuscular injection of 25 mg. daily for five days. These courses are repeated as the patient's condition demands. The dose of 6-Mercaptopurine (Purinethol) is 2·5 mg. per kilogram per day, given by mouth, for up to six weeks in a course. 5-Fluorouracil should be given intravenously in a dose of 15 mg. per kilogram of body weight, up to a maximum of one gram, stopping immediately any gastrointestinal symptoms appear.

The alkalating agents, which are radiomimetic compounds, act by combining with compounds within the cell which are essential to mitosis and metabolism and thus deprive the cell of the use of some of its enzymes and nucleoproteins. These include nitrogen mustard (Mustine), Chlorambucil (Leukeran), Melphalan (Alkeran L-Phenyl-Alanine Mustard), Thiotepa (Triethylene Thiophosphoramide) and Cyclophosphamide (Endoxana). Nitrogen mustard, which is used extensively in the treatment of Hodgkin's disease, carcinoma of the bronchus, lymphosarcoma and leukaemia, is usually given intravenously (0·1 mg. per kilogram of body weight per day up to a maximum of 8 mg.) It is seldom used in the treatment of ovarian neoplasm, except for local perfusion which is not usually possible in this particular disease. Chlorambucil is given by mouth (0·2 mg. per kilogram of body weight per day) for a course of from three to six weeks, repeated again after a six-week gap. Some remarkable results have been obtained in the treatment of ovarian carcinoma by Chlorambucil. Melphalan may also be given by mouth (2–35 mg. per day up to a total dose of 200 mg.) or intravenously in single doses of 1 mg. per kilogram of body weight. This drug is of particular value in the treatment of melanoma, dysgerminoma and fibrosarcoma. Thiotepa has been extensively used in the treatment of carcinoma of the ovary and is usually given intravenously in a dose of from 2–30 mg. per week. Thiotepa may also be injected into the abdominal cavity at operation, when usually the dose is 60 mg. Cyclophosphamide may also be injected into the peritoneal cavity at operation (200 mg.). For systemic treatment the course may be started by giving an intravenous injection of from 100–200 mg. per day up to a total of 3 Gms. and then maintaining treatment by oral administration of from 50 to 150 mg. per day continuously.

The Antibiotics

Actinomycin-D (Cosmogen) may not be much help in the treatment of carcinoma of the ovary, but certainly has a place in the treatment of chorion-epithelioma and sarcoma. It is given by intravenous injection in a dose of 0·5 mg. per day for five days. Ulceration not uncommonly occurs at the site of injection.

Plant Products

Velbe (Vinblastine sulphate) is a plant product which prevents the spindle stage of mitosis and is often very effective against anaplastic neoplasms. It is given intravenously with an initial dose of 0·1 mg. per kilogram of body weight, followed by weekly doses with increments of 0·05 mg. until the white cell count has been lowered to 3,000, after which the dose is maintained at one increment less than the maximum attained.

DANGERS

All these chemotherapeutic agents are extremely toxic to both normal as well as malignant cells and the art of administering a chemotherapeutic agent is to destroy malignant cells whilst still preserving the non-malignant cells. The bone marrow is probably the most vulnerable of the non-malignant tissues so that depression of the bone marrow is an inevitable result of chemotherapy. A careful record must therefore be kept of haemoglobin and white cell count, as well as platelet levels both before and during treatment, and according to the intensity of the course of treatment adopted these indices should be recorded either each day or each week.

The cells of the hair follicles are also very vulnerable to certain cytotoxic agents, so that loss of hair is frequently associated with their administration. This is a side effect particularly noticeable with Cyclophosphamide but is almost completely unknown with other alkalating agents such as Chlorambucil.

The intestinal mucous membrane is also a very active tissue and damage to this may result in gastro-intestinal symptoms such as nausea, anorexia, vomiting, abdominal discomfort and diarrhoea.

Patients being treated by chemotherapeutic agents require very careful and sympathetic handling, since most of them are aware of the reason for their treatment. Profound anaemia must be treated by blood transfusion. If the white cell count drops below 3,000 treatment should usually be discontinued temporarily, and if the white cell count is lowered below 1,000 it may be a wise precaution to provide the patient with antibiotic therapy to offset the danger of severe infection. Iron and vitamin supplements should be given continuously.

Cytotoxic agents must never be given during pregnancy. It is obvious from their mode of action that they will damage or maim the foetus, giving rise to congenital abnormalities if they do not in fact actually kill the foetus in utero.

29 Inflammations of the Uterine Appendages

INFLAMMATIONS OF THE FALLOPIAN TUBES AND OVARIES. SALPINGO-OÖPHORITIS

Introduction

Most inflammations of the Fallopian tubes and ovaries are the result of an ascending infection such as complicates gonorrhoea, septic abortion or puerperal sepsis. The inflammation, though mainly affecting the Fallopian tube, always involves the ovary coincidentally and is almost invariably bilateral. It is customary, therefore, to consider inflammations of the tubes and ovaries together, rather than to deal with each organ separately. The only exception to this involvement of both tube and ovary is seen in mumps where the ovary may be selectively attacked.

Aetiology

There are several natural barriers to the ascent of bacteria from the vagina to the endometrium and to the Fallopian tubes. The acidity of the vagina inhibits the growth of pyogenic organisms which may enter the vagina through the introitus, the cervical canal has a relatively small lumen which is normally filled by a plug of alkaline mucus and the ciliary movement in the uterus and cervical canal is directed downwards and discourages the spread of non-motile organisms to the cavity of the uterus (Fig. 421). This natural protective mechanism is impaired during menstruation and after abortion and childbirth, because the cervical canal becomes dilated, the protecting epithelium of the endometrium is shed, and raw surfaces are left in the cavity of the uterus. The post-partum and post-abortion genital tract is also likely to have suffered local trauma which provides a portal of entry for infection. Reduction in the acidity of the vaginal contents lead to a more favourable environment for the growth of pyogenic bacteria. After abortion and childbirth, the puerperal uterus is undergoing involution and the resistance of its tissues to infection is probably lower than at any other time. It is well known clinically that the majority of infections of the uterus and appendages occur either after abortion or childbirth, while gonococcal salpingo-oöphoritis almost always arises immediately after menstruation.

In addition to the factors already mentioned, direct infection of the cavity of the uterus is brought about by intrauterine manipulations during childbirth, by the evacuation of retained products after abortion, by operations for inducing abortion, and by such intrauterine manipulations as curettage and removal of myomatous polypi.

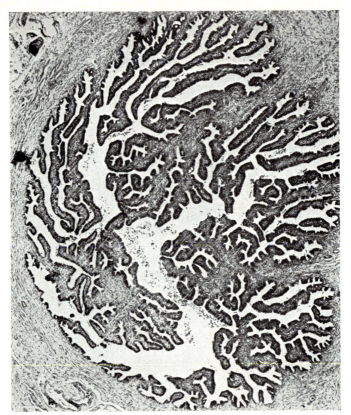

Fig. 420. Normal Fallopian tube between isthmus and ampulla. Note the convolutions of the plicae. (× 36.)

(1) *Direct ascending infection* of the tube by continuity of the mucous membrane occurs in gonorrhoea and it is usually possible to demonstrate in the examination of operation specimens an endometritis and an endosalpingitis which eventually involves all parts of the Fallopian tube. The lining mucosa of the tube is first attacked and it is only later that the wall of the tube becomes infiltrated. It is the end results of the destruction of the tubal mucosa which lead to tubal obstruction and infertility. Extra-uterine gestation results from partial obstruction of the tubal lumen. With virulent infections the inflammation spreads to the pelvic peritoneum, and as the result of suppurative pelvic peritonitis an abscess may form in Douglas's pouch.

(2) *The pyogenic infections* which result from post-abortional and puerperal sepsis reach the Fallopian tube by a different method. In these the infection passes from a primary focus of infection, usually a septic endometritis or infected placental remnant, by way of the lymphatic and blood vessels through the myometrium to the broad ligament, producing a broad ligament

cellulitis. The Fallopian tube is thus involved from without—an exosalpin-gitis—and the tubal wall is primarily involved in an interstitial salpingitis. The mucosa may be largely spared and the intra-luminal exudate may be insufficient to cause a pyosalpinx which is so common a feature of gonococcal endosalpingitis where intra-luminal damage and exudate are extreme.

(3) Although ascending infections comprise the majority of inflam-mations of the appendages, this may occur *by direct spread from the peritoneal cavity*. In appendicitis, particularly when the appendix is lying in the pelvic position, the right appendage may become involved by direct spread, and by the same mechanism left salpingo-oöphoritis complicates diverticulitis

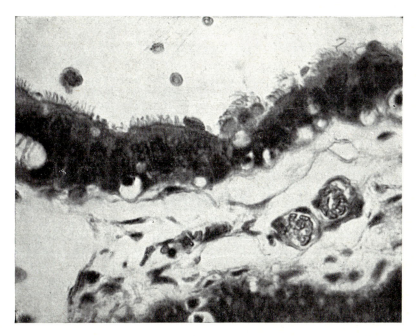

Fig. 421. High power view of tubal epithelium. Note the cilia. ($\times$ 670.)

of the sigmoid colon. Other forms of peritonitis may lead to inflammations of the appendages, and in almost any type of general peritonitis the outer surfaces of the Fallopian tubes and ovaries are infected.

(4) *Associated with intrauterine contraceptive devices.* It is most unlikely that such devices, either metal or plastic, will cause an infection but they may be indirectly responsible for a tubal infection. First, organisms may be carried into the uterus when the device is introduced, hence the reason for strict asepsis and for eliminating any cervical infection prior to insertion. Secondly, if any infection is already present in the uterus or subsequently gains access to the uterine cavity, the presence of a foreign body will un-doubtedly make it more severe and therefore predispose to ascending infection of the Fallopian tubes.

(5) *Blood stream infections* are best exemplified by tuberculosis of the appendages. In tuberculosis of the Fallopian tubes two forms are recognised: perisalpingitis, when the tubes are involved by infection from the peritoneal cavity; and endosalpingitis, when the infection is carried by the blood stream. The primary focus of the tuberculosis is usually the lung. A primary tuberculosis of the Fallopian tube may become secondarily infected and this secondary infection naturally modifies the primary picture, i.e. it may produce a pyosalpinx.

Organisms. The organisms which cause the infection are the gonococcus, the streptococcus haemolyticus, the streptococcus faecalis, the E. coli and the staphylococcus. Infections with other organisms, apart from the tubercle bacillus, are rare.

Pathological Anatomy

Acute Salpingitis. In acute salpingitis the Fallopian tube is swollen, oedematous, and hyperaemic with visible dilated vessels on the peritoneal surface. There is always some degree of serous exudation in the peritoneal cavity around the Fallopian tube. One of the most important signs of acute salpingitis is the discharge of seropurulent fluid from the abdominal ostium of the tube. This sign is of the greatest importance at laparotomy as without it there is no justification for diagnosing primary salpingitis. The peritoneal

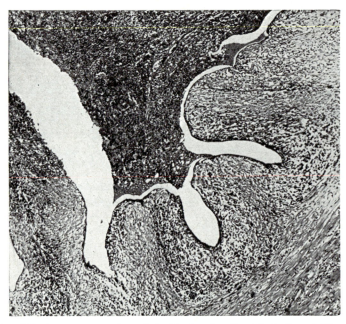

FIG. 422. Acute suppurative salpingitis showing the tubal plicae infiltrated with inflammatory cells, with desquamation of the surface epithelium and a transudation of inflammatory cells into the lumen of the tube. (× 48.)

surfaces of the Fallopian tubes may be inflamed in any form of peritonitis which involves the pelvic peritoneum. In acute salpingitis the fimbriae around the abdominal ostium are swollen and oedematous and covered with exudate.

If the tube is removed and examined microscopically in ascending infections the plicae are oedematous, infiltrated with leucocytes and plasma cells and the capillaries are dilated. Round-cell infiltration spreads into the muscle and subserous layer. As the result of the inflammatory infiltration of the plicae there is an exudation of leucocytes into the lumen of the tube. The epithelial cells covering the plicae become desquamated in places, so that inflammatory exudate is discharged directly into the lumen of the tube. In the process of healing adjacent plicae becomes adherent where the surface epithelium has been shed, so that crypts and pockets are formed in the Fallopian tube which may subsequently be the cause of ectopic gestation (see Fig. 422 and compare with the normal in Fig. 420).

Two forms of acute salpingitis are recognised, namely: the **catarrhal** and the **suppurative.** The catarrhal variety comprises those of moderate severity when pus formation in the lumen of the tube is of a minor degree; in the suppurative the infection is intense, and pus either accumulates in the lumen of the tube or is discharged through the abdominal ostium into the peritoneal cavity and causes a pelvic peritonitis. Gangrenous acute salpingitis is unknown because the Fallopian tube has a double blood supply, from the uterine end by way of the tubal branch of the uterine artery and at the fimbriated extremity and along its whole length by branches from the ovarian artery.

Both appendages are affected simultaneously, as the Fallopian tubes lie symmetrically with respect to the uterus and with ascending infections there is no reason why one tube should be infected rather than the other. Unilateral salpingo-oöphoritis is, however, seen as the result of either appendicitis or diverticulitis, and only rarely in puerperal cases. Although both tubes show histological evidence of bilateral inflammation, it is often found on clinical examination and at operation that one side is more seriously involved than the other.

In the acute stage the ovary is infected simultaneously with the Fallopian tube, partly from direct infection of its peritoneal surface and partly from lymphatic spread by way of the lymphatics of the mesosalpinx and mesovarium. With catarrhal salpingitis the ovary becomes swollen, vascular and oedematous. Its peritoneal surface is first covered by exudate and subsequently surrounded by adhesions. The Graafian follicles become larger than normal. In suppurative salpingitis small abscesses may develop in the substance of the ovary, and they are particularly apt to form in ripening follicles and in young corpora lutea. The end-result of such multiple abscesses is either the formation of an enlarged ovary studded with abscesses of this kind, or the abscesses may fuse with a pyosalpinx to form a tubovarian abscess. Some ovarian abscesses are lined by ragged yellow tissue and are regarded as corpus luteum abscesses. The yellow tissue often consists mainly of pseudolutein cells. It is not established definitely that all such abscesses are formed in a corpus luteum.

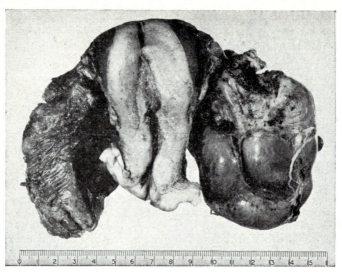

FIG. 423. Bilateral tubovarian abscess. It was impossible at operation to define or separate the ovaries from the tubes.

In acute suppurative salpingitis the plicae around the abdominal ostium become oedematous, so that the lumen of the tube is much reduced at the fimbriated end, which causes a retention of the exudate. Moreover, the intense inflammation around the fimbriated extremity causes an exudation which leads to adhesions, and these adhesions close the outer end of the Fallopian tube. The interstitial portion of the tube becomes closed by the oedema of the mucous membrane so that finally the tube becomes distended with pus, forming a pyosalpinx. The most distensible part of the tube is the ampullary region, which is also the most movable. In consequence the outer part of the tube becomes more distended than the isthmus and falls downwards behind the broad ligament. The shape of the distended tube resembles that of a retort. An acute pyosalpinx of this kind is surrounded by adhesions which fix it to the back of the broad ligament, the ovary, the sigmoid colon, adjacent coils of ileum and the posterior surface of Douglas's pouch. The wall is thickened and the tube is tense with the pent-up fluid (Figs. 423–425).

In acute salpingitis there is some degree of inflammation of the pelvic peritoneum and even with mild infections free serous fluid is found in the pelvis. With virulent infections pus forms in the pelvis partly as a result of the inflammation of the peritoneum itself, but also from the discharge of pus from the abdominal ostium of the infected tube. Fairly large collections of pus may accumulate in Douglas's pouch and can be detected by vaginal examination through the posterior fornix. These pelvic abscesses sometimes discharge into the rectum.

End-Results of Inflammation of the Appendages. Although acute inflammation of the appendages is frequently of an extremely severe degree, a spreading general peritonitis is a very uncommon complication except with streptococcal infections developing after abortion or during the puerperium. The pelvic peritoneum forms the lowest part of the peritoneal cavity, and not only is it probable that the pelvic peritoneum has a high resistance to infection but its situation helps to localise the infection.

In most acute inflammations of the appendages, it is standard practice to treat the patient conservatively with adequate chemotherapy in the hope that complete control of the infection will be achieved with resolution of the inflammatory process before irreparable damage to the tubal mucosa

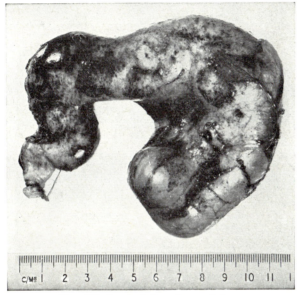

FIG. 424. A retort-shaped pyosalpinx.

results. If an abscess has already formed, it will be localised to the pouch of Douglas and, should it fail to resolve, it is a simple matter to drain it by a local incision in the posterior fornix—the operation of posterior colpotomy.

In many acute inflammations of the appendages there is no subsequent abscess formation in the pelvis so that operation is unnecessary, but even with mild catarrhal cases there is always permanent damage to the tubes and ovaries. This may take the form of membranous adhesions surrounding the Fallopian tube, which may lead to sterility, or the tubal plicae may become adherent and, by the formation of pockets, may be responsible for the subsequent development of ectopic gestation. If a pyosalpinx or tubovarian abscess has formed during the acute stage as soon as the active inflammation subsides, the pus contained in such abscesses becomes sterile within six weeks or sooner after the initial attack.

It is customary to classify chronic salpingo-oöphoritis as follows:
Hydrosalpinx.
Pyosalpinx.
Chronic interstitial salpingitis.
Tubovarian cyst and tubovarian abscess.
The tuberculous forms.

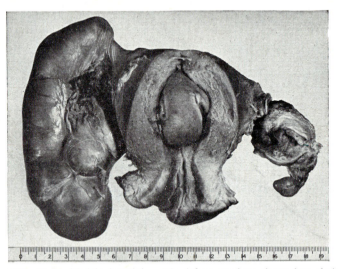

Fig. 425. Right-sided hydrosalpinx. The left appendage shows less obvious but well marked chronic salpingitis.

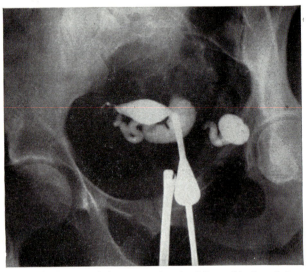

Fig. 426. Hysterosalpingogram showing bilateral hydrosalpinx.

In **hydrosalpinx,** the fimbriated end of the Fallopian tube is closed and the tube is distended with clear fluid. The interstitial end of the tube is curiously enough not always closed since it is often possible to demonstrate a hydrosalpinx by hysterosalpingography (Fig. 426), when the dye passes quite readily into the cavity of the hydrosalpinx. A hydrosalpinx is usually covered by membranous adhesions which fix it to the ovary and to the pelvic peritoneum. This is, however, not invariable since a hydrosalpinx can undergo torsion which would be manifestly impossible if it were always adherent. The wall is thin and the tubal plicae are flattened out. In the region of the abdominal ostium the fimbriae are indrawn so that the outer surface of the hydrosalpinx is smooth and rounded. The abdominal ostium is probably closed by adhesions around the fimbriae, so that the wall of a hydrosalpinx in this situation consists of these adhesions and not of the muscle wall of the tube.

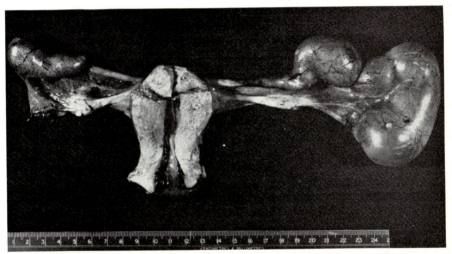

Fig. 427. An unusual cause of hydrosalpinx. The patient had been sterilised by partial salpingectomy of the isthmic portion of the tube. There is a large hydrosalpinx on the left side and a smaller one on the right which clearly shows the site of tubal ligation.

A hydrosalpinx is retort-shaped and it may form a tumour as much as 15 cm. in diameter. The condition is often bilateral (Figs. 425–428). A hydrosalpinx must be distinguished from a fimbrial cyst. A hydrosalpinx represents a retention cyst of the Fallopian tube; it is not associated with active inflammation but represents the end-results of a previous acute salpingitis. The condition of hydrops tubae profluens, or intermittent hydrosalpinx, when the tube intermittently discharges its contents into the uterus, has been described. In this rare condition, a clear serous and often copious discharge periodically floods the vagina. The diagnosis can only be made with accuracy if a tense tumour has been previously identified in the pouch of Douglas and if the tumour disappears when the patient is examined after the watery fluid has been discharged.

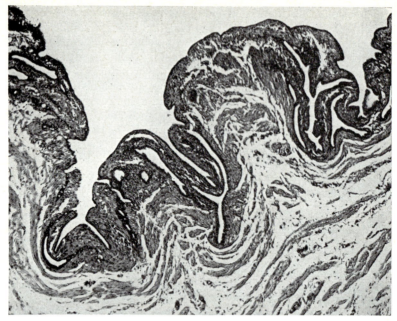

FIG. 428. The wall of a hydrosalpinx. Note the flattening of the plicae. (× 60.)

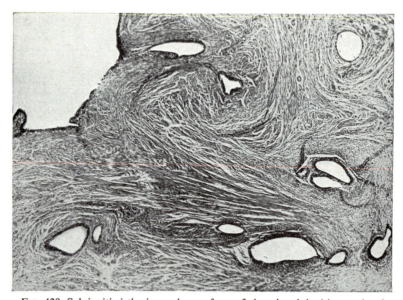

FIG. 429. Salpingitis isthmica nodosa, a form of chronic salpingitis associated with down-growths of the tubal epithelium into the muscle wall. These isolated epithelial islands should be compared with those seen in adenomyosis. The lumen of the tube lies above and to the left. (× 40.)

A chronic **pyosalpinx,** on the other hand, is thick-walled, surrounded by dense adhesions and filled with pus. The inner wall is replaced in part by granulation tissue.

In chronic **interstitial salpingitis** the wall of the Fallopian tube is thickened and fibrotic, and there may be small collections of pus either in the muscle wall or beneath the peritoneum, but there is no accumulation of pus in the lumen of the tube, which is therefore not palpably distended. The clinical importance of fibrosis is that it impedes or destroys the muscular movements of peristalsis and provides one more explanation for ectopic gestation.

In **tubovarian cyst** a hydrosalpinx communicates with a follicular cyst of the ovary, while with tubovarian abscess a pyosalpinx communicates with an ovarian abscess. In both types it is usually difficult to identify normal ovarian tissue in any part of the swelling.

The **tuberculous** forms have already been described in Chapter 10. Salpingitis **Isthmica Nodosa** (see Fig. 429) has been discussed on page 703.

Symptoms and Diagnosis

The onset of acute salpingo-oöphoritis is marked by the development of abdominal pain. The pain is situated in the lower abdomen below the umbilicus, and as both tubes are usually infected simultaneously the pain is bilateral. It is often quite accurately localised both by the patient and the examiner to a point 1 in. above and midway between the extremities of Poupart's ligament. The pain is of a severe degree and is induced partly by inflammation of the pelvic peritoneum and partly by distension of the Fallopian tubes and ovaries. The pain can be distinguished from that of acute appendictitis because there is never a history of central abdominal pain subsequently localised to the right iliac fossa. Fever is often well marked, the temperature rising to 103° or 104° F. with a considerable leucocytosis. The pulse rate is raised and in severe cases may be as high as 120. Nausea and vomiting are not so characteristic as in appendicitis, but in severe cases a history of vomiting can usually be obtained. The tongue is, however, always dirty and the patient looks toxic.

Menstrual irregularities are extremely common, particularly in the acute stage. With ascending infections an endometritis precedes the inflammations of the appendages, so that the menstrual period is heavy and prolonged, also perhaps for this reason patients develop uterine bleeding at times when a menstrual period is not expected and this uterine bleeding is often profuse and prolonged. These menstrual irregularities are extremely common in inflammations of the appendages and may cause great difficulty in diagnosis, as prolonged uterine bleeding is also a feature of ectopic gestation.

Some degree of vaginal discharge is always present if the infection is ascending in type. The discharge may be caused by gonorrhoea or it may be derived from the infected lochia of septic abortion or puerperal sepsis. It follows that the vaginal discharge should be investigated carefully when the diagnosis of inflammation of the appendages is made.

A carefully obtained history is important in diagnosis. Recent delivery or abortion will suggest the possibility of pelvic infection. Inflammations of the appendages occur after an interval which varies with the virulence of the infecting organism, the severity of any local trauma and the resistance of the host. For example, a clostridial infection resulting from a criminal abortion appears within a matter of hours whereas a low-grade intrauterine sepsis from retained products of gestation may not reach the tube for ten to fourteen days. Sometimes there is difficulty in obtaining an accurate history. For example, after an illegal abortion patients are often reluctant to admit that they have been pregnant and may give a menstrual history which is deliberately inaccurate.

In gonorrhoea a history of vaginal discharge associated with scalding micturition and vulvitis may be elicited.

Physical examination of the abdomen shows the signs of distension combined with tenderness and rigidity below the level of the umbilicus. It is relatively rare for an abdominal tumour to be palpated in acute salpingo-oöphoritis. At a later stage, if a large pelvic abscess develops or if large pyosalpinges form, a tender fixed abdominal tumour may be palpated arising from the pelvis, especially if omentum or loops of bowel are adherent. On vaginal examination, in ascending infections a purulent vaginal discharge is always present and the cervix should be examined with a speculum to demonstrate that the discharge emanates from the cervical canal and also to demonstrate the threads of a plastic intrauterine device. Swabs are taken for culture. The patient is then examined bimanually and the physical signs vary according to the severity and duration of the infection. In the early acute phase, the only constant physical sign is that of acute local tenderness in the fornices, so severe as to prevent the identification of the individual viscera. The diagnosis is then made by circumstantial evidence rather than by feeling the inflamed appendages. In fact, it is unlikely at this stage that they will be palpable. At a later date, swollen tender appendages can be palpated lateral to the uterus. The swollen appendages always tend to be prolapsed behind the uterus so that their lower borders can be felt in Douglas's pouch through the posterior fornix. If the patient is easy to examine the retort-shape of the pyosalpinx can be recognised. If, however, much abdominal tenderness and rigidity are present an accurate bimanual examination may be impossible. If a pelvic abscess has formed pus accumulates in Douglas's pouch to form an indurated swelling with softening in the middle. A large abscess produces bulging of the posterior vaginal wall and the fluctuating swelling can also be identified by rectal examination.

Chronic Salpingo-oöphoritis. The symptoms of chronic salpingo-oöphoritis are often indefinite, though the history of a previous acute pelvic inflammatory disease should always indicate the likelihood of the diagnosis. The main complaint is vague pain localised in the lower abdomen associated with chronic backache. Vaginal discharge is a constant symptom and is caused not by an intermittent discharge of pus through the interstitial portion of the tube into the uterus, but by an associated chronic cervicitis. The menstrual periods are apt to be excessive and sometimes the menstrual rhythm is irregular. Most patients complain of dyspareunia because the swollen appendages are prolapsed behind the uterus and form tender swellings in Douglas's pouch. Infertility may also be a complaint and is, in fact, the main reason for the diagnosis which is made after investigations for tubal patency. There is sometimes a history of congestive dysmenorrhoea. If extensive adhesions have formed in the pelvis the patient may complain of vague pains in the abdomen related to distension of the rectum and bladder. The debilitating symptoms of women suffering from chronic salpingo-oöphoritis react upon the general health so that such patients become depressed and show emotional disturbances.

Recurrent attacks of acute inflammation are liable to occur in chronic salpingo-oöphoritis when it has been incompletely treated. Some are due to reinfection with the gonococcus.

Pelvic examination in chronic salpingo-oöphoritis is always easier than in the acute stage of the disease. The appendages are found to be tender, thickened and fixed and an associated fixed retroversion is a very common finding. With hydrosalpinx and pyosalpinx the typical retort-shape can be distinguished and the position of the swelling with its lower pole attached to the back of the uterus is characteristic. A hydrosalpinx is tense, thin-walled, and fixed, whereas a fimbrial cyst is more movable and not so tense. A pyosalpinx is often hard and firm and may be mistaken for a myoma. Fixity due to the presence of adhesions is an important sign in chronic inflammation of the appendages and helps to differentiate the swelling from a myoma or ovarian cyst.

Differential Diagnosis of Acute Salpingo-oöphoritis

(1) **Acute Appendicitis.** It is important to distinguish between acute appendicitis and acute inflammation of the appendages. In appendicitis the abdominal pain, at first centred around the umbilicus, subsequently becomes localised to the right iliac fossa, whereas in acute salpingo-oöphoritis the pain is from the first in the lower abdomen and situated on each side of the mid line. In appendicitis tenderness and rigidity are localised to the right iliac fossa except when general peritonitis has developed. In appendicitis a bout of vomiting often coincides with the onset of the central abdominal pain and though vomiting can occur with acute salpingitis it is not such a well-marked feature. With appendix abscess a tumour can be felt in the iliac fossa and it is usually possible to insert the examining fingers below the level of the swelling. In acute adnexal inflammations tenderness and rigidity are present on both sides of the mid-line and except with large pelvic abscesses it is unusual for an abdominal swelling to be found. Distension is commonly present, however, even with localised pelvic peritonitis. The distinction between the two conditions is established by pelvic examination. In acute salpingo-oöphoritis a purulent vaginal discharge is present and the swollen oedematous Fallopian tubes should be palpated in Douglas's pouch.

(2) **Ectopic Gestation.** There is often difficulty in distinguishing between ectopic gestation and acute salpingo-oöphoritis, as in both conditions there is a history of severe abdominal pain associated with the presence of a swelling in the pelvis. Moreover, in acute salping-oöphoritis patients frequently suffer from continuous uterine bleeding. Another difficulty is that salpingo-

oöphoritis may complicate illegal abortion and only a history of a missed period may be obtained. In inflammations of the appendages there is usually a considerable pyrexia, whereas in ectopic gestation a temperature above 100° is hardly ever seen. In salpingo-oöphoritis the signs are those of an infection so that the patient has a furred tongue, the abdominal tenderness is intense and there is well-marked leucocytosis.

(3) **Diverticulitis** may present a clinical picture very similar to that of acute salpingo-oöphoritis. The condition, however, usually arises in obese women about the age of 50 and the abdominal signs and pelvic swelling are limited to the left side. It may be possible to move the uterus independently of the pelvic tumour. A barium enema will establish the diagnosis.

(4) **A twisted ovarian cyst** gives rise to sudden severe pain, associated with some degree of shock, in a previously fit woman. There is usually no significant previous history at all. The immediate severity of the condition is obvious and dramatic, and the physical signs, if carefully elicited, are different from those of acute salpingo-oöphoritis.

A twisted ovarian cyst usually forms an abdominal tumour, although small cysts are sometimes restricted to the pelvis. A twisted cyst is not accompanied by severe pyrexia or by vaginal discharge and the outline of the tumour is circumscribed. With a twisted ovarian cyst the tenderness is localised, unilateral and extreme.

(5) **Endometriosis** in which rupture and leakage of the tarry contents have occurred can be confused with pelvic inflammatory disease. In this complication of endometriosis, there is a fixed, tender mass in the pouch of Douglas, possibly menorrhagia and congestive dysmenorrhoea, and acute local tenderness in the lower abdomen. There is, however, less or little fever, no vaginal discharge and no suggestive history.

Chronic Salpingo-oöphoritis. The physical signs found in chronic salpingo-oöphoritis are usually elicited without difficulty, but are not always easy to interpret. Ectopic gestation and diverticulitis present rather similar pictures and myomata and ovarian cysts may also give rise to difficulty. In chronic salpingo-oöphoritis the swellings are usually bilateral, tender and fixed and the history obtained is of the greatest importance in establishing the diagnosis.

Treatment

Acute Salpingo-oöphoritis. General Considerations. The treatment of acute salpingo-oöphoritis should be conservative in almost every instance with a few exceptions which will be considered later. Conservative treatment with the correct antibiotic in adequate dosage can be expected to limit the infection to the pelvis and to promote complete resolution of the inflammation so that, in a number of patients, ultimate fertility has been unimpaired. If, however, laparotomy has been performed under a mistaken diagnosis, as does sometimes happen, the manipulation of the pelvic viscera should be kept to a minimum, swabs only taken from the ostia of the tubes and pouch of Douglas and, in the acute phase of the disease, the abdomen should be promptly closed as soon as the diagnosis of salpingitis is obvious and no drainage used. Chemotherapy can be relied upon to control the infection.

Any manipulation or disturbance of the pelvic viscera can spread the localised pelvic peritonitis to the upper abdomen and even an enthusiastic pelvic examination can do this in the out-patient clinic or ward.

Apart from the risk of dissemination of the infection, surgical intervention by the abdominal route is unsound in principle unless the source of infection is removed, and this would necessitate not only the removal of both Fallopian tubes but also both ovaries, as they are almost always simultaneously infected. Such a drastic procedure is to be condemned, especially as many of these patients are young women. Simple drainage of the pelvis following laparotomy with conservation of the appendages is unnecessary, as the pelvic peritoneum is capable of dealing with the infection, and even if a pelvic abscess develops it will usually become localised to the pouch of Douglas, when it can be evacuated through the posterior vaginal wall. The most important point in the treatment of acute salpingo-oöphoritis is that it is exceptional for the infection to involve the general peritoneal cavity, so that conservative treatment can be confidently undertaken with small risk of an acute general peritonitis developing. The only exception is perhaps with acute salpingo-oöphoritis complicating septic abortion when general peritonitis and even septicaemia may develop. This complication should first be treated vigorously with chemotherapy and antibiotics and surgical intervention reserved for any subsequent complications such as the formation of a chronic tubo-ovarian abcess or the rare and sinister advent of intestinal obstruction.

Conservative Treatment. The diagnosis must be made with precision before conservative treatment is undertaken and it is particularly important to exclude appendicitis.

As in all inflammations the first essential is complete rest. The patient is kept in bed in the most comfortable position, which is usually semi-recumbent. The bowels should be emptied with a mild aperient or glycerine enema. Dry heat to the lower abdomen is often a great help to the patient in relieving pain. The authors have abandoned the traditional hot douche, a relic of the pre-antibiotic era. It is always disturbing, occasionally dangerous as patients have been scalded, demands a considerable degree of nursing skill and nursing time, and achieves nothing that sedatives and chemotherapy do not more easily and comfortably effect.

The abdominal pain can be relieved by the administration of such drugs as aspirin and codeine. The opium derivatives should be used with caution, particularly if there is any doubt as to the diagnosis.

Treatment by antibiotics is governed by the sensitivity of the responsible organisms to a specific drug, but while awaiting the report from the laboratory it is certainly justifiable to give penicillin and streptomycin empirically. A high vaginal or cervical swab is taken and the organisms typed against the various antibiotics. If a gonococcal infection is suspected a urethral swab should also be taken. The sensitivity reports and the clinical response of the patient will determine what antibiotic should be used and the duration of treatment.

Almost all patients with acute salpingo-oöphoritis respond well to this conservative therapy, and it is remarkable how large swellings regress. Unless an abscess forms in the pelvis the patient is usually relieved of symptoms and is able to get up a few days after the temperature and pulse have returned to normal. The process of resolution is assessed by abdominal and pelvic examination as well as the patient's symptoms.

If a pelvic abscess forms, it usually points in Douglas's pouch and may empty itself spontaneously by bursting into the rectum, an eventuality which is best avoided. It is better to drain the abscess by the operation of posterior colpotomy, which consists of the incision of the posterior vaginal wall immediately posterior to the cervix and the evacuation of the pus. A piece of corrugated drain is passed into the abscess cavity and sutured with catgut to the margins of the incision in the vaginal wall. It is unsatisfactory, however, to drain a pyosalpinx by the vaginal route and care must be taken to ensure that the swelling in the posterior fornix is a collection of pus located in the pouch of Douglas and not the lower pole of the large pyosalpinx. It may be fairly said, in summary, that the treatment of acute salpingo-oöphoritis is always conservative except in the following circumstances:

(1) Acute spreading peritonitis resistant to a full dosage of chemotherapy.
(2) Where the infection follows a criminal abortion in which the possibility of intra-abdominal damage is suspected, e.g. to the bowel. This situation may complicate (1) above.
(3) The presence of signs of intestinal obstruction which is fortunately rare.
(4) When the diagnosis is in doubt; e.g. it is better to operate on a patient suspected to have acute appendicitis and discover the true diagnosis to be salpingitis.
(5) The drainage of a pelvic abscess by posterior colpotomy hardly counts as more than an extension of conservative treatment and has been discussed.

Chronic Salpingo-oöphoritis

If an acute salpingo-oöphoritis leads to the formation of a chronic pyosalpinx the pyosalpinx should be removed by abdominal operation. The best results are obtained if the patient is treated conservatively for about a fortnight, after which the infection becomes strictly limited to the pelvis and the risk of spread to the general peritoneal cavity is small. Some surgeons before resorting to surgery prefer to give a second course of antibiotics, if the results of the first have been disappointing. A change of antibiotic agent is often rewarded by the resolution of a previously obstinate mass. If resolution does not occur after such conservative methods laparotomy is then more certainly indicated. The operation is often extremely difficult because the Fallopian tubes are adherent to the back of the uterus and the broad ligament and also the omentum and intestines may be fixed firmly by adhesions. After the abdomen has been opened the intestines are packed away with swabs soaked in warm saline or dilute aqueous flavine solution, strength 1:1,000, diluted with sterile water to 1:5,000, and the omentum and intestines are separated from the tubal swellings. The distended Fallopian tubes with the ovaries are then separated from the back of the uterus. The operator should effect the separation by starting from below and working upwards. The affected appendages are then excised and the pedicles tied with catgut. It is very rarely necessary to drain the pelvis. Some surgeons prefer to remove the uterus if the adnexa of both sides are being removed. This drastic operation should be reserved for patients near the menopause. In younger patients even if both tubes must be removed it is almost always possible to save a part of one ovary and the uterus. The psychological benefits of this conservative treatment outweigh the advantages of hysterectomy and bilateral salpingo-oöphorectomy.

It should be emphasised that since the introduction of chemotherapy, the severity of salpingo-oöphoritis has been reduced and the operation of salpingo-oöphorectomy for this condition are now extremely rare.

The treatment of a hydrosalpinx is exactly similar to that of a chronic pyosalpinx though the symptoms and signs are less obvious and the necessity for surgery less urgent.

Apart from these two examples of chronic salpingo-oöphoritis, namely pyosalpinx and hydrosalpinx, where the physical signs of a fixed pelvic swelling indicate surgical treatment, there is the less obvious and surgically important one of chronic interstitial salpingitis which, perhaps, is better termed chronic pelvic inflammatory disease. This usually produces a well recognised syndrome of ill-health, physical and psychological, with pelvic pain, backache, congestive dysmenorrhoea, menorrhagia, dyspareunia and sterility. This formidable array of symptoms is not always present in its entirety but some or several are usually combined. The past history of a known salpingo-oöphoritis, gonorrhoea, septic abortion or puerperal fever is most helpful in diagnosis. The physical signs on pelvic examination are often uninstructive apart from a tender, fixed retroversion and some thickening and fixity in the fornices laterally. There is often evidence of old parametritis in that the parametrium feels thickened and rigid.

The patient outlined above will have had a full course or several courses of antibiotics, short-wave diathermy and other physiotherapy and, in fact, all conservative treatment will have been exhausted. There is everything to be said for radical surgery and very little against it, except the youth of the patient. There is only one certain cure for this patient and that is total hysterectomy and bilateral salpingo-oöphorectomy with conservation of any healthy ovary that can be reasonably salvaged. If, for reasons of her youth and because the patient demands the retention of her uterus or is very keen to conceive, this radical surgery is not considered justifiable, the alternative is to perform a laparotomy, remove what tube and ovary is hopelessly disorganised and save the better appendage, after freeing all adhesions. The uterus will be ventro-suspended by some modification of Gilliam's operation and, if necessary, a salpingostomy operation performed to free the obstructed tubal ostium. Owing to the general diseased state of the pelvic organs, this operation rarely results in a successful conception and even less frequently if the tube is damaged irreparably by chronic interstitial salpingitis or endosalpingitis. The risk of an extrauterine gestation is a real one if pregnancy should occur after conservative surgery. The depressing aspect of conservative surgery in chronic salpingo-oöphoritis is that it fails to relieve the patient's symptoms and, sooner or later, the radical operation of pelvic clearance becomes inevitable.

The indications for surgery in chronic salpingo-oöphoritis are, therefore:

(1) In a young woman who is keenly anxious to do everything possible to conceive, some conservative operation such as freeing of adhesions, ventrosuspension of the uterus, unilateral salpingo-oöphorectomy, if necessary, and salpingostomy if the fimbrial end of the remaining tube is blocked.

(2) Total hysterectomy and bilateral salpingo-oöphorectomy if both tubes and ovaries are hopelessly disorganised. If some ovary that is healthy can be retained and the patient is young, this should be done. If even this conservation is impracticable any subsequent menopausal symptoms can be controlled quite effectively by oestrogen.

The patient more likely to qualify for this more radical surgery is one:

(a) in whom, in spite of all conscientiously applied conservative treatment, symptoms and signs persist;

(b) who suffers periodic acute exacerbations of a chronic salpingo-oöphoritis, in spite of conservative treatment;

(c) who is nearing the menopause or is over 40 years of age.

If it has been found necessary to excise both ovaries and the patient is young, the patient should be carefully observed for several months and the appearance of the symptoms of a surgical menopause noted. It is a surprising fact that even young women who have lost both ovaries do not necessarily suffer from menopausal flushes, obesity and psychological upset and in such patients no treatment is indicated. The opposite results may be expected in many cases and severe symptoms of ovarian deficiency may be most distressing to the patients. Synthetic oestrogen in small regular maintenance dosage by mouth, such as stilboestrol 0·5 mg. daily, is most useful for these patients and some authorities recommend the intramuscular implantation of 25–50 mg. of oestrogen in pellet form. This implantation can be repeated as required, usually in twelve to eighteen months. The pellets consist of oestradiol benzoate. The authors know of several patients in whom the implants have been most effective and who periodically request a repeat when they feel the recurrent symptoms of oestrogen deficiency.

30 Diseases of the Broad Ligament, Fallopian Tubes and Parametrium

BROAD LIGAMENT CYSTS

BROAD ligament cysts are fairly common. With the exception of parovarian cysts, they rarely attain a size greater than 25 mm. in diameter.

Anatomical Considerations

Vestigial remnants of the Wolffian duct (mesonephric duct) are seen in the broad ligament, lying between the Fallopian tube and the hilum of the ovary. The mesonephric duct extends from the outer aspect of the ovary, parallel to the Fallopian tube in an inward and downward direction until it enters the myometrium in the region of the cervix. Its lowermost limit is the region of the hymen. For some reason, the lower half is called Gartner's duct which is confusing. Cysts of Gartner's duct occurring in the vagina have been described elsewhere. The student should appreciate that mesonephric duct, Wolffian duct and Gartner's duct are one and the same structure.

Associated with the mesonephric duct and opening into it are the tubules of the upper part of the Wolffian body, the epoöphoron or parovarium (sometimes called the organ of Rosenmüller). These are situated in the broad ligament adjacent to the hilum of the ovary. These mesonephric tubules are sometimes called Kobelt's tubules. In addition to these mesonephric tubules which connect with the mesonephric duct, a number of blind isolated tubular remnants are seen near the inner border of the ovary; these constitute the paroöphoron.

The lining of the mesonephric duct is a non-ciliated, low columnar epithelium. The lining of the mesonephric tubules is low columnar or cuboidal and both ciliated and non-ciliated cells are present in it.

Cysts may arise in the broad ligament from both the mesonephric duct and its tubules. These cysts are either small and pedunculated or intraligamentary, lying between the leaves of the broad ligament where they may attain a considerable size, up to 15 cm. or even bigger. Large cysts are, however, rare. Some idea of the derivation of these cysts can be obtained from a study of their lining epithelium. Mesonephric duct cysts are never lined with ciliated epithelium, whereas cysts of the mesonephric tubules may be.

Whatever their exact derivation, it is reasonable to call them all parovarian cysts since they lie adjacent to the ovary, between it and the tube, but always separate and easily defined from the ovary itself.

PAROVARIAN CYSTS

Parovarian cysts are extraperitoneal cysts lying in the broad ligament adjacent to the ovary, below the Fallopian tube. The tube is stretched and flattened over the top of the cyst which tends to enlarge in a lateral direction so that it may lie to the side of and above the ovary. Small parovarian cysts are extremely common and are often found at operation without their presence having previously been suspected. They may, however, form tumours as large as 15 or even 30 cm. (6 or 12 in.) in diameter. The cysts are usually

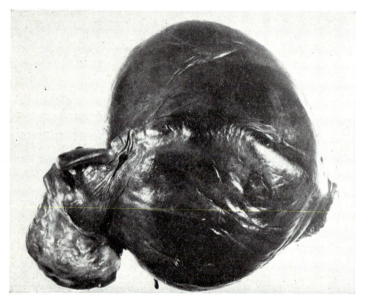

Fig. 430. A parovarian cyst which had undergone torsion involving also the appendages. Note the ovary to the left and the Fallopian tube passing over the cyst. This specimen comes from one of the author's house surgeons who assisted him during a long operating list, at the end of which she asked her chief to examine her because she had been in some considerable pain for the last few hours. The specimen is presented as a testimony to the superior fortitude of women and in all humility by her surgeon.

unilocular, containing clear fluid, their walls being smooth, thin and translucent. Sometimes a few loculi are present, and papillomata, similar to the stationary papillomata of papillary cystadenomata of the ovary, may be scattered over the inner surface of the cyst. Unlike ovarian cysts, the wall of a parovarian cyst frequently contains smooth muscle as do the mesonephric tubules.

Parovarian cysts are sometimes confused with ovarian cysts at operation. A parovarian cyst should be identified because the ovary is separate from the cyst and because both the Fallopian tube and the ovarian fimbria are stretched over the convexity of the swelling. Moreover, the cyst is extraperitoneal. The nomenclature "fimbrial cyst" is misleading, as the tumours do not arise from the fimbriae of the tube and its use should be abandoned in favour of parovarian cyst which is more correct both clinically and embryologically. Parovarian cysts are usually diagnosed on clinical examination as ovarian cysts and their true nature is only disclosed at operation. As they can undergo torsion, they are also misdiagnosed as twisted ovarian cysts (Fig. 430).

Treatment. Parovarian cysts must be treated surgically by removal at abdominal operation. A delicate incision is made in the peritoneum over the cyst from which it is reflected by blunt dissection. A finger is then swept round the cyst between it and its bed until it is sufficiently free to be enucleated. Only a few small vessels will need ligation or diathermy coagulation in the cyst bed and it is unnecessary to provide drainage. This surgical treatment preserves both the ovary and the Fallopian tube. A large parovarian cyst may displace the ureter and this structure is always at some hazard during its removal. It should, therefore, be identified before anything is clamped or cut, and if it cannot be visualised or felt in the vicinity of the cyst it should be traced down from the pelvic brim where it is always easily recognised.

Apart from the larger parovarian cysts which are obvious on clinical examination, small, often multiple, cysts situated in the region of the mesonephric tubules may be found at operation as an incidental discovery. If minute, they need no treatment but, if bigger than 0·5 cm. can be enucleated.

Cyst of the Hydatid of Morgagni

These cysts are of no clinical significance. They take the form of minute cysts attached to one or other tubal fimbriae. They have been regarded as paramesonephric in origin, i.e. a derivative of the Müllerian system. They do not need removal unless the pedicle is long and attenuated.

It is not uncommon to find small cysts in the region of the broad ligament and Fallopian tube which belong to none of the groups already mentioned. They have no clinical importance, but are of some interest pathologically. Small subperitoneal cysts frequently develop after pelvic peritonitis and are most common on the peritoneal surface of the tube and the posterior layer of the broad ligament. Quite frequently the serosal surface is studded with small sago-like bodies—perhaps 2 mm. in diameter of which perhaps 20 or 30 may be identified. They are of no significance whatever and should be disregarded. Very rarely an accessory tube may become distended as the result of closure of its abdominal ostium.

TUMOURS OF THE FALLOPIAN TUBE

Neoplasms of the Fallopian tube are extremely rare and the only types which need description are adenocarcinoma and chorion-epithelioma.

Primary adenocarcinoma of the tube is an extremely rare growth and comprises only 0·1–0·3 % of all malignant tumours of the genital tract. Over 500 cases have been reported in the literature to date (Novak). It is chiefly encountered in the postmenopausal patient, half of whom will be nulli-parous. The earliest symptom is a characteristic amber-coloured discharge, which is subsequently followed by bleeding. Pain is a common symptom and quite frequently is severe. The tumour is an adenocarcinoma composed oi villous-like processes, which are surrounded by malignant cells. The tumour is bilateral in about a third of cases and has a high degree of malignancy, with rapidly developing metastases in the peritoneum and omentum accompanied by ascites. In most respects it simulates ovarian cancer in its method of spread and in its metastatic deposits. The high malignancy of the tumour is shown by the bad 5-year cure rate (25%) and the frequent recurrence after operation. The condition is diagnosed with difficulty, as the clinical picture

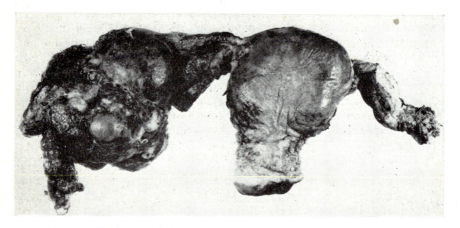

FIG. 431. Carcinoma of the Fallopian tube. One Fallopian tube containing papillary growth lies to the left. Between it and the uterus lies the corresponding ovary, while the opposite tube and ovary lie to the right.

is similar to that of carcinoma of the ovaries. It is extremely rare for the diagnosis to be made before operation, which is usually undertaken on the diagnosis of an ovarian tumour. Operation consists in removal of both tubes, both ovaries, and the uterus (Fig. 431) followed by pelvic irradiation. In recurrent cases cytotoxic drugs may be indicated.

Chorionepithelioma of the Fallopian tube may arise in the tube as a result of ectopic gestation (32 reported cases), where the parallel incidence of hydatidiform mole has been well authenticated, or it may form by metastasis from a primary growth of the uterus.

Secondary carcinoma of the Fallopian tube. This is much more common than primary carcinoma of the tube and the usual primary focus is the ovary or the uterine body. The method of spread is by lymphatic permeation rather than by direct implantation on the tubal mucous membrane. This latter method of invasion is reasonable since it is not unusual to find masses of malignant cells in the tubal lumen when hysterectomy has been performed for cancer of the endometrium. Intra-luminal spread of endometrial cancer must be accepted as one pathway of malignant invasion from the primary endometrial focus to the peritoneal cavity. This is the rationale of tying or clamping the tube as an integral step in the operation of hysterectomy for malignancy of the body of the uterus in order to eliminate this mode of spill of cancer cells.

Swellings of the Fallopian Tube

The Fallopian tube may become distended with clear serous fluid, forming a hydrosalpinx, or with pus causing a pyosalpinx. Both swellings have already been described in the previous chapter. At other times the Fallopian tube becomes distended with blood, forming a haematosalpinx.

A **haematosalpinx** arises most frequently in ectopic gestation, particularly in tubal mole (see page 410). Haematosalpinx is found not uncommonly in the Fallopian tube of the opposite side in cases of ectopic gestation, when regurgitant blood from the uterus into the Fallopian tube is prevented from spreading into the peritoneal cavity by adhesions around the abdominal ostium. A haematosalpinx may also develop as the result of vaginal or cervical atresia, when menstrual blood accumulates in the uterus and regurgitates back into the Fallopian tube, the abdominal ostium of the tube becoming closed by adhesions. Vaginal atresia is due to partial or complete failure of canalisation, while cervical obstruction is usually the result of trachelorrhaphy, amputation of the cervix, cauterisation or, occasionally, a malignant growth. Sometimes a hydrosalpinx undergoes torsion, becomes filled with blood and gives rise to a haematosalpinx.

AFFECTIONS OF THE BROAD LIGAMENT AND PARAMETRIUM

Haematoma. Haematoma of the broad ligament and parametrium may result from an ectopic gestation which ruptures extraperitoneally into the broad ligament. Large haematomata develop in consequence of rupture of the uterus or cervix during childbirth. They may arise after dilatation of the cervix, when the cervix may split and the uterine vessels be wounded. The condition sometimes develops in cases of concealed accidental haemorrhage. A broad ligament haematoma tends to spread extraperitoneally and may track upwards and cause a swelling above Poupart's ligament and very exceptionally it may spread to the perinephric region. Haematoma of the broad ligament is not uncommonly encountered after abdominal or vaginal hysterectomy where a vessel has escaped the clamp or ligature and retracted into the cellular tissues of the broad ligament. Such a haematoma may attain considerable size and later become infected. Pain, raised pulse rate and fever ensue. It is usually evacuated spontaneously from the vaginal wound and its drainage can be encouraged by a digital exploration of the broad ligament through the vaginal vault. As a possible cause of unexplained fever after hysterectomy its presence should always be excluded by vaginal examination. The authors are well aware of the danger of anticoagulant therapy indicated for phlebo-thrombosis in the causation of broad ligament haematoma following hysterec-tomy. During the course of therapy a very considerable retroperitoneal haemorrhage may occur, severe enough to demand blood transfusion. Cessation of anticoagulant drugs is usually all that is indicated, but it may be several weeks before the swelling is completely absorbed.

Parametritis. Parametritis, first described by Matthews Duncan, is a cellulitis of the tissues of the parametrium. Well-marked parametritis almost invariably follows childbirth or abortion, when the parametrium is infected from lacerations of the vaginal portion of the cervix and of the vaginal vault or from lacerations of the lower uterine segment. Some degree of parametritis is present in all acute infections of the uterus and Fallopian tubes and in established carcinoma of the cervix. The cases which are of clinical importance are those complicating childbirth and abortion. The condition causes symptoms at the beginning of the second week when the patient complains of pain in the hypogastrium and back. The temperature is raised to about 102° F., the pulse rate being raised in the same proportion. The inflammation of the pelvic cellular tissue leads to the development of a large indurated swelling in the pelvis. In the early stages the uterus is pushed to the opposite side and the indurated swelling of the parametrium extends from the uterus to the lateral wall of the pelvis and fixes the uterus in the pelvis. It is impossible to separate the uterus from the swelling, because the parametrium extends to the wall of the uterus. The parametric effusion spreads backwards along the uterosacral ligaments, but it may also track upwards and point above Poupart's ligament. On rare occasions the effusion may point in the perinephric region, in the ischiorectal fossa and even in the buttock, having tracked through the greater sciatic foramen. Suppuration in parametritic effusions is uncommon, and even if the effusion points and has to be incised, it is rare for frank pus to be evacuated. As the effusion is extraperitoneal, symptoms of peritoneal irritation are absent, but rectal symptoms may arise as the result of inflammation involving the rectum.

Most parametric effusions subside under conservative treatment, but they are followed by scarring of the parametrium which causes chronic pelvic pain. The scarred tissue draws the uterus over to the affected side and the thick scar tissue is readily palpated on bimanual examination.

Parametritis is usually complicated by some degree of pelvic thrombo-phlebitis with its risk of pyaemia, pulmonary infarction and extension to the lower extremities to produce "white leg". This clinical syndrome is especially common if the responsible organism is the anaerobic streptococcus. Almost all parametritic effusions lie lateral to the uterus and vagina, where the parametrium is most plentiful, but on rare occasions an anterior parametritis develops situated between the cervix and anterior vaginal wall posteriorly and the bladder and urethra anteriorly. The treatment of parametritis consists in rest in bed, local heat and a full course of the correct antibiotic. The treatment is similar to that described in the treatment of acute salpingo-oöphoritis in Chapter 29.

TUMOURS OF THE BROAD LIGAMENT AND PARAMETRIUM

The commonest tumours are myomata arising in the uterus and spreading laterally, but myomata may arise independently of the uterus and lie in the uterosacral ligament or even in the round ligament.

Sarcomata of the broad ligament are very rare tumours and may present clinical physical signs similar to those of a myoma. Sometimes it is possible to remove them surgically, otherwise they are treated with radiation.

Lipomata of the broad ligament and the parametrium are occasionally encountered and may form very large swellings. In most cases they are enucleated without difficulty.

Retroperitoneal Tumours. These are included in this chapter because laparotomy may be indicated for an obscure fixed tumour where the exact nature is not pre-operatively diagnosed. Its retroperitoneal situation may not be obvious and it may be mistaken for an ovarian or broad ligament tumour, the former fixed by adhesions, the latter immobile because of its retroperitoneal origin.

These retroperitoneal tumours may be classified as follows:

(1) *Congenital.* Ectopic pelvic kidney, demonstrable by intravenous pyelography if this has been, as it should be, performed. Such a kidney, unless hydronephrotic, calls for no treatment and a urologist should be consulted. Meningoceles, sacro-coccygeal dermoids and teratomata are other rare examples of retroperitoneal pelvic tumours of this type.

(2) *Rare tumours of neurogenic origin*, neurofibromata and tumours arising from the spinal meninges.

(3) *Solid tumours arising from the bony pelvis*—oesteoma, chondroma and sarcoma.

(4) *A miscellaneous group of mesodermal origin* not arising from the bony pelvis, fibroma, myoma and lipoma. Included in this group are those tumours which cannot be histologically classified and all metastatic tumours.

When faced with a retroperitoneal tumour the most thorough pre-operative investigations—I.V.P. and barium enema, etc. are indicated. Diagnosis may be possible only by laparotomy and biopsy. Sometimes the tumour is encapsulated and easy to enucleate at operation. Two dangers are ever present (1) the ureter which must as always be identified before any attempt at removal of the tumour; (2) *Large vessels* of the hypogastric system may obtrude into the operative field and these must be individually identified and secured. If haemostasis is indifferent the tumour bed, after removal of the growth, should be drained by a separate stab incision, so that the drain track is retroperitoneal. If the tumour is irremovable by operation, x-radiation therapy may be an alternative.

31 Proctological Aspects of Gynaecology

The close parochial boundaries of urology, gynaecology and proctology must always be artificial when a mere matter of a centimetre or two separates the one from the other. Surely a gynaecologist should be a pelvic surgeon and while not trespassing on the precincts of his two pelvic colleagues he should be competent to diagnose those conditions of his sister specialities for which he is so often primarily consulted. For example, we have stated without reservation that a proper pelvic examination of the genital tract includes a rectal examination and the use of a proctoscope and it would amount to negligence if an alleged postmenopausal haemorrhage due to a carcinoma of the rectum were missed simply because the gynaecologist did not deign to soil his glove by performing a rectal examination. In support of this attitude it is incontrovertible that many urological symptoms are presented in the first place to the gynaecologist and he should be able accurately to diagnose these before referring them to his urological confrère. Narrow specialisation is a particular menace of the gynaecologist and he should firmly resist the temptation to concentrate on the genital tract to the exclusion of the other symptoms of which the patient is the owner. This catholic outlook will certainly enhance the interest of his practice and will enable him to solve many of the obscure problems with which his patient may present him.

   1. **Congenital Defects.** As most gynaecologists are also obstetricians the examination of the neonate is still part of their province and before the paediatrician takes over the care of the newborn they will be expected to make an intelligent assessment of the product of their and their patient's labours. Certain congenital defects of the proctodaeum are recognised and most of these are due to failure of the septum which divides the cloaca from the urogenital sinus. The rarest variety is where there is a true common cloaca into which the three pelvic systems open. A more frequent modification is where the hind gut terminates in a perineal or vaginal opening; in other words there is a congenital fistula of recto-perineal or recto-vaginal type. These fistulous openings as a rule are adequate for the passage of meconium and later of faeces and as a baby grows a reasonable sphincteric control is acquired largely by virtue of levator tone. Provided there is no undue constriction of the outlet no surgery is required and many such patients will marry and bear children. Stenosis obviously provides one indication for corrective surgery. When these patients reach childbearing age a confinement which may involve a third degree perineal tear is a real hazard and this may require delivery by Caesarean section. Corrective surgery for this type of congenital fistula is always somewhat disappointing, for the simple reason that although it is not difficult to transplant the rectum into its proper place

it is almost impossible to reconstitute the normal external sphincter. The patient therefore is left with her original symptom, imperfect control of flatus and faeces.

Imperforate anus is a more obvious neonatal defect and this, when diagnosed, calls for expert paediatric surgery.

2. Traumatic Conditions Affecting the Ano-Rectum

(a) *Associated with child-birth injuries.* Third degree tears and recto-vaginal fistulae have already been considered on page 275 and these need no further comment here.

(b) *Operation injuries of the rectum* which usually result in a recto-vaginal fistula may occur after a posterior colporrhaphy, an abdominal or vaginal hysterectomy, but are most likely to result from extensive operations for genital tract malignancy, less so for endometriosis, tuberculosis and pelvic inflammatory disease. A recto-vaginal fistula following a Wertheim or similar operation may well be not so much the result of surgery as a recurrence of the growth. Biopsy of the fistulous edge is, therefore, always indicated before reparative treatment.

(c) *Radiation fistula* is always a sinister possibility of radiation therapy, particularly when used in the more advanced stages of cervical cancer.

(d) *Criminal abortion* performed by the amateur or unskilled does not as a rule damage the rectum, though this is a possibility if the uterus is retroverted.

(e) *The rare impaling injuries* where some sharp object enters the posterior vaginal wall constitute a menace to the adjacent rectum and this possibility, if suspected, will demand laparotomy and perhaps temporary colostomy.

3. Inflammatory Conditions

(a) *Acute.*

1. Gonorrhoeal proctitis should always be excluded by a rectal swab in all patients with overt or suspected genital and urinary tract gonococcal infection.

2. *Trichomoniasis,* which so often complicates and accompanies gonorrhoea, though not affecting the rectum should be therefore investigated as (1) above.

3. *Moniliasis,* essentially a genital tract infection, may be derived from the bowel and is occasionally found on the perianal skin. This is particularly liable to be one source of the infection after the use of broad spectrum antibiotics. The bowel should not be overlooked as a reservoir of recurrent otherwise inexplicable reinfections. The patient should be treated with oral nystatin if intestinal moniliasis is suspected or proven.

(b) *Chronic Inflammatory Conditions of the Perianal Region.* Many of these can be explained as chronic epithelial dystrophies and give rise to the same symptoms, e.g. pruritus, as those occurring in the vulva. Leukoplakia and lichen sclerosus are good examples and as the vulval and anal condition are so often interrelated it is natural for the gynaecologist to treat both. Though not strictly chronic inflammatory these conditions are included here.

In children threadworm infestation is common and certainly is one cause
of pruritus. In the adult a fungus infection with tinea is always a possibility,
especially if the interdigital clefts of the toes or fingers are involved by the
epidermophyton.

(c) *Chronic Inflammatory Conditions of the Sigmoid and Colon.* Diverticulosis and diverticulitis are an ever-present differential diagnosis in all
gynaecological patients; in fact this disease is as frequently diagnosed in the
first place by the gynaecologist as by the physician or surgeon. It is one common cause of pain in the left lower quadrant for which the innocent ovary
may be incriminated. It provides, if presenting as a fixed inflammatory mass,
one differential diagnosis from tubo-ovarian inflammatory disease and ovarian
neoplasm. In the right lower quadrant Crohn's disease affecting the ileo-
caecal region behaves in a similar way.

4. Neoplastic Conditions Affecting the Recto-Sigmoid

(a) *Carcinoma of the rectum* may be confused with bleeding from genital
tract disease, especially in the postmenopausal patient. Every year the present
authors diagnose one or two unsuspected rectal cancers in their gynaecological out-patients and it is to be emphasised that these patients often present
themselves with symptoms unrelated to the intestinal tract.

(b) *Carcinoma of the sigmoid* is probably the commonest intestinal new
growth to be confused with that of the ovary. In both there is a fixed mass
in the left lower quadrant and only sigmoidoscopy and a barium enema will
reveal the correct diagnosis. Even with these diagnostic refinements a high
lying colonic growth may only be ultimately diagnosed at laparotomy.

5. Other Rectal Conditions Seen in Gynaecological Practice

(a) *Prolapse.* It is not rare to see a procidentia of the rectum associated
with the sister genital tract procidentia. This is especially so with frail,
elderly patients. The two conditions are almost exactly parallel even to the
extent of ulceration and bleeding. Quite a length of rectum may protrude—in
fact it may be larger than the associated utero-vaginal procidentia. The condition is often self-reducing at rest but if the patient is asked to cough or strain
down the eversion becomes obvious. It is not so much the rectal prolapse that
disturbs the patient as the incontinence of flatus and faeces.

If carefully examined the rectal prolapse is found to be associated with a
hernia of Douglas' pouch as well as a utero-vaginal prolapse. In fact, the
pelvic floor is entirely deficient and the levatores ani incompetent so that the
whole of the pelvic contents are involved in the descensus.

The best results for the cure of this rectal and genital prolapse will be
obtained by a combined operation performed by both proctologist and
gynaecologist and the technical details of the bowel operation are best left
in the hands of the former. Notwithstanding this statement a thorough
gynaecological pelvic floor repair goes more than half-way to control the rectal
prolapse and occasionally cures it and the genital prolapse at the same
time.

(b) Apart from actual rectal prolapse a number of gynaecological patients complain of *incompetence of the anal sphincter*. Many of these also suffer from genital tract prolapse and a few from obstetric third degree tears. These defects are naturally gynaecological problems and have been fully discussed in a previous chapter (Chapter 11). Most prolapse patients with a rectocele and a relaxed perineum suffering from rectal incontinence can be controlled by a carefully performed colpo-perineorrhaphy with special reference to the levator and external sphincter sutures.

(c) *Haemorrhoids*. It is not our intention to trespass on the surgical treatment of this very common condition, but merely to observe that very many gynaecological patients, particularly after a confinement, are found to have symptom-producing piles. Quite frequently they do not realise the true nature of their complaint and regard it as some form of genital prolapse. Piles may be regarded as one of the dubious privileges of maternity and because of this common association are frequently first seen by the gynaecologist. The two varieties most likely to be seen are:

(1) *The thrombosed, painful perianal haematoma*, tense and exquisitely tender which hardly permits the sufferer to sit down. This may or may not be, but usually is, associated with internal piles. It quite often occurs in pregnancy and is then best treated with rest, sedatives, frequent hot baths, an ointment containing cortisone combined with a local anaesthetic and can be expected to resolve in a few days. It can be equally and more expeditiously dealt with by evacuation of the clot under local anaesthesia. Any internal piles can be dealt with later.

(2) *Prolapsing interno-external piles* whose main presenting symptom is bleeding. The primary situation is at 3, 7 and 11 o'clock, but secondary piles may develop in the intervening areas. The treatment of this condition is referral to a surgeon who specialises in proctology. Only the rash gynaecologist operates on a prolapse and then performs a haemorrhoidectomy as an encore. The two operations should always be performed at separate sittings with a decent interval intervening.

(3) 1 and 2 as stated may co-exist where a prolapsing interno-external pile is strangulated by spasm of the sphincter. This is particularly liable to occur in pregnancy or the puerperium. Treatment is as for (1) with perhaps local infiltration of the sphincter with a long-acting anaesthetic.

(4) *Anal Tags*, the end result of thrombosed perianal haematoma, may cause irritating local symptoms and consciousness of their presence. Local excision and attention to any internal piles may be required.

(d) *Fissure in Ano*. This is again an essentially proctological problem but the gynaecologist may be called upon to diagnose it in the first instance, as it quite often appears in the puerperium. It is a minute fissure situated posteriorly and is extremely painful during defaecation or rectal examination. Starting as an acute condition, if untreated it can become chronic and owing to the fear of pain on defaecation leads to voluntary constipation when not unnaturally the passage of a hard stool aggravates the condition. It is quite simple to diagnose by passing a very small Sim's speculum with the open side of the blade directed posteriorly. Treatment consists of local injection and stretching of the sphincter followed by daily dilatation of the anal canal with an anal dilator which has been previously smeared with local anaesthetic. The chronic variety may require excision.

(e) *Pruritus ani* has already been mentioned as a coincident of pruritus vulvae. It is seen with chronic fungus infection, threadworms in young patients and the chronic epithelial dysplasias of the vulval and anal region. Regrettably, simple excision of the vulva for the latter, while controlling the pruritus vulvae is often exchanged for the more intractable pruritus ani. The treatment of the two conditions is often simultaneous and surgery is usually disappointing. As good results as any may be obtained by bathing and washing after every motion using a non-irritant, non-scented soap, elimination of any bowel infection by tinea, threadworms or moniliasis and an anti-inflammatory ointment such as 1% hydrocortisone cream. Anti-histamines may be useful.

(f) *Radiation proctitis.* This is quite a common complication of all forms of radiation treatment to the genital tract, especially a full local application of radium given for carcinoma of the cervix. The condition develops in two ways. (1) As an immediate inflammatory reaction of the bowel at the time of treatment or soon after. The manifestations are an acute proctitis with diarrhoea and discharge from the rectum. (2) A late result, sometimes many months after the initial inflammation, is an avascular necrosis of the anterior rectal wall with the formation of an indurated ulcer. It has a smooth base, the edges are not heaped up as in a carcinoma and it may cause bleeding. It can be extremely painful. On inspection and palpation it is usually possible to make the correct diagnosis, though a small punch biopsy may be needed. Cytology can be helpful. One serious possible complication is a recto-vaginal fistula and this always suggests the grave possibility of malignant recurrence. Treatment is by bland irrigations of hamamelis and hydrocortisone and only a few will require colostomy. This operation is naturally obligatory if a fistula develops or seems likely to do so.

(g) *Endometriosis* of the bowel has already been dealt with in Chapter 27. Owing to the generous calibre of the rectum it is most unlikely to cause obstruction in this region and its symptoms are mainly irritative but in the sigmoid it can and does cause obstruction and its differentiatal diagnosis from carcinoma of the colon is difficult (*vide supra* page, 698).

6. Functional Disorders of the Large Bowel

Perhaps these are as important to the gynaecologist as any condition in this chapter. Pride of place must be given to colon spasm, which seems to be a disorder of the modern age. It is essentially a stress condition and can be regarded as a flatulent dyspepsia of the colon. The patient is aged between 30 up to well after the menopause, and the peak incidence is around the menopause itself. The patient is either introspective and thin or frustrated and fat. She is almost invariably constipated and this is sometimes aggravated by punishing her colon with periodic and powerful purgatives. In her diet carbohydrate and tea play a large aggravating part. Her pain is perfectly genuine and she can usually localise it over the left colon and the left lower quadrant is tender. The spasm causes a distension of the colon in whole or in part, and the caecum can often be appreciated as inflated and tender. The spastic area in the left colon can be rolled under the examining finger and patients always confirm that the examiner has found the spot. In this essentially functional disorder the clinician must not fall into the trap of affixing a psycho-somatic label until he has excluded the possibility of organic disease, notably a carcinoma of the colon or diverticulosis. The latter is quite a likely finding in an obese woman at or after the menopause and is incidental to the spastic colon. As one of the patient's main complaints is abdominal swelling she may be initially referred with a diagnosis of ovarian cyst. This, if the patient is obese, may be difficult to refute without examining her under an anaesthetic. A barium enema is the most certain method of confirming what is plainly an easy clinical diagnosis and excluding any organic disease of the colon.

Treatment is mainly dietetic with carbohydrate restriction, some simple bland aperient such as isogel, and if the discomfort disturbs the patient an antispasmodic such as buscopan. Last and most important is the control and elimination of stress, if this is ever possible, which is unfortunately unlikely. With an intelligent patient, and most with colon spasm are, a frank, sympathetic and tactful explanation of the mechanism of the condition will do more than drugs to control it and it may be possible for the observant and patient practitioner to disclose the hidden cause which is operative. For example, the patient may have an undisclosed fear that the gaseous distension of the colon at her particular age can only signify the diagnosis of inoperable cancer.

Glossary

Glossary

ABORTION—Latin, *aboriri*—the prefix *ab* suggests an abnormal or premature expulsion + *oriri*, to be born, or to arise; cf. origin.

ACROMEGALY—Greek, *acron*, extremity + *megalos*, big.

ADENO—a prefix associating a condition with a gland—Greek, *aden*, *adenos*, hence:

ADENOMYOMA—Greek, *aden*, gland; *mus*, muscle and *oma*, tumour—a glandular tumour with or in muscular tissue.

ADENOMYOSIS—the suffix *osis* suggests a morbid process often associated with hyperplasia but not cancer; cf. endometriosis and stromatosis.

ADNEXA—Latin, plural of *adnexum* = appendage. In gynæcology, the tube and the ovary.

ADRENAL—Latin, *ad*, near to, + *ren*, the kidney.

ADRENOGENITAL (syndrome), a condition in which the adrenal gland causes a (usually) masculinising effect on the female genitalia.

ADRENOTROPIC—adrenal + Greek, *trope* = a turning toward or influence upon, e.g. adrenotropic hormone of pituitary influences the adrenal gland causing hyperplasia.

ALLANTOIS—Greek, *allas*, *allantos*—literally a sausage, hence a sac.

AMENORRHŒA—Greek, *a*, no; *men*, month; *rheein*, to flow = no menstrual loss.

ANDROGEN—Greek, *aner*, *andros*, male; *gen*, verb root, meaning to produce = masculinising.

ANOREXIA—Greek, *a*, none; *orexis*, appetite.

ANOVULAR—Greek-Latin hybrid—literally, no *ovulum*, diminutive of *ovum* = egg.

ANTEFLEXION—Latin—forward bending.

ANTEVERSION—Latin—forward turning.

ANURIA—Greek-Latin hybrid—no urine.

APLASIA—Greek—*a*, not; *plassein*, to form = failure of tissues to grow.

ARRHENOBLASTOMA—Greek—*arren*, male; *blastanein*, to grow; *oma*, suffix—tumour. A masculinising tumour.

ASCHHEIM-ZONDEK (German gynæcologists: Selmar Aschheim, born 1878; Bernhardt Zondek, born 1891).

ASPERMIA—Greek—*a*, none; *sperma*, seed.

ATRESIA—Greek—*a*, no; *tresis*, literally, a hole or canal bored out = non-canalisation.

AUVARD, Alfred. French gynæcologist (born 1855).

AVELING, James. British obstetrician (born 1825; died 1892).

BARTHOLIN, Casper (1655–1738). Danish anatomist.

BEHCET, Hulusi (1889–1948). Turkish dermatologist (Istanbul).

BOWEN, John T. (1857–1941). American dermatologist.

BRENNER, Fritz. Contemporary German pathologist.

CALL-EXNER. Friedrich von Call (1844–1917), Austrian physician; Siegmund Exner (1846–1925), Austrian physiologist.

CARDINAL—Latin, *cardo*, *cardinis*—a hinge; hence, something on which everything hinges or depends = vitally important.

CARNEOUS—Latin, *caro*, *carnis*—flesh = fleshy.

CARUNCLE—diminutive of *caro* = a little fleshy tumour. (Also CARUNCULA—Æ.)

CERVIX—Latin, neck.

CHORION—Greek, skin. *Frondosum* (Latin) leafy or villous; *læve* = smooth.

CLITORIS—Greek, *kleitoris*. The derivation of this word is obscure. *Kleitos*—renowned or famous; *Kleio*—to close; this has the same root as *kleis*—a key or bar.

CLOACA—Latin, a drain or sewage pipe.

CLOQUET, Jules Germain (1790–1883). French surgeon.

CŒLOM—Greek, a hollow place or cavity.

COITUS—Latin, *con* = together; ire, to go = conjunction.

COLPO—Greek, *colpos*—a fold or hollow = vagina, hence :

COLPECTOMY—excision of vagina.

COLPOCLEISIS—Greek, *cleisis*, closing = obliteration of vagina.

COLPORRHAPHY—Greek, *raphe*; stitching of . . .

COLPOSTAT—Greek, *statos*; standing in position, e.g. something which keeps an applicator (radium) in position in the vagina.

COLPOTOMY—Greek, *temnein;* to cut—incision of the posterior vaginal fornix.

CORNU—Latin, horn.

CORONA—Latin, crown.

CORPUS—Latin, body.
   ALBICANS—of white = scar tissue.
   LUTEUM—yellow.

CORTEX—Latin, bark or outer surface.

CRUS or CRURA (plural)—Latin, leg.

CRYPTOMENORRHŒA—Greek, *cryptos*, hidden + menstruation—e.g. menstrual bleeding occurring internally with no external loss.

CUSCO, Edouard Gabriel (1819–1894). French surgeon.

CYSTOCELE—Greek, *custis*, a sac or bladder; *cele*, a hernia.

CYTOTROPHOBLAST—Greek, *cutos*, cell, *trophe*, nourishment; *blastos*, growth. The cellular inner layer of the trophoblast.

DECIDUA—Latin, *deciduus* (*de—cadere*)—that which falls off or is shed.

DERMOID—Greek, *derma*, skin; *eides*, like = resembling skin.

DETRUSOR—Latin, *de*, out; *trudere*, to push = expulsive.

DISCUS—Latin, disc.

DÖDERLEIN, Albert (1860–1941). German gynæcologist.

DOUGLAS, James (1675–1742). Scottish anatomist emigrated to London.

DYS—Greek, prefix = bad, painful, difficult, disordered or diseased as opposed to eu— which means everything good and proper. Hence:

DYSMENORRHŒA—painful periods.

DYSPAREUNIA—difficult or painful coitus. (*para*—together; *eune*—couch or bed).

ECTOPIA—IC—Greek, displacement.

ECTROPION—Greek, *Ek*, out; *trepein*, to turn = eversion.

EMBRYO—Greek, *en*, inside; *bruein*, to grow.

ENDOCERVICITIS—Greek/Latin hybrid, *endos*, (Greek), inside; *cervitis* (Latin), inflammation of the neck (of womb).

ENTEROCELE—Greek, *enteron*, gut; *cele*, hernia.

EPIMENORRHŒA—Greek, prefix *epi*— = on or upon; hence, added to or excessive.

EPISPADIAS—Greek, *epi-*, upon or above; *spadon*, a tear—hence an opening above the normal urinary meatus.

EPOOPHORON—Greek, above the oophoron, eggbearer or ovary. A body situated above the ovary.

EROSION—Latin, an eating away; ulcer.

FALLOPIUS (Gabriello Fallopio) (1523–1562). Italian anatomist.

FASCIA—Latin, sheet or band.

FERGUSSON, Sir William (1808–1877). British surgeon.

FIBROID—Latin/Greek hybrid—*fibra* (Latin), a fibre; *eidos* (Greek), like. (Slang term for leiomyoma.)

FIBROMYOMA—Ditto.

FIMBRIA—Latin, fringe.

FISTULA—Latin, a little pipe or flute.

FOLLICLE—Latin, little bag or sac.

FORCEPS—Latin, *forcipis*, plural *forcipes* = pincers. Forceps is a singular noun and the strictly correct plural is forcipes, but usage has anglicised the word out of all Latin recognition. (Hence, a pair of forceps, the forceps were or was applied.)

FOSSA—Latin, a ditch or shallow depression.

FOTHERGILL, William Edward (1865–1926). Manchester gynæcologist and repairer of prolapse.

FOURCHETTE—French from Latin, *furca* = a little fork or U-shaped fold.

FRANKENHÄUSER, Ferdinand (died 1894). German gynæcologist.

FRIEDMAN, Maurice. Contemporary American physician.

FUNDUS—Latin, the base or bottom (curiously, often the top, e.g. the upper part of the uterus or bladder)—that part of a hollow viscus farthest from the opening, e.g. cervical canal or urethra.

GARTNER, Hermann Trechow (1785–1827). Danish anatomist and surgeon.

GILLIAM, David Tod (1844–1923). American gynæcologist.

de GRAFF, Regner or Reijnier (1641–1673). Dutch physician and anatomist.

GRANULOSA—Latin, *granulum*, a small particle or grain.

HERMAPHRODITISM—Greek, *Hermes*, the messenger of the Gods, a mischievous, essentially masculine character + *Aphrodite*, Goddess of Love. A condition in which an individual possesses characteristics of both sexes.

HILUM—plural HILA—Latin, i.e., that part of an organ where its main blood supply enters.

HILUS—plural HILI—Latin, the point of attachment of a seed to its parent vessel.

HODGE, Hugh Lenox (1796–1873). Gynæcologist at Philadelphia.

HOGBEN, Lancelot Thomas (born 1895). Professor of Zoology at Birmingham.

HORMONE—Greek, *horman*, to excite. A chemical substance capable of exciting specific target organs.

HYALINE—Greek, *halos*, glass.

HYDATIDIFORM—Latin, *hydatis*, a drop of water; fluid vesicle.

HYDROPS—Greek, dropsical.

HYDROSALPINX—Greek, a tube filled with watery contents.

HYMEN—Greek, probably *humen*, a membrane, rather than *Hymen*, the God of marriage.

HYPO—A Greek prefix meaning "under" and signifying deficiency or subnormality, e.g. hypoplasia, under-development.

HYSTERO—Greek, *hustera*, the womb. The Greek adjective, *husteros*, means last or lowest.

INFUNDIBULUM—Latin, a funnel—hence infundibulo-pelvic = the ligament which joins the fimbriated extremity of the tube to the pelvis.

INSUFFLATION—Latin, *in-suf-flare*—to blow into a cavity, e.g. Fallopian tube.

INTERSTITIAL—Latin, *inter*, between; *sistere*, to set. Those structures lying between, e.g. interstices.

INTROITUS—Latin, *intro*, inside; *ire*, to go = entrance.

INVERSION—Latin, *in*, into; *vertere*, to turn = a turning into or inside out.

ISTHMUS—Greek = a narrow srtip of land (or tissue) connecting two greater continents or tissues, e.g. the narrow part of the tube connecting the ampulla with the uterus.

KERATINISATION—Greek, *kera*, horn. Usually the deposition of scleroprotein in the outer layers of the skin.

KRAUROSIS—Greek, *krauros* = dry. A dry, shrivelled appearance of the vulva.

KYMOGRAPH—Greek, *kuma*, wave; *graphein*, to write. The recording of an undulation in e.g. the Fallopian tube.

LABIUM (singular), LABIA (plural)—Latin = a lip.
Majus = the greater. Minus = the lesser.

LAMINA—Latin, a thin plate or layer.

LAMINARIA—Latin, a genus of seaweed, seatangle.

LAWRENCE-BEIDL-MOON Syndrome.
   T. C. Lawrence (1830–1874), British ophthalmologist: A. Beidl (1869–1933), endo-
   crinologist in Prague; R. C. Moon (1844–1914), ophthalmologist in Philadelphia.
LE FORT—Leon Clement Le Fort (1829–1893). French surgeon with a leaning towards
   orthopædics.
LEVATOR—Latin, a lifter up of anything.
LEUKOPLAKIA—Greek, *leukos*, white; *plax*, plate. The presence of white patches or plaques
   on the tongue, cheeks or, in gynæcology, the vulva.
LIBIDO—Latin, sexual desire.
LICHEN—Greek, *leichen*, a moss. A flat, papular or patchy skin condition.
LITHOPÆDION—Greek, *lithos*, a stone; *pædion*, a child. A petrified fœtus.
LUTEIN—Latin, *luteus*, yellow. Any lipochrome.
LUTEOTROPIN—Latin, *luteus*, Greek—*trepein*, a hormone of the pituitary which influences
   luteinisation of the corpus luteum and, incidentally, is a galactagogue.

MACKENRODT, Alwyn Karl (1859–1925). A German gynæcologist.
MEIGS, Joe Vincent (born 1892). Gynæcologist in Boston, Mass.
MENO—Greek, *men*, month. This prefix denotes a relationship to menstruation, e.g. menarche,
   beginning of; menopause, end of; menorrhagia + *regnunai*, to erupt = excessive
   menstruation, etc.
MENSTRUAL, MENSTRUATION—Latin, appertaining to the month.
MESO—Greek, situated in the middle or appertaining to the mesentery of any organ, i.e.
   that fold of peritoneum which attaches a particular organ to the cœlom, e.g. mesovarium.
   mesocolon and mesentery.
META—Greek, beyond, over, above. A prefix which denotes alteration or superiority.
METAPLASIA—Greek, *plassein*. A change or alteration in tissue form.
METASTASIS—Greek, *meta* + *stasis* = situation. A change or alteration in situation. Of
   cancer, a secondary deposit beyond the primary growth.
METR—Greek, prefix from *metra* = womb; e.g. metrorrhagia, an excessive or pathological
   bleeding from the uterus.
MICTURITION—Latin, *micturire*, to pass urine.
MITTELSCHMERZ—German, literally, middle pain.
MOLE—Latin, *moles* = a mass. Hence, carneous mole = a fleshy mass.
   Hydatidiform mole = a mass composed of dropsical cysts.
   Vesicular = hydatidiform.
MORGAGNI, Giovanni Battista (1682–1771). Italian anatomist and pathologist.
MÜLLER, Johannes Peter (1801–1858). German physiologist. Of all the distinguished Müllers,
   Johannes, Heinrich, Hermann, Rudolf, Peter, Friedrich and Edward—to Johannes
   should be given the credit for discovering the Müllerian duct.
MYCOTIC—Greek, *muces* = fungus. Any disease caused by a fungus.
MYO—Greek, prefix from *mus* = muscle. Hence, myometrium, muscle of the womb.
   Myoma, a tumour of the muscle (usually) of the womb, and myomectomy, the
   enucleation of such a tumour by a cutting operation.

NABOTH, Martin (1675–1721). Anatomist of Saxony. (Not to be confused with the owner
   of the Old Testament vineyard.)
NAPIER, Alexander Disney Leith (1844–1926). British gynæcologist.
NUCK, Anton (1650–1692). Dutch anatomist.

OBTURATOR—Latin, a flat structure which closes an opening.
ŒSTRUS—Latin, a gadfly. Hence, the temporary excitation of the sexual urge or the periodic
   heat of lower animals. As a prefix, œstro-, e.g.
ŒSTROGEN—any substance which produces œstrins or, more generically, which produces
   changes associated with ovarian activity.
OLIGO—Greek, prefix = scanty or infrequent, e.g. oligomenorrhœa or oligospermia.
OOPHORON—Greek, *oophoros* = egg producing, or ovary. Hence, oophoritis, an inflamma-
   tion of the ovary, and oophorectomy, removal of the ovary.
OVUM—Latin, egg. Hence, ovary.

PARA—Greek, beyond, beside, in addition to, supplementary. Hence, paroophoron, parovarian (hybrid Latin and Greek), parametrium (literally, beside the uterus), paracolpos, paravaginal, parametritis, etc.

PELVIS—Latin, a basin.

PERI—Greek, prefix = around or about, e.g. perimetrium = the serosal covering of the uterus.

PERIN(A)EUM—Greek, *perineos* = Hippocratic term for the space between urethra and anus

PESSARY—Greek, *pessos* = oval stone used for playing the classical version of draughts. Latin, *pessarium* = a foreign body (originally and probably, a stone) placed in the vagina to prevent prolapse.

PFLÜGER, Edward Friedrich Wilhelm (1829–1910). German physiologist in Bonn.

PITUITARY—Latin, adjectival of pituita or phlegm, i.e. the organ that secretes phlegm or mucus. (Phlegm was regarded by the old physicians as one of the four humours, which were blood, phlegm, choler and melancholy.)

PLACENTA—Latin and Greek, *plax*, a flat plate and *placœis*, plate-like.

POLY—Greek, prefix from *polus* = many or excessive.

POLYPUS—Greek, *polus* = many; *pous:* foot = many-footed. This is a peculiar name to give a structure which usually has only one foot or pedicle, but anatomists are seldom logical and rarely classical scholars. Students should, therefore, be charitable.

PORTIO—Latin, part. Portio vaginalis of the cervix = that part which protrudes into the vagina as opposed to the supravaginal part.

PRIMORDIAL—Latin, *primus*, first, and *ordiri*, to begin = original, fundamental or primeval, e.g. follicle.

PROCIDENTIA—Latin, literally, a falling out or forwards = *pro*, forwards and *cadere*, to fall.

PROLAPSE—Latin, *pro*, forwards or before; *labi*, to fall as above, or slip (e.g. to lapse from grace).

PRURITUS—Latin, *prurire*, to itch.

PSAMMOMA—Greek, *psammos*, sand. A tumour containing calcareous granules.

PSEUDO—prefix denoting false, e.g. pseudo-cyesis, a bogus pregnancy.

PUDENDAL—appertaining to those parts of the body of which one should be modestly ashamed, e.g. external genitalia (originated from the eating of the apple of the tree of knowledge (Old Testament, Genesis). Before this occasion, there were no pudendals.

PUERPERAL—Latin, *puer*, a child; *parus*, bearing. Cf. oviparous, viviparous, multiparous.

PYO—prefix denoting the presence of pus in any organ. Cf. pyosalpinx, pyometra and empyema. Greek, *pyon*, pus.

RETINACULUM—Latin, a halter = a structure which retains an organ in its place, e.g. Mackenrodt's ligament.

RETROFLEXION—Latin, a bending back.

RETROVERSION—Latin, a turning back.

REVERDIN, Albert (1881–1929). A Swiss surgeon in Geneva.

ROSENMÜLLER, Johann Christian (1771–1820). A German anatomist in Leipsig.

SALPINX—Greek, a trumpet. The female's oviduct. Hence, salpingitis = inflammation of the tube; salpingography = demonstration of tube by radiology; salpingoophoritis = inflammation of tube and ovary; salpingostomy = a permanent opening in the tube.

SARCOMA—Greek, *sarx* = flesh; *oma* = tumour.

SCHAUTA, Friedrich (1849–1919). An Austrian gynæcologist in Vienna.

SCHILLER, Walter (born 1887). Emigré pathologist who spent his later years in Chicago.

SCLEROCYSTIC—Greek, *scleros* = hard; *kustis* = bladder. A disease of the ovary characterised by a thick capsule and the presence of several cysts.

SEROSA—Latin, *Serosus*. Producing or containing serum, e.g. peritoneum.

SIMMONDS, Maurice (1885–1925). Hamburg physician who described a disease due to atrophy of the pituitary.

SIMS, James Marion (1813–1883). Gynæcologist in New York who invented the position and speculum for repairing a vesico-vaginal fistula. The original model is supposed to have been modified from a bent teaspoon.

SKENE, Alexander J. C. (1838–1900). Physician in New York.

SPECULUM—Latin, a mirror.

SPHINCTER—Greek, *sphinkter* = a binder or sling.

STROMA—Greek, a covering, hence the tissue which forms the groundwork or basis of any organ.

STRUMA—Latin, goitre.

SUBINVOLUTION—Latin, *sub* = less than. Involution = restoration to normal.

SYNCYTIOTROPHOBLAST—Greek, *syn* = together; *kutos* = cell (i.e. a multi-nucleated mass of protoplasm); tropho = appertaining to nutrition; blast = Greek root for growing. Multinucleated mass of chorionic cells.

TAUSSIG, Frederick Joseph (born 1872). Gynæcologist in St. Louis.

TELANGIECTASIA—Greek, *telos* = end; *aggeion* = vessel; *extasis* = stretching out or dilatation. Dilatation of the end vessels or capillaries—lymphatic, venous or arteriolar.

TENT—Latin, *tenta—tendere* = to stretch. An expandable plug for dilating an orifice.

TERATOMA—Greek, *teras* = monster; *oma* = tumour. A tumour containing incompletely developed elements of the human body.

TESTOSTERONE—Greek/Latin hybrid, *testis* (Latin) = testicle; sterol from *stereos* (Greek) = solid; *oleum* (Latin) = oil. Steroids are cholesterol-like compounds containing the cyclopentenophenanthrene ring.

THECA—Greek, a repository, hence a case or sheath, i.e. of a tendon or of the spinal cord.

TRACHELORRHAPHY—Greek, *trachelos* = a neck; *raphe* = stitching. Stitching of the cervix.

TRICHOMONAS—Greek, *thrix* = hair; *monas* = a unit. An organism with flagella or hair-like antennæ.

TROPHOBLAST. See Synctiotrophoblast (above).

TUNICA—Latin, tunic or covering.

TURNER, Henry Hubert (born 1892). American endocrinologist of Oklahoma City.

URACHUS—Greek, *aurachos;* the urinary canal of a fœtus.

URETER—Greek, *oureter.*

URETHRA—Greek, *oureo;* to urinate.

UTERUS—Latin, counterpart of (Greek) *husteros.*

VAGINA—Latin, a sheath, usually of a sword.

VESICA—Latin, bladder. Hence, vesicular = a little bladder.

VESTIBULE—Latin, entrance-hall.

VOLSELLUM—Latin, forceps with prehensile hooks.

VULVA—Latin, possibly from *valva* = a folding door.

WALDEYER, Wilhelm von (1836–1921). German anatomist in Berlin.

WERTHEIM, Ernst (1864–1920). Gynæcologist in Vienna.

WOLFF, Casper Friedrich (1733–1794). German anatomist and embryologist.

Index

Index

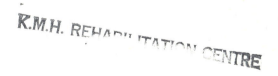

PRINTED IN GREAT BRITAIN BY THE WHITEFRIARS PRESS LTD.
LONDON AND TONBRIDGE